Medical Professionalism

Medical Professionalism

Theory, Education, and Practice

Edited by

GIA MERLO, MD, MBA, MED

Clinical Professor of Psychiatry

NYU Grossman School of Medicine, New York University

THOMAS D. HARTER, PHD

Director

Department of Bioethics and Humanities, Emplify Health System

OXFORD
UNIVERSITY PRESS

OXFORD
UNIVERSITY PRESS

Oxford University Press is a department of the University of Oxford. It furthers the University's objective of excellence in research, scholarship, and education by publishing worldwide. Oxford is a registered trade mark of Oxford University Press in the UK and certain other countries.

Published in the United States of America by Oxford University Press
198 Madison Avenue, New York, NY 10016, United States of America.

Library of Congress Cataloging-in-Publication Data
Names: Merlo, Gia, author. | Harter, Thomas D., author.
Title: Medical professionalism : theory, education, and practice /
Gia Merlo, MD, MBA, MEd and Thomas D. Harter, PhD.
Description: New York, NY : Oxford University Press, [2025] |
Includes bibliographical references and index.
Identifiers: LCCN 2024020187 | ISBN 9780197640814 (hardback) |
ISBN 9780197640838 (epub) | ISBN 9780197640821 (updf) | 9780197640845 (digital online)
Subjects: LCSH: Medicine—Vocational guidance. | Medical ethics.
Classification: LCC R690 .M39 2024 | DDC 610.69—dc23/eng/20240522
LC record available at https://lccn.loc.gov/2024020187

DOI: 10.1093/med/9780197640814.001.0001

Printed by Integrated Books International, United States of America

MIX
Paper
FSC FSC® C183721

Contents

PART B UNDERSTANDING AND EDUCATING FOR MEDICAL PROFESSIONALISM ALONG THE CONTINUUM OF PHYSICIAN PRACTICE

PART C PROFESSIONALISM IMPLEMENTATION IN CLINICAL PRACTICE

Illustrations

Figures

Tables

Boxes

Foreword

Preparing for the Future by Building on the Past

What has been termed the "professionalism movement"[1] is now almost three decades old, having been initiated by the American Board of Internal Medicine in the 1990s under the heading of Project Professionalism.[2] The stimulus for specifically addressing the issue of professionalism at the time clearly originated both from the general public and within the medical profession. Both were concerned with the conduct of individual physicians and the organizations representing medicine. There was no mystery in identifying the factors that were influencing both the profession and physicians. Medicine had been transformed from a cottage industry that gradually became science based and therefore essential to the welfare of every citizen and to society.[3] It came to consume an ever-increasing percentage of the gross domestic product in every country. Because of its importance, in large parts of the developed world access to healthcare became a right of citizenship, thus leading to pressures for the state to establish national health plans. In the United States, its traditional social contract made this direction difficult, and the corporate sector assumed responsibility for much of the organization and funding of healthcare.[3,4] These foundational events had transformative effects on the structure and organization of healthcare systems throughout the world, on the practice of medicine, and on the expectations of physicians, patients, and society.[5,6] These forces disrupted the traditional relationship between medicine and society that for generations had been based on the activities of individual physicians treating individual patients. Essentially, the social contract between medicine and society was being altered, and this relationship was examined, almost for the first time.[5] It was rapidly determined that the relationship depended on the concept of professionalism.[5,6] Professionalism was not an inherent right of the medical profession. Individual physicians and the profession were granted professional status, including autonomy in practice, status, and prestige and considerable financial rewards along with the privilege of self-regulation. In return, they were expected to demonstrate honesty and integrity in their activities, be governed by codes of ethics, place the interests of patients and society above their own, address issues of societal concern, and self-regulate with rigor and integrity. Professional status was established by laws and regulations, and its maintenance depended on physicians meeting reasonable societal expectations. This they would do by acting professionally. Essentially society used the professions as a means of delivering the complex and essential services that it required.[6]

Early investigators and commentators in the field, heavily influenced by its evolution in the Anglo-American world, searched for universal and relatively stable definitions and understandings of professionalism and its role in society.[7] The globalization of healthcare rendered this concept untenable as professionalism is a social construct.[8,9] Different cultures, national beliefs, and religions all led to the presence of differing social contracts and hence differing interpretations of the meaning of professionalism.[8,9] This actually led to a deeper understanding of the concept. To its credit, this book reflects well on the past changes in our understanding of professionalism and looks forward to the future changes that, while difficult to predict, are inevitable.

An important challenge that, once again, is well documented in this book relates to the growing discrepancy between the expectations of the parties to the social contract and the reality of the practice of medicine in healthcare systems that are being challenged throughout the world.[10] From the point of view of individual physicians, they feel themselves to be losing autonomy as they are forced to practice in either a heavily commercialized sector or one in which national health plans increasingly direct their activities. [10,11] In the United States, some physicians feel compelled to become entrepreneurs in a competitive marketplace, a situation that poses challenges to the traditional value systems of the healer.[3] The great increase in number of physicians actually employed in or by large organizations is a further deterrence to the traditional autonomy enjoyed by independent practitioners. There thus is a growing yearning on the part of physicians to return to the professionalism of yesteryear—a condition that Hafferty has termed "nostalgic professionalism."[1] Clearly this will not occur. A further challenge results from medicine's well-publicized failures of self-regulation as well as resistance to change in the system that have tarnished its collective reputation.[3,6,10] In short, physicians appeared to be acting unprofessionally and the organizations representing them have often failed to understand that representing professionals imposes limitations in both attitudes and activities.[12] The profession's devotion to the welfare of individual patients and to society was questioned, and a growing perception developed that the profession, through its representatives, was tending to establish or maintain control over the medical marketplace, including who could enter practice, the nature and standards of that practice and discipline.[13] These criticisms tended to support George Bernard Shaw's earlier comment that the professions represented a conspiracy against the laity.[14]

While medicine's response to these existential threats was multifactorial, a major thrust involved using its educational establishments to formally address the issue of professionalism on the assumption that if physicians entering practice understood professionalism and embraced its values and attitudes, their behaviors would improve.[15] This important book is part of this ongoing and still relevant activity. It is worth emphasizing how necessary it is to continually address these issues. The literature on the subject, which, as noted, goes back over two decades, has been both significant and impactful, but we have come to realize the importance of context. What work has been previously produced addressed issues relevant to their place and time, and many were correct and impactful. However, healthcare systems have evolved rapidly, funding mechanisms have changed, educational theory in medicine has progressed enormously, and we have come to better understand the importance of wellness, diversity, and equity as we address the relationship between medicine and society. Thus the analyses and solutions proposed in the past must be constantly re-examined. This book, which takes an extraordinarily comprehensive approach to analyzing both current society and professionalism, provides an insightful analysis into today's world, building upon what has gone before.

However, it must be emphasized that some core issues remain unchanged. As is outlined in the text, professionalism serves as the basis of medicine's social contract with society. As this contract evolves, so must professionalism. Another unchanging element relates to its importance. While the details of today's healthcare system and of the nature of the professionalism expected may alter, professionalism is of great importance to both medicine and society. For medicine this is straightforward. Its practitioners are granted a privileged position in society, substantial financial and nonfinancial rewards, and the benefits of self-regulation.[3,4] Thus any change in professional status has the potential to diminish the role and status of the physician. However, one can postulate that it is even more important to society. As Sullivan pointed out: "Neither economic incentives, nor technology, nor administrative control has proved an effective surrogate for the commitment to integrity invoked in the ideal of professionalism."[6] This integrity can be neither imposed nor legislated. It must come from within each practicing physician, a fact that is largely responsible for the evolution in our thinking on how best to produce a true professional. Until the intervention of the American Board of Internal Medicine, professionalism was not taught explicitly. It was acquired as a result of the process of socialization that takes place throughout the continuum of medical education.[16] Behavior patterns, attitudes, and beliefs are acquired from respected mentors and role models. It depends in part on shared value systems, a situation that certainly was present for much of medicine's history when a reasonably homogeneous profession served equally homogeneous societies. The threats to professionalism and the profession's initial failures to respond highlighted the fact that relying on mentors and role models alone was no longer sufficient, and a consensus arose that professionalism must be taught explicitly. Educational practices that dictated specific objectives needed to be established, definitions developed, and methods of teaching and assessment began to emerge.[17] The emphasis was on developing a cognitive base and providing periods of reflection so that attitudes and behaviors could be incorporated into the self. This thrust was essentially codified when licensing and certifying bodies of virtually all educational programs began to require the presence of effective teaching and assessment of professionalism as a condition of program approval. The emphasis was on producing observable behaviors that would ensure professional conduct.[18]

A new status quo emerged and, due to the impact of the regulatory bodies, is still largely in force. However, individuals interested in medical education began examining the process of identity formation that had occupied those in developmental psychology for many years.[19,20] If proper professional behavior, including characteristics such as integrity needed to come from within, it became apparent that the teaching of professionalism was in fact a means to an end, with assisting learners to develop their own professional identity emerging as the proper objective.[21] This concept was not new. In 1957, Merton's introduction to the first book examining the sociology of medical education stated that it was the purpose of medical education to produce individuals who possess not only the knowledge and skills necessary for practice, but also a professional identity so that they came to "think act and feel like physicians." [21,22] This concept has had traction in recent years, and we appear to be in a period of transition where identity formation becomes a principal goal of medical education, a principal recommendation of the Carnegie Foundation report on the future of medical education.[23]

Inextricably linked to the concept of professional identity formation is the social learning theory community of practice. This theory, originally developed by Lave and Wenger,[24] states that those wishing to join a community of practice such as medicine do so voluntarily and in the process of becoming members, acquire the identity of community members. Implicit in this act is the acceptance of the core values of the community. Medicine has been described as a landscape of communities, in concluding the global medical community, its specialties, and local departments.[25]

As will be apparent to those who read this book, directing this poses problems for medicine's educational establishments. Different educational methods are necessary to engage learners in the development of their own identities,[26] and the problem of assessment of progress toward that identity has yet to be properly addressed in a way that can be implemented on a large scale.[27] Regulatory bodies thus far have not embraced the concept because they are required to actually assess whether this educational objective has been achieved, and, as noted, methods are not yet available. Furthermore, there is general agreement that there is not one professional identity that is required of all learners. While it took time for us to fully understand much about professional identity and its formation, there is now absolute certainty that each individual must be permitted to retain their own personal identity as they become professionals.[24,28] Thus, identity formation is a concept that is meant to be inclusionary rather than exclusionary. An examination of medicine's past performance provides a striking example of Bourdie's suggestion that social structures tend to reproduce themselves, including a continuation of both positive and negative aspects as well as power relationships. [29,30,31,32] The exclusion of women and other minorities from medicine's communities of practice for generations has been striking and, while acknowledged, is only now being addressed. Each learner in the health sciences must be able to feel a part of the community and remain who they are throughout the process of socialization.

Two final points deserve emphasis. First, never in the history of humankind have healers possessed a greater capacity to prevent human disease, to alter its course, and to enrich the quality of life of each individual citizen. Our ability to make this statement has been totally dependent on changes that have occurred in the biomedical and psychosocial field in the last few generations. It is ironic that in the face of this situation, trust in the professions, medicine, and healthcare systems is much lower than it has been historically.[27] Second, there is also absolute agreement that the future will hold further changes of at least equal impact and significance, and that medicine's educational institutions must prepare learners to be able to adapt to changes, which will include an unpredictable healthcare system as well as additional diagnostic and therapeutic tools. One need not be overly concerned with this issue. The current generation of students and residents have already been forced to adapt to multiple changes in both medicine and ever-changing methods of communication and have shown themselves to be brilliantly resilient in their capacity to do so.[28] What should concern us more is not change and how to adjust to it. There have been healers throughout recorded history who have adapted to change, and this tradition will undoubtedly continue into the infinite future. The principal challenge is not what will change but what must remain unchanged. We are the stewards of the historical role of the healer, a role that has for generations shaped the identity of physicians and dictated their role in society and their relationship to the society that they must serve. Those aspects that give meaning and joy to the practice of medicine and satisfaction to patients and society must be preserved, and it will be difficult to identify them and to ensure their survival in organizational systems that often threaten them. The values and attitudes that must be preserved are encompassed by the word *professionalism*. This book, which is comprehensive and timely, can offer guidance as we plan for a future that will be very different from the present but must include the commitment to integrity and competence that is inherent in the word professionalism.

Note: This Foreword represents the last collaboration between the author and his beloved wife and partner of 62 years. She was an equal participant in all of our joint contributions and in the conception of this work, but sadly passed away before it was completed. It is dedicated to her memory with love and gratitude.

Richard L. Cruess, MD
Institute for Health Sciences Education
Lady Meredith House
McGill University

References

1. Wear D, Kuczewski MG. The professionalism movement: can we pause? *Am J Bioethics.* 2004;4:1–10.
2. American Board of Internal Medicine (ABIM). *Project Professionalism.* Rev. ed. 1999. https://medicinainternaucv.wordpress.com/wp-content/uploads/2013/02/project-professionalism.pdf
3. Star, P. *The Social Transformation of American Medicine.* 2nd ed. Epilogue. Basic Books; 2016.
4. Krause E. *Death of the Guilds: Professions, States and the Advance of Capitalism, 1930 to the Present.* Yale University Press; 1996.
5. Cruess RL, Cruess SR. Expectations and obligations: professionalism and medicine's social contract with society. *Perspect Biol Med.* 2008;51:579–598.
6. Sullivan W. *Work and Integrity: The Crisis and Promise of Professionalism in North America.* 2nd ed. Harper Collins; 2005.
7. Brennan T, et al. Medical professionalism in the new millennium: a physician charter. *Ann Int Med.* 2002;136:243–246; *Lancet.* 2002;359:520–522; *Eur J Int Med.* 2002;13:215–220; *Med J Aust.* 2002;177:208–212.
8. Ho M-J. Culturally sensitive medical professionalism. *Acad Med.* 2013;88:1014.
9. Al-Eraky MM, Chandratilake M. How medical professionalism is conceptualized in Arabian context: a validation study. *Med Teach.* 2012;34:S90–S95.
10. Cruess RL, Cruess SR. Professionalism, communities of practice, and medicine's social contract. *J Am Board Fam Med.* 2020;33:S50–S56.
11. Hafferty FW, Castellani B. A sociological framing of medicine's modern-day professionalism movement. *Med Ed.* 2009;43:826–828.
12. Pellegrino ED, Relman A. Professional medical associations: ethical and practical guidelines. *JAMA.* 1999;282:1954–1956.
13. Larson. M. *The Rise of Professionalism: A Sociological Analysis.* University of California Press; 1977.
14. Shaw, B. *Introduction to "Own the Doctor's Dilemma."* Penguin Books; 1946:75. (Original published 1911)
15. Cruess SR, Cruess RL. Professionalism must be taught. *BMJ.* 1997;7123:1674–1677.
16. Hafferty FW. Socialization, professionalism, and professional identity formation. In: Cruess RL, Cruess SR, Steinert Y, eds. *Teaching Medical Professionalism: Supporting the Development of a Professional Identity.* Cambridge University Press; 2016:43–68.
17. Cruess R, Cruess S. Teaching professionalism: general principles. *Med Teach.* 2006;28: 205–208.

18. Irby DM, Hamstra SJ. Parting the clouds: three professionalism frameworks in medical education. *Acad Med.* 2016;91:1606–1611.

19. Erikson EH. *The Lifecycle Completed.* Norton; 1982.

20. Kegan R. *The Evolving Self: Problems and Process in Human Development.* Harvard University Press; 1982.

21. Cruess RL, Cruess SR, Boudreau JD, Snell L, Steinert Y. Reframing medical education to support professional identity formation. *Acad Med.* 2014;89:1446–1451.

22. Merton RK, Reader LG, Kendall PL, eds. *The Student Physician: Introductory Studies in the Sociology of Medical Education.* Harvard University Press; 1957.

23. Cooke M., Irby DM, O'Brien C. *Educating Physicians: A Call for Reform of Medical School and Residency.* Jossey-Bass; 2010.

24. Cruess RL, Cruess SR, Boudreau JD, Snell L, Steinert Y. Reframing medical education to support professional identity formation. *Acad Med.* 2014;89:1446–1451.

25. Wenger-Trayner E, Wenger-Trayner B. Learning in a landscape of practice. In: Wenger-Trayner E, Fenton-O'Creevy M, Hutchison S, Kubiak C, Wenger-Trayner B, eds. *Learning in a Landscape of Practice: A Framework.* Routledge; 2015:13–31.

26. Wald H. Professional identity (trans)formation in medical education: reflection, relationship, resilience. *Acad Med.* 2015;90:701–706.

27. Cruess SR, Cruess RL. Development of a professional identity. In: Swanwick T, O'Brien B, Forrest K, eds. *Understanding Medical Education.* 3rd ed. John Wiley & Sons;2019:239–254.

28. Kalet A, Buckvar-Keltz L, Harnik V, et al. Measuring professional identity formation early in medical school. *Med Teach.* 2017;39:255–261.

29. Frost HD, Regehr G. "I am a doctor": negotiating the discourses of standardization and diversity in professional identity construction. *Acad Med.* 2013;88:1570–1577.

30. Bourdieu P, Passeron J-C. *Reproduction in Education, Society, and Culture.* 2nd ed. Sage Publishing; 1990.

31. Mechanic D. In my chosen doctor I trust. *BMJ.* 2004;329:1418–1419.

32. Fenwick T. Social media in medical professionalism: rethinking the debate and the way forward. *Acad Med.* 2014;89:1331–1334.

Preface

Gia Merlo and Thomas D. Harter

While medical professionalism as a field of academic study has a relatively a short history, what was obvious to us in the wake of the book *Principles of Medical Professionalism* (Oxford University Press; 2021) is that there are multiple approaches to addressing medical professionalism, and that the field has been developing in very divergent ways. The vision for this book early on was to capture and highlight these differences with the goal to further the dialogue to bring these diverse perspectives together. Having two people with different backgrounds and who view medical professionalism through different lenses—one a physician and clinical psychiatrist (Merlo), the other an academic philosopher and clinical ethicist (Harter)—serve as editors of this book seemed a perfect means to attain this vision. Although we approach medical professionalism from different angles, we both embrace ideas and the ideals that are foundational to the field, and we both want to ensure that the field continues to flourish and that the conversations about medical professionalism—as highlighted in this book—do not become stagnant.

This volume started as a collaborative phone call between Merlo and Harter shortly after the publication of *Principles*. Merlo recognized more needed to be said about both the origins of medical professionalism as a field and discipline and about how the field has been expanding in vibrant, yet different, directions. During that initial conversation there was an understanding that while *Principles* serves as a concise, easy-to-read text directly targeting physicians, the literature on medical professionalism—and the field overall—would benefit from a larger, comprehensive volume that brought these various perspectives on medical professionalism together across the full spectrum of the field with different points of view from contributing authors. We envisioned this book to include the spectrum of theory, education, and clinical applications of medical professionalism. In the spirit of this vision, Harter and Merlo agreed to go on this editing journey together.

One of the most significant strengths of this volume is including authors whose primary disciplines are fundamentally different in how they conceptualize medical professionalism. Strong advocates of medical ethics see medical professionalism as evolving from and as a subdiscipline of medical ethics, yet, for example, professional identity formation theorists and researchers view medical professionalism as its own unique discipline, separate from any other, including medical ethics. Overly reductionistic constructs are often addressed in the medical professionalism literature, but in order for the discipline of medical professionalism to continue its vibrant flourishing, it is essential to bring these divergent views together to identify and understand core definitions and concepts, as well as appreciate the unique values found among the different perspectives of what medical professionalism is and what it is not.

As Doukas and Fins discuss in Chapter 2, the fields of medical professionalism and medical ethics overlap. It is, from their perspective, impossible to consider one without the other since both fields are oriented around the notions that medical care requires clinical competence, a pledge to act for the benefit of the patient, and an implicit social contract that requires physicians to be self-regulating stewards of the profession. Yet, as we address in the Introduction, whereas medical ethics is broadly applicable across all healthcare disciplines, the field of medical professionalism is less broad and rightly applicable only to medical doctors. Although the terms *medical professionalism* and *healthcare professionalism* are now often interchanged and the term medical professionalism is occasionally used in reference to any medical provider, medical professionalism and healthcare professionalism are conceptually different. As noted in the Introduction, the reason for this difference primarily can be traced to the unique training of medical doctors compared to other healthcare professions, as well as the special fiduciary bond that is inherent to patient-physician relationships. The foreword by Sylvia and Dick Cruess carefully considers these similarities and differences in how medical professionalism has evolved amid these various perspectives of the field and offer their own perspective on how the field should continue to develop moving forward. They emphasize that although context matters in the ongoing analysis and educational endeavors of medical professionalism—and that the field of medical professionalism should evolve in relation to the changes in medicine's social contract with society—it is important to recognize that the core issues related to medical professionalism are bedrock, yet not exclusionary. The field of medical professionalism, therefore, cannot and should not experience a paradigm shift with changing social attitudes or each time a new professionalism challenge emerges calling into question old ways of thinking about professionalism. Instead, the field should broaden its conceptual field of vision to be inclusive of new perspectives, while remaining anchored to its core identity as a healing profession that exists for the benefit of society and individual patients.

To accomplish our vision of creating a diverse, comprehensive volume that pulls together authors from various medical and academic disciplines, we broke the continuum of medical professionalism into three general categories: its theoretical underpinnings, how professionalism is communicated and taught to learners, and professionalism in practice. As we began to consider professionalism in practice, we realized and appreciated that there are at least two distinct types of implementation concerns: those at the individual practice level and those at the organizational level at the interface of patients, physicians, *and* organizational leaders and administrators. This led us to the decision to organize this volume into four parts with a total of thirty-seven chapters. We aimed for an integrative approach, seeking authors with expertise either in the field of medical professionalism, medical ethics, or in their respective disciplines or with a chosen topic.

Together these contributing authors provide a wealth of knowledge and robust dialogues along the spectrum of medical professionalism that no one author or small group of authors could narrate alone. They are thought leaders from universities or academic medical centers with top-rated programs or departments in medical professionalism or medical ethics, clinicians at top health centers, or key figures with organizations such as the Accreditation Council for Graduate Medical Education, the Academy for Professionalism in Health Care, or the National Institutes of Health. Perhaps most important, the contributing authors are representative of the thousands of teachers, innovators, and influencers in healthcare who have been entrusted to learn, teach, and hold themselves, their colleagues, and their institutions accountable to the highest levels of patient-centered care.

There are two additional pieces of this book that merit special mention. Part of our aim was to capture the dynamic realities of medical professionalism as physicians live it. This is hard to achieve amid an intellectual and analytical endeavor. Tom Inui helped us achieve this aim by offering to write personal narratives—the stories of being a doctor grappling with medical professionalism issues at the clinician and administrative levels of patient care—as epilogues to each part of this text. Inui also penned the prologue, which illustrates, through his work transforming professionalism cultures in academic health sciences, the importance of personal reflection in the development of one's medical professionalism. We hope these pieces provide readers a more complete engagement with the material.

Second, we asked a team of writers who are futurist healthcare innovators to write a conclusion to this volume. Here, our goal was not to pause, reflect on, and provide a synopsis of the work covered in this volume, but offer a glimpse of where the future of medical professionalism may be headed. The authors of this chapter look at several different "tensions" that the field of medical professionalism will soon need to contend with as part of its continued growth and maturation.

Just as important as it is to note what we included in this volume and why, it is also important to note what we did not include in this book. While there were other topics of importance to the current and future state of medical professionalism education and training, we could not find authors to write on these topics for the book. We simply did not have the capacity to write the chapters ourselves, including assessments of technological innovation on patient care; managing scarce resources, especially during health calamities; the termination of patient care; and healthcare professionalism in different disciplines. Regarding this last topic—expanding the scope of this volume to include multiple other disciplines would have made this volume significantly lengthier, and we are not in a position to speak about with any authority since many other healthcare disciplines already have well-developed professionalism frameworks. Likewise, including other disciplines would have required either electing which disciplines to include and exclude from the volume or attempt to have this volume be an all-inclusive of other healthcare disciplines; neither strategy seemed ideal or practical. While we did include chapters from authors outside North America, including Goh and her team from Singapore and de Carvalho-Filho and his team from the Netherlands and Brazil, this volume does not include nuanced perspectives of medical professionalism that might be seen in other countries outside of North America. We hope any future editions of this text will be able to address some of these limitations.

Medical professionalism as a discipline is required to be taught as part of accreditation requirements in medical schools and residencies across North America. As this book demonstrates, there are multiple ways to think about and integrate medical professionalism theory, education, and practice into one's professional life. We hope that beyond providing foundational material for learners at all levels, whether students just entering the medical profession, those in graduate medical education programs, or independent practicing physicians, the lessons about medical professionalism in this book are embraced with curiosity and passion, allowing readers to expand their knowledge and challenge assumptions and ways of thinking and overcome individual obstacles to achieve transition and growth in the professionalism development.

Ultimately, as editors and contributing authors, we appreciate our personal and professional growth through this process. In seeking to expand on key constructs and add new perspectives to the literature, neither of us anticipated how much change and growth we would experience in our professional lives and friendship through editing this book. For that, we express thanks and gratitude to each other, all of our contributing authors, and our readers.

Acknowledgments

Gia Merlo and Thomas D. Harter

The process of conceptualizing, reconceptualizing, proposing, combing through the literature, identifying leaders in medical professionalism, and ultimately editing this volume has been a labor of love involving dozens of colleagues, friends, contributing authors, and family. We owe a sincere debt of thanks and gratitude to all of them. This volume would not exist without their support.

We decided that involving all the contributing authors in helping shape the direction of the book was most beneficial for the field for the sake of completeness and inclusivity. In that spirit, we embarked on meeting with each of the contributing authors—in some cases multiple times—to share our vision, to engage with them in dialogue about their contributions, and to heed their suggestions to create this comprehensive work that encompasses the spectrum of medical professionalism from its theoretical underpinnings to its implementation in practice. Especially insightful and helpful in this process were Sylvia and Dick Cruess, Tom Inui, Elizabeth Gaufberg, and Ayelet Kuper. We want to acknowledge Tom Inui's vision and contribution of the narrative sections and prologue. For their ongoing conversations and support, we would like to particularly thank Sylvia and Dick Cruess, who began writing the foreword together, while Dick Cruess saw it to completion after her passing.

With all the conversations and excitement created around this book, and the desire to produce a volume that covers such a broad set of topics within medical professionalism, the co-editors felt it necessary to engage in weekly meetings, where we hashed out all the decisions about the direction of the book and came to a place of understanding. The work on this book over the last three years would not have been possible without the support of our work colleagues at both the New York University Grossman School of Medicine, Emplify Health and the Gundersen Medical Foundation. Members of the Academy for Professionalism in Health Care also served as a sounding board for this project and many of the chapters in this book, specifically, David Doukas, Fred Hafferty, Elizabeth Kachur, Dennis Novack, Preston Reynolds, and John Spandorfer.

We are thankful to the publishing team at Oxford University Press, especially Andrea Knobloch for her belief and helpful suggestions in the project early on, and to Emma Hogdon for helping bring this project to completion.

We are especially grateful to our families and friends for their support throughout our careers and in the process of creating this book.

Acknowledgments

About the Editors

Gia Merlo, MD, MBA, MEd

Gia Merlo is a clinical professor of psychiatry at the New York University (NYU) Grossman School of Medicine, and a fellow of the American College of Lifestyle Medicine. Merlo recently published a textbook *Lifestyle Nursing* (Taylor & Francis/CRC Press; August 2022) that expands lifestyle medicine (an evidence-based approach in preventing, treating, and—oftentimes—reversing chronic diseases) to nursing. Her first book, *Principles of Medical Professionalism* (Oxford University Press; 2021), stresses the importance of physician wellness, the need to address the social determinants of health, as well as the need to address chronic diseases with prevention. In December, 2023, Merlo published *Lifestyle Psychiatry: Through the Lens of Behavioral Medicine* (Taylor & Francis/CRC Press; 2023). Merlo is the associate editor of the *American Journal of Lifestyle Medicine*. She is a contributing author of the American College of Lifestyle Medicine (ACLM) curriculum *Lifestyle Medicine 101* and of the board review course *Foundations to Lifestyle Medicine*.

Merlo is a part of the Psychiatry Faculty Group Practice at NYU Grossman School of Medicine and sees patients at NYU Langone Health Psychiatry, 1 Park Avenue, New York, NY. She completed her master of education in health professions at Johns Hopkins University School of Education in August 2022 and is currently an adjunct faculty at Johns Hopkins helping students in the program complete their capstone projects. Merlo has served on the board of directors of many nonprofits over the years, including Academy of Professionalism in Health Care (APHC) and is currently on the board of directors of Plant-Powered Metro of New York (PPMNY) and the advisory board of the Global Positive Health Institute (GPHI). She is founding chair of the American Psychiatric Association's Lifestyle Caucus, creating curricular content for psychiatrists on lifestyle interventions. She has been involved in clinician care and medical education for nearly 30 years in professional development and mental health, particularly for healthcare professionals.

Before joining NYU, Merlo was an associate dean of health professions at Rice University. She also taught medical students, residents, and fellows at Baylor College of Medicine, where she was a 2017–2019 Master Teacher Fellow. She has served on the faculty at the University of Pennsylvania School of Medicine, Baylor College of Medicine, Rice University, Texas Children's Hospital, and Children's Hospital of Philadelphia.

Thomas D. Harter, PhD

Thomas (Tom) Harter is the director of the Department of Bioethics and Humanities with Emplify Health and an adjunct assistant professor with the Department of Clinical Research and Leadership with the School of Medicine and Health Sciences with the George Washington University. Harter recently published a chapter on Atul Gawande for *Contemporary Physician Authors: Exploring the Insights of Doctors Who Write* (Cambridge University Press; 2021), exploring the professional and personal impacts of Gawande's narrative writings. Harter's recent journal articles include an argument for tolerating conscientious objections in medicine (HEC Forum; 2021), a survey of physicians about treatment decision-making capacity in cases of withholding and withdrawing treatment and suicide (AJOB Empirical Bioethics; 2021), and a discussion of financial vulnerability and organizational ethics stemming from the COVID-19 pandemic (*American Journal of Bioethics*; 2020).

Harter provides ethics education programs and workshops for a variety of health profession audiences at all different training levels within Emplify Health, as well as with local, national, and international audiences and universities. Harter chairs both the Gundersen Lutheran Institutional Review Board and the Emplify Health Ethics Committee and works to develop institutional policies and practices, staff education, and patient and community education with a special focus on medical professionalism, advance care planning, community engagement, and medico-industry relationships. On joining Emplify Health in 2012 (then known as Gundersen Health System), he was tasked with creating a formal medical professionalism curriculum for their internal medicine residency program.

Harter served on the Board of Directors with the Academy for Professionalism in Health Care (APHC) from 2016–2024 and served as APHC president from 2020 to 2022. He recently served on the Wisconsin Department of Health Services COVID-19 vaccine allocation committee (2020–2021), is the current board Secretary for the Association of Bioethics Program Directors (2024–2027), and most recently helped form the newly established Bioethics Network of the Upper Midwest.

Before joining Emplify Health, Harter studied philosophy at the University of Tennessee, specializing in medical ethics and business ethics, and gained formal training in clinical ethics as a fellow with the Cleveland Fellowship in Advanced Bioethics at Cleveland Clinic.

Contributors

Julie L. Agris, PhD, JD, LLM
Assistant Professor
Shepard Broad College of Law, Nova Southeastern University

Amy Alexander, MD
Clinical Assistant Professor
Department of Psychiatry & Behavioral Sciences
Stanford University School of Medicine

Peter Angelos, MD, PhD
Department of Surgery and
MacLean Center for Clinical Medical Ethics
The University of Chicago

Jay Baruch, MD
Professor of Emergency Medicine
Alpert Medical School of Brown University
Brown Emergency Medicine

Elliott Louis Bedford, PhD
Ascension St. Vincent (Indiana); Ascension Via Christi (Kansas)
Marian University College of Osteopathic Medicine

Judy Bolstad, JD, MA
Assistant Dean, Faculty Affairs and Learning Innovation
Assistant Professor, Department of Bioethics, Humanism and Policy
Roseman University College of Medicine

Timothy P. Brigham, MDiv, MS, PhD
Chief of Staff and Chief Education Officer
Accreditation Council for Graduate Medical Education

Pier Bryden, MD, MPhil, FRCPC
Associate Dean, Clinical Affairs and Professional Values
Associate Professor, Department of Psychiatry
Temerty Faculty of Medicine, University of Toronto

Leon Budrie, MD, MS
Center for Medical Ethics and Health Policy, Baylor College of Medicine

Nathan Carlin, PhD
Director of the McGovern Center for Humanities and Ethics
McGovern Medical School

Joseph Carrese, MD, MPH, FACP
Professor of Medicine
Core Faculty, Johns Hopkins Berman Institute of Bioethics
Johns Hopkins University

Brian S. Carter, M.D., FAAP
Chairman and Sirridge Endowed Professor of Medical Humanities & Bioethics
University of Missouri-Kansas City School of Medicine
Bioethics Center, Children's Mercy-Kansas City

Vanika Chawla, M.D, FRCPC
Staff Psychiatrist
Department of Psychiatry, Ross Memorial Hospital

Lynden (Lindsay) Crowshoe, MD, CCFP
Assistant Dean, Indigenous Health
Associate Professor, Family Medicine
Cumming School of Medicine, University of Calgary

Richard L. Cruess, MD
Emeritus Professor, Institute for Health Sciences Education
Lady Meredith House
McGill University

Marco Antonio de Carvalho Filho, MD, PhD
Professor of Research in Health Profession Education
University Medical Center Groningen, University of Groningen

Janet de Groot, MD, FRCPC
Professor, Psychiatry, Oncology and Community Health Sciences
Cumming School of Medicine, University of Calgary

Edison Iglesias de Oliveira Vidal, MD, MPH, PhD
Associate Professor of Geriatrics, Botucatu Medical School
São Paulo State University (UNESP)

David J. Doukas, MD
James A. Knight Chair of Humanities and Ethics in Medicine,
Director, Program in Medical Ethics and Human Values,
Professor, Department of Family and Community Medicine
Tulane University School of Medicine
Integrated Ethics Program Officer, Southeast Louisiana Veterans Health Care System, and Clinical Ethics Liaison, VISN 16, US Department of Veterans Affairs

Jason T. Eberl, PhD
Hubert Mäder Chair in Health Care Ethics
Professor of Health Care Ethics and Philosophy
Director, Albert Gnaegi Center for Health Care Ethics
Saint Louis University

Laura Edgar, EdD
Senior Vice President, Competencies, Milestones, and Faculty Development
Accreditation Council for Graduate Medical Education

Rachael Essig, MD
Department of Surgery
MacLean Center for Clinical Medical Ethics
The University of Chicago

Joshua M. M. Faber, MD
Department of Emergency Medicine
New York-Presbyterian, Columbia University Irving Medical Center,
Weill Cornell Medical Center

Christopher P. Fagundes, PhD
Professor
Rice University

Joseph J. Fins, MD, MACP, FRCP
E. William Davis, Jr., MD, Professor of Medical Ethics
Chief, Division of Medical Ethics
Professor of Medicine, Weill Cornell Medical College
Solomon Center Distinguished Scholar in Medicine, Bioethics, and the Law
Visiting Professor of Law, Yale Law School

Renato Soleiman Franco, MD, PhD
Adjunct Professor at the Graduate Program in Bioethics and Medical School
Pontifical Catholic University of Paraná (PUCPR)

Thomas H. Gallagher, MD, MACP
Professor, Department of Medicine and Department of Bioethics and Humanities

S. Monty Ghosh, MBT, MSc, MPH, MD, FRCPC
Assistant Professor, University of Alberta
Assistant Professor, University of Calgary

Tyler S. Gibb, JD, PhD
Associate Professor
Department of Medical Ethics, Humanities, and Law,
Western Michigan University Homer Stryker MD School of Medicine

Marin Gillis, PhD, LPh
Senior Executive Dean, Faculty Affairs and Learning Innovation
Professor, Department of Bioethics, Humanism and Policy
Roseman University College of Medicine

Suzanne Goh, MBBS, MEd
Assistant Professor
Associate Dean, Medical Curriculum
Duke-NUS Medical School
Department of Paediatric Endocrinology
KK Women's & Children's Hospital

Christine Grady, RN, PhD
Department of Bioethics, Chief,
Clinical Center,
National Institutes of Health

F. W. Hafferty, PhD
Senior Fellow, Center for Ethics, Professionalism, and the Future of Medicine
Office of the President and Chief Executive Officer, Accreditation Council for Graduate Medical Education

Thomas D. Harter, PhD
Director
Department of Bioethics and Humanities, Emplify Health and Gundersen Medical Foundation
Medical Director of Clinical Ethics, Emplify Health
Past President, Academy for Professionalism in Health Care

Nathan Houchens, MD
Medicine Service, Veterans Affairs Ann Arbor Healthcare System
Department of Internal Medicine, University of Michigan Medical School

Thomas S. Inui, ScM, MD, FACP
Retired Professor of Medicine
Indiana University, Harvard, University of Washington
Member Emeritus, National Academy of Medicine

Elizabeth Krajic Kachur, PhD
Director
Medical Education Development
Global Consulting

Rachel H. Kowalsky, MD, MPH
Associate Professor, Division of Pediatric Emergency Medicine, Department of Emergency Medicine and Pediatrics, New York Presbyterian Weill Cornell Medicine and Cornell Center for Health Equity

Lalit Kumar Radha Krishna, PhD, MD, FRCP, MRCP
Division of Supportive and Palliative Care
National Cancer Centre, Singapore
Yong Loo Lin School of Medicine, Singapore
Duke-NUS Medical School, Singapore
Health Data Science, University of Liverpool
Palliative Care Institute Liverpool
Academic Palliative & End of Life Centre
University of Liverpool
PalC, The Palliative Care Centre for Excellence in Research and Education, Singapore

Ayelet Kuper, MD, DPhil, FRCPC
Scientist and Associate Director, The Wilson Centre
University Health Network/University of Toronto
Professor, Department of Medicine
Temerty Faculty of Medicine, University of Toronto

Justin Lam, MD, FRCPC
Assistant Professor, Division of Paediatric Hospital Medicine
Department of Paediatrics,
Schulich School of Medicine and Dentistry
Children's Hospital - London Health Sciences Centre

Ariel Lefkowitz, MD, CM, MEd, FRCPC
Education Lead,
Division of General Internal Medicine, Sunnybrook Health Sciences Centre
Scholar, The Wilson Centre, University Health Network/University of Toronto
Assistant Professor, Department of Medicine, Temerty Faculty of Medicine, University of Toronto

Cheryl C. Macpherson, PhD
Department of Clinical Skills
St. George's University, Grenada

Jerry M. Maniate, MD, MEd, FRCPC
Founding Director, Equity in Health Systems (EqHS) Lab
Affiliate Researcher, Bruyere Research Institute
Associate Professor, Department of Medicine & Department of Innovation in Medical Education
University of Ottawa
Vice-Chair of Member Support, Department of Medicine, University of Ottawa

M. A. Martimianakis, PhD
Professor, Department of Paediatrics
Director of Medical Education Scholarship
Associate Director Collaborations and Partnerships
University of Toronto

Gia Merlo, MD, MBA, MEd
Clinical Professor of Psychiatry
New York University Grossman School of Medicine
Associate Editor, *American Journal of Lifestyle Medicine*

Kelly N. Michelson, MD, MPH
Northwestern University Feinberg School of Medicine

Henry J. Michtalik, MD, MPH, SFHM
Assistant Professor
Division of Hospital Medicine
Department of Medicine, Johns Hopkins University
Johns Hopkins Bayview Medical Center
Collaborative Inpatient Medicine Service

Parth K. Modi, MD, MS
Department of Surgery, University of Chicago Medicine
The MacLean Center for Clinical Medical Ethics, University of Chicago Medicine
Assistant Professor of Surgery, Section of Urology
University of Chicago Medicine and Biological Sciences

Mantoa Mokhachane, FC (Paeds) SA, PGDip (HSciEd), PhD
Director, Unit for Undergraduate Medical Education, School of Clinical Medicine
Faculty of Health Sciences, University of Witwatersrand

Marie Nicolini, MD, PhD
Kennedy Institute of Ethics, Georgetown University
Center for Biomedical Ethics and Law, KU Leuven University

David Ozar, PhD
Emeritus Professor
Philosophy Department
Loyola University Chicago

Morag Paton, PhD
Associate Director, Maintenance of Certification & Education Consultation Services, Continuing Professional Development
Temerty Faculty of Medicine, University of Toronto

Ryan Pferdehirt, D. Bioethics, HEC-C
Rosemary Flanigan Chair, The Center for Practical Bioethics
Vice President of Ethics Services, the Center for Practical Bioethics
Assistant Professor of Bioethics, Kansas City University

LTG Ronald Place, MD
Director
Defense Health Agency

Saleem Razack, MD, FRCPC
Department of Pediatrics, Critical Care Medicine, British Columbia Children's Hospital
Centre for Health Education Scholarship, University of British Columbia

Michael J. Redinger, MD, MA
Associate Professor
Department of Medical Ethics, Humanities, and Law, and Psychiatry,
Western Michigan University Homer Stryker MD School of Medicine

P. Preston Reynolds, MD, PhD, MACP
Professor, Department of Medicine, University of Virginia School of Medicine

James M. Rippe, MD
Professor of Medicine, UMass Chan Medical School
Editor in Chief, *American Journal of Lifestyle Medicine*
Founder/Director, Rippe Lifestyle Institute

Steven Rosenzweig, MD
Professor, Emergency Medicine (Hospice and Palliative Medicine)
Director, Professionalism Education
Director, Office of Community Engagement
Drexel University College of Medicine

Shiva Sarraf-Yazdi, MD, MEd, MBA
Associate Professor
Vice Dean of Education
Duke-NUS Medical School

Nathan R. Selden, MD, PhD
Dean, Oregon Health & Science School of Medicine
Campagna Chair of Pediatric Neurosurgery
Oregon Health & Science University

Annie Simpson, MD
The University of New Mexico Health Sciences Center
Professor Emeritus, Medicine and Geriatrics
Previously Rust Professor of Ethics
Associate Vice-Chancellor African American Health
Director Institute of Ethics, Chair—Bioethics Committee
Executive Director Black Health Resource Center

Eric A. Singer, MD, MA, MSFACS, FASCO
The Dave Longaberger Endowed Chair in Urology
Professor of Urology and Bioethics
Divisions of Urologic Oncology and Bioethics
The Ohio State University College of Medicine and Wexner Medical Center

Armaan Singh, BA
Department of Surgery, University of Chicago Medicine

Carlos S. Smith, DDA, MDiv, FACD
Associate Dean, Inclusive Excellence, Ethics, and Community Engagement
Assocaite Professor, Department of Dental Public Health and Policy
VCU School of Dentistry

John Spandorfer, MD
Roger Daniels Associate Dean for Professionalism in Medicine
Professor of Medicine
Sidney Kimmel Medical College of Thomas Jefferson University

COL Steven G. Sugden, MD, MPH, MSS
Assistant Professor (Clinical)
Huntsman Mental Health Institute
University of Utah Spencer Fox Eccles School of Medicine
Command Surgeon
76th Operational Response Command
Fort Douglas

Chad M. Teven, MD, MBA, FACS
Northwestern University Feinberg School of Medicine

Jason Adam Wasserman, PhD, HEC-C
Professor, Foundational Medical Studies
Director of Student Professionalism
Oakland University William Beaumont School of Medicine

Andrew A. White, MD
Professor, Department of Medicine
University of Washington

Cynthia R. Whitehead, MD, PhD, CCFP, FCFP
Director and Scientist, The Wilson Centre
BMO Financial Group Chair in Health Professions Educational Research
University Health Network/University of Toronto
Professor, Department of Family and Community Medicine
Temerty Faculty of Medicine, University of Toronto

Mark Wicclair, PhD
Adjunct Professor of Medicine
Center for Bioethics and Health Law, University of Pittsburgh
Professor of Philosophy, Emeritus, West Virgina University

Albert W. Wu, MD, MPH
Fred and Juliet Soper Professor
Director, Center for Health Services and Outcomes Research
Johns Hopkins Bloomberg School of Public Health

Tasha R. Wyatt, PhD
Vice Chair of Research, Center for Health Professions Education,
Department of Health Professions Education
Uniformed Services University of the Health Sciences

Prologue

Professionalism and the Stories of Our Lives

Thomas S. Inui

In the health professions, a "curriculum vitae" (CV) usually refers to a document in a standardized format, compiling information that includes a current address, telephone number, email address, place of birth, undergraduate and graduate degrees, postdoctoral training, fellowships, licensure, certification, and—if applicable—academic appointments and/or other professional positions. In a standard CV, there is also room for listing awards and a personal bibliography. The deeper literal meaning of *curriculum vitae* is, of course, not entirely well captured by this itemization, but instead we could also understand CV to refer to how, what, where, and when we have *learned* in the course of our lives.

My CV dutifully documents the milestones of my life as I moved through five universities, four academic ranks, and eight health systems and produced 353 papers/books/chapters in the course of 53 years. The large majority of my publications are peer-reviewed research papers, but 23 of the publications[1–23] have incorporated personal *stories*, including 33 narratives of events in my life from which I have learned a great deal when making choices and taking actions that I hoped might add up to a virtuous life. I chose to write and publish stories that were personal in nature not because I imagined I was a role model for others, but because my own life is the one I understand best and automatically have "permission" to share its "interiors." Creating this storyline over time has certainly not been the product of self-adulation. A substantial fraction of the stories are accounts of *mistakes* I have made, perhaps because these are the events in my life that I most vividly recall—sometimes in my conscious reflections, many in the liminal space between my daytime mind and sleep, and, indeed, often in my dreams (alas).

Throughout my career, I have kept "floating lists" of events that I might choose one day to write about. In my own experience, it has been important to commit these recollections to a written form whether or not I intend to publish them. Most of the time an event or a situation "makes the list" at first simply because it was associated with a strong emotional reaction—anger, horror, joy, sadness, confusion, shame, regret, or grief. Writing these events, even as a crude first draft, organizes them in my mind, clarifies why they have been emotionally stirring, and reveals the essential elements of the experience as well as the chaff that can be discarded as the story is reduced to its essential form. In some important way, the stories have revealed to me what has been most valuable in my life in medicine, how sources of meaning have welled up like springs of cool water in the sometimes arid land, what I can contribute at my best, what needs to change to permit my greatest contribution going forward, what I need and consume, and how I stand in critical interactions with others (patients, colleagues, team members, friends, and family) and how I am affected by organizational environments, policies, and systems. The stories have been about choices and actions in caring for patients, teaching, doing research, struggling with death and dying, learning from success and failure, trying to communicate in difficult situations, recognizing a spiritual life, or expressing love. When I have shared these stories in lectures, presentations, organizational newsletters, and peer-reviewed publications, I have done so in hopes of illuminating dark corners in our professional lives, sharing thoughts, touching hearts, and encouraging others to contribute their own stories in an effort to co-create a shared narrative, a crazy quilt, or a storyboard of our professional and/or organizational community.

In the late 1960s, when I had my clinical skills training at Johns Hopkins, one of the skill-building exercises was a group session in the operating rooms (ORs) of the Women's Clinic for learning the fundamentals of the pelvic exam. The days chosen were ones on which the Resident Service had "EUA" (examination under anesthesia) procedures, often a prelude to dilatation and curettage of women for excessive uterine bleeding. We changed into scrubs in the dressing room, masked up, and entered the designated OR, some of us in the OR for a first time. I don't recall that we had any information about the patients. I do remember that a large woman in scrubs was clearly in charge of all our movements. She referred to us as "young students" and didn't introduce herself. I didn't cover myself with glory in this exercise. Twenty-six years later, I wrote about it for the *Annals of Internal Medicine*[8] as follows (reprinted with permission):

Fainting before the First Pelvic Exam
In the dark.

Her legs in stirrups and draped.
At first furtive glance looking
Like a settee covered for winter.
She was easily mistaken for furniture.

To green-gowned novitiates
The OR was a whirl—
Bottles of blood on the wall.
Sucking, hissing sounds,
And cutlery set at side table—
A ritual in the making.
Heady vapors ablated my smell,
And breathing labored through
The dampening mask.
Glasses steam; two senses gone.

Suddenly that clank,
And with an eerie low hum.
Labial parts flare incandescent.
Strangely disembodied and
Frothy brown with betadyne prep.
Queuing now we wait to press for the
Too large uterus, the possible mass.
Soft belly and searching fingers
Pressing hard enough to hurt,
Except for the anesthesia.

Waiting, the question
Forms itself.
Did she know of our pressing need.
The logic for this occasion?
Was she asked.
And did she also want us?
Players in the spotlight's glare.
Rehearsing now for far-off
Tasks and times,
Tech talk stage left.

Wait.
But why is the air so thin, the
Wait so long in a dizzying dead space?
My turn comes to feel, but
Wait . . . slipping down, hissing all around . . .
Slide back into a grey hollow-headed night.
"Good lord young doctors,"
Says the mother tech,
"One of you has passed!"

Examination under anesthesia.[1]

Why did I choose to write this prose poem in 1994? In retrospect, I can only speculate. I was helping to create OSCEs (objective, structured, clinical exercises) for medical students and residents at the University of Washington; I had been elected to the National Board of Medical Examiners and was active in the Association of American Medical Colleges (AAMC) as we moved toward emphasizing competencies rather than sheer knowledge. As a primary care internal medicine residency program director, I was aware that that these residents' skills in pelvic examinations and Pap (Papanicolaou) tests were demonstrably inadequate. Half of the Pap test results reported the presence of no cervical cells, suggesting that we were fishing blindly with spatulas hoping to encounter the cervix somewhere. I was trying, without much success, to decide how a pelvic exam OSCE might reasonably be created (A manikin? Standardized/teaching patient?). I had been stunned to learn, from firsthand accounts, that the faculty wives at one new medical school had volunteered to teach pelvic exam skills. In the midst of all this cognitive turmoil, I wrote.

I hoped that this story, indeed I hoped that all my stories, might provoke others to thoughtfulness, their primary function for me. As the stories usually came to me, none of them had a definitive conclusion, or—heaven forbid—a moral. In fact, I have been satisfied to leave listeners and readers with more live *questions* than advice or conclusions. The questions I hope others will ask are those I have asked myself. After engaging with one of my stories, for example, I hope that we can fruitfully ask:

1. Who in this story can I see as myself?
2. From the point of view of whomever you have chosen, what do you bring to the situation that makes these events possible?

3. Who else in this story (or its organizational or cultural context) influences this story?
4. Where/what in this story is "the good," the value, the virtue, the "North Star" or the principle we might seek to preserve?
5. What, then, ought I do?

Let's try this analytic approach out on "Fainting Before the First Pelvic Exam."[8]

1. Persons: do you identify with the patient, the student, the tech, other (such as the clinician whose patient this is)?
2. What do I bring: patient/lack of informed consent, history of victimization or powerlessness; student/naivete, assumption of privilege, need to know/prepare, peer pressure, fear of failure?
3. Organizational context: academic hospital training culture, usual procedures, history of "residency service" for poverty/minority patients?
4. The "good": training to competence, informed consent, efficient educational exercises? Are these values in competition?
5. What ought I do/say/think? The student escapes by swooning. Are there some circumstances students and others (e.g., patients) are placed in by our academic organizations that are "no exit" situations? Should these situations prevail at all? Sometimes? Only under specific circumstances? What circumstances?

There are other questions that a reading of the poem might provoke, of course. Many hinge on closer inspection of the language of this poem. From what you know or could surmise, would it be possible to ask what race the patient is or is likely to be? What is the role of race, gender, and hierarchy in this situation? Who sets the rules for "what we do around here?" What does use of the word "furniture" suggest? Similarly, what contexts do the words "novitiates" and "cutlery" each invoke? What do the phrases "mother tech" and "pressing needs" mean or invoke? Does any aspect of the experience suggest a violation, even a rape? What does the lead tech mean by "passed"? Is this a reasonable use of an operating room in a teaching hospital? If the OR charges are levied by time, would it be reasonable to add the minutes for this activity to the patient's bill?

All of the questions I have listed (and more of your own choosing) might be on your mind after reading "On Fainting." The initial five questions recommended above are ones borrowed from literary or sacred text exegesis. They apply as well to any stories we tell one another about our experiences in the healthcare environments in which we live and work. They are especially applicable because the health professions and our organizations express a "calling" to serve. As Robert Coles observed,[24] we are compelled to tell and share such stories because they build a firm foundation for our *moral* development. If you doubt this set of assertions, try to conduct such an exegesis of the first story that comes to your mind about an event or situation you have encountered that you believe taught you something about professionalism or professional values. This story need not be about a particularly important occasion or seminal event—just one that has lodged itself in your store of memories and pops up as "top of mind." Take a 3-by-5 card or a blank sheet of paper and write for 5 minutes to record the story in brief. Artistry is not essential. Explore this story with our set of questions, see what you learn about your life, your organization, your colleagues, patients, values, guiding principles, and spiritual pillars. Make your own floating list. Start storytelling now. *Ars longa, vita brevis. The art is long; life is short.*

References

1. Inui TS. Oh Calcutta! President's editorial. *Soc Gen Intern Med Newsl.* 1987;9(4):2–3.
2. Inui TS. Just so stories. President's editorial. *Soc Gen Intern Med Newsl.* 1987;10(1):2.
3. Inui TS. Sephadex, my Sephadex: discovering the process of inquiry. President's editorial. *Soc Gen Intern Med Newsl.* 1987;10(5):2.
4. Inui TS. Our work, our selves. President's column. *Soc Gen Intern Med Newsl.* 1988;11(1):2.
5. Inui TS. Tiger, tiger. President's column. *Soc Gen Intern Med Newsl.* 1988;11(2):2, 6.
6. Inui TS. Though Sydenham fled the plague: 1988 SGIM Presidential Address. *J Gen Intern Med.* 1988;3:566–571.
7. Inui TS. In mid-life [prose]. *J Gen Intern Med.* 1991;6(5):444.
8. Inui TS. On fainting before the first pelvic exam [poetry]. *Ann Intern Med.* 1992;117(2):167.
9. Inui TS. And the dead shall be raised [prose]. *J Gen Intern Med.* 1992;7(5):565.
10. Inui TS. What would Sir William Osler think of internal medicine today? *Ann Royal Coll Phys Surg Can.* 1994;27(2):103–108.
11. Inui TS. A turning point for the ballerina—exploring an epidemiologic association [prose]. *Med Encounter.* 1995;11(2):9–10.
12. Inui TS. The land speaks [prose]. *GilChrist Lett.* Fetzer Institute 2001;Winter(January):1–2.
13. Inui TS. On belonging and beginning [prose]. *GilChrist Lett.* Fetzer Institute 2001;Spring (April):5–6.
14. Inui TS. Communion at the supper table [prose]. *GilChrist Lett.* Fetzer Institute 2001;*Summer*(August):6–10.
15. InuiTS.Comingunbidden[prose].GilChristLett.FetzerInstitute2001;Fall(November):5–8.
16. Inui TS. The length of our journey: care near the end of life. *Sufi.* 2002;Spring(53):8–11.
17. Inui TS. Foreword: we shall all be well-served. In: Carr PL, Bickel J, Inui TS (eds), *Taking Root in a Forest Clearing: A Resource Guide for Medical Faculty.* Boston University School of Medicine; 2003:10–13.
18. Inui TS. *A Flag in the Wind: Educating for Professionalism in Medicine.* Association of American Medical Colleges; February 2003.
19. Inui TS. Recollection and mindfulness in medicine: Southern Illinois University School of Medicine commencement. 2004. Aspects: 5. Full version at https://www.siumed.edu/pubs/SIUaddress04. pdf
20. Inui TS. Learning to save lives [prose]. *J Gen Intern Med.* 2005;20(7):670–671.
21. Inui TS. Dr. Harvey and the ballistic glasses. *Acad Med.* 2007;82(8):756.
22. Inui TS. Garlands. In: *Reflections: Voices of Hope in Our Community.* Indiana University School of Medicine; August 2008:ii–iii.
23. Inui TS, Inui TS. An intergenerational reflection on the first night on call—*plus ca change, plus le meme chose? J Grad Med Educ.* 2010;2(1):4–6.
24. Coles R. *The Call of Stories: Teaching and the Moral Imagination.* Houghton Mifflin Company; 1989.

References

PART A

WHAT DO WE MEAN BY MEDICAL PROFESSIONALISM?

Definitions, Theory, and Scope

1
Introduction
What Is and Is Not Medical Professionalism?

Thomas D. Harter and Gia Merlo

Key Points

- Although many of the concepts and topics discussed within the realm of medical professionalism can be extrapolated to other health professions, medical professionalism is distinct from healthcare professionalism and is applicable only to medical doctors.
- The narrative prologue and epilogues to each section of this textbook provide readers the opportunity to combine the teaching elements of each section with lived experiences.
- This chapter describes the overall structure of the textbook, previewing the chapters in each section.

What is and is not medical professionalism? Does—or should—the concept cover all allied health professionals or only medical doctors? Is it purely sociological in nature, encompassing a set of beliefs, rules, or codes to be followed; or does it have an objective, ontological existence that is witnessed and described through the personality dispositions, attitudes, and behaviors of medical professionals? Can professionalism be taught and if so, how? How is medical professionalism tied to, yet distinct from, medical ethics and how should the ties between the two fields be addressed? What does medical professionalism look like in practice at the individual level and at the organizational level?

During the initial brainstorming sessions about the text—working to identify what we wanted to, needed to, and should say about medical professionalism—these were some of the orientation questions that were pondered. These questions remain the driving force of the architecture and content of this volume.

Initially, the possibility of writing a text on medical professionalism that was broad enough to encompass all the different health professions was considered. However, it quickly became apparent that not only was this task too big but also that it was wrongheaded. To be all inclusive, it would be necessary to acknowledge and include the perspectives of all health care professionals. Electing to be all inclusive therefore would mean either having to identify a limited number of professionalism topics and make sure each health profession was represented in our treatment of the topic, or not be inclusive of *all* the health professions, but rather decide which health professions ought to be included and which should not. Neither strategy seemed appropriate because the consequence of either meant likely failing to adequately represent the broad spectrum of health professions or creating a volume so large it would be nearly unreadable. Furthermore, there was an underlying recognition and appreciation that many health professions already have their own professionalism standards, practices, and education.

In this regard, it is clear that the general concepts and topics within the scope of medical professionalism expand beyond the borders of medical doctors and that there are multiple professionalisms that guide health care practices. Those who work in the space of health care professionalism sometimes use the term "medical professionalism" as a catch-all to encompass clinical providers such as nurses or physician assistants. Given that the terms "medical" and "healthcare" are commonly treated as synonymous and often are interchanged in general conversations, it makes sense that some consider "medical professionalism" as synonymous with "health care professionalism." Certainly, too, if one thinks of health care professionalism as being a spectrum, medical professionalism is a slice of that spectrum. This is important to keep in mind when going through the chapters of this text. There is little doubt that many of the topics covered, particularly in parts C and D, could be extrapolated to encompass some—if not all—other health care professions. However, given the limitations of being all inclusive of the health professions, this volume refers to "medical professionalism" rather than "health care professionalism" and treats the concept and term "medical professionalism" narrowly, applying only to medical doctors.

Beyond the practical concerns with attempting to be inclusive of all health professions, there is another reason to narrowly focus on medical professionalism as applicable only to medical doctors. Simply, medical doctors have the highest educational and practice standards of all the health professions, and they experience the greatest patient care burdens. This is not to diminish the practical and emotional investment of other health care professionals in patient care. Especially as the delivery of patient care has evolved to be multidisciplinary and specialized, all health care providers are expected to develop the expertise relevant to their chosen fields to provide exemplary patient care. Likewise, no health care provider is exempt from experiencing the emotional burdens and personal sacrifices that come with caring for patients. However, to be an independent practicing physician requires earning the highest educational degrees possible, having the most clinical contact hours, as well as undergoing residency training beyond earning a medical degree.[1] The financial costs to become a medical doctor is the highest of all the all the health professions.[2,3] Medical doctors also bear the ultimate responsibility for treatment decision outcomes.

With respect to this latter point about medical doctors being responsible for patient care outcomes, there is a special, fiduciary bond that exists between medical doctors and patients. Medical doctors are granted a variety of privileges; they are permitted to offer and provide a plethora of treatments and interventions and are well-compensated for their efforts. Patients must trust in both the abilities and intentions of their medical doctors. In exchange, medical doctors are expected to act in their patients' best interests, even if there are personal costs for doing so.[4,5]

It is the special, fiduciary bond between patients and medical doctors—the colloquial patient-physician relationship—that is the cornerstone of this text. More accurately, it is the changing nature of this bond tied to the evolution of what it means or may mean to be a medical professional, as well as the ways in which this bond can be jeopardized, that is the corner stone of this text. What is evident and unchanged is that medical doctors continue to have deep-rooted obligations to their patients. The ways in which medical doctors develop and express professionalism, however, is changing. Health care that is responsive to the needs of the communities in which care is provided requires diversity of cultural practices, ways of thinking, and ways of interacting with patients. Medical doctors who all look, think, and act the same hinders diverse patient care.

This is all to say that there is no singular, cemented ontological idea of medical professionalism. There is no single pathway toward cultivating or being a medical professional. One might even counter that it is unprofessional to argue for a monolithic, unchanging conceptualization of medical professionalism and only a single way to be a medical professional, as this fails to appreciate the ever-changing complexity of what it means to be healthy and what it means to provide health care within a society, as well as the unique dynamics present in each patient-physician relationship.

Yet, while there might not be a single way to think about and cultivate medical professionalism, there remain some fundamental aspects of medical professionalism that remain unchanged. Notably, the commitment of medical doctors toward patient well-being serves as the ultimate compass for directing us toward understanding medical professionalism. A doctor's ability to care for patients demands that the doctor's conduct never jeopardizes the health of those patients and, perhaps most important, never irreparably damages their fiduciary bond.

A Pathway Forward

This text is structured to fully explore the robust complexities of medical professionalism, from its theoretical roots to implementation in practice. The goal is to provide a layering effect that walks readers through the life cycle of medical professionalism from antiquity to its contemporary state, showing its bedrock pieces while addressing its evolution regarding various practice concerns. There are two special features to highlight before delving into the overall structure of the text.

Narrative Epilogues

It is one thing to engage in an intellectual assessment of medical professionalism, it is another to experience it. The stories of *being* a medical doctor are just as crucial—if not more so—as the analytical process of thinking about the intricacies of medical professionalism education and practice. A common theme throughout many of the chapters of this volume is the importance of reflection in both the teaching of medical professionalism and the personal cultivation of one's behaviors toward being a medical professional. Thomas Inui, MD, spent much of his career working to enhance and transform professionalism culture in the academic health sciences by focusing on the interface between the academic, normative aspects of becoming a medical doctor and the lived experiences that make-up the informal—and sometimes hidden—curriculum. Inui offers a prologue to this volume that illustrates the importance of reflecting on the lived experience as a crucial element of medical professionalism development. Each section also concludes with an epilogue written by Inui that are his personal reflective writings from becoming and being a medical doctor that span the course of his career. These pieces tie together the lessons of the respective section in which they appear and offer an opportunity for readers to combine the key teachings of each section with a narrative element, allowing for a more complete engagement with the material.

A Different Kind of Conclusion

As much as this volume attempts to account for the ever-changing nature of medical professionalism, it still represents only a snapshot of where the field is at present. Recognizing this limitation and appreciating the non-static state of medical professionalism education and any number of potential—yet presently unknown—challenges to medical professionalism, a concluding chapter was wanted that did not just summarize the text and highlight key points. Instead, the goal was to have a conclusion that focuses on the possible future state of medical professionalism. The authors of this chapter take a futurist view of medical professionalism and task readers with considering multiple tensions likely to disrupt the current state of medical professionalism education, research, and practice, while addressing several innovative ways to navigate those tensions. Taking lessons from chapters in this text, the authors look to expand the bedrock notion of medical professionalism being tied just to patient care, and rather consider medical professionalism as tied to communities—both physical and digital—in which medical professionals are also members. Here, medical professionalism is considered beyond the attitudes and behaviors of medical doctors toward patients and instead encompasses the ideas that medical professionalism also involves how medical doctors care for themselves and their colleagues and how they engage with their communities as advocates and allies for social changes in promoting the health and well-being of all persons.

Overall Structure

The literature on medical professionalism is vast. However, there are three main tracks of in the field:

1. Conceptual: works that focus on the philosophical understanding of "medical professionalism," or works that provide ethical evaluations of the concept as tied to medical practice.
2. Teaching and assessment: works that assess the ways and means for teaching and evaluating medical professionalism across the spectrum of medical care.
3. Practical or practice issues: works that evaluate the ethics or expected application of a particular practice or set of practices such as work hours reform for surgeons, burnout and resiliency in residency, resource stewardship, cultural competence, human subjects research, issues at the interface of human resources with ethical practice or at the interface of medical professionalism, ethics and the law.

Most works in medical professionalism tend to be nuanced and provide deep, rich analysis but within a limited practice scope. Of all the literature on medical professionalism, none attempt to meld together these three tracks of medical professionalism into a cohesive volume as delivered by the field's leading experts.

This text provides a comprehensive, four-part look at the three tracks of medical professionalism—the conceptual, educational, and the practical—in a single resource from the world's leading experts in medical professionalism. It is intended for independent practicing physicians, physician trainees, residents, fellows, health professions educators, administrators and directors in health organizations, and policymakers.

Part A: Theory

This section focuses on the definitions, theoretical underpinnings, and scope of medical professionalism. Doukas and Fins explore the symbiotic relationship between medical professionalism and medical ethics via a historical assessment of both concepts. While noting that medical ethics and medical professionalism did not develop simultaneously, Doukas and Fins demonstrate how they have become intractable intertwined in the recognition of the importance of clinical competence and pledge to the beneficial care of patients. de Groot, Simpson, and Crowshoe discuss the integration of equity, diversity, inclusion, and accessibility as essential to professional identity formation (PIF). They analyze codes of ethics from an indigenous perspective in demonstrating how medical professionalism can address historical inequities within healthcare. Lam, Martimianakis, and Hafferty propose a framework to integrate the formal, informal, and hidden curriculum to help socialize medical students toward becoming medical professionals. Here, the hidden curriculum is considered and treated as a powerful teaching tool for educators and researchers to anticipate and analyze curricular misalignments in ways that further promote PIF. Baruch and Kowalski consider the importance and role of arts and humanities in medical professionalism development. They demonstrate how incorporation of arts and humanities in all facets of medical education and practice provide a lens by which doctors can better navigate moral tensions that naturally arise in the practice of medicine. de Carvalho-Filho, Franco, and Vidal take readers through an exploration of the social contact between the medical profession and society, highlighting reciprocal duties and obligations. They further explore how changing dynamics within societies might, however, make the social contact metaphor insufficient to address medical professionals' responsibilities and accountabilities to the societies in which they practice. This problem can be addressed, they argue, by combining the social contract metaphor with cultural humility to create a professionalism of solidarity. Last, Ozar provides a philosophical perspective of medical professionalism that explores the cognitive and affective learning outcomes associated with medical professionalism education toward helping learners achieve an aspiration level of professionalism development.

Part B: Understanding and Educating for Medical Professionalism

This section explores different ways to understand and educate for medical professionalism along the continuum of medical practice. Gillis and Bolstad describe challenges to providing continuing professional development education to clinician educators in ways that meaningfully translate to undergraduate medical education. They propose utilizing concepts within PIF to guide developmental efforts for clinical educators toward their professional identities as *educators*, noting that preceptors should be prepared and supported as role models for students and that merely changing professionalism curriculums in insufficient in teaching medical professionalism. Chawla and Alexander explore unique considerations in medical professionalism education for underrepresented medical students, notably first-generation physicians, international medical students, and LGBTQ+ physicians, those with disabilities, and those who are considered racial and ethnic minorities. They carefully review bias in current educational constructs and identify opportunities for inclusivity and diversity within medical student education. Kachur provides a review of approaches to developing medical professionalism assessment tools. Here, Kachur highlights that assessment of medical professionalism in medical school is just as crucial as the education itself and that assessment is multifactorial and needs to be responsive to the changing landscapes of healthcare and medical professionalism education. Goh, Krishna, and Sarraf-Yazdi provide an assessment of the current state of PIF education, with a focus on reflective portfolios, while further noting how PIF can be difficult to assess given its deeply individualized nature. Rosenzweig discusses the challenges and risks associated with teaching empathy in medical school sans compassion. It is argued that teaching and cultivation of compassion is distinct from empathy and is central to professional formation. Brigham, Edger, and Seldon help pivot the conversation by discussing the transition from medical student to professional by providing an empirical look at how professionalism education—particularly via ACGME milestones—changes professional behavior over time. Here they discuss the purpose and impact of the ACGME's milestones in the continuum of professionalism education and development.

Part C: Implementation in Clinical Practice

One of the unique and important aspects of this volume is addressing medical professionalism in clinical practice. As the chapters in this section show, there are many different practice scenarios in which the appropriate application of medical professionalism is unclear. Fagundes, Merlo, and Rippe begin this section by providing an in-depth assessment of how it is essential to medical professionalism for physicians to incorporate lifestyle medicine into their clinical practices for the sake of patient care. Wicclair turns the lens of medical professionalism back to physicians and discusses the challenges to medical professionalism posed when physicians have conscientious objections to treatment, while offering strategies to managing conscientious objections in alignment with medical professionalism. Merlo then provides an exploration of the challenges doctors might experience at the interface of clinical practice and spirituality, both in terms of respecting patients' spiritual, religious, or cultural beliefs, as well as doctors respecting their own belief systems when those systems conflict with their professional training. Eberl and Bedford take the idea of challenges at the interface of spirituality and clinical practice and focus the lens on providing care in Catholic health systems. Angelos and Essig explore some of unique aspects of providing care during volunteer or mission work, in which there are often prevalent cultural differences, while discussing strategies for managing those differences that support professional and ethical practice. Place and Sugden address how medical professionalism is treated within military medical practices with a focus on the distinction between wartime and peacetime practices and among military and civilian populations. Carlin focuses on the application of humanities literature—namely Shem's *The House of God*—in the development of communication practices that affect professional identity formation, particularly in graduate medical education. Carter and Pferdehirt extrapolate the ideas of communication as tied to medical professionalism by exploring physician communication with patients, families, and the parents of minor patients. Ghosh explores medical professionalism in connection with the care of vulnerable populations, namely persons experiencing homelessness, persons who have experienced trauma or persons with histories of substance use disorder. Caresse and Merlo address how concern for one's well-being is an essential feature of medical professionalism. Spandorfer takes on the ever-changing and ever-challenging struggle with social media, highlighting the potential benefits to the doctors and medical profession in general, but also the potential pitfalls and risks to medical professionalism at both the clinician and organizational levels. Houchens addresses professionalism personification and attire and the potential stereotypes, biases, discrimination and microagressions that can occur from patients and physicians based on how physicians look, speak and dress. Grady and Nicolini review and address ethical and professionalism challenges that occur at the interface of clinical practice and medical research, and what it means for clinician-scientists to act professionally in their dual roles.

Part D: Implementation at the Organizational Level at the Interface of Physicians and Administrators

The final section of this volume explores in detail the kinds of professionalism challenges that occur for physicians at the organizational level. Even in cases in which medical doctors have their own private practices, the issues explored in this section are applicable to their responsibilities as administrators of their practices. Michelson, Teven, and Farber begin by addressing why and how medical professionalism challenges at the organizational level are different and logistically more difficult to manage than professionalism challenges at the clinical practice level. Whereas physicians' primary obligations are to their specific patients, organizations have obligations and responsibilities to a wider group of stakeholders including patients, employees, communities, and partner organizations. Harter explores what it means—or may mean—for physicians to express and develop professionalism in their roles as employees. By assessing what expectations employers and physicians have toward one another, Harter identifies core concepts and values that ground obligations between physicians and their employers, as well as potential employment threats physician professionalism. Gallagher and White address professionalism concerns related to physician retirement. Citing literature that demonstrates a link between physician age and patient outcomes, Gallagher and White argue that the medical profession is obligated to self-regulate aging physicians for the sake of patient safety. Michtalik and Wu address why and how it is imperative of medical professionalism for health care organizations to develop resiliency programs for the sake of physicians experiencing moral distress and burnout. Gibb, Wasserman, and Redinger examine the role for remediation of unprofessional conduct. Taking a skill-based approach to professionalism, they note that professionalism requires supportive organizational environments and argue for a just culture framework to address cases of medical professionalism lapses. Smith, Reynolds, and Razack address discrimination and racism within medical learning environments and argue that the current and future states of health professions education are obligated to prioritize diversity, equity, inclusion, belonging and justice as essential elements of PIF and care delivery. Razak builds on this argument by further exploring what it means to have an inclusive medical professionalism and how to create inclusive medical learning and care environments that account for those who are underrepresented or structurally marginalized within medicine. Agris assess medical professionalism at the organizational level through the lens of health law, noting how health law can have unintended consequences that sometimes impede medical professionalism. Here, recommendations and strategies are offered to address the identified obstacles. Singer and Modi examine the impacts on medical professionalism resulting from financial relationships between physicians and industry and offer guidance for the management of these relationships. Lastly, Macpherson and Budrie analyze the ties between health and the natural environment. Here they argue that being environmentally conscious and active aligns with medical professionalism, while providing examples of how physicians and health care organizations can be advocates for environmental stewardship.

References

1. Chekijian SA, Elia TR, Horton JL, et al. A review of interprofessional variation in education: challenges and considerations in the growth of advanced practice providers in emergency medicine. *AEM Educ Train.* 2020;5(2):e10469. doi:10.1002/aet2.10469
2. Craig CK, Holmes JH, Carter JE. Return on investment of advance practice medical degrees: NPs vs. PAs. *J Am Acad Physician Assist.* 2017;30(6):35–38.
3. Kraus MB, Hasan SH, Buckner-Petty SA, et al. Out-of-state students at state medical schools and increasing medical education debt. *Acad Med.* 2023;98(5):595–605.
4. Merlo G. *Principles of Medical Professionalism.* Oxford University Press; 2021.
5. Medical Professionalism Project. Medical professionalism in the new millennium: a physicians' charter. *Lancet.* 2002;359(9305):520–522.

2

The Evolution and Symbiosis of Medical Ethics and Professionalism

David J. Doukas and Joseph J. Fins

Key Points

- Medical ethics and professionalism are interdependent constructs that co-developed over the course of medicine's evolution.
- The essential touchstone of medicine is caring for the patient, predicated on competence in skills and knowledge, the recognition that patient interests supersede physician self-interest, and that the collective medical enterprise is an implicit social contract founded on patient-directed trust.
- The history of medical professionalism is a relatively new concept, introduced by John Gregory and Thomas Percival, founded on precepts from Bacon and Hume.
- The concept of the medical contract is minimalist in its construction and is better described by a covenant, with an initial promise, sustained by a trusting relationship, and with aspirations to excellence and fidelity.

Introduction

In this chapter, we assert that medical ethics is a necessary foundational predicate to professionalism. However, professionalism was not a social construct extant at the creation of the healing art. Professionalism was a relatively contemporaneous development in the nineteenth century, rooted in the collective ethical considerations of physicians in their care of society at large and the subsuming of their own interests to those of their patients. Medical professionalism is a foundational concept grounded on knowledge and skills, the promotion of patient benefit with the rejection of self-interest, excellence in comportment, and a covenant of trust with society. Professionalism's implicit social contract binds both the *ethics* (through character and personal behavior) of the individual practitioner and the *professionalism* of physicians collectively. The intersection and interdependence of medical ethics and medical professionalism are key to understanding the relationship between the physician and society and the distinction between the ethical obligations of the physician and the medical community writ large. Metaphorically, the relationship of ethics and professionalism in medicine is not unlike the holistic, dualistic nature of the DNA strand. For the whole to function, both ethics and professionalism components must have integrity and be linked with each other. The intersection of medical ethics and medical professionalism is key to the ongoing nurtured relationship between the physician, the medical profession, and society. To understand the interdependence of medical ethics and medical professionalism, we need to turn to the history of medicine, the basis of medical ethics, and the evolution of professionalism.

Medical Ethics and Professionalism From Antiquity

Although ethics and professionalism are linked in our conception of the physician's and the profession's obligations and responsibilities, ethics pre-dates professionalism in the history of medicine. Since antiquity, the central ethical consideration was the ethical duty of beneficence toward the patient as conveyed by the physician's requisite virtues in the care of the patient. The physician promoted the betterment of patient's health-related interests and the mitigation of harm to the patient.

In Hippocratic times, this practice was based on an oath-based promise to put the primacy of the patient's welfare first (implicitly) above the physician's self-interest and to practice honorably in the service of that good. Physicians were admonished to practice within their abilities and to withdraw in favor of those who were more expert, again in order to serve the patient thusly: "have two special objects in view with regard to disease, namely, to do good or to do no harm," as summarized in *The Epidemics*.[1,2] The primary intention of practice was the well-being of the patient—help and at least do not make things worse (balancing ethical principles of beneficence and non-maleficence). The primary motivation of practice for the physician was the physician's care for the patient. The motivation for the patient was to protect and promote their own interests during the vulnerability of illness.

Outside the Western tradition, the regulation of physician beneficence was dictated by a set of regulatory rules within a faith-based construct in Islamic medicine.[3] In Chinese medicine, there was a flourishing of virtue-based care emphasizing patient benefit.[4] The approaches of cultures around the world regarding medicine were distinctly different, but the common ethical thread on humankind's practice of medicine, whether by duty or virtue-based argument, is that the physician's mandate was to benefit the patient.

Beneficence was closely linked to competence. The physician was expected to acquire knowledge based on observational facts accumulated by the teacher of the apprentice, who would then utilize these observations to assist the patient. Additionally, aspects of skill-based competence were expected to be acquired during this apprenticeship. Whether we are talking about Hippocratic medicine or that in the twenty-first century, this concept of possessing both knowledge and skills exemplified a dedication to scientific, although imperfect, observations needed to treat the patient.[5–7]

Early medicine constituted a time of coherence between medical ethics and what could be considered, at best, nascent professionalism. This concept of medical ethics, based on beneficence and competence, was codified as a commitment among a group as an oath in which knowledge would be passed to future generations and utilized for the benefit of the patient while preventing harm befalling them.

This embryonic version of professionalism is not what we would recognize as professionalism today. Here, the commitment of these early healers was to the craft and to the guild of the assembled healers, not an agreement with society. Each healer was operating on their own within the Hippocratic oath, bound to the guild that they had created with clear devotion of care to the patient and the promotion of their guild.

For over two millennia, healers of medicine did what they could do with the little knowledge that observational practice afforded them to help patients in the best way that they could deduce. The scientific basis of medicine shifted far beyond what could be directly observed. Despite being well intended, physicians of the Hippocratic order were hampered in their patient care with a meager knowledge base of science. To this day, the science of our profession struggles valiantly to catch up to the healing requisite in our art—witness the exertions to address the scientific and clinical challenges of the COVID-19 pandemic in the face of great suffering.

More troubling, patient-centered beneficence did not always rule the day, however. Regrettably, especially at times of grave health peril such as epidemics and pandemics, fear of their morbidity and mortality would prompt some physicians to shirk their responsibilities of assisting patients, instead departing the cities to go off to the countryside—including Galen from Rome in the second century AD.[8] Boccaccio wrote of this during the plague in *The Decameron*.[9] This abandonment of patients at a time of great social need harmed the public's perception of medicine. Some cities even responded by offering contracts to physicians to serve in times of plague, with economic incentives for their increased risk.[8] One might observe that this gesture feeding the physician's self-interest was impure to the altruism theme one would desire in a plague doctor, but desperation in the face of departing physicians was a powerful inducement for these benefactors.

These healers lacked adherence to a social contract or trust-based responsibility.[10] Without that social-moral layer of responsibility, these physicians were not yet what we would term *medical professionals*, as they had no adherence to the implicit contract of rejecting concepts of self-interest in order to promote patient benefit and societal trust. Over time this deficiency would come back to affect unfavorably both medicine and society's perception of it.

The Enlightenment and Rise of Professionalism

The late eighteenth century represents the emergence of professionalism and evolution of medical ethics in a way that would be familiar to the modern eye. Jay Katz, for example in *The Silent World of Doctor and Patient*, writes of how the Age of Enlightenment, with influences from Bacon and Hume, ushered in a new valuation of the physician-patient relationship with the realization that physicians utilize "openness and candor."[11] Nonetheless, there was a dynamic tension with Hippocratic era prohibitions regarding reticence and omission of candid details that could defeat hope. The time period from the late eighteenth to the early nineteenth century saw changes regarding physician obligations of candid communication, even though such truthfulness would be consigned to circumstances *in extremis* (i.e., at times of "impending death"). This conflict of being a truth-bearer while also being a "minister of hope" made truth-telling problematic for the practicing physician.[12] Nevertheless, it opened the door to future considerations of disclosure by physicians and the eventuality of informed consent that would begin to shape medical ethics in the following centuries. The view that science and the humanities were antithetical domains was a paradox. It was the achievements of science and the rise of the scientific method that ultimately compelled physicians to use critical thinking skills of the humanities (cultivated with philosophy art, narrative, and history) conveyed via humanistic virtues to share information with patients regarding prognoses and, subsequently in informed consent, the risks and benefits of therapeutic interventions.[13] This evolution would manifest into the fostering of the doctor-patient relationship and the end of the silent world of doctor and patient that had reigned in medicine until the start of the Enlightenment.

While this constituted progress in the practice of medicine improving scientific knowledge and its application to patient care and its dissemination through increasingly organized efforts in medical education, there was a negative side to these advances. As medicine became more beneficial, it became commodified. Medicine's practice became a free market entity, with the competitive force, and the associated challenges to integrity, that one might expect. This change led to fierce competition that became unsavory between physicians. This discord of self-interest and competition between physicians tarnished the perception that physicians operated for the benefit of the patient and society. The Hippocratic notion of guild, which itself has been characterized as a way to advance the Hippocratic school in the marketplace, did not preclude and might have even fostered self-interest of the guild in the marketplace.[14] Something more was needed that extended beyond the individual and spoke to a broader ethos or professionalism for all practitioners.

The birth of modern professionalism can be traced to two key individuals, as cited by Katz above, and Laurence McCullough: John Gregory and Thomas Percival.[10,11,15,16] They helped to articulate rules of ethics and professional boundaries that would guide more modern practice. In the late nineteenth century, Scotland's John Gregory nurtured the evolution of scientific medicine by promoting the coherence of medical ethics with a commitment by the physician to society at large. It was Gregory's writings and lectures on sympathy and his disparagement of "the corporation spirit" that served as a bellwether change against self-interested physicians.[14] Practitioners who valued their revenue rather than their patients were suspect, and Gregory's promotion of "sympathy" counters this distrust.[10,14] McCullough asserts that Gregory "invented the ethical concept of medicine" premised on both Bacon and Hume.[10]

This connection between the group of medical professionals and society allowed for a truer sense of professionalism than had ever been utilized before in that the expectation of the physician was to act as an entrusted agent for the patient's interests. It was at this time that Gregory promoted the notion of transparent and rigorous, evidence-based (i.e., experiential) medicine.[10] Further, Gregory advocated that beneficence in its conduct must also be extended to self-abnegation, in which self-interest would be eschewed. As time passed, Gregory's lectures were disseminated widely, first in the United Kingdom, then the United States and beyond.

Thomas Percival was then the next carrier of the torch promoting competence coupled with patient-directed beneficence. Thomas Percival's argument of medicine's provision as a "public trust" to benefit the patient first and foremost promoted the evolution of medicine as a profession—rather than a self-interested person promoting their own interests primarily or as a guild member protecting the guild's interests.[10,16,17] This public trust is an implied contract to provide excellence in knowledge and skills in the care of all patients and one that no one physician owns. This connection between the group of medical professionals and society allowed for a truer sense of professionalism than had ever been utilized before. The expectation was that each physician serves as a self-critical practitioner whose authority could then be entrusted to the patient's care.

As a result of Percival's dedication, a code of ethics was formulated in the United Kingdom in 1794 and expanded in 1803. These writings then served as the framework for the American Medical Association (AMA) Code of Ethics just a few decades later in 1847 in the United States.[18] The evolution of the concept of medical professionalism was due to the incorporation of the concept of the public trust of the physician with its implied social contract. With this maturation, medical professionalism became conceptualized within the social order as a way to describe a group of physicians and their collective responsibilities to society both ethically and sociologically. This evolution led to the professionalism embodied in medical specialty societies such as the American College of Physicians and their attestations of professionalism.[19] This model is in stark contrast to the Hippocratic guild concept whereby professionalism is a model of individual physicians who cohere to common goals but operate independently of each other while promoting the guild's interests.

Professionalism and Medical Education: The Impact of Flexner

Even as professional societies were emerging early in the twentieth century, discord between medical ethics and professionalism emerged in the context of broad efforts at educational reform prompted by the vast (commercial) proliferation of medical educational institutions geared toward maximal profit in order to churn out new physicians. Regrettably, these physicians had very little in the way of knowledge, scientific skills, or critical thinking rigor. Medical education's bleak and self-interested economic stance with extraordinarily dubious quality and scientific integrity was the backdrop of what necessitated Abraham Flexner's famous 1910 report to the Rockefeller Foundation calling for scientifically informed medical education modeled on the experience of Johns Hopkins.[20,21]

What Flexner's report emphasized was the need to redouble efforts and medical education toward the importance of science. He proposed a vast curricular change in which students would have clinical exposure to patients after a two-year basic science immersion in scientific method and critical thinking. He also proposed a huge reduction in the number of medical schools, which resulted in many schools closing, but far from his idyllic goal. Further, with this closure and consolidation of medical schools, the vast majority of schools training and serving African Americans were outright closed, thereby worsening healthcare inequity in a segregated United States.

Unfortunately, American medicine missed Abraham Flexner's premise found in his other writings, that medical ethics and humanities coupled with sound role modeling were necessary to the contemporary medical professional—that "colleges need to set premedical requirements for sound liberal humanistic education."[22(p320)–24] Abraham Flexner believed that the medical educational efforts in the wake of his report missed his intended mark. He opined this medical school reform process had concentrated *only* on science while entirely leaving out the humanities and was "sadly deficient in cultural and philosophic background."[21,22(p319),25,26] US schools restructured medical education for students to think like a scientist and to abstract basic science to clinical medicine with the recognition of the importance of patient care and apprenticeship. However, in their zeal of promoting science in medicine, medical education left medical ethics and humanities by the wayside.

Medicine in the United States thereby had made its educational commitment to "medicine as science." The result of this is that the promotion of all things scientific and technological minimized aspects of humanistic care and contact between physician and patient and family. Osler rebuffed this effort in 1919, asserting that "Twin berries on one stem, grievous damage has been done to both in regarding the Humanities and Science in any other light than complemental."[27(p4),28] But medicine's viewpoint had so singularly focused on the physician as a scientist that the underpinnings of ethics and its incorporation into professionalism remained only implicit in the wake of the Flexnerian medical school reform. As apprenticeship was now passé, comportment—a key aspect of professionalism driven by adept role modeling—was now placed in jeopardy. These changes were an attempt to articulate not only an educational mandate (with its scientific bias) but also the need for competence—which does play an essential role in professionalism.

The Modern Era and Medical Education

The result of this contraction and the structure of how new physicians were formed ultimately resulted in discord for professionalism and medical ethics 60 years later. Beginning with the confluence of social upheaval, civil rights, questions in the minds of the public regarding the rectitude of using all technological discoveries in medical care, and multiple ethical wrongs something finally gave way. Cataclysmic ethical breaches such as findings at the Nuremberg trials and the US public's recoil on learning of the Tuskegee Public Health Service experiment resulted in a contemporary worldwide shift toward the development of a new discipline, that of bioethics.[29]

Slowly at first, but with rapidity, medical schools incorporated curricula of medical ethics, in parallel with the development of centers and departments devoted to ethics and humanities. However, the challenge in teaching the medical learner the concept of benefiting another person outside of themselves is daunting. Self-effacement is a virtue far removed from the self-absorbed, hypercompetitive drive to enter medical school. Therefore, to become a professional, trainees required a firm foundation in medical ethics and humanities, and most will not bring these qualifications. As a result, concepts of deontology, virtue ethics, care ethics, and casuistry became (unevenly) part of the modern lexicon of medical ethics education. A modern era touchstone regarding some of the ethical underpinnings that can and should be part of medical education are found in the DeCamp report.[30]

The DeCamp report laid out curricular goals for medical ethics and framed basic concepts and approaches in deontological ethics. It laid out minimalist expectations of educational requirements in medical ethics for medical schools and residencies. The report also contributed to the comportment expectations of professionalism, as it laid out the requirement of training in "interaction skills" by an ethicist, clinician, or appropriate specialist in the area. The report therefore serves as a benchmark for contemporary professionalism, despite its lack of discussion regarding the social contract between medicine and society, and its trust-based underpinnings. The DeCamp report's decoupling of professionalism's concepts of public trust and its implied contract of the medical professional leads us to recommend a refinement of how medical professionalism is articulated in contemporary practice. It spoke to the ethical duty and virtue of beneficence and care coupled with socially acceptable comportment and an implicit contract that exists between the healthcare profession and society.

DeCamp noted that "the basic moral character of medical students has been formed by the time they enter medical school" and that "a medical-ethics curriculum is designed not to improve the moral character of future physicians but to provide those of sound moral character with the intellectual tools and interactional skills that will give moral character its best behavioral expression." [30(p253)] As inferred from DeCamp, the purpose of medical school and residency education is therefore not to create ethical agents de novo, but instead to refine well-selected candidates who have entered medical school with the capacity to behave morally. However, there is no validated method of "virtuous candidate selection"—medical schools receive fallible human beings with widely variable social, cultural, religious, and philosophical backgrounds. Some argue that indeed candidates entering medical education may not have the necessary components of critical thinking skills in ethics and humanities prior to their arrival.[31–33] The list of objectives in the DeCamp report is very basic (given its modest goals) and details key concepts in medical ethics, such as informed consent, capacity, treatment refusal, confidentiality, and other essential concepts for early medical ethics education.

To be clear, the DeCamp report was a helpful starting point. However, it did not link how medical ethics was instrumental to professionalism formation or the essential roles of medical humanities. It did note the importance of "interactional skills" but did not opine on the importance of comportment in patient care. As a result, it was an ethics-bound document, dissociated from how the medical learner evolves into a medical professional. Given the ongoing forces in medicine, this narrow view would not be sufficient or sustainable. At roughly the same time, the practice of medicine was changing.

The social change in the 1960s spurred the founding of Medicare and Medicaid, designed to help the elderly and disenfranchised, respectively. Within two decades, healthcare insurance companies would attempt to exert market forces on the practice of medicine and on individual practitioners through "managed care." The inherent conflicts of interest that would soon emerge, coupled with a resurgence of physician competition that had not been seen since Percival, resulted in great tumult. Physicians began to question their own place within the medical profession. Society itself began to question whether medicine could be trusted in the social contract in which it was engaged. Perhaps an emblematic editorial cartoon of the time best portrayed a patient's plight: A woman is giving birth in a convertible at a drive-through in order to facilitate her swift (and economical) return to home. The lack of compassion *to* the patient coupled with the desire for revenue *from* the patient catalyzed a huge shift of opinion for society. Medicine had lost its way—again.

As a result, medical professionalism required a reboot, a re-engagement of the medical ethics to the societal implicit contract of all physicians. This reboot was offered by the American College of Physicians-American Board of Internal Medicine (ACP-ABIM) charter as a commitment to professionalism in medical education. Implicit within the response of organized medicine to the shortcomings is that we must clean our own house or else the government may take away our own self-regulatory function.

More recently, per the Project to Rebalance and Integrate Medical Education (PRIME project) of 2010–2012, we assert that medical professionalism has three key components: (1) The attainment of clinical knowledge, skills, and competence in order to practice; (2) the use of sound, evidence-based clinical knowledge and skills to promote the patient's health-related best interests while keeping one's own self-interest systematically secondary; and (3) sustaining the societal trust of this agreement as a public trust rather than as a guild.[31–33] Underlying this commitment is the requisite training toward the building of that knowledge and skill set and a responsibility to nurture and apply virtue to accomplish professionalism's ends.[34] Medical professionalism is grounded on a sound foundation of medical ethics and medical humanities (thereby promoting critical thinking skills), coupled with excellence in comportment, and advocacy of the primacy of patient benefit in the social contract.

When the practice of medicine strays far from its ethical duty to the patient benefit with its endpoint of individual patient and societal betterment, professionalism suffers. When medicine integrates medical ethics, comportment, and the social contract into its education and practice, it can acknowledge, accept, and promote the responsibility that comes with being a medical professional.

Reform at this time was an attempt to achieve coherence between medical ethics and expectations of what it meant to be a professional. Professionalism was more than a moral responsibility of the individual physician; it was also the assemblage of all of those physicians in their service to their patients and collectively to society. Change began with the Association of American Medical Colleges' (AAMC's) Medical Schools Objectives Project emphasizing aspects of knowledge, virtue, and competency in medical education.[35] (AAMC, 1998) Subsequently, the Accreditation Council for Graduate Medical Education (ACGME), followed by the Liaison Committee on Medical Education (LCME) and the Accreditation Council for Continuing Medical Education (ACCME), each promulgated (and subsequently revised) the general competencies, one of which specifically articulated the competency of professionalism.[36–38]

However, many authors noted that there was an ethical backbone that existed throughout the general competencies.[39] Each specific competency had a focus on a facet of professionalism formation. In one of the seminal publications that were the fruit of the PRIME project, the 2015 Romanell report (going far beyond the DeCamp report from thirty years earlier) had a much broader scope conceptualizing the physician's place in medicine as a steward of the inherent trust of the implied social contract with responsibilities that are undertaken as a member of our profession that not only are patient centered, but also require self-effacement, rejection of self-interest, and the recognition of the importance of interprofessionalism and self-care.[40] Efforts to promote medical ethics and professionalism were also recognized as extending far beyond philosophy into other areas of humanities, such as history, literature, the arts, law, and the social sciences.[14,41]

The concept of professionalism identity formation (PIF) has arisen in the last two decades to address how education should be integrated via psychological and sociological bases.[42–45] Irby and Hamstra point out how three intersecting frameworks paint a fuller picture of what professionalism education must address to be successful.[46] Those frameworks are virtue based, behavior based, and PIF. The "virtue-based" framework requires education in the knowledge and critical thinking skills that bring to bear medical ethics (duty, virtue, casuistry, and more) to set the stage for habituation of moral reasoning and actions that routinize their future application in practice. The "behavior-based" framework (often through role-modeling) informs how one acts and applies these actions to measurable competencies and milestones, allowing for personal growth through critical and positive feedback. The PIF framework describes the socialization process by which the individual physician engages a learning community to nurture one's own maturation through positive (and resilience from negative) role-modeling.[46] Curricular evolution will need to account for the incorporation of these distinct frameworks in undergraduate and postgraduate medical education and during the entire course of one's medical career.

Conceptual Issues

Despite all this progress, conceptual challenges remain relating to the role of the individual physician and the broader profession of medicine within which practice is nested. This is the social contract that warrants our work as physicians and that motivates the good that we do to better society. Medical ethicist Robert Veatch detailed this as a multilevel contract between the patient, the medical profession, and the society writ large.[47]

Veatch also made a modest proposal to have an interactive process of the expectations and limitations of the social contract between individuals and society. Yet, there has not been a town hall, policy, or poll that has ever truly captured what it means for a physician to care for patients and the expectation of patients in the duties and virtues of acting as a physician for an individual and as an agent of society. We have an *implicit* contract between medicine and society, but regrettably, we do not have an *explicit* consensual contract.

Indeed, it is this social contract between physicians as a group that transcends the individual and speaks to the collective, recognizing the responsibility to serve the public's welfare and to reject one's self-interest. This means that physicians act as fiduciaries for their patients and in doing so must promote the care of patients and the whole of society as a public trust. In this way, obligations transcend an individual's oath and become a standard to which all must adhere.

Of course, there is no professional obligation in the aggregate if individuals do not themselves act ethically. This linkage cannot be severed. One cannot be a professional if one does not act ethically, and a physician cannot be ethical if the physician departs from norms or educational mandates dictated to them by organized medicine. A physician, for example, who did not stay current with medical education or licensure would be both incompetent and dangerous, breaching both the principles of beneficence and non-maleficence.

Conceptually, viewing this dynamic is best understood as a covenant that *binds* the individual to something bigger than themselves. This transcends the contractarian arguments of Veatch and is transformed by the covenantal framework of William F. May, who instead stated that the relationship between physician and patient and society requires an articulated initial promise, nurtured with accumulating trust, with ongoing expectations of fidelity in the future relationship between the parties.[48,49] A contract's standing in medical professionalism is an important first step as an obligation with minimal expectations. May's covenant is an aspirational relationship that strives to build on the promise of adherence to a corpus of knowledge and of norms, tasking the physician to build trust with individual patients and the broader society, and amplified by larger expectations of fidelity and excellence.

Whereas contracts exist in the setting of distrust and stipulate minimal expectations, a covenant is something that is larger and more aspirational in nature. Regrettably, the language of covenant has been incorporated into neither the broader understanding of professionalism nor organizational structures that often constrain professionalism at the level of the individual practitioner. Thus, covenant language has had a limited impact situating the obligations of physicians to society in the minimalist expectations of contracts. For example, the writings of Herbert Swick and the ACP-ABIM charter spoke to a societal contract to exist between the medical profession and society, perhaps worried that covenant carried a religious overtone.[50,51] Unfortunately, there has not been true engagement between the public and physicians to struggle with the role responsibilities of the physician in working with patients.

Here we invoke covenant in a secular vein and speak to the patient-physician-society construct and reciprocal obligations.[52,53] Physicians choose to become doctors as individuals and take on obligations individually, but they also become part of a collective that generates and enforces those mutual expectations and responsibilities. One cannot be a doctor in isolation. From practice in the medical home, to complex medical care in a tertiary care hospital, or of the public health in the face of a pandemic, medicine is a collective enterprise made up of ethical practitioners working in and sustained by the broader professional community. One cannot exist in isolation from the other. Like all covenants, the relationship is reciprocal, whereby each is dependent on the other.

The relationship between ethics and professionalism is symbiotic, with each component dependent on the other. To view ethics as distinct from professionalism is to mistake comportment for ethics because it fails to contextualize overt individual behavior against broader and deeper norms and values that are grounded in the profession and not the individual. Ethical practice means far more than the superficial social veneer of persons interacting with one another. Instead, ethics and professionalism are the actualization of duty and virtue directed toward the benefit of the patient, their caregivers, their family—and ultimately all of society. Ethics requires virtue and civility in the care of others; these attributes are necessary but not sufficient as they are only skin deep.

From a regulatory and collective point of view, it is only possible to regulate behaviors and comportment, and this is why this veneer is so problematic. We cannot know what truly motivates behavior, and thus we are left with a paradox. Comportment requires virtue and civility in the care of others. Some think that comportment is ingrained, yet medical students do not enter their education with a full knowledge of virtue and care ethics and its application to the benefit primarily on the patient's behalf. Comportment is a clear individual responsibility of every medical learner and medical professional, and yet in professionalism programs in medical centers and residency programs, it is often comportment that is the basis of the vast majority of complaints of "lack of professionalism." Despite all the regulation from outside (what the profession might require) of demonstrated behaviors, we are still left with the shrouded personal refuge of one's inner commitments. If the values, attitudes, and beliefs within one's own moral core do not align with promoting patient and societal care, they can only be challenged, reproached, or remediated by self-regulation, which is the cornerstone of professional and personal ethics.

There is no sure way to appreciate intent and motivation. The best we can do as educators is to inculcate trainees during their formative period with the solemnity of what they are preparing to do, based on the duties owed and the virtues displayed to patients.[54,55] Here, the pre-Flexnerian norm of role modeling is essential. In order to understand the method and manner of the physician-patient interaction, the learner must listen, observe, and emulate positive role models. Contrariwise, the learner must be able to identify the negative influence of negative role models (of the hidden curriculum) who lack key elements of respect, beneficence, and care. The evolution that should take place over medical school and residency could be evaluated prior to entry into medical practice using available undergraduate medical education and graduate medical education established metrics.

Medical education from medical school through residency and continuing medical education must instill the emulation of sound, excellent role models that demonstrate how to interact with patients, families, and others in healthcare. This modeling requires not only sound mentorship by identifiable protégé-mentor pairs but also all persons who are interacting with others in the healthcare system. This translation of knowledge and skills into behavior has instrumental outcomes of enhanced patient care, interprofessionalism, and the reduction of errors.[33,50,56] It is in the formulation of comportment as part of the professionalism mosaic that mentorship is key. All healthcare learners need excellent mentors in order to serve as role models to complete the professionalism formation process. The challenge in our system is that such role models must see and acknowledge their intrinsic value even if the system itself does not reward them for their critical need.

Conclusion

The future of medical professionalism and the role of medical ethics require that we proactively encourage feedback between medical professionalism and medical ethics. One cannot have professionalism in medicine without medical ethics, just as one cannot have medical ethics and lack medical professionalism (see the past history of medicine noted above). There needs to be a greater conversation and critical interrogation of organized medicine to question how medical ethics is integrated into medical professionalism. This should include members of the medical profession as well as members of society, including all strata, particularly the disenfranchised. In relationships, power often dictates who rules in a particular social interaction, and in medicine there is an inherently greater state of power held by the physician in both knowledge and lack of vulnerability compared to the patient. There needs to be a more even playing field to allow for a peer-to-peer conversation to take place and for constructive feedback and remodeling to occur over time.

In this chapter, we discussed how medical ethics and medical professionalism are interdependent on one another. We discussed how medicine has been transformed over the last two and half millennia from a group of healers who attempted to help their patients on an individual basis to a collection of medical professionals who ascribed to common goals and a societal contract that sets aside self-interest for the promotion of patient interest, benefit, and care. This evolution of a nascent professionalism to the professionalism that is now extant in medicine and society benefits the collectivity of patients, physicians, and society.

References

1. Hippocrates. *The Genuine Works of Hippocrates.* Adams F, trans. Sydenham Society; 1849.
2. Hippocrates. *Hippocrates.* Smith WD, trans. Harvard University Press; 1994.
3. Arawi TA. The Muslim physician and the ethics of medicine. *J IMA.* 2010;42(3):111–116. doi:10.5915/42-3 -5403
4. Tsai DF. Ancient Chinese medical ethics and the four principles of biomedical ethics. *J Med Ethics.* 1999;25(4):315–321. doi:10.1136/jme.25.4.315
5. Galen. *On the Natural Faculties.* Brock AJ, trans. Harvard University Press; 1916. Ser. The Loeb Classical Library, 71.

6. Brain P. Galen on the ideal of the physician. *S Afr Med J.* 1977;52(23):936–938.
7. Schiefsky M. *Hippocrates on Ancient Medicine.* Brill; 2018.
8. Fox DM. The politics of physicians' responsibility in epidemics: a note on history. *Hastings Cent Rep.* 1988;18(2):5. doi:10.2307/3562420
9. Boccaccio G, McWilliam GH. *The Decameron.* Penguin Classics; 1996.
10. McCullough LB, Percival T. *Thomas Percival's Medical Ethics and the Invention of Medical Professionalism.* Springer Nature; 2022.
11. Katz J. *The Silent World of Doctor and Patient.* Johns Hopkins University Press; 2002.
12. Fins JJ. Truth telling and reciprocity in the doctor-patient relationship: a North American perspective. In: Bruera E, Portenoy RK, eds. *Topics in Palliative Care.* Vol 5. Oxford University Press. 2001:81–94.
13. Fins JJ, Pohl B, Doukas DJ. In praise of the humanities in academic medicine. *Camb Q Healthc Ethics.* 2013;22(4):355–364. doi:10.1017/s0963180113000200
14. Chervenak FA, McCullough LB, Hale RW. Guild interests: an insidious threat to professionalism in obstetrics and gynecology. *Am J Obst Gynecol.* 2018;219(6):581–584. doi:10.1016/j.ajog.2018.09.007
15. Percival T. Medical Ethics, or a Code of Institutes and Precepts, Adapted to the Professional Conduct of Physicians and Surgeons. London: Russell and Johnson; 1803. In: Pellegrino ED, ed. *Medical Ethics by Thomas Percival.* Gryphon Editions; 1985:1–246. The Classics of Medicine Library.
16. Gregory J. Lectures on the Duties and Qualifications of a Physician. London (United Kingdom): W. Strahan and T. Cadell; 1772. In: Gregory J, McCullough LB, eds. *John Gregory's Writings on Medical Ethics and Philosophy of Medicine.* Kluwer Academic Publishers. 1998:161–245 .
17. Patuzzo S, Goracci G, Ciliberti R. Thomas Percival. Discussing the foundation of medical ethics. *Acta Biomed.* 2018;89(3):343–348. doi:10.23750/abm.v89i3.7050
18. American Medical Association. *Code of Medical Ethics: Adopted by the American Medical Association at Philadelphia in May 1847 and by the New York Academy of Medicine in October 1847.* Printed for the Academy of Medicine by H. Ludwig & Co; 1848.
19. Fins JJ, Snyder Sulmasy L. Ethics and professionalism: professing and living our principles. In: Tooker JT, Dale DC, eds. *Serving Our Patients and Profession: A Centennial History of the American College of Physicians, 1915–2015.* American College of Physicians, 2015:199–217.
20. Flexner A. *Medical Education in the United States and Canada: A Report to the Carnegie Foundation for the Advancement of Teaching.* Carnegie Foundation for the Advancement of Teaching; 1910.
21. Bonner TN. *Iconoclast: Abraham Flexner and a Life in Learning.* Johns Hopkins University Press; 2002.
22. Doukas DJ, McCullough LB, Wear S. Reforming medical education in ethics and humanities by finding common ground with Abraham Flexner. *Acad Med.* 2010;85(2):318–323. doi:10.1097/acm.0b013e3181c85932
23. Doukas DJ, McCullough LB, Wear S. Re-visioning Flexner: educating physicians to be clinical scientists and humanists. *Am J Med.* 2010;123(12):1155–1156. doi:10.1016/j.amjmed.2010.05.027
24. Zelenka MH. *The Educational Philosophy of Abraham Flexner: Creating Cogency in Medical Education.* Edwin Mellen Press; 2008.

25. Flexner A. *Letter to Simon Flexner, 18 May 1925.* Simon Flexner Papers, Manuscript Division, Library of Congress Washington, D.C.; 1925.

26. Flexner A. *Medical Education: A Comparative Study.* Macmillan; 1925.

27. Osler W. The old humanities and the new science: the presidential address delivered before the Classical Association at Oxford, May, 1919. *BMJ.* 1919;2(3053):1–7. doi:10.1136/bmj.2.3053.1

28. Fins JJ. In memoriam: Dr. Edmund Pellegrino's legacy: secure in the annals of medicine. *Kennedy Inst Ethics J.* 2014;24(2):97–104. doi:10.1353/ken.2014.0014

29. Jonsen AR. *The Birth of Bioethics.* Oxford University Press; 2003.

30. Culver CM, Clouser KD, Gert B, et al. Basic curricular goals in medical ethics. *N Engl J Med.* 1985;312(4):253–256. doi:10.1056/nejm198501243120430

31. Doukas DJ, McCullough LB, Wear S. Medical Education in Medical Ethics and Humanities as the Foundation for Developing Medical Professionalism. *Acad Med.* 2012;87(3):334–341. doi:10.1097/acm.0b013e318244728c

32. Doukas DJ, McCullough LB, Wear S, et al. The challenge of promoting professionalism through medical ethics and humanities education. *Acad Med.* 2013;88(11):1624–1629. doi:10.1097/acm.0b013e3182a7f8e3

33. Doukas DJ, Kirch DG, Brigham TP, et al. Transforming educational accountability in medical ethics and humanities education toward professionalism. *Acad Med.* 2015;90(6):738–743. doi:10.1097/acm.0000000000000616

34. Brody H, Doukas D. Professionalism: A framework to guide medical education. *Med Educ.* 2014;48(10):980–987. doi:10.1111/medu.12520

35. Association of American Medical Colleges. *Report I: Learning Objectives for Medical Student Education: Guidelines for Medical Schools.* Association of American Medical Colleges; 1998.

36. Accreditation Council for Graduate Medical Education. Common program requirements, 2022. ACGME. Accessed October 14, 2022. https://www.acgme.org/What-We-Do/Accreditation/Common-Program-Requirements/

37. Accreditation Council for Continuing Medical Accreditation. Accreditation criteria, 2022. ACCME. Accessed October 14, 2022. https://accme.org/accreditation-rules/accreditation-criteria

38. Liaison Committee on Medical Education. Standards, publications, & notification forms. LCME. 2022. Accessed October 18, 2022. https://lcme.org/publications/

39. Doukas DJ. Where is the virtue in professionalism? *Camb Q Healthc Ethics.* 2003;12(2):147–154. doi:10.1017/s0963180103122037

40. Carrese JA, Malek J, Watson K, et al. The essential role of medical ethics education in achieving professionalism. *Acad Med.* 2015;90(6):744–752. doi:10.1097/acm.0000000000000715

41. Shapiro J, Nixon LL, Wear SE, Doukas DJ. Medical professionalism: what the study of literature can contribute to the conversation. *Philos Ethics Humanit Med.* 2015;10(1):1–8. doi:10.1186/s13010-015- 0030-0

42. Cruess RL, Cruess SR, Boudreau JD, Snell L, Steinert Y. Reframing medical education to support professional identity formation. *Acad Med.* 2014;89(11):1446–1551. doi:10.1097/ACM.0000000000000427

43. Cruess RL, Cruess SR, Boudreau JD, Snell L, Steinert Y. A schematic representation of the professional identity formation and socialization of medical students and residents: a guide for medical educators. *Acad Med.* 2015;90(6):718–725. doi:10.1097/ACM.0000000000000700

44. Cruess SR, Cruess RL, Steinert Y. Supporting the development of a professional identity: general principles. *Med Teach.* 2019;41(6):641–649. doi:10.1080/0142159X.2018.1536260
45. Sawatsky AP, Huffman BM, Hafferty FW. Coaching versus competency to facilitate professional identity formation. *Acad Med.* 2020;95(10):1511–1514. doi:10.1097/ACM.0000000000003144
46. Irby DM, Hamstra SJ. Parting the clouds: three professionalism frameworks in medical education. *Acad Med.* 2016;91(12):1606–1611. doi:10.1097/ACM.0000000000001190
47. Veatch RM. *Theory of Medical Ethics.* Basic Books; 1981.
48. May WF. Code, covenant, contract, or philanthropy? *Hastings Cent Rep.* 1975;5(6):29. doi:10.2307/3560994
49. May WF. *The Physician's Covenant: Images of the Healer in Medical Ethics.* John Knox Press; 2002.
50. Swick HM. Toward a normative definition of medical professionalism. *Acad Med.* 2000;75(6):612–616. doi:10.1097/00001888-200006000-00010
51. ACP-ABIM Foundation; European Federation of Internal Medicine. Medical professionalism in the new millennium: a physician charter. *Ann Int Med.* 2002;136(3):243. doi:10.7326/0003-4819-136-3-200202050-00012
52. Doukas DJ. Autonomy and beneficence in the family: describing the family covenant. *J Clin Ethics.* 1991;2(3):145–153.
53. Fins JJ. From contract to covenant in advance care planning. *J Law Med Ethics.* 1999;27(1):46–51. doi:10.1111/j.1748-720x.1999.tb01435.x
54. Fins JJ. Vowing to care. *J Pain Symptom Manage.* 2002;23(1):54–57. doi:10.1016/s0885-3924(01)00387-6
55. Doukas DJ, Ozar DT, Darragh M, de Groot JM, Carter BS, Stout N. Virtue and care ethics & humanism in medical education: a scoping review. *BMC Med Educ.* 2022;22(1):1–10. doi:10.1186/s12909-021-03051-6
56. Kirk LM, Blank LL. Professional behavior—a learner's permit for licensure. *N Engl J Med.* 2005;353(25):2709–2711. doi:10.1056/nejme058275

3
From Codes and Ethics to Professional Identity Formation and Beyond
An Equity, Diversity, Inclusion and Accessibility Perspective

Janet de Groot, Lynden (Lindsay) Crowshoe, and Annie Simpson

Key Points

- Indigenous perspectives on ethical listening have the potential to support relational learning from Indigenous and Western perspectives on professionalism.
- Inviting patients and allied health professionals in addition to physicians will support the development of truly inclusive medical ethics and codes of professionalism.
- Professional identity formation theory and education require greater attention to equity, diversity, inclusion, and accessibility and intersectional experiences.
- Undergraduate and postgraduate medical education for professional resistance is needed to enhance the capacity to address social injustice and health inequities.

Introduction

To better uphold medicine's social contract, the medical profession acknowledges the need for a more diligent integration of equity, diversity, inclusion, and accessibility (EDIA) perspectives and practices. Traditionally, the social contract refers to the implicit and explicit obligations and expectations between society and the field of medicine. [1] In this context, professionalism is rooted in the social contract, meaning that physicians should provide patient care with compassion, respect, duty, and integrity,[2] while also engaging in self-regulation and contributing to the public good.[1] In return, society grants physicians autonomy and the privilege of self-regulation, which ensures the profession's competency, as well as financial and nonfinancial rewards.[1]

Professionalism faces the challenge of addressing the complexities inherent in a social contract that respects and recenters relationships with historically disadvantaged and dispossessed populations. Critiques of the social contract metaphor as perpetuating privilege and lacking a solid theoretical foundation have prompted recommendations for a more proactive approach.[3] These recommendations call for addressing social determinants of health, health inequities, and the adverse dynamics between racialized communities and the healthcare system that contribute to inequities in access to care and health outcomes.[4,5] To overcome these challenges, it is essential to take tangible actions aimed at promoting health equity.

In this chapter, we examine the evolution of professionalism and explore how EDIA can be integrated into the medical field. The medical literature presents three professionalism frameworks,[6] including the earliest informed by virtue ethics,[7,8] followed by a behavior/outcome-based model,[9,10] and more recently, a professional identity formation (PIF) framework.[11,12] The behavior-based model (Accreditation Council for Graduate Medical Education [ACGME], Canadian Medical Education Directives for Specialists [CanMEDS]) outlines expectations and has been the preferred framework for evaluating medical learners' competencies and milestones. Professional codes of conduct and ethics, consistent with the behavior-based framework, explicitly define physicians' societal obligations, including legal requirements. However, codes of conduct are constructed within a particular time and context and are subsequently reconstructed over time to adapt to social changes.[13] (We provide a case example of the evolution of the American Medical Association (AMA) Code of Ethics[14] to illustrate the current inclusion of EDIA directives.)

Contemporary medical education literature emphasizes the importance of PIF in medical trainees' education.[15] This movement emerged as an effort to shift the competency-driven discourse to one that considers what it means to be a physician, recognizing that one is not born a physician.[12] Theorization about physician professional identity highlights two processes: first, individual psychological and adult developmental growth and, second, a process of socialization.[11,12] During the psychological developmental process, medical students and postgraduate learners are anticipated to internalize and be motivated by the values of the medical profession, rather than simply following a code that defines behaviors.[11]

We explore the concept of PIF in the context of socialization with the medical community and the growing recognition of the importance of integrating EDIA. In doing so, we conclude the chapter by examining the idea of professional resistance, which involves critiquing and/or preventing the recurrence of social injustice.[16] Professional resistance to injustice is balanced by affirmatively expressing what is needed, doing so intentionally and proportionately, and seeking constructive solutions.[16] This chapter includes a critical literature review that identifies the role of power and privilege and the notable absences of EDIA perspectives in PIF. We discuss professional resistance as a means to further integrate EDIA perspectives into professionalism and the practice of medicine.

Reflexivity

As coauthors, we engaged in reflexivity[17] to describe our relationship to the content area and the writing of this chapter. As coauthors, we include perspectives as a Canadian settler and clinician-researcher, a Canadian Indigenous clinician-researcher, and an African American academic physician.

Dr. Janet de Groot is a first-generation Dutch settler to Canada and a psychiatrist and professor of psychiatry, oncology, and community health sciences. She is the inaugural associate dean, equity and professionalism, Cumming School of Medicine, University of Calgary (2008–2017). Her work as a clinician-researcher is in psychosocial oncology and psychosocial aspects of palliative care. As a medical educator, she engages in collaborative research on professionalism, vulnerability, and collective moral resilience. She and Dr. Crowshoe are collaborating on a theater-based education innovation for postgraduate trainees to address Indigenous racism in healthcare education.[18] She and Dr. Simpson are in an Executive Leadership in Academic Medicine (ELAM) study group continuing since 2012.

Lynden Crowshoe, MD, is a member of Piikani First Nation, associate professor in the Department of Family Medicine and assistant dean, Indigenous Local and Global Health, Cumming School of Medicine, University of Calgary. In **research**, he bridges multiple disciplines of knowledge, including health, clinical, social sciences, professional health education, and Indigenous ways of knowing. In **health education**, he provides input on Indigenous health education policy and programming within national organizations (Association of Faculties of Medicine and the College of Family Physicians of Canada) and leads health education innovation initiatives for medical and health research learners within his home institution and across Canada.

Annie R. Simpson, MD, is a professor emeritus of medicine/geriatrics. She was also the Rust professor of ethics; associate vice-chancellor for African American health; director of the Institute for Ethics; chair of the Bioethics Committee; and executive director of the Black Health Resource Center. She has tremendously informed this chapter, not only in her writing and recommendations for reading but also in discussions over the past decade with the first author and other members of a women's leadership group. Her focus on how we share human nature is tremendously valuable.

We aim to honor Canada's Truth and Reconciliation Commission (2015)[19] calls to action to redress the impact of residential schools and colonization and calls to action in healthcare. To engage with differences, including different ethical perspectives between societies or communities, Indigenous legal scholar Willie Ermine describes the necessity for an ethical space where the construction of diversity and differences occur.[20] In that space, members of Western and Indigenous communities engage in ethical listening to support reconciliation and decolonization and the removal of colonial structures and uncover assumptions, which adversely influence relationships.[20] In this chapter, we aim to engage with our diverse lived experiences and the literature to move toward reconciliation and decolonizing codes and ethics and PIF. Further, we are informed by the *Advancing Health Equity Guide* jointly developed by the AMA and the Association for American Medical Colleges.[21] The guide urges recognition and reconciliation regarding the injustices of both genocide and forced labor. In addition, the contributions of people of African descent and of Indigenous peoples to medicine and sciences are recognized.

Codes, Ethics, and Professionalism

Ethics and medical professionalism must be informed about, or inclusive of, all peoples to be useful as codes for medical learners and physicians and the patients and populations they serve. This requires inclusive engagement of diverse physicians, patients, and allied health professionals in writing codes and ethics. Further, in referring to the social contract as the basis of professionalism, it is essential to recognize that society is not homogeneous. Further, members of society have extensive access to scientific knowledge, and many question science. In this regard, society has become more polarized in relation to healthcare and the practice of medicine. We need a greater understanding of the diverse health needs of the communities in which we live and serve and how to effectively communicate about health to people of different backgrounds. This understanding is required to fulfill our commitments to social justice.

Hippocratic Oath

The Hippocratic oath, considered the earliest known code of ethics for physicians, provided ethical guidance for the application of medical knowledge.[22] It outlines physicians' responsibility to society and was traditionally recited by new medical graduates as a way to express gratitude to their teachers and connect them to the larger community of physicians.

Contemporary medical graduation ceremonies now often include revised forms of the oath to reflect the numerous and ongoing changes in the practice of medicine and knowledge from medical science. The rights of patients, including rights to confidentiality, privacy, and consent, now take precedence over the original Hippocratic oath's principle of beneficence, which focused on doing good for the sick. The principle of "do no harm" is of greater consequence today. During Hippocrates's time, few therapeutic interventions were available. Today, physicians must consider numerous interventions and medications, each with its benefit and risk. Further, patient harm may be due to system failures.[23] Thus, physician commitments include recognition of the complexity of healthcare, the role of interprofessional teams and the social determinants of health.[23]

Formal Medical Ethics

In the late eighteenth century, during an epidemic, Britain's Manchester Fever Hospital closed due to political discord and disrespectful behavior among its doctors with divergent beliefs and values. In response, Dr. Thomas Percival was invited to develop a means of avoiding similar events in the future. Drawing from the works of John Gregory and Thomas Gisborne, Percival and his colleagues developed a document that emphasized physicians' duty and responsibility to their patients, a focus consistent with the Hippocratic oath. However, they also addressed the need for respectful physician engagement. The resulting book, *Medical Ethics; or, a Code of Institutes and Precepts, Adapted to the Professional Conduct of Physicians and Surgeons* (1803),[24] marked the first use of the phrases "medical ethics" and "profession."[25,26]

AMA Code of Medical Ethics

A few decades later, the AMA established a Code of Medical Ethics to provide a standardized set of rules and standards for medical professionals.[14] Gradually, the recitation of the Hippocratic oath during medical school graduation ceremonies became more common to reassure the public and distinguish the medical profession from other healing professions as well as establish a claim for higher stature.[27] The role of exclusion was evident. Traditionally, the public and those in other health professions were not invited to contribute to medicine's codes of ethics. However, public criticism contributed to a change in the code of ethics that would more fully obligate physicians to treat those with human immunodeficiency virus (HIV).[28,29]

Professional Education That Supports the AMA Code of Ethics

The current AMA Code of Ethics' detailed attention to the "Physician Exercise of Conscience" is clearly valuable, yet leaves interpretation to individual members. Although language opposing racial and ethnic discrimination is written into the AMA Code of Ethics, it appears overshadowed by the language applied to gender discrimination and sexual harassment. The latter two seem to be taken more seriously, requiring mandatory training aimed at eradicating gender bias and sexual harassment. Still, impact is limited, as such educational principles are not always followed.[30]

Educational efforts to address institutional culture are increasingly being made.[31] It is recognized that ethics and professionalism cannot be limited to the physician-patient dyad alone but must also occur at an organizational level. In this context, leadership is necessary in supporting change, and organizations are held accountable for addressing sexual harassment within their ranks.[31]

Transforming institutional culture regarding implicit or unconscious bias—assumptions about and ingrained differential behavioral responses to men and women—requires educational interventions that draw on learning theory and organizational change principles in the STEMM (science, technology, engineering, mathematics, medicine) programs.[32,33] The aim is to bring tacit knowledge to conscious awareness and facilitate intentional behavioral change.[31]

More recently, members of the medical profession acknowledge the systemic inequities arising from stereotyping and "white privilege," the unearned advantages and biases associated with color and race.[34] To address these biases, additional competency training is required. In one example, a study of over 8,500 medical faculty at one school found lasting effects in competencies for bias reduction three months after a three-hour workshop.[35]

Medical education often fails to demonstrate or teach that race is a social construct, not a biological determinant.[36,37] Therefore, employing antiracism training may be a necessary competency in support of the public good. To this end, antiracism is also recommended as a foundational competency within the CanMEDS framework that includes the professional role, to ensure medical educators and learners actively engage in antiracism activity.[38]

Need for an International Publishing Code of Ethics

There is a call for an international publishing code of ethics to address historical scientific racism,[39] as numerous articles and books have been published based on scientific racism, even in high-impact journals. The recommended code would provide guidance for editors in handling pseudoscientific or racist articles. This could include disclaimers for such articles that remain accessible as historical documents.[39]

Unified Health Professions Code

Codes of medical ethics may be revised in response to societal and cultural changes. With the increasing emphasis on team-based healthcare, efforts to flatten the hierarchy of healthcare and community engagement with patients, families, and partners, a transdisciplinary code of ethics has been proposed.[40,41] This initiative, which emerged from the 2013 Institute of Medicine Global Forum on Health Professional Education, was accompanied by additional recommendations. Meaningful transdisciplinary professionalism requires new institutional frameworks that also engage the public in defining, debating, and revising standards and expectations for healthcare professionals. A principle of reciprocity regarding mutual obligations was considered essential between healthcare professionals, individuals, and society.[41] Ongoing effort from the Global Forum includes the exploration of a culture of respect, fairness, and antiracism in health professions education in connection with the National Academies of Science, Engineering, and Medicine.[42]

The Role of Codes

Public codes of medical ethics aim to foster trust between patients and healthcare providers, as well as support collegial behaviors with other healthcare providers.[26] Examples are the Canadian Medical Association Code of Ethics and Professionalism[9] and the Physician Charter on Professionalism,[43] accepted by over 130 organizations. They highlight the values, attitudes, and responsibilities of the medical profession, including a commitment to patient care, social justice, and improving access to care.

However, codes do not address the specifics of cases where there is uncertainty.[28] During the recent coronavirus pandemic declared in early 2020, public health and hospital organizational policies were quickly drawn up, often without consideration of the impact on the structurally stigmatized. The policies failed to consider implications for the cognitively impaired or those marginalized by culture or language. A Canadian study of postgraduate trainees found many reported experiences of "structural distress," that is, a sense of powerlessness related to barriers in care provision for individuals who were structurally vulnerable early in the pandemic.[44]

Newer Ethical Framings

Ethical theories that shape professionalism and medical ethics have undergone a shift from individual-focused perspectives to a greater emphasis on relational aspects and the delivery of healthcare in teams. One such theory, virtue ethics, centers on cultivating moral qualities such as integrity, honesty, altruism, and moral reasoning to foster professionalism.[45] Care has been deemed a virtue. However, recent feminist framings of an ethic of care,[46,47] highlight its relational nature, where moral reasoning takes place within relationships.

The concept of vulnerability in ethical accounts "is a characteristic that positions us as humans in relation to one another."[48] The limits and uncertainty that is part of medicine may increase feelings of vulnerability among healthcare professionals.[48,49] Further, as healthcare providers and trainees negotiate the different values, goals, and understandings of patients and their families, they may experience moral distress, particularly in high-acuity situations where the healthcare provider feels constraints in acting in a way they believe is most appropriate for the patient.[50] However, within intentionally developed communities of practice of healthcare providers that may be composed of interprofessional healthcare providers, vulnerability is implicit within the reflective process, and shared wisdom can support valuable innovations.[51] The role of communities of practice also reflects the greater focus on relational practice within professionalism.[1,51]

Of interest, vulnerability is also linked to the concept of resilience. That is, vulnerability supports connection, and through trust and communication, contributes to the group's capacity to develop innovative solutions that support resilience.[51] In this regard, a new concept has been proposed, "collective moral resilience" that emphasizes relationships and the process of dialogue to support moral resilience.[51] In addition, patients' relationships support their healthcare decision-making, which healthcare providers may not be taught to recognize. Hedlin describes understanding how a patient changed from choosing a DNR (do not resuscitate) order when alone to canceling the DNR order when family arrived, in the context of relational autonomy.[52] That is, patients will also integrate new information with the support and guidance of close family members to ultimately make their own decisions.

Professional Identity Formation

Definition and Role in Medical Education

Professional identity formation is increasingly considered central to medical education.[11,15,53] PIF is defined as integrating or interweaving a profession's knowledge, skills, values, and behaviors within or in interaction with one's preexisting personal values and identity.[54,55] Interweaving highlights potential tensions between personal and professional identities. Volpe and coauthors' scoping review of PIF among trainees in the helping professions, including medical students and residents, found a paucity of attention to sociocultural elements, including but not limited to race, gender, sexual orientation, and socioeconomic status.[55]

Structural Barriers to Entering the Profession and Within the Profession

Medicine has historically been predominantly comprised of white males. "To produce more Black male doctors, start by acknowledging bias," states an article published by Andis Robeznieks in July 2021.[56] In the article, the author quotes Clyde Yancy, MD, vice dean for diversity, equity, and inclusion at Northwestern University Feinberg School of Medicine. "What chills me is—I think about the number of Black men that went into medical school with me in 1978 is the same number that enrolled in 2016."[56]

PIF and Intersectionality

Mount and colleagues (2022) call for an intersectional approach to PIF.[54] Intersectionality highlights multidimensional identifications, including, but not limited to, race and gender.[57] In Crenshaw's original description of intersectionality and discrimination among Black women, identification with two or more forms of difference was associated with greater disadvantage than the sum of each disadvantage or even erasure.[57] Recent medical learner and physician narratives describe the erasure of aspects of their personal identity, including race, sexual orientation, gender, and disabilities, to be accepted.[58,59] That is, learners are pressed to engage in "covering" behaviors, efforts to minimize attention to stigmatized identities or identities that differ from the dominant identity.[59]

An intersectional approach aims to consider psychological, developmental growth, and the socialization that occurs in relationships throughout medical training. In one school, medical students collaborated with faculty members to revise professionalism orientation sessions for new medical students in order to add consideration of diverse personal identities and their influence on professional identity development.[60] Within small-group sessions, students discussed case examples that fostered empathy and allyship for the diversity of medical learners.[60] Many participating medical students expressed a desire to retain personal identity related to cultural backgrounds and personal values. The facilitators and authors recommended a longitudinal PIF curriculum including plans to prevent the erasure of valued personal identities.[60]

As indicated in the introduction, PIF is considered complementary to the competency discourse.[12] However, Frost and Regehr, using a social constructivist lens, assert that the discourse on training standardization is in tension with that of diversity.[61] Recommendations for a unified competency-based medical education[62] have been associated with concern that standardizing or benchmarking favors majority voices and potentially harms those who have been marginalized.[63] Throughout medical training, individuals define for themselves and in relation to standards what it means to become a physician, along with continued growth of one's personal identity, which may include intersectional identities.[11,64]

Professional Identity Formation, Socialization, and Relationships

Among medical students, socialization through relationships in healthcare strongly influences PIF.[2] Influential relational experiences occur with patients, peers, residents, physicians in practice, and other health professionals.[12] Wyatt and colleagues advocate for more attention to ways of being and becoming a physician that are neither validated nor actively silenced within healthcare and training.[65] Further, they state that marginalized and racialized medical students, residents, and physicians are often faced with addressing sociohistorical contexts, including discrimination in negotiating the development of their professional identity. Dedicated Indigenous mentors of Indigenous students in the health sciences provide valuable time, critical thinking, and emotional and mental resources that are unacknowledged by academic health centers.[66] Among Black Canadian medical students, some described being called on by Canadian medical leaders to review antiracism statements.[67] The lack of Black leaders and faculty members contributed to this extra, unacknowledged burden.[67]

Transitions occur in medical careers, representing a change from one type of work to another.[68,69] Kay, Berry, and Coles describe several transition periods in undergraduate medical education that include entering medical school and beginning clerkship.[70] Entering medical school often requires a focus on individual achievement in relation to school marks and building a curriculum vitae. From the time one enters medicine, a collective identity may be developed. At the University of Calgary Cumming School of Medicine, a collective PIF is promoted through the naming of each class. Further along in clinical care, teams of healthcare providers, including physicians, contribute to excellence in healthcare. Thus, PIF moves from an individual focus on obtaining entry into medicine to subsequently recognizing and identifying oneself as a healthcare team member.

Kay and colleagues utilized conceptual change theory to explore how triggers, which have also been referred to as crises or rites of passage, introduce cognitive discontinuities in how medical students see themselves.[70] Jarvis-Selinger and colleagues suggest that what sparks a medical student to reflect on who they are or are becoming can be considered catalysts.[71] Using social-cognitive theory to analyze medical student experiences, they found catalysts are often more relational (e.g., talking to laypersons and teaching another medical student how to scrub), than is often described.[71] Further, with the demands of medical school, medical students may experience losses in conceptualizing what they had anticipated in becoming a doctor. Beagan describes almost half of medical students experiencing "a loss of who they were."[72] Some experiences may leverage medical students' decisions in choosing a specialty.[70] Residents who described successfully addressing professionalism challenges, such as providing feedback to peers or colleagues about unprofessional behavior, often described feeling more like a leader or no longer a student and identified improved patient care outcomes or peer professional behavior.[50]

Appropriate responsibility for patient care with some level of autonomy for trainees is found to be important to PIF.[71,73] A simulation study prompted a sense of autonomy and responsibility for patient care through decision-making that affected the patient outcome and found many students responding to the *unfamiliar and disorienting* situation with a changed professional sense of themselves.[65] With debriefing, the medical students described shifting from a focus on their individual performance to the aim of learning to enhance patient care and identifying gaps in that knowledge.

Without relatable role models or mentors, medical learners from underrepresented minority groups may be more vulnerable in navigating transitions.[63,66] Furthermore, bias and discrimination toward medical students and residents by patients or members of the healthcare team can lead to a diminished sense of belonging among the learners unless support and opportunities to be heard and believed are provided.

Mentorship is salient to medical career development generally; most likely, it is especially important within healthcare systems that have structural inequities. To define mentoring behaviors for Indigenous health science students, experienced Indigenous health sciences research mentors and allies compared Indigenous mentoring strategies with non-Indigenous mentoring strategies.[66] The researchers observed that "Indigenous mentors practice relationalism," highlighting interconnectedness and interdependent relationships.[66] Further, an Indigenous mentorship approach intentionally provides a mentee-centered focus, ensuring interactions are not top-down to ensure that mentees develop their own goals. Self-advocacy is encouraged, and mentors advocate for the trainees when the latter are not present.[66] Importantly, Indigenous mentorship fosters

Indigenous identity, promoting connection to community. For Indigenous students less connected to their heritage, mentors role-model Indigenous protocols and etiquette. In place of traditional Indigenous protocols, mentors practice Indigenous etiquette with more listening than speaking and allowing for silence. Mentoring has the potential to support Indigenous students' professional identities in aversive healthcare training environments that include stereotypes of First Nations people[34] and significant health inequities due to discrimination.[74]

The Indigenous mentoring model can be utilized by both Indigenous and non-Indigenous mentors of Indigenous health sciences and medical students. The mentee-centered approach could also usefully inform the mentorship of most medical students. Learning from the Indigenous practice of relationalism may also inform Western perspectives of healthcare generally.

Recently, the Black Physicians of Canada founded a national racially concordant mentorship program for residents, fellows, and early career physicians who less commonly had mentors compared to cohort medical students.[75] The mentoring program was developed to support professional development and how to negotiate race-related barriers in careers. Given the value of identity-concordant mentors, educational and institutional leaders are encouraged to provide faculty development and mentor training to support and mentor equity-deserving trainees with different identities than one's own.[76]

Communities of practice are proposed to foster collective moral resilience.[51] This model has potential for groups who work to address structural racism or discrimination in healthcare. In developing a project to address anti-Indigenous racism in medicine, awareness of embodied experiences was important to recognizing injustice, and residents learned more about becoming an ally.[18]

Culture of Medicine and Professionalism

Recently, Schrewe and Martimianakis emphasized the need for a deeper consideration of the culture of medicine.[77] That is, current formulations of professional identity often do not account for the increasing diversity and intersectionality of those who enter medicine. Race, abilities, gender identities, and the numerous other aspects of identity, including intersectionality and prior life and career experience, are not often considered in medical trainees' socialization. As an example of intersectionality, in a single-institution qualitative study, the qualities of rurality, history of immigration, or race were more prominent in some medical students' intersectional personal identities than was identification with "not coming from advantage" prior to entry into medicine.[78]

Certainly, experiences among equity-seeking groups in medicine highlight aversive experiences within medicine. Mistreatment and discrimination within medicine during training is more commonly reported by LGB (lesbian, gay, bisexual) students than their heterosexual peers and is partly associated with burnout.[79] Further, students who are transgender or non-binary (TGNB) often do not disclose their identity due to fears of discrimination.[76]

Professional Identity, Wellness, and Meaning

Strategies to support the wellness of students, residents, and physicians are complicated by the medical culture of perfectionism that stigmatizes disabilities.[62] Further,

Stergiopolous and colleagues found that medical students self-identifying with a disability experience tensions between the *good student* and the *good patient* roles or identities.[80] That is, a good medical student manages their studies while maintaining a social life with limited sleep requirements and physical exercise. In contrast, a good patient limits activities to support performance. Medical students who self-identify with disabilities describe intersectional identities that support advocacy, communication, and compassion. Stergiopolous and coauthors make the case for greater awareness among medical educators that disabilities are part of the complexity of being human.[80]

There are increasing calls to improve institutional or organizational cultures rather than focus on individual strategies to address the high rates of burnout and distress among medical students and residents as well as physicians.[81-83] Toubassi and colleagues propose that grounding trainees in the meaningfulness of their work while developing a professional identity may also promote well-being.[84] Meaning is described to include the coherence of one's past, present, and imagined future and purpose with a clear sense of one's goals and significance in doing work that matters.[84-86] Each element of meaning supports well-being and resilience. Further, the concept of purpose is consistent with that of mission in Baarnhorn and coauthors' multilevel professional framework.[87] During the COVID-19 pandemic, physicians who found new meaning in their work conveyed constructive adaptation, in contrast to physicians who experienced disruption and discord during the pandemic.[88] This novel framework, with attention to meaning making in the course of PIF, requires further exploration and assessment for its implementation.

This chapter focuses on the experiences of medical students and residents. We acknowledge social injustice often occurs even for more senior equity-deserving colleagues, who may also experience discrimination in their healthcare careers.

Professional Resistance, Critical Consciousness, and Solidarity

Ellaway and Wyatt recently recommended medical students be educated for a principled approach to professional resistance to oppose social injustices, including structural racism and misogyny.[16] Their work highlights a tension that arises from the need to remain part of the healthcare system while also resisting injustice or moral wrongs within that system. In this regard, Hafferty and colleagues indicate that physicians require skills and knowledge to "disrupt" the system and contribute to identity formation.[89] Further, Ellaway and Wyatt propose that professional resistance requires an approach that is affirmative—*for* something rather than against—deliberate, intentional, proportionate, and constructive in seeking solutions.[16]

Education for professional resistance is consistent with Freire's stance that education contributes to heightened awareness of the need for social justice.[90] Kumagai and Lypson further propose that for medical education to prepare physicians to treat diverse populations requires medical students and residents to develop critical consciousness as an orientation.[91] Critical consciousness is described as "reflective awareness of the differences in power and privilege and the inequities that are embedded in social relationships."[91(p783)] This awareness supports physicians' capacity to both recognize medicine's social, cultural, and historical context *and* to actively identify social injustice and work to find solutions for societal problems that may adversely affect healthcare.

An illustration of critical consciousness is provided with the professional role description in the Family Practice CanMEDS Indigenous Health Supplement.[92] This supplement highlights the importance of working alongside Indigenous patients and communities to contribute to the process of decolonization. Decolonization involves dismantling the remnants of colonial power present in various parts of society, including government, culture, education, and healthcare.[93] Within this framework, learners are "urged to be fully aware of and address the oppression, power imbalance, and racism that is often re-enacted within health care."(p42) To accomplish this, individuals must engage in deep self-reflection, particularly regarding their own perspectives that may stem from "power and privilege held by virtue of profession and societal position."(p43)

Razack and colleagues describe the importance of a professionalism of solidarity with patients, whereby recognizing structural inequities within healthcare systems includes mutual commitment with communities to address societal factors that may perpetuate health inequities.[94] Recently, we found that residents identified several professionalism challenges, including managing interprofessional conflicts to ensure optimal patient care, providing informal feedback to peers regarding perceived unprofessional behavior, and attending to personal and preceptor wellness. However, residents did not report taking action to address social injustice or foster greater social responsibility.[50] Although a single medical school study, its findings suggest the need for further education and support to cultivate attitudes and skills related to professional resistance.

As physicians acknowledge their profession (like others in most professions in this imperfect world) encompasses and contributes to inequities, medical professionalism requires we work toward achieving greater social justice within our field. One example is confronting the historical practice of forced or coerced sterilization of Indigenous women, which was enabled from 1928 to 1976 by Canada's Sexual Sterilization Act.[95] Lawsuits indicate that the practice persisted until recent times.[96] A path forward includes working alongside Indigenous communities to reform healthcare system policies, systems, and individual practices to ensure safe sexual healthcare (among other changes and mitigations that may address known and potential harms) and uphold reproductive rights. Additionally, we must recognize and build on the strengths of Indigenous women in this process.[95]

Closing

This chapter engages in professional resistance by providing a critical perspective on the limited attention given to EDIA considerations in current codes of ethics and how PIF is conceptualized. Further, we emphasize the importance of drawing on Indigenous perspectives to foster a more relational and nonhierarchical model of mentoring for PIF.

Physicians of color, as well as some white female physicians and doctors whose appearance for some reason does not match the commentator's "doctor stereotype" have encountered comments like: "You don't look like a doctor." What impact might that sort of statement yield in the context of one's overall acceptance as a professional and developing a professional identity?

When we examine medicine's long-standing image of the white male of a certain age and appearance as most representative of the profession and the embodiment of professionalism, the question is raised whether this image has tainted the persona of the medical profession, revealing an incongruity between the perceived and actual diversity of who practices medicine. As stereotypes often do, it may contribute to the perpetuation of discriminatory practices.

Frameworks and ideals for the medical profession and professionalism ought to be inclusive and foster a sense of belonging through language that supports, welcomes, and helps all physicians and medical students develop their professional identity. Moreover, we also need mentoring programs that actively support the personal identities of Indigenous individuals, people of color, and those with disabilities to ensure true inclusivity within the profession.

References

1. Cruess RL, Cruess SR. Professionalism, communities of practice, and medicine's social contract. *The Journal of the American Board of Family Medicine.* 2020;33(Supplement):S50–S56. doi:10.3122/jabfm.2020.S1.190417
2. Cruess SR, Cruess RL. Professionalism as a social construct: The evolution of a concept. *Journal of Graduate Medical Education.* 2016;8(2):265–267. doi:10.4300/jgme-d-16-00102.1
3. Rockich-Winston N, Taylor TR, Richards JA, White D, Wyatt TR. "All Patients Are Not Treated as Equal": Extending Medicine's Social Contract to Black/African American Communities. *Teaching and Learning in Medicine.* 2021;34(3):238–245. doi:10.1080/10401334.2021.1902816
4. Dzau VJ, Laitner MH, Balatbat CA. Has traditional medicine had its day? The need to redefine academic medicine. *The Lancet.* 2022;400(10361):1481–1486. doi:10.1016/s0140-6736(22)01603-8
5. Manca A, Gormley GJ, Johnston JL, Hart ND. Honoring medicine's social contract: A scoping review of critical consciousness in medical education. *Academic Medicine.* 2020;95(6):958–967. doi:10.1097/acm.0000000000003059
6. Irby DM, Hamstra SJ. Parting the clouds: Three professionalism frameworks in medical education. *Academic Medicine.* Dec 2016;91(12):1606–1611. doi:10.1097/acm.0000000000001190
7. Brody H, Doukas D. Professionalism: A framework to guide medical education. *Medical Education.* 2014;48(10):980–987. doi:10.1111/medu.12520
8. Doukas DJ. Promoting professionalism through virtue ethics. *Am J Bioeth.* Jan 2019;19(1):37–39. doi:10.1080/15265161.2018.1545879
9. Association CM. *CMA Code of Ethics and Professionalism*; 2018.
10. Lesser CS, Lucey CR, Egener B, Braddock CH, 3rd, Linas SL, Levinson W. A behavioral and systems view of professionalism. *JAMA.* 2010;304(24):2732–2737. doi:10.1001/jama.2010.1864
11. Cruess RL, Cruess SR, Boudreau JD, Snell L, Steinert Y. Reframing medical education to support professional identity formation. *Academic Medicine.* 2014;89(11):1446–1451. doi:10.1097/acm.0000000000000427
12. Jarvis-Selinger S, Pratt DD, Regehr G. Competency is not enough. *Academic Medicine.* 2012;87(9):1185–1190. doi:10.1097/ACM.0b013e3182604968
13. Hodges B. Professional identities of the future: Invisible and unconscious or deliberate and reflexive. In: Cruess RL, Cruess SR, Steinert Y., ed. *Teaching medical professionalism supporting development of a professional identity formation* (2nd ed). Cambridge University Press; 2016:chap 19.
14. Association AM. *Code of Medical Ethics*; 2017.

15. Cooke M ID, O'Brien BC. *Educating physicians: A call for reform of medical school and residency.* Jossey-Bass; 2010.
16. Ellaway RH, Wyatt TR. What role should resistance play in training health professionals? *Academic Medicine.* 2021;96(11):1524–1528. doi:10.1097/acm.0000000000004225
17. Rankl F, Johnson GA, Vindrola-Padros C. Examining what we know in relation to how we know it: A team-based reflexivity model for rapid qualitative health research. *Qual Health Res.* Jun 2021;31(7):1358–1370. doi:10.1177/1049732321998062
18. Merner E BE, Roach P, Grimminck R, Crowshoe L, de Groot JM, Descottignies M. A Novel Pedagogical Project to Spur Decolonization in Medical Education. Paper presented at: International Congress on Academic Medicine; April 17, 2023; Quebec. Session Indigenous Health - Humanities in Medicine.
19. Truth and Reconciliation Commission of Canada: Calls to Action. 2015.
20. Ermine W. The ethical space of engagement. *Indigenous Law Journal.* 2007;6:193–203.
21. Colleges. AMAaAoAM. Advancing Health Equity: Guide on Language, Narrative and Concepts. 2021. Accessed June 12, 2024. ama-assn.org/equity-guide
22. Sioutis S, Reppas L, Bekos A, Limneos P, Saranteas T, Mavrogenis AF. The HIPPOCRATIC Oath: Analysis and Contemporary Meaning. *Orthopedics.* Sep-Oct 2021;44(5):264–272. doi:10.3928/01477447-20210819-08
23. Walton M, Kerridge I. Do no harm: is it time to rethink the Hippocratic Oath? *Med Educ.* Jan 2014;48(1):17–27. doi:10.1111/medu.12275
24. Thomas P. Medical Ethics, Or a code of Institutes and Precepts, Adapted to the Professional Conduct of Physicians and Surgeons. vol Third Edition. Oxford; 1803.
25. Baker RB CA, Emanuel L, Latham SR (editors). The American Medical Ethics Revolution: How the AMA's Code of Ethics has transformed physicians relationships to patients, professionals, and society. Johns Hopkins University Press; 1999.
26. AR J. A short history of medical ethics. Oxford University Press; 2000.
27. Scheinman SJ, Fleming P, Niotis K. Oath Taking at U.S. and Canadian Medical School Ceremonies: Historical Perspectives, Current Practices, and Future Considerations. *Academic Medicine.* 2018;93(9):1301–1306. doi:10.1097/acm.0000000000002097
28. London AJ. Self-Defeating Codes of Medical Ethics and How to Fix Them: Failures in COVID-19 Response and Beyond. *The American Journal of Bioethics.* 2020;21(1):4–13. doi:10.1080/15265161.2020.1845854
29. Huber SJ, Wynia MK. When pestilence prevails...physician responsibilities in epidemics. *Am J Bioeth.* Winter 2004;4(1):W5–11. doi:10.1162/152651604773067497
30. Russell HA, Sanders M, Nofziger A, et al. Addressing Sexual Harassment and Gender Bias: Mandatory Modules Are Not Enough. *Fam Med.* Apr 2023;55(4):253–258. doi:10.22454/FamMed.2023.488622
31. Carnes M, Devine PG, Isaac C, et al. Promoting institutional change through bias literacy. *Journal of Diversity in Higher Education.* 2012;5(2):63–77. doi:10.1037/a0028128
32. Kaatz A, Carnes M. Stuck in the out-group: Jennifer can't grow up, Jane's invisible, and Janet's over the hill. *J Womens Health (Larchmt).* Jun 2014;23(6):481–484. doi:10.1089/jwh.2014.4766
33. McIntosh P. *White privilege: unpacking the invisible knapsack.* Peace and Freedom; 1989:10–12.
34. Ly A, Crowshoe L. 'Stereotypes are reality': addressing stereotyping in Canadian Aboriginal medical education. *Medical Education.* 2015;49(6):612–622. doi:10.1111/medu.12725

35. Carnes M, Sheridan J, Fine E, Lee YG, Filut A. Effect of a Workshop to Break the Bias Habit for Internal Medicine Faculty: A Multisite Cluster Randomized Controlled Study. *Acad Med.* Oct 1 2023;98(10):1211–1219. doi:10.1097/acm.0000000000005271

36. Nuru-Jeter AM, Michaels EK, Thomas MD, Reeves AN, Thorpe RJ, Jr., LaVeist TA. Relative roles of race versus socioeconomic position in studies of health inequalities: A matter of interpretation. *Annu Rev Public Health.* Apr 1 2018;39:169–188. doi:10.1146/annurev-publhealth-040617-014230

37. Richeson JA, Sommers SR. Toward a social psychology of race and race relations for the twenty-first century. *Annu Rev Psychol.* 2016;67:439–463. doi:10.1146/annurev-psych-010213-115115

38. Osei-Tutu K, Ereyi-Osas W, Sivananthajothy P, Rabi D. Antiracism as a foundational competency: Reimagining CanMEDS through an antiracist lens. *CMAJ.* Dec 19 2022;194(49):E1691–e1693. doi:10.1503/cmaj.220521

39. Ben-Cheikh I, Beneduce R, Guzder J, et al. Historical Scientific Racism and Psychiatric Publications: A Necessary International Anti-racist Code of Ethics. *The Canadian Journal of Psychiatry.* 2021;66(10):863–872. doi:10.1177/07067437211020613

40. Bedzow I, Wynia M. Ethical Training Can Turn an "Ought" to a "Can". *Am J Bioeth.* May 2020;20(4):73–75. doi:10.1080/15265161.2020.1730517

41. Wynia MK, Kishore SP, Belar CD. A unified code of ethics for health professionals: insights from an IOM workshop. *JAMA.* Feb 26 2014;311(8):799–800. doi:10.1001/jama.2014.504

42. National Academies S, Engineering Medicine. Exploring a Culture of Fairness, Respect, and Anti-racism Through Diversity, Equity, and Inclusion in Health Professions Education: A Workshop Series; 2022.

43. Medical professionalism in the new millennium: a physician charter. *Ann Intern Med.* Feb 5 2002;136(3):243–246. doi:10.7326/0003-4819-136-3-200202050-00012

44. Sukhera J, Kulkarni C, Taylor T. Structural distress: experiences of moral distress related to structural stigma during the COVID-19 pandemic. *Perspectives on Medical Education.* 2021;10(4):222–229. doi:10.1007/s40037-021-00663-y

45. Doukas DJ, Ozar DT, Darragh M, de Groot JM, Carter BS, Stout N. Virtue and care ethics & humanism in medical education: a scoping review. *BMC Med Educ.* Feb 26 2022;22(1):131. doi:10.1186/s12909-021-03051-6

46. Tronto JC. An ethic of care. Generations. *Fall* 1998;22(3):15–20.

47. Edwards SD. Three versions of an ethics of care. *Nurs Philos.* Oct 2009;10(4):231–240. doi:10.1111/j.1466-769X.2009.00415.x

48. Delgado J, de Groot J, McCaffrey G, Dimitropoulos G, Sitter KC, Austin W. Communities of practice: acknowledging vulnerability to improve resilience in healthcare teams. *Journal of Medical Ethics.* 2021;47(7):488–493. doi:10.1136/medethics-2019-105865

49. Tomkow L, Prager G, Worthing K, Farrington R. In critique of moral resilience: UK healthcare professionals' experiences working with asylum applicants housed in contingency accommodation during the COVID-19 pandemic. *Journal of Medical Ethics.* 2024;50(1):33–38. doi:10.1136/jme-2022-108632

50. De Groot JM, Kassam A, Swystun D, Topps M. Residents' transformational changes through self-regulated, experiential learning for professionalism. *Canadian Medical Education Journal.* 2021;doi:10.36834/cmej.70234

51. Delgado J, Siow S, de Groot J, McLane B, Hedlin M. Towards collective moral resilience: the potential of communities of practice during the COVID-19 pandemic and beyond. *Journal of Medical Ethics.* 2021;47(6):374–382. doi:10.1136/medethics-2020-106764

52. Hedlin M. The Web We Weave. *N Engl J Med.* Dec 2 2021;385(23):2119–2121. doi:10.1056/NEJMp2109820

53. RK M. Some preliminaries to a sociology of medical education. vol The Student Physician. Introductory studies in the sociology of medical education. Harvard University Press; 1957.

54. Mount GR, Kahlke R, Melton J, Varpio L. A Critical Review of Professional Identity Formation Interventions in Medical Education. *Academic Medicine.* 2022;97(11S):S96–S106. doi:10.1097/acm.0000000000004904

55. Volpe RL, Hopkins M, Haidet P, Wolpaw DR, Adams NE. Is research on professional identity formation biased? Early insights from a scoping review and metasynthesis. *Medical Education.* 2019;53(2):119–132. doi:10.1111/medu.13781

56. Robeznieks A. To produce more Black male doctors, start by acknowledging bias. American Medical Association. June 7, 2024. Accessed June 12, 2024. https://www.ama-assn.org/education/medical-school-diversity/produce-more-black-male-doctors-start-acknowledging-bias

57. Crenshaw K. Demarginalizing the intersection of race and sex: a black feminist critique of antidiscrimination doctrine, feminist theory and antiracist politics. *University of Chicago Legal Forum.* 1989;1(8):139–167.

58. AbdelHameid D. Professionalism 101 for Black Physicians. *New England Journal of Medicine.* 2020;383(5). doi:10.1056/NEJMpv2022773

59. Tsai J. Diversity and inclusion in medical schools: The reality. Scientific American Blog Network blog. 2018. https://www.scientificamerican.com/blog/voices/diversity-and-inclusion-in-medical-schools-the-reality/

60. Bhatia-Lin A, Wong K, Legha R, Walker VP. What Will You Protect? Redefining Professionalism Through the Lens of Diverse Personal Identities. *MedEdPORTAL.* 2021. doi:10.15766/mep_2374-8265.11203

61. Frost HD, Regehr G. "I AM a Doctor." *Academic Medicine.* 2013;88(10):1570–1577. doi:10.1097/ACM.0b013e3182a34b05

62. Ryan MS, Blood AD, Park YS, Farnan JM. Competency-Based Frameworks in Medical School Education Programs: A Thematic Analysis of the Academic Medicine Snapshots, 2020. *Acad Med.* Nov 1 2022;97(11s):S63–s70. doi:10.1097/acm.0000000000004912

63. Wyatt TR, Balmer D, Rockich-Winston N, Chow CJ, Richards J, Zaidi Z. "Whispers and shadows": A critical review of the professional identity literature with respect to minority physicians. *Medical Education.* 2020;55(2):148–158. doi:10.1111/medu.14295

64. Cruess RL, Cruess SR, Boudreau JD, Snell L, Steinert Y. A schematic representation of the professional identity formation and socialization of medical students and residents: a guide for medical educators. *Academic Medicine.* Jun 2015;90(6):718–725. doi:10.1097/acm.0000000000000700

65. Wyatt TR, Rockich-Winston N, Taylor TR, White D. What Does Context Have to Do With Anything? A Study of Professional Identity Formation in Physician-Trainees Considered Underrepresented in Medicine. *Academic Medicine.* 2020;95(10):1587–1593. doi:10.1097/acm.0000000000003192

66. Murry AT, Barnabe C, Foster S, et al. Indigenous Mentorship in the Health Sciences: Actions and Approaches of Mentors. *Teaching and Learning in Medicine.* 2021;34(3):266–276. doi:10.1080/10401334.2021.1912610

67. Kalifa A, Okuori A, Kamdem O, Abatan D, Yahya S, Brown A. "This shouldn't be our job to help you do this": Exploring the responses of medical schools across Canada to address anti-Black racism in 2020. *CMAJ.* Oct 24 2022;194(41):E1395–e1403. doi:10.1503/cmaj.211746

68. Atherley A, Teunissen P, Hegazi I, Hu W, Dolmans D. Longitudinal exploration of students' identity formation during the transition from pre-clinical to clinical training using research poetry. *Med Educ.* Jul 2023;57(7):637–647. doi:10.1111/medu.14998

69. Soo J, Brett-MacLean P, Cave MT, Oswald A. At the precipice: a prospective exploration of medical students' expectations of the pre-clerkship to clerkship transition. *Adv Health Sci Educ Theory Pract.* Mar 2016;21(1):141–162. doi:10.1007/s10459-015-9620-2

70. Kay D, Berry A, Coles NA. What Experiences in Medical School Trigger Professional Identity Development? *Teach Learn Med.* Jan-Mar 2019;31(1):17–25. doi:10.1080/10401334.2018.1444487

71. Jarvis-Selinger S, MacNeil KA, Costello GRL, Lee K, Holmes CL. Understanding Professional Identity Formation in Early Clerkship: A Novel Framework. *Academic Medicine.* Oct 2019;94(10):1574–1580. doi:10.1097/acm.0000000000002835

72. Beagan BL. Neutralizing differences: Producing neutral doctors for (almost) neutral patients. *Soc Sci Med.* Oct 2000;51(8):1253–1265. doi:10.1016/s0277-9536(00)00043-5

73. Wyatt TR, Kleinheksel AJ, Tews M. Linking Patient Care Ownership and Professional Identity Formation through Simulation. *Teaching and Learning in Medicine.* 2020;33(2):164–172. doi:10.1080/10401334.2020.1813583

74. McLane P, Barnabe C, Mackey L, et al. First Nations status and emergency department triage scores in Alberta: A retrospective cohort study. *Canadian Medical Association Journal.* 2022;194(2):E37–E45. doi:10.1503/cmaj.210779

75. Egbedeyi O, El-Hadi H, Madzima TR, Semalulu T, Tunde-Byass M, Swaleh R. Assessing the need for Black mentorship within residency training in Canada. *CMAJ.* Oct 31 2022;194(42):E1455–e1459. doi:10.1503/cmaj.212124

76. Cook TE, Dimant OE, Novick R, et al. Gendered Expectations: Strategies for Navigating Structural Challenges in Support of Transgender and Nonbinary Trainees in Academic Medicine. *Academic Medicine.* 2020;95(5):704–709. doi:10.1097/acm.0000000000003202

77. Schrewe B, Martimianakis MA. Re-thinking "I"dentity in medical education: genealogy and the possibilities of being and becoming. *Advances in Health Sciences Education.* 2022;27(3):847–861. doi:10.1007/s10459-022-10095-w

78. Conway-Hicks S, de Groot JM. Living in two worlds: Becoming and being a doctor among those who identify with "not from an advantaged background". *Current Problems in Pediatric and Adolescent Health Care.* 2019;49(4):92–101. doi:10.1016/j.cppeds.2019.03.006

79. Samuels EA, Boatright DH, Wong AH, et al. Association Between Sexual Orientation, Mistreatment, and Burnout Among US Medical Students. *JAMA Network Open.* 2021;4(2). doi:10.1001/jamanetworkopen.2020.36136

80. Stergiopoulos E, Fernando O, Martimianakis MA. "Being on Both Sides": Canadian Medical Students' Experiences With Disability, the Hidden Curriculum, and Professional Identity Construction. *Academic Medicine.* 2018;93(10):1550–1559. doi:10.1097/acm.0000000000002300

81. Ruzycki SM, Lemaire JB. Physician burnout. *Canadian Medical Association Journal.* 2018;190(2):E53–E53. doi:10.1503/cmaj.170827

82. West CP, Dyrbye LN, Erwin PJ, Shanafelt TD. Interventions to prevent and reduce physician burnout: a systematic review and meta-analysis. *Lancet.* Nov 5 2016;388(10057):2272–2281. doi:10.1016/s0140-6736(16)31279-x

83. Cohen JS, Leung Y, Fahey M, et al. The happy docs study: a Canadian Association of Internes and Residents well-being survey examining resident physician health and satisfaction within and outside of residency training in Canada. *BMC Research Notes.* 2008;1(1). doi:10.1186/1756-0500-1-105

84. Toubassi D, Schenker C, Roberts M, Forte M. Professional identity formation: linking meaning to well-being. *Adv Health Sci Educ Theory Pract.* Mar 2023;28(1):305–318. doi:10.1007/s10459-022-10146-2

85. Heintzelman SJ, King LA. Life is pretty meaningful. *Am Psychol.* Sep 2014;69(6):561–574. doi:10.1037/a0035049

86. King LA, Hicks JA. The Science of Meaning in Life. *Annu Rev Psychol.* Jan 4 2021;72:561–584. doi:10.1146/annurev-psych-072420-122921

87. Barnhoorn PC, Houtlosser M, Ottenhoff-de Jonge MW, Essers G, Numans ME, Kramer AWM. A practical framework for remediating unprofessional behavior and for developing professionalism competencies and a professional identity. *Med Teach.* Mar 2019;41(3):303–308. doi:10.1080/0142159x.2018.1464133

88. Butler CR, Wong SPY, Vig EK, Neely CS, O'Hare AM. Professional roles and relationships during the COVID-19 pandemic: a qualitative study among US clinicians. *BMJ Open.* Mar 25 2021;11(3):e047782. doi:10.1136/bmjopen-2020-047782

89. Hafferty FW, Michalec B, Martimianakis MA, Tilburt JC. Alternative Framings, Countervailing Visions: Locating the "P" in Professional Identity Formation. *Acad Med.* Feb 2016;91(2):171–174. doi:10.1097/acm.0000000000000961

90. Paulo F. Pedagogy of the Oppressed. Bergman Ramos M. 30th Anniversary Edition ed. Continuum International Publishing Group; 2005.

91. Kumagai AK, Lypson ML. Beyond cultural competence: critical consciousness, social justice, and multicultural education. *Acad Med.* Jun 2009;84(6):782–787. doi:10.1097/ACM.0b013e3181a42398

92. Crowshoe L. Professional. In: Kitty D FS, ed. CanMEDS-FM Indigenous Health Supplement. The College of Family Physicians of Canada; 2020.

93. Kitty D FS. CanMEDS-FM: Indigenous Health Supplement. The College of Family Physicians of Canada; 2020.

94. Razack S, de Carvalho Filho MA, Merlo G, Agbor-Baiyee W, de Groot J, Reynolds PP. Privilege, social justice and the goals of medicine: Towards a critically conscious professionalism of solidarity. *Perspect Med Educ.* Mar 2022;11(2):67–69. doi:10.1007/s40037-022-00699-8

95. Leason J. Forced and coerced sterilization of Indigenous women: Strengths to build upon. *Can Fam Physician.* Jul 2021;67(7):525–527. doi:10.46747/cfp.6707525

96. The scars that we carry: forced and coerced sterilization of persons in Canada. Part II / Standing Senate Committee on Human Rights; the Honourable Salma Ataullahjan, chair, the Honourable Wanda Thomas Bernard, deputy chair; 2022.

4

Socialization and the Hidden Curriculum in Medical Professionalism

Justin Lam, M. A. Martimianakis, and F. W. Hafferty

Key Points

- Medical professionalism curricula and training primarily developed in the 1990s as a way to combat the perceived erosion of medical professionalism in physicians' practices.
- The formal, informal, and hidden curricula of medical professionalism education continue to impact physician practices beyond medical training.
- The socialization around medical professionalism education now needs to focus on the incorporation of diversity, equity, and inclusion (DEI) initiatives.

Introduction

Much effort has been made to teach professionalism effectively because professionalism is a fundamental part of medicine's contract with society. This professionalism contract gives the profession financial and social privileges, as well as its independence to self-regulate. However, professionalism is a negotiable construct that evolves with shifting socio cultural values. This has resulted in countervailing messages about what it means to be a good professional; these messages complicate learner socialization to a professional identity. Moreover, professionalism is learned and internalized in the interstitial spaces between the classroom and the clinic—or between what is formally taught versus informally or even invisibly conveyed by the many structures and processes of the educational environment. Learners unavoidably experience educational tensions as they attempt to reconcile their prior understandings of what constitutes (in an ideal sense) respectful, ethical, and compassionate care with what is espoused and practiced as professionalism within the complexities and lived experiences of in-the-moment patient care decisions. Competing versions of professionalism also make it challenging to teach and evaluate professionalism effectively. In short, if medicine is to better fulfill its promise to train competent physicians who serve the public, then helping medical educators to better navigate the hidden spaces between "the ideal" and "the real" is essential.

In this chapter, we first explore the theoretical relationships between the concepts of hidden curriculum, socialization, and professionalism and show how educational culture, structure, and process contribute to the production of professional identities. Next, we briefly review the history of medical professionalism in North America, describing how the perceived problem of an eroding medical professionalism in the 1990s led to the creation of a formal professionalism curriculum for medical training.[1,2] We argue that the educational project of formally teaching professionalism was experienced by learners and faculty as being in tension with the hidden curriculum effects of this period. This tension transmitted tacit messages about what operationally constitutes professional behaviors. Specifically, we argue that there is friction between these dueling professionalisms: a more idealized and nostalgic rendering of professional values and a more pragmatic professionalism grounded in the structure and processes of medical work, which reflect the "actual" values and professional identities practiced in clinical medicine. We also explore how alignments and misalignments between formal educational experiences and informal and tacit socialization of learners can lead to varied outcomes and indeed socialize students along a professionalism spectrum, from normalized to deviant, from nostalgic to expedient.

Finally, we consider how ideas of diversity, equity, and inclusion (DEI) in medical education might impact professionalism education given that professionalism is and always has been a negotiable social construct that evolves as social demands on medicine change. In teaching an ever-evolving professionalism, we posit that it is essential to attend to both formal and hidden curricula dimensions simultaneously rather than only planning the former and reacting to the latter. We then demonstrate the utility of the hidden curriculum as an analytic tool for anticipating and investigating curricular misalignments and for connecting individual experiences to structural factors.

An Overview of Key Concepts

Socialization is the process that transforms first -year medical students from laypeople into medical professionals through the internalization of professional values and norms. There is an important distinction to be made here: to be socialized is to become, to embody. It is insufficient to just perform, even though it may be through performance of expected behaviors that socialization initially takes root. A powerful lever in the socialization process is role modeling. Watching an insider to a group (in our case the profession of medicine), particularly someone in authority, behave a certain way delivers important messages about expectations associated with group membership. Therefore, to be deliberate about socializing learners into a profession requires teachers to go beyond outlining the expected behaviors associated with professionalism. Educators must appreciate their role in imparting values, attitudes, and expertise as they go about their practice of medicine. Role modeling goes beyond what is explicitly stated as important and also appears in the implicit messages transmitted to learners through the butt of jokes, the venting of frustrations, or what gets prioritized in practice. This intentional or unintentional role modeling greatly influences what learners come to appreciate as the formal professionalism curriculum of their school.[3]

The formal, informal, and hidden curricula are one of many conceptual lenses through which medical educators and researchers can explore and understand the socialization process.[4] The formal curriculum is an institution's intended teaching for students that takes place in formal settings and covers predetermined topics. The informal curriculum consists of idiosyncratic, deliberate, opportunistic, and sometimes unplanned instruction by a teacher to a student.[4] The informal curriculum often occurs as just- in -time teaching in clinical environments. The hidden curriculum consists of tacit influences that operate at the level of structure and culture and consists of implicit messages around what is valuable and important.[5] The formal, informal, and hidden curricula interact in ways that both conflict and align to influence student socialization into medicine. In the context of professionalism education, the ideals and operationalization of professionalism in medical education is a socializing mechanism that informs professional identity formation in students. And while socialization is a complex process with many contributing parts and mechanisms, our focus in this chapter is specifically on the role of the formal, informal, and hidden curricula and how they influence the socialization of medical students. And in doing so, we consider the formal/informal curricula together as forms of deliberate teaching, in contrast with the hidden curriculum.

It is also important to recognize that there are additional contextual factors beyond the purview of medical training programs that influence how professionalism is conceptualized and operationalized through the hidden and formal curricula in formal medical education.[6] For example, the different roles of patient insurance coverage and its impact on care provision in Canadian and American healthcare systems highlight how professionalism, while similar conceptually, might transmit different lessons to students training in clinical settings.[7,8] In the United States, insurance determines where a patient might seek care and by whom they might be seen. In Canada, there are fewer issues related to access to healthcare on the basis of insurance coverage given the nearly universal healthcare system. These specific structural differences cultivate different expectations in both patients and physicians as to what constitutes good care and how this is expressed through professionalism.

Another example of an external influence on how professionalism is conceptualized and operationalized is the mandates around efficiency in patient care, measured in lengths of stay, patient outcomes, and resource stewardship. The influence of this bureaucratic rationality in healthcare institutions is a feature of the learning environment that is beyond the control of a medical training program and is often villainized in medical education as subsuming trainees into a dehumanizing approach to work, with downstream implications for care.[9] Other contextual factors that might influence socialization to professionalism include factors inside the institution—funding, leadership structure, mission and value statements, donor funding—and outside as well, such as industry involvement within and outside a healthcare organization; local, regional, and national legislation; and professional organizations.

Finally, while formal/informal and hidden curricula predominantly impact learner socialization to professionalism, they are still relevant to independently practicing physicians due to their involvement in medical education. Physicians who work with learners, regardless of whether they do so at an academic health center (AHC), private clinic, or other location, are active contributors to both the formal/informal and hidden curricula in the learning environment and transmit values to learners around what they consider to be professional. There is potential here for a looping effect of cultural reproduction, where graduates of a training program at an AHC could return as staff physicians and transmit the professional values that were transmitted to them during their training. A disruption effect is also possible, where a newly graduated staff physician might have resisted their socialization throughout their training and instead transmits new or different values to their trainees through the hidden curriculum. Recognizing the many contextual influences on the conceptualization and operationalization of professionalism, the formal and informal medical school professionalism curricula form only part of the potential equation in socializing students to professionalism. Therefore, examining the interplay between formal, informal, and hidden curricula is crucial.

The Creation of a Hidden Curriculum: How Medical Professionalism Became a Medical Education Problem

Scholars both outside and within medicine have been fascinated by the history of medical professionalism. Though some histories of professionalism span millennia back to ancient Greece,[6] the emergence of more contemporary professionalism concerns, and consequently medicine's modern-day professionalism movement, is linked to the social and industrial transformation of Western medicine during the 1980s and 1990s.[1,10] Outside of medicine, sociologists of the professions critically examined the relationship between medicine and society,[11] including professionalism's role in medicine's professional project and dominance over the division of labo r in healthcare,[12,13,14,15] as well as the effects of widespread sociopolitical, technological, and economic change on medicine's identity as a profession and the subsequent effects on the professional identity formation of doctors.[16] Did professionalism go hand in hand with caring well for patients or did it fulfill some other role altogether, such as elevating medical work to a vocation or establishing the boundaries of self-regulation and authority to control how care was organized and delivered? Sociologists took a structurally focused stance,[14,15,17] framing the professionalism crisis as individuals adapting to increasingly prominent market and bureaucratic logics in medicine.[13] Within medicine, the professionalism issue was also taken quite seriously. Scholars noted that with the advent of neoliberalism came an incursion of the market in the matters of medicine,[6,18] contributing to widespread individualism, a focus on efficiency, and maximizing productivity and profit through corporate management at the expense of individual morality and patient centeredness.[1]

The solution to the crises of professionalism and the so-called return to the professionalism of the past mirrored a contemporaneous shift from selecting for personal character in admissions toward training desirable characteristics in medical students.[19] This shift made it possible for educational interventions to emerge as the proposed solution for the "rising crisis" of medical professionalism. Professionalism as a training goal was formalized into medical education in the 1990s[20] with a discourse of nostalgia emerging in scholarly writing related to professionalism. Professionalism took many forms, including the creation of organizations for professionalism, medical school and residency program curricula, programming, evaluation systems, institutional policies, and new dedicated leadership positions. Other examples of this formalization included the creation of the Arnold Gold Foundation in 1988, white coat ceremonies,[21] and calls to develop medical student professionalism by governing medical training bodies such as the American Board of Internal Medicine,[22] Association of American Medical Colleges (AAMC),[23] and the Accreditation Council of Graduate Medical Education (ACGME).[20,24] A plethora of professionalism documents followed, including codes, charters, and competency frameworks.[22,23,24,25,26] Ironically, this formalization process obscured the origins of the professionalism movement as a response to the complex web of socio political and economic relationships that made caring a lucrative occupation in contemporary society.

In these ways, professionalism was constructed as a central responsibility of medical education and accrediting bodies. Professionalism was conceptualized as a list of "traditional" desirable attributes that were integral to the caring of the patient, such as altruism, honesty, integrity, and ethical behavior, which has been termed by some as "nostalgic professionalism."[27] The logic was as follows: If adequately taught to students, this list of professional competencies would generate the best possible doctors. Teaching these competencies would then grant the profession all the benefits of being a self-regulating occupation: autonomy, control over the structure and object of work, prestige, and financial rewards.[6]

The formal and informal professionalism curricula were intended to create a standardized, more transparent, and explicit investment in developing the behaviors, attitudes, and practices associated with good care. However, these very acts of formalization that brought professionalism into the classroom contrasted with the socializing influences predominantly from the clinical environment, captured in the literature as hidden curriculum effects. The influence of socialization was of course not new.[16] If anything, prior to the formalization of professionalism into medical curricula, students had always learned professionalism in the clinical environment through role modeling and immersion into medical culture. What was new is that these hidden curriculum effects were now experienced as a disjuncture between a cut -and- dried code of conduct that did not reflect the messiness of a "real doctor" doing "real clinical work."

The formalization of professionalism therefore led to an unprecedented learning environment: For the first time in medical education, students were learning about how to become medical professionals from three curricula.[15] These three dominant educational forces—the formal and informal curricula backed by the authority of professional organizations and the hidden curriculum powered by the pre existing culture and structure of the medical profession—were not always aligned in the values they imparted on students. Misalignments would lead to tensions for students, as they had to navigate expectations of training associated with nostalgic professionalism.[28] These misalignments would arise during formal evaluations of their performance as well as in the day-to-day expectations of their supervisors during informal teaching moments or when learners were involved in the delivery of care as part of a practiced professionalism.[7] These conflicting tensions in professionalism evaluation not only had consequences for students, but also resulted in professionalism workarounds to shoehorn on-the-ground professionalism practices to game formal professionalism requirements, which point to a misalignment between formal/informal and hidden curricula. In the next section of this chapter we explore how the tensions between formal, informal, and hidden professionalism curricula impact student socialization.

Dueling Professionalisms

Given that many sociopolitical factors beyond formal medical school curricula *additionally* influence how professionalism is conceptualized and operationalized through the hidden curriculum, let us now consider how the formal, informal, and hidden curricula impact the socialization of medical students into the professions. We begin with an examination of the different ways formal, informal, and hidden curricula alignments and misalignments create tensions in the socialization of medical trainees to professionalism specifically. We argue that while the formal, informal, and hidden curricula can at times align, it is in their misalignment that we get due ling professionalisms that socialize students along a spectrum of professionalism that by and large reproduce existing medical culture.

Importantly, the hidden curriculum concept does not have a valence[5] and is not inherently "good" or "bad," "positive" or "negative"—that is, even with the values that it transmits to students, it is not inherently a force for inhumane, unethical care, or a force for empathetic, patient-centered care. Rather, it is the effects that arise from the embodiment and performance of these values learned through the formal, informal, and hidden curricula that can have positive or negative outcomes on individuals and environments. However, the hidden curriculum concept has been used by scholars to draw attention to predominantly negative effects on learners. For example, humanism and empathy are upheld as core values of the formal curriculum. The hidden curriculum concept, however, is often described as having negative socialization effects that erode these values in student physicians.[9] We argue that it is just as important to recognize the *alignments* between the formal and hidden curricula of professionalism, even though they often appear in the literature as successful mentorship,[29,30] good role modeling of professionalism,[31] or humanism in highly regarded medical education programs.[32] Importantly, because curricular alignments are the medical education system working as planned, they are less often labeled or thought of as hidden curricular phenomena. Through these alignments and misalignments, hidden curriculum effects can have positive or negative impacts on medical student socialization.

The core tension experienced by students lies between the socialization forces generated by aligned and misaligned formal, informal, and hidden professionalism curricula. On the one hand, professionalism curricular alignments have been problematized by some as socializing students to a "nostalgic professionalism"[33] that fails to reflect evolving societal values. Conversely, professionalism curricular misalignments produce two effects: First is the conflict for learners as they negotiate incongruent ideas of what constitutes a professional physician. Second, these misalignments socialize students to what we term a "practical professionalism." The word *practical* refers to a version of professionalism that exists at the interface of professed, ideal-type values and everyday work of practicing physicians, complete with its workarounds to manage the tensions between bureaucratic, market, and professionalism forces in modern care provision. For example, students may be taught in the formal professionalism curriculum that all patients are deserving of equitable care, and that equity is an important value of their medical school. Once on their clinical rotations, they observe that most of the patients they see in their outpatient clinic are intersectionally marginalized—uninsured, racialized, low socioeconomic status, precariously employed—which contrasts the relatively privileged and insured patients seen by their attending physicians.[34] Furthermore, they observe that there are certain VIP patients that are cared for only by attending physicians.[35] In this way, conflicting messages stemming from formal, informal, and hidden curricular misalignments can generate tension in the learner socialization process, as learners must respond to both forms of professionalism if they are to be successful.

Neither learners nor faculty are blank slates or empty vessels that blindly accept the teachings of professionalism curricula. However, existing power dynamics and hierarchy within the learning environment make these lessons difficult for learners to resist, at least openly. It is therefore challenging for educators to predict which values learners will adopt and embody during their socialization to medical professionalism and which they will exercise agency in rejecting and resisting. What is certain is that the choices that faculty make to either resist or reinforce professionalism expectations impact what learners adopt as necessary attitudes, behaviors, and practices for succeeding in their training, and for practicing medicine after graduation.[36] We can expect that learners at the end of their socialization process will land somewhere along the spectrum between the ideal and practiced professionalisms professed by formal and hidden professionalism curricula. Therefore, although the formal/informal and hidden curricula are conceptually diametrically opposed to each other, in practice, formal and hidden curricula effects mix to socialize learners along a spectrum of acceptable and unacceptable attitudes, behavio rs, and practices.

Where students land on the spectrum of professionalism is distinct from how professional they are evaluated to be. Most often the *evaluation* of student professionalism is based on a nostalgic view of professionalism that has informed the standards set out in competency frameworks. Yet students may be required to adopt a "practical professionalism" while on the wards, resulting in behaviors, attitudes, and practices that contradict formal teaching. As a result, they run the risk of being labeled or assessed as unprofessional, while in practice of acting in ways that meet socially accepted demands for diligent, empathic care. Indeed, the same learner may theoretically be praised for dealing with patient complaints briskly and not holding up clinic flow and subsequently be evaluated as lacking professionalism toward patients when judged in relation to formal expectations. Being labeled unprofessional can have significant ramifications for future career prospects and individual mental health, especially for learners from marginalized or non dominant backgrounds.[37,38,39] However, misalignments do not always lead to poor learner outcomes because socialization is a result of a complex interplay between structure, culture, and personal agency. We explore this further in the final section of this chapter.

While there may be conceptual tension between what is taught and learned through the formal, informal, and hidden curricula, students may not experience this tension in practice and might not perceive hidden curricular lessons as problematic. For example, core ACGME professional standards emphasize the importance of cultural proficiency and humanism in caring for patients, which informs and motivates aspects of the formal curriculum.[40] Consequently, in clinical skills courses, a medical student learns about the social history and the importance of cultural safety and empathetic statements. This teaching may be reinforced during rounds when a patient asks to integrate an alternative medicine practice with their hospital treatment and the attending uses the opportunity to speak about the value of holistic approaches to care. On their clinical rotation, however, the same medical student takes a thorough medical and social history with a patient, only to be berated by their senior resident: "Why are you wasting my time! Just get to the important stuff."[41] Here, they learn from this hidden curriculum to omit the social history, to try to focus on the core issues as quickly as possible; their patients often don't complain to them about it either. In short, students learn implicitly that being a good professional also means prioritizing efficiency. And even though this example harbors conceptual tension between formal, informal, and hidden professionalism curricula, the learner does not always experience this tension. Instead, learners might view this discrepancy as learning the way things are in practice, especially if the implications for the quality of patient care are not immediately evident. Identifying such conceptual tensions is still important though since a lack of attention to the social determinants and culturally safe care can detrimentally impact healthcare outcomes.[42,43]

So far, we have briefly overviewed how perceived ailments in medical professionalism led to a solution based in medical education. In its original conception, the formal professionalism curriculum was proposed as the solution to a moral crisis in the medical profession. However, as we have argued, in the process of formalizing the teaching of professionalism, the interplay between explicit and tacit socializing influences was obscured. We have laid out how the formal and hidden curricula can align or misalign and how this tension is a dominant force in the socialization of medical trainees onto a spectrum, between the ideals of nostalgic professionalism and practical professionalism, and how this could lead to evaluations that deem learners as professional or unprofessional.

We are, however, at yet another turning point in how we define, conceptualize, and operationalize professionalism that has been sparked by the medical education project of increasing DEI in our profession. The core problem is that the values encapsulated by professionalism curricula may not represent well the needs of all patients. Moreover, the most pressing challenge in contemporary medical education is to socialize students to new aspects of professionalism that integrate an appreciation of DEI. This shift in socialization goals impacts our existing conceptual framework for how the formal, informal, and hidden curricula contribute to identity formation in medical trainees and points to the utility of attending to hidden curriculum effects not as problems to be solved, but as opportunities for educating learners more fully. We explore this, and its implications, in the final section of this chapter.

A New Professionalism

What happens when existing professional values no longer reflect societal expectations? And how do new values, such as those espoused by DEI movements in medical education, become incorporated into what it means to be professional? In recent years, the medical profession has reckoned with systemic anti-Black and anti-Indigenous racism in healthcare and society,[44,45,46,47] structural health inequities in access to care and health outcomes,[48,49,50,51] gender inequities,[52] and the historical complicity of the medical profession with the colonization and oppression of marginalized groups and communities of color.[53] In turn, there have been significant DEI-related reform efforts in medical education, including culture change efforts to improve representation in medicine and equity and inclusion in the learning environment.[54,55,56]

The DEI efforts in medical education have sparked reconsideration of what professionalism means both within medicine and in relation to broader issues of social justice.[57] To address this, medical educators and students alike have asked for what we term a "new professionalism." This new professionalism is a foil to "nostalgic professionalism" and incorporates DEI and social justice values into the formal professionalism curriculum, exemplified by calls to incorporate resistance and critical consciousness in conceptualizing professional behavio rs and practices.[58,59] What preparation for DEI-informed practice means and looks like is still being negotiated and defined and includes tensions around the physician's role as an advocate.

A DEI lens makes visible the negotiated nature of the construct of professionalism.[11] The starting point for applying the DEI lens is that what counts as professionalism is contestable, and developing professional competencies is an act of power—legitimizing some socio cultural perceptions of what counts as professionalism over others. Although the tenets of nostalgic professionalism might appear enshrined as evergreen traits, we have shown previously how these professional values were actually socially constructed into an educational problem and then integrated into the educational and organizational structures of medicine at a specific period of time.[60] The International Ottawa Conference Working Group on Professionalism captures the breadth of professionalism constructs and the ever-shifting expectations associated with being a professional.[61] In the North American context, the social construction of professionalism has been rendered invisible by the passage of time, in the way that "structures, as they last, acquire an objective character that actors can read as obligatory." [17(p29)] However, one only needs to look to past expansions of the medical division of labor, for example through internal differentiation by specialization, bureaucratization, and academicization, to see how professionalism has evolved.[62]

Since professionalism is a negotiable construct, we can imagine what transforming education for professionalism might achieve, at least as an ideal, if not also in practice. The possibility for transforming professionalism sets the stage for continuous renovation (or as one might say, quality improvement) as the social contract between the medical profession and society evolves. Transformation demands disruption of the status quo, which will require significant investment of time and effort and will inevitably generate tension and conflict before a new professionalism culture emerges from the settling dust.[63] In the remainder of this chapter, we explore how it might be possible to socialize students to new DEI-related, or other, aspects of professionalism. Such an undertaking is practically complex, but worthwhile and important given the stakes—at the systems level, the future of professions; at the individual level, the experience of all learners, but especially of those from marginalized backgrounds. We conclude with the educational implications of inviting students from diverse backgrounds into the profession and of encouraging all students to exercise agency in educational reform, and end with recommendations for how to use the hidden curriculum as an analytic tool to anticipate and analyze hidden curriculum problems.

Socializing Against the Grain of Power: The Possibility of Incorporating and Teaching DEI Aspects of Professionalism

As DEI initiatives seek to include students from under-represented? backgrounds in the medical profession and prepare medical students for DEI-informed practice, we are suddenly striving simultaneously toward different socialization goals. On the one hand, medical education continues as always to socialize students to the medical profession. On the other hand, medical education is attempting something new: to socialize a generation of physicians that is not intended to conform to senior role models. Thus, professionalism—(a) as it is currently conceptualized and operationalized, (b) as a socializing force that reproduces medical culture, and (c) as a significant contributor to the overall socialization of medical students—may face challenges transmitting new values to students.

Historically, professionalism has socialized students into a value system that is both Eurocentric and androcentric. Since its formalization in the 1990s, socialization for professionalism through medical education has been a project of normalization through the transmission of core values and neutralization of socio cultural differences to reproduce an image of the profession as a political.[64,65] These socialization processes in medical education have relied on *current* physicians (often educated at a different time and cultural place) passing on their expertise and experience to the younger generation through formal, informal, and hidden curricula.

However, the socialization process around DEI-related aspects of professionalism is now flipped: Rather than reproducing physician culture, its aim is to socialize a new generation of physicians who embody DEI-related aspects of professionalism not previously embodied by the profession. In other words, the existing mechanisms of socializing trainees through the downward exercise of power (from those with more power [faculty] to those with less power [trainees]) through the formal, informal, and hidden curricula is disrupted as the medical education system confronts a topic with relatively less professional expertise and experience. In fact, such efforts to incorporate DEI-related professionalism into medical education have resulted in phenomena like a conscripted curriculum, where students from historically under represented backgrounds have been tasked with educating their often more senior peers and supervisors against the grain of power, with the added impossible expectation that their experience represents their background.[66] This educational phenomenon leads to increased tension for learners and contributes to feelings of isolation, exclusion, and burnout. Thus, socializing for this new DEI-related professionalism complicates an already complex socialization mechanism for professionalizing trainees and requires a consideration of power and hierarchy.

Moreover, when implementing educational interventions to socialize students to a new professionalism, educators and scholars must attend not only to the formal and informal curricula , but also the hidden curriculum and their alignment. As we show in examples throughout this section, changing the formal curriculum without a strategy to shift the hidden curriculum worsens conceptual and experiential misalignment and tension for learners. Let us consider this: While socializing students to DEI-related professionalism seemingly requires education against the grain of power, the formal, informal, and hidden curricula continue to socialize students to both nostalgic and practical professionalisms. Therefore, medical educators must now contend with how these socializing forces—to DEI-related, nostalgic, and practical professionalisms—might align or misalign and how the additional socialization to a DEI-related professionalism through formal curriculum might exacerbate misalignments with hidden professionalism curricula. In other words, as DEI-related professionalism becomes formalized into medical education, it is also just as, if not more, important to attend to relevant hidden curriculum from existing medical culture and structure as well.

Developing any formal curriculum must account for how power circulates downward.[67] In practice, this could mean focusing formal/informal curricula efforts where power is concentrated: on faculty development to empower and educate those in positions of power to transmit DEI values. Paying equal attention to the hidden curriculum means that this focus on faculty education cannot fall solely on medical educators or physicians within academic hospitals, but must involve all physicians regardless of their involvement in medical education to maximize the alignment between formal/informal and hidden curricula. In these efforts, it is especially important to target those who feel ambivalent about the relevance of DEI to their work as they may be the ones that otherwise intentionally or unintentionally are transmitting values, behavio rs, and practices to learners that are the most misaligned with formal learning objectives.

Consultative expertise drawn from within, or alternatively from outside of the medical profession, may be required to inform a formal curriculum where there is a dearth of internal expertise to address DEI priorities. Furthermore, it is essential to center the experiences of students and physicians from marginalized backgrounds in the development of such a formal curriculum for these new aspects of professionalism. However, medical educators must avoid exacting a minority tax on faculty or the conscription of student experts within the profession by ensuring fair compensation and judicious, coordinated consultation efforts.[66,68] Moreover, while there are common elements to medical culture, there are many different medical subcultures that vary by institution, specialty, and geography that transmit subtly different values to learners. Particularly relevant to the evolution of professionalism through a DEI lens, while one specialty at a particular site may be culturally more open to new ideas from learners, another specialty may demand that learners conform without resistance.

In addition, from an epistemic standpoint, while many frameworks and programming aimed at addressing DEI issues have been constructed through the lens of rationalism (rational dialogue, reasoning through discussion),[69,70,71,72] these topics oftentimes also invoke strong emotions of discomfort. For addressing DEI priorities, solutions framed through the lens of rationality alone are insufficient without concurrent consideration through the lens of theorized emotion, such as pedagogies of discomfort.[73]

Shifting Professionalism and Learner Implications

As we consider how to shift the definition of professionalism to incorporate new DEI elements, we must attend to how these shifts might differentially affect trainees based on their intersectional identities.[74,75,76,77] The tensions we described above experienced by learners when there is misalignment between formal, informal, and hidden curricula are likely to have a more significant negative impact on trainees from historically marginalized backgrounds. We now explore how the hidden curriculum can be used as an analytic tool to explore implications for learner discrimination and harassment policies, evaluation of professionalism, as well as issues of burnout and attrition.[78,79,80,81,82,83,84,85,86,87,88]

As much as the hidden curriculum is an educational mechanism for socializing students to professionalism, it is also an important analytic tool for health professions education researchers to interrogate how individual experiences are linked to and influenced by education structures such as curriculum and policy. For example, medical students from social sciences and humanities and other under represented backgrounds have long felt that their knowledge was not valued interpersonally but also structurally; they learned these lessons from the way the curriculum was structured, the attendance at classes depending on the topic, by what was examined on tests or discussed at the bedside—these hidden curriculum effects could be traced back to the very structure of undergraduate medical education.[36] In this way, the concept of the hidden curriculum can serve as a useful heuristic for detecting and analyzing individual—or specific group—experiences related to a combination of cultural and structural issues. In the context of our conceptual framework laid out above, the hidden curriculum as an analytic tool can be helpful to anticipate curricular misalignments and other potential challenges of shifting professionalism values.

Learner Discrimination and Harassment Policies

As medical education pays renewed attention to learner mistreatment, medical training programs have revisited existing harassment policies, and language related to discrimination and harassment has been incorporated into what it means to be professional in the workplace. Scholars have noted the conceptual tension in these policies as they are on the one hand meant to legally protect the institution and on the other hand preserve the safety of learners that that seek justice for wrongdoing.[89] This duality in policy focus/intent translates to a hidden curriculum. For example, learners might notice elements of institution centeredness in how issues of discrimination are handled in contrast to the professed learner-centered policies that are advertised.[89] They may subsequently adopt maladaptive learning behaviors, such as staying silent in instances of learner mistreatment or accepting harassment and discrimination from peer or faculty. In other words, for learners from vulnerable groups, socialization effects that validate a partial uptake of DEI imperatives can lead to behaviors such as learner self-censoring and avoidance to disclose discrimination they have experienced or have observed during patient interactions for fear of reprisal.

Evaluating Professionalism

Incorporating DEI values into professionalism also has implications for how professionalism is evaluated in medical education. A hidden curriculum around evaluating professionalism teaches students what behaviors, attitudes, and practices are deemed valuable or important in the care of patients based on what is commented on, examined, or evaluated by their teachers, with non evaluated aspects forming a type of null curriculum[90,91] that is, elements of learning that are deemed not important. For example, a medical school that does not evaluate learner advocacy on rotation in training evaluation reports (ITERs) transmits a hidden curriculum that nullifies the importance of advocacy compared to other professional roles. From this vantage point, the formal and hidden curricula socialize students to various healthcare roles and scripts of how a doctor should speak, act, dress, and value.

Furthermore, as new DEI-related aspects of professionalism are integrated into the formal curriculum, and students adopt the values and associated behaviors of this "new professionalism," they are at risk of being labe led as unprofessional by their preceptors through the lenses of either nostalgic or practical professionalism.[92,93] For example, DEI-related professionalism could value greater physician advocacy around disrupting structural issues that impact the health of their patients, such as the systemic anti-Black and anti-Indigenous racism seen in the COVID-19 pandemic or in policing across North America. Students, feeling supported by a formal curriculum that espouses the values of new professionalism, may be perceived and evaluated as unprofessional in learning environments where such advocacy-directed activities are not seen as "professional" by their supervisors or where values around what constitutes "appropriate advocacy" are misaligned.[94] In particular, students from marginalized backgrounds, whose experiences are used to inform the tenets of new professionalism, are more likely to participate and express these values and are therefore more at risk of being labeled as unprofessional and undisciplined, which could have significant consequences in their training experience. This again speaks to the importance of aligning formal and hidden curricula in any educational initiative or policy change as a key part of shifting professional values and indeed any other educational reform.

Learner Burnout

Learner burnout is linked to DEI-related learning experiences and could be potentially worsened by integrating DEI principles into professionalism formal curriculum without also changing the learning environment. As an example, let us say that a medical training program surveys their learners and finds that there is a 40% rate of discrimination and harassment experienced by learners across the learning environment. In response to this, the medical training program establishes DEI-related programming, policy, and formal curriculum with good intentions to improve the learning environment and socialize students to DEI-related aspects of professionalism. Faculty development is also an area of focus, but progress is slow and uptake among departments is inconsistent.[95,96] Faculty development projects often take several years to get off the ground and implement, with change—if any—happening gradually, further leaving trainees to face hidden curriculum cross messaging. A repeat survey is performed a couple years later to measure progress and shows similar rates of discrimination and harassment. Moreover, learners report worsened burnout compared to previous experience. Experiences of institutional betrayal stemming from worsening misalignment between the hidden and formal curricula could contribute to the phenomenon in this example[97] and highlights the importance of shifting both formal and hidden curricula simultaneously in culture change work. As change in the formal curriculum gets underway and institutions more strongly profess the importance of DEI-related aspects of professionalism, a lack of change in what learners experience in practice creates the conditions for learner distress.

Addressing both formal and hidden curricula in educational change is easier said than done. After all, creating formal curricular interventions is arguably much easier than the work of shifting the culture and structures that give rise to hidden curriculum effects. In other words, by deciding that the crisis of professionalism was an educational problem that could be fixed simply by teaching it to students—without also changing the practiced culture of professionalism—the medical profession created a hidden curriculum problem for itself. While there is a growing recognition of the importance of structural and culture change, it is understandable why the focus so far has been to create curriculum as a solution because the tools to effectively shift culture are much more resource intensive and challenging to implement. In addition, changing structure requires a broader health system approach that is beyond the control of the educators tasked with the job of reforming how patients experience care.

Positive Effects of Hidden Curriculum and Learner Agency

As much as hidden curriculum misalignments can have negative impacts on learner socialization, they can also be productive and have a positive impact. For example, in cases of formal curricula that are out of date, the hidden curriculum can be a powerful socializing force. For instance, some healthcare institutions are developing DEI-related mandates related to revising curriculum content to address epistemic racism and discrimination. One such example is the removal of clinical content from formal curricular materials that promote conceptualization of race as a biological construct, such as stopping the use of race-corrected estimated glomerular filtration rate (eGFR).[98] Such initiatives, when authorized and celebrated by institutional leadership, also contribute to educational culture reform more broadly. Watching said changes unfold socializes medical trainees toward desired DEI-related professionalism goals, such as refusing to reproduce clinical practices they encounter on the wards that premise race as a biological construct. Other examples of DEI-related reforms that have led to positive hidden curriculum effects include having diverse representation on committees and hospital leadership, non segregated care based on insurance status or other identifiers, and institutional support for staff to celebrate non-Eurocentric holidays.[99] These sort of initiatives signal openness and inclusivity and can be harnessed to shape the formal curriculum to align the outcomes of medical student socialization, and vice versa, toward new aspects of professionalism.

Furthermore, this chapter would be incomplete without addressing the role of learner agency in resisting curricular misalignments.[59,100] Indeed, trainees enter medical training with personal values and motivations that inform their professional identity formation. Learners hold these values to varying degrees using them as guiding beacons while wading through the waters of training; these beacons may stay afloat throughout residency or submerge under choppy waters, only to re-emerge later on. While learners are not tabula rasa and resist socializing forces of both the formal and hidden curricula,[101] they can only do so to the degree where they can still be considered professional and a member of the profession by their peers and teachers.[102]

Conclusion

Professionalism is at the core of the medical profession's social contract with society, a contract that gives physicians autonomy when it comes to the structure and content of its work—which includes the training of future physicians. Near the end of the twentieth century, professionalism was deemed to be under threat, and the prevailing response by the profession was to make it the job of medical education to teach professionalism to future doctors. Furthermore, by incorporating the tenets of what could best be described as a "nostalgic" version of professionalism into formal curricula in medical schools without considering the socializing effects of learning through practicing medical work, learners were left trying to negotiate differences between the taught professionalism and the practiced professionalism they experienced in clinical settings. Finally, despite the misalignments described in the literature between nostalgic and practical professionalism, both serve to reproduce a dominant white, male, Eurocentric approach to healthcare work. Medical education's role in reinforcing a value system for healthcare that meets the needs of society requires deliberate attention to how DEI imperatives challenge traditional approaches to teaching professionalism.

In this chapter, we proposed a relational framework of how the formal and hidden curricula socialize medical students to duel ing professionalisms. Furthermore, we highlighted how these curricula predominantly are mechanisms for reproducing existing medical culture due to the way power circulates through medical education as a part of the enculturation process.

Finally, we demonstrated how the hidden curriculum—in the context of our framework—can be a powerful analytic tool for medical educators and researchers alike to anticipate and analyze curricular misalignments. By examining the implications for learner socialization through phenomena like learner mistreatment policies, evaluation of professionalism, and burnout, we demonstrate how attention to hidden curriculum effects can connect individual experiences to issues at the level of structure and culture.

References

1. Relman AS. The new medical industrial complex. *N Engl J Med.* 1980;303(17):963–970.
2. Relman AS. Education to defend professional values in the new corporate age. *Acad Med.* 1998;73(12):1229–1233.
3. Hafferty FW. Professionalism and the socialization of medical students. In: Cruess RL, Cruess SR, Steinert Y, eds. *Teaching Medical Professionalism* 2nd ed. Cambridge University Press; 2008:53–70.
4. Wear D, Skillicorn J. Hidden in plain sight: the formal, informal, and hidden curricula of a psychiatry clerkship. *Acad Med.* 2009;84(4):451–458. https://doi.org/10.1097/ACM.0b013e31819a80b7
5. Hafferty W. Beyond curriculum reform: confronting medicine's hidden curriculum. *Acad Med.* 1998;73(4):403–407.
6. Cruess RL, Cruess SR. Teaching professionalism: general principles. *Med Teach.* 2006; 28(3):205–208. https://doi.org/10.1080/01421590600643653
7. Ginsburg S, Regehr G, Hatala R, et al. Context, conflict, and resolution: a new conceptual framework for evaluating professionalism. *Acad Med.* 2000;75(10):S6–S11.
8. Ho MJ, Yu KH, Hirsh D, Huang TS, Yang PC. Does one size fit all? Building a framework for medical professionalism. *Acad Med.* 2011;86(11):1407–1414. https://doi.org/10.1097/ACM.0b013e31823059d1
9. Martimianakis MA, Michalec B, Lam J, Cartmill C, Taylor JS, Hafferty FW. Humanism, the hidden curriculum, and educational reform: a scoping review and thematic analysis. *Acad Med.* 2015;90(11):S5–S13. https://doi.org/10.1097/ACM.0000000000000894
10. Starr P. *The Social Transformation of American Medicine.* Basic Books; 1982.
11. Martimianakis MA, Maniate JM, Hodges BD. Sociological interpretations of professionalism: interpretations of professionalism. *Med Educ.* 2009;43(9):829–837. https://doi.org/10.1111/j.1365-2923.2009.03408.x
12. Freidson E. Professional dominance and the ordering of health services. In: Manners RA, ed. *Professional Dominance: The Social Structure of Medical Care.* Routledge; 1970:127–164. https://doi.org/10.4324/9781315127491-5
13. Freidson E. *Professionalism: The Third Logic.* Polity Press; 2001.
14. Abbott AD. *The System of Professions: An Essay on the Division of Expert Labor.* University of Chicago Press; 1988. http://site.ebrary.com/id/10991090
15. Witz A. *Professions and Patriarchy.* Routledge; 1992.
16. Hafferty FW. Academic medicine and medical professionalism: a legacy and a portal into an evolving field of educational scholarship. *Acad Med.* 2018;93 (4):532–536. https://doi.org/10.1097/ACM.0000000000001899
17. Larson MS. Professions today: self-criticism and reflections for the future. *Sociologia, Problemas e Práticas.* 1970; (88):27–42. https://doi.org/10.7458/SPP20188814796

18. Hafferty FW. Professionalism and commercialism as antitheticals: a search for "unprofessional commercialism" within the writings and work of American medicine. In: Parsi K, Sheehan M, eds. *Healing as Vocation: A Medical Professionalism Primer*. Rowen and Littlefield; 2006:35–59.

19. Whitehead CR, Hodges BD, Austin Z. Dissecting the doctor: from character to characteristics in North American Medical Education. *Adv Health Sci Educ Theory Pract.* 2013;18(4):687–699. https://doi.org/10.1007/s10459-012-9409-5

20. Wear D, Kuczewski MG. The professionalism movement: can we pause? *Am J Bioeth.* 2004;4(2):1–10. https://doi.org/10.1162/152651604323097600

21. Wear D. On white coats and professional development: the formal and the hidden curricula. *Ann Intern Med.* 1998;129(9):734–737. https://doi.org/10.7326/0003-4819-129-9-199811010-00010

22. Project Professionalism. American Board of Internal Medicine. 1995. https://medicinainternaucv.files.wordpress.com/2013/02/project-professionalism.pdf. Accessed: May 4, 2022.

23. Physicians for the twenty-first century. Report of the Project Panel on the General Professional Education of the Physician and College Preparation for Medicine. *J Med Educ.* 1984;59 (11 Pt 2):1–208.

24. ACGME/ABMS Outcome Project: toolbox of assessment methods. Accreditation Council on Graduate Medical Education and American Board of Medical Specialties. 2000. https://medicine.llu.edu/sites/medicine.llu.edu/files/docs/acgme_toolbox_of_assessment_methods_2000.pdf.Accessed May 4, 2022.

25. Project of the ABIM Foundation, ACP–ASIM Foundation, and European Federation of Internal Medicine. Medical professionalism in the new millennium: a physician charter. *Ann Intern Med.* 2002;136(3):243–246. https://doi.org/10.7326/0003-4819-136-3-200202050-00012.

26. Swick HM. Toward a normative definition of medical professionalism. *Acad Med.* 2000;75(6):612–616. https://doi.org/10.1097/00001888-200006000-00010.

27. Castellani B, Hafferty FW. The complexities of medical professionalism: a preliminary investigation. In: Wear D, Aultman JM, eds. *Professionalism in Medicine: Critical Perspectives.* Springer US; 2006:3–23. https://doi.org/10.1007/0-387-32727-4_1

28. Hafferty FW. In search of a lost cord: professionalism and medical education's hidden curriculum. In: Wear D, Bickel JW, eds. *Educating for Professionalism: Creating a Climate of Humanism in Medical Education.* University of Iowa Press; 2000:11–34.

29. Bonifacino E, Ufomata EO, Farkas AH, Turner R, Corbelli JA. Mentorship of underrepresented physicians and trainees in academic medicine: a systematic review. *J Gen Intern Med.* 2021;36(4):1023–1034. https://doi.org/10.1007/s11606-020-06478-7

30. Choi AMK, Moon JE, Steinecke A, Prescott JE. Developing a culture of mentorship to strengthen academic medical centers. *Acad Med.* 2019;94(5):630–633. https://doi.org/10.1097/ACM.0000000000002498

31. Bickel JW, Wear D. *Educating for Professionalism: Creating a Culture of Humanism in Medical Education.* University of Iowa Press; 2000.

32. Doukas DJ, McCullough LB, Wear S. Perspective: medical education in medical ethics and humanities as the foundation for developing medical professionalism. *Acad Med.* 2012;87(3):334–341. https://doi.org/10.1097/ACM.0b013e318244728c

33. Hafferty FW, Levinson D. Moving beyond nostalgia and motives: towards a complexity science view of medical professionalism. *Perspect Biol Med.* 2008;51 (4):599–615. https://doi.org/10.1353/pbm.0.0044

34. Vinekar K. Pathology of racism — a call to desegregate teaching hospitals. *N Engl J Med.* 2021;385(13):e40. https://doi.org/10.1056/NEJMpv2113508

35. Tilburt J, Stout J, Hafferty FW. If academic medical centers won't stop growing VIP care, they can, at least, offset its harms. *Health Aff* blog. November 4, 2021. doi: 10.1377/hblog20211029.791317. https://www.healthaffairs.org/content/forefront/if-academic-medical-centers-won-t-stop-growing-vip-care-they-can-least-offset-its-harms. Accessed July 7, 2022.

36. Lam JTH, Hanson MD, Martimianakis MA. Exploring the socialization experiences of medical students from social science and humanities backgrounds. *Acad Med.* 2020;95(3):401–410.

37. Fenton R. The first (Black) fellow. *Medium* blog. January 26, 2022. https://medium.com/@rfentonmd/the-first-black-fellow-48634bba0fe4. Accessed February 7, 2022.

38. Papadakis MA, Hodgson CS, Teherani A, Kohatsu ND. Unprofessional behavior in medical school is associated with subsequent disciplinary action by a state medical board. *Acad Med.* 2004;79(3):244–249.

39. Attilus J. Why I left Boston residency program. *Medium* blog. May 17, 2022. https://medium.com/@jonasattilus/why-i-left-boston-residency-program-9ee2b12ed006. Accessed July 19, 2022.

40. Professionalism Competencies — ACGME. Accreditation Council for Graduate Medical Education. May 2008. https://www.acgme.org/globalassets/PDFs/commonguide/IVA5e_EducationalProgram_ACGMECompetencies_Professionalism_Explanation.pdf. Accessed June 1, 2022.

41. Good BJ. *Medicine, Rationality and Experience: An Anthropological Perspective.* Lewis Henry Morgan Lectures. Cambridge University Press; 1993. https://doi.org/10.1017/CBO9780511811029

42. Behforouz HL, Drain PK, Rhatigan JJ. Rethinking the social history. *N Engl J Med.* 2014;371(14):1277–1279. https://doi.org/10.1056/NEJMp1404846

43. DiMatteo MR. Social support and patient adherence to medical treatment: a meta-analysis. *Health Psychol.* 2004;23(2):207–218. https://doi.org/10.1037/0278-6133.23.2.207

44. Sharma M, Kuper A. The elephant in the room: talking race in medical education. *Adv Health Sci Educ Theory Pract.* 2017;22(3):761–764.https://doi.org/10.1007/s10459-016-9732-3

45. Dryden OS, Nnorom O. Time to dismantle systemic anti-Black racism in medicine in Canada. *CMAJ.* 2021;193(2):E55–E57. https://doi.org/10.1503/cmaj.201579

46. Mpalirwa J, Lofters A, Nnorom O, Hanson MD. Patients, pride, and prejudice: exploring Black Ontarian physicians' experiences of racism and discrimination. *Acad Med.* 2020;95 (11S):S51–S57. https://doi.org/10.1097/ACM.0000000000003648

47. Boatright D, Ross D, O'Connor P, Moore E, Nunez-Smith M. Racial disparities in medical student membership in the Alpha Omega Alpha honor society. *JAMA Intern Med.* 2017;177(5):659. https://doi.org/10.1001/jamainternmed.2016.9623

48. Bailey ZD, Krieger N, Agénor M, Graves J, Linos N, Bassett MT. Structural racism and health inequities in the USA: evidence and interventions. *Lancet.* 2017;389 (10077):1453–1463. https://doi.org/10.1016/S0140-6736(17)30569-X

49. Bailey ZD, Feldman JM, Bassett MT. How structural racism works — racist policies as a root cause of US racial health inequities. *N Engl J Med.* 2021;384(8):768–773. https://doi.org/10.1056/NEJMms2025396

50. Fawzy A, Wu TD, Wang K, et al. Racial and ethnic discrepancy in pulse oximetry and delayed identification of treatment eligibility among patients with COVID-19. *JAMA Intern Med.* 2022;182(7):730–738. https://doi.org/10.1001/jamainternmed.2022.1906

51. Hoffman KM, Trawalter S, Axt JR, Oliver MN. Racial bias in pain assessment and treatment recommendations, and false beliefs about biological differences between Blacks and whites. *Proc Nat l Acad Sci USA.* 2016;113(16):4296–4301. https://doi.org/10.1073/pnas.1516047113

52. The Editors. Lawmakers v. the scientific realities of human reproduction. *N Engl J Med.* 2022;387(4):367–368. https://doi.org/10.1056/NEJMe2208288

53. Zaidi Z, Partman IM, Whitehead CR, Kuper A, Wyatt TR. Contending with our racial past in medical education: a Foucauldian perspective. *Teach Learn Med.* 2021;33(4):453–462. https://doi.org/10.1080/10401334.2021.1945929

54. Wingard D, Trejo JA, Gudea M, Goodman S, Reznik V. Faculty equity, diversity, culture and climate change in academic medicine: a longitudinal study. *J Nat l Med Assoc.* 2019;111(1):46–53. https://doi.org/10.1016/j.jnma.2018.05.004

55. Viruell-Fuentes EA, Miranda PY, Abdulrahim S. More than culture: structural racism, intersectionality theory, and immigrant health. *Soc Sci Med.* 2012;75(12):2099–2106. https://doi.org/10.1016/j.socscimed.2011.12.037

56. Mostow C, Crosson J, Gordon S, et al. Treating and precepting with RESPECT: a relational model addressing race, ethnicity, and culture in medical training. *J Gen Intern Med.* 2010;25 (suppl 2, 8605834):S146–S154. Erratum in: *J Gen Intern Med.* 2010;25(11):1257. https://doi.org/10.1007/s11606-010-1274-4

57. Goddard VCT, Brockbank S. Re-opening Pandora's box: who owns professionalism and is it time for a 21st century definition? *Med Educ.* 2023;57(1):66–75. https://doi.org/10.1111/medu.14862

58. Kumagai AK, Lypson ML. Beyond cultural competence: critical consciousness, social justice, and multicultural education. *Acad Med.* 2009;84(6):782–787. https://doi.org/10.1097/ACM.0b013e3181a42398

59. Ellaway RH, Wyatt TR. What role should resistance play in training health professionals? *Acad Med.* 2021;96(11):1524–1528. https://doi.org/10.1097/ACM.0000000000004225

60. Fournier V. The appeal to "professionalism" as a disciplinary mechanism. *Sociol Rev.* 1999;47(2):280–307. https://doi.org/10.1111/1467-954X.00173

61. Hodges BD, Ginsburg S, Cruess RL, et al. Assessment of professionalism: recommendations from the Ottawa 2010 conference. *Med Teach.* 2011;33 (5):354–363. https://doi.org/10.3109/0142159X.2011.577300

62. Adams TL. Self-regulating professions: past, present, future. *J Prof Organiz* 2016;4(1):70–87. https://doi.org/10.1093/jpo/jow004

63. Shim RS. Dismantling structural racism in academic medicine: a skeptical optimism. *Acad Med.* 2020;95(12):1793–1795. https://doi.org/10.1097/ACM.0000000000003726

64. Beagan BL. Neutralizing differences: producing neutral doctors for (almost) neutral patients. *Soc Sci.* 2000;51(8):1253–1265. https://doi.org/10.1016/s0277-9536(00)00043-5

65. Taylor JS. Confronting "culture" in medicine's "culture of no culture." *Acad Med.* 2003;78 (6): 555–559.

66. Olsen LD. The conscripted curriculum and the reproduction of racial inequalities in contemporary US. Medical Education. *J Health Soc Behav.* 2019;60(1):55–68. https://doi.org/10.1177/0022146518821388

67. Foucault M. *Discipline and Punish: The Birth of the Prison.* Pantheon Books; 1977.

68. Hirshfield LE, Joseph TD. "We need a woman, we need a Black woman": gender, race, and identity taxation in the academy. *Gender Educ.* 2012;24(2):213–227. https://doi.org/10.1080/09540253.2011.606208

69. Kumagai AK, Wear D. "Making strange": a role for the humanities in medical education. *Acad Med.* 2014;89(7):973–977. https://doi.org/10.1097/ACM.0000000000000269

70. Kuper A, Boyd VA, Veinot P, et al. A dialogic approach to teaching person-centered care in graduate medical education. *J Grad Med Educ.* 2019;11(4):460–467. https://doi.org/10.4300/JGME-D-19-00085.1

71. Sukhera J, Watling CJ, Gonzalez CM. Implicit bias in health professions: from recognition to transformation. *Acad Med.* 2020;95(5):717–723. https://doi.org/10.1097/ACM.0000000000003173

72. Sukhera J, Watling CJ. A framework for integrating implicit bias recognition into health professions education. *Acad Med.* 2018;93(1):35–40. https://doi.org/10.1097/ACM.0000000000001819

73. Boler M. *Feeling Power: Emotions and Education.* Routledge; 1999.

74. Crenshaw K. Demarginalizing the intersection of race and sex: a Black feminist critique of antidiscrimination doctrine, feminist theory, and antiracist politics [1989]. In: Bartlett KT, Kennedy R, eds. *Feminist Legal Theory.* Routledge; 2018:57–80. https://doi.org/10.4324/9780429500480-5

75. Eckstrand KL, Eliason J, St. Cloud T, Potter J. The priority of intersectionality in academic medicine: *Acad Med.* 2016;91(7):904–907. https://doi.org/10.1097/ACM.0000000000001231

76. Muntinga ME, Krajenbrink VQE, Peerdeman SM, Croiset G, Verdonk P. Toward diversity-responsive medical education: taking an intersectionality-based approach to a curriculum evaluation. *Adv Health Sci Educ.* 2016;21(3):541–559. https://doi.org/10.1007/s10459-015-9650-9

77. Monrouxe LV. When I say . . . intersectionality in medical education research. *Med Educ.* 2015;49(1):21–22. https://doi.org/10.1111/medu.12428

78. Eaton JE, Reed DA, Aboff BM, et al. Update in internal medicine residency education: a review of the literature in 2010 and 2011. *J Grad Med Educ.* 2013;5(2):203–210. https://doi.org/10.4300/JGME-D-12-00238.1

79. Ayyala MS, Chaudhry S, Windish D, Dupras D, Reddy ST, Wright SM. Awareness of bullying in residency: results of a national survey of internal medicine program directors. *J Grad Med Educ.* 2018;10(2):209–213. https://doi.org/10.4300/JGME-D-17-00386.1

80. Leisy HB, Ahmad M. Altering Workplace Attitudes for Resident Education (A.W.A.R.E.): discovering solutions for medical resident bullying through literature review. *BMC Med Educ.* 2016;16 (127). https://doi.org/10.1186/s12909-016-0639-8

81. Mustapha Taj, Ho Y, Andrews JS, Cullen MJ. See no evil, hear no evil, stop no evil: institutional-level tracking to combat mistreatment of residents and fellows. *J Grad Med Educ.* 2019;11(5):601–605. https://doi.org/10.4300/JGME-D-19-00218.1

82. Kulaylat AN, Qin D, Sun SX, et al. Perceptions of mistreatment among trainees vary at different stages of clinical training. *BMC Med Educ.* 2017;17(1):14. https://doi.org/10.1186/s12909-016-0853-4

83. Premkumar A, Whetstone S, Jackson AV. Beyond silence and inaction: changing the response to experiences of racism in the health care workforce. *Obstet Gynecol.* 2018;132(4):820–827. https://doi.org/10.1097/AOG.0000000000002868

84. Moutier C, Cornette M, Lehrmann J, et al. When residents need health care: stigma of the patient role. *Acad Psychiatry.* 2009;33(6):431–441. https://doi.org/10.1176/appi.ap.33.6.431

85. Underman K, Hirshfield LE. Detached concern?: emotional socialization in twenty-first century medical education. *Soc Sci Med.* 2016;160:94–101. https://doi.org/10.1016/j.socscimed.2016.05.027

86. Lockman JL, Schwartz AJ, Cronholm PF. Working to define professionalism in pediatric anesthesiology: a qualitative study of domains of the expert pediatric anesthesiologist as valued by interdisciplinary stakeholders. *Paediatr Anaesth.* 2017;27 (2):137–146. https://doi.org/10.1111/pan.13071

87. Nagler A, Andolsek K, Rudd M, Sloane R, Musick D, Basnight L. The professionalism disconnect: do entering residents identify yet participate in unprofessional behaviors? *BMC Med Educ.* 2014;14 (60). https://doi.org/10.1186/1472-6920-14-60

88. Jennings ML, Slavin SJ. Resident wellness matters: optimizing resident education and wellness through the learning environment. *Acad Med.* 2015;90(9):1246–1250. https://doi.org/10.1097/ACM.0000000000000842

89. Sukhera J, Goez H, Brown A, Haddara W, Razack S. Freedom from discrimination or freedom to discriminate? Discursive tensions within discrimination policies in medical education. *Adv Health Sci Educ.* 2022;27(2):387–403. https://doi.org/10.1007/s10459-022-10090-1

90. Jones TW. Creating a longitudinal environment of awareness: teaching professionalism outside the anatomy laboratory. *Acad Med.* 2013;88(3):304–308. https://doi.org/10.1097/ACM.0b013e318280f075

91. Eisner EW. *The Educational Imagination: On the Design and Evaluation of School Programs.* 2nd ed. Macmillan; 1985.

92. Hardouin S, Cheng TW, Mitchell EL, et al. RETRACTED: prevalence of unprofessional social media content among young vascular surgeons. *J Vasc Surg.* 2020;72(2):667–671. https://doi.org/10.1016/j.jvs.2019.10.069

93. Singh N -K. Translating ideals into practice: a pragmatic approach to advocacy for medical trainees. *Acad Med.* 2022;97(6):771–772.

94. Lee JH. The weaponization of medical professionalism. *Acad Med.* 2017;92 (5):579–580.

95. Hafler JP, Ownby AR, Thompson BM, et al. Decoding the learning environment of medical education: a hidden curriculum perspective for faculty development. *Acad Med.* 2011;86(4):440–444. https://doi.org/10.1097/ACM.0b013e31820df8e2

96. Leslie K, Baker L, Egan-Lee E, Esdaile M, Reeves S. Advancing faculty development in medical education: a systematic review. *Acad Med.* 2013;88(7):1038–1045. https://doi.org/10.1097/ACM.0b013e318294fd29

97. Watson-Creed G. Gaslighting in academic medicine: where anti-Black racism lives. *C M A J.* 2022;194(42):E1451 –1454. https://doi.org/10.1503/cmaj.212145

98. Vyas DA, Eisenstein LG, Jones DS. Hidden in plain sight—reconsidering the use of race correction in clinical algorithms. *N Engl J Med.* 2020;383(9):874–882.

99. Lam JTH, Giroux RJP. Resident equity, diversity, and inclusion committee: a mechanism for programmatic change. *Acad Med.* 2022;97(6):770. https://journals.lww.com/academicmedicine/Fulltext/2022/06000/Resident_Equity,_Diversity,_and_Inclusion.12.aspx

100. Hafferty FW, Michalec B, Martimianakis MA, Tilburt JC. Resistance and radicalization: retraining professionals for the modern era. In: Byyny RL, Papadakis MA, Paauw DS, Pfeil SA, eds. *Medical Professionalism Best Practices: Professionalism in the Modern Era.* Alpha Omega Alpha Honor Medical Society; 2017:59–72.

101. Fergus KB, Teale B, Sivapragasam M, Mesina O, Stergiopoulos E. Medical students are not blank slates: positionality and curriculum interact to develop professional identity. *Perspect Med Educ.* 2018;7(1):5–7. https://doi.org/10.1007/s40037-017-0402-9

102. Cribb A, Gewirtz S. *Professionalism. Key Themes in Health and Social Care Series.* Polity Press; 2015.

5

The Foundational Importance of Arts and Humanities in Medical Professionalism

Rachel H. Kowalsky and Jay Baruch

Key Points

- This chapter examines medical professionalism through the lens of the arts and humanities.
- Emphasis is placed on narrative-based skills such as hearing, seeing, empathy, and managing uncertainty and demonstrates that, first, these are cornerstones of medical professionalism, and, second, that their career-long evolution is a function of engagement with the arts and humanities.
- The application of humanities content and pedagogy to social justice is discussed. Suggestions are given for modes of curricular integration.

The Health Humanities and Medical Professionalism

The humanities is a transdisciplinary field that spans the arts, literature, history, sociology, psychology, philosophy, and spirituality. As such, it provides a foundational lens through which we can understand, interrogate, and develop medical professionalism.

If medicine is an applied science, professionalism is the means of application, *the way in which* we care for others. It is the embodiment of values and ideals that have been agreed on, at least in theory, by patients, doctors, and society. But this agreement, while an important starting point, is aspirational. Twenty-first-century medicine requires uneasy compromise between conflicting values and objectives that may change across context and time.

Using the humanities as a platform for investigation and reflection, trainees and seasoned physicians alike can navigate the moral tensions—the need to work fast, to be all-knowing, to connect to each patient with empathy and cultural humility, to be flexible, and to accept uncertainty—inherent in medical practice.

The humanities go where our science textbooks and hospital bylaws do not. They go straight to the heart of who we are, who our patients are, and why we have found ourselves together on a certain day and time.

Rationale and History

The importance of the humanities in medicine has been recognized for centuries. From deities such as Apollo and Lugh,[1] to "trance tellers" who heal with story,[2] to legends told for healing,[3] the two disciplines have always been intertwined. In fact, it may be appropriate to consider them as a single entity, fractured artificially by the advent of modern science.[4]

The term "medical humanities" was coined in 1947 by historian and chemist George Sarton when he wrote of a deceased colleague: "His death . . . is a sad blow to the medical humanities."[5(p127)] In 1952, Case Western Medical School added medical history to its curriculum, and in 1967, the first Department of the Humanities was created at Penn State College of Medicine. In 1973, the Institute for the Medical Humanities at the University of Texas Medical Branch followed suit. The nascent field was reinforced by a report prepared for the Hastings Center in 1984: The Place of Humanities in Medicine.[6]

In the 1990s, the concept of narrative emerged as an important aspect of the medical humanities with Katherine Montgomery Hunter's "Doctors' Stories: The Narrative Structure of Medical Knowledge."[7] The concept was reframed as the discipline of narrative medicine and championed by physician and literary scholar Dr. Rita Charon, who brought the concept to a wider audience. Charon wrote: "A disciplined and rigorous understanding of how stories work and what narrative actions reveal about their participants help to comprehend clinical care."[8(p1)] Narrative medicine has been engaged as a means to support the development of residency competencies, including professionalism.[9]

In 1998, the Association of American Medical Colleges (AAMC) published a series of learning objectives for medical student education, which combined statements about professionalism (physicians must "bring to the study and practice of medicine those character traits, attitudes, and values that underpin ethical and beneficent medical care") with the pedagogy of the humanities ("They must understand the history of medicine, the nature of medicine's social compact," and "the ethical precepts of the medical profession.").[10p(4)]

The connection between the medical humanities and professionalism was reinforced at the turn of the century with the formation of the American Society of Bioethics and Humanities, which includes in its mission statement the promotion of "professional development and collegiality among people engaged in all of the endeavors related to clinical and academic bioethics and the health-related humanities."[11p(4)] Scholar Anne Hunsaker Hawkins advanced new theories of knowledge acquisition and advocated for the inclusion of cultural studies in the medical humanities, broadening the scope of the field and its applicability to professionalism.[12,13]

Since then, multiple frameworks have been published regarding the humanities in medical education. In 2009 Shapiro et al.[14] proposed a three-point pedagogical definition of medical humanities education: (1) using methods and content from the humanities to investigate illness, pain, disability, suffering, healing, and therapeutic relationships; (2) employing these methods in teaching health professions students to be more self-aware and humane; and (3) working collaboratively across disciplines. Ultimately, they wrote: "Medical humanities aim to improve health care by influencing its practitioners to refine and complexify their judgements in clinical situations, based on a deep and complex understanding of illness, suffering, personhood, and related issues."[14(pp.192-193)]

The use of the visual arts to support observation, interpretation, and meaning-making in medicine was described by several groups in the early 21st century[15,16] notably Schaff et al. who designed an Art and Medicine Focus Experience based upon contemporary art. They wrote that this art form (as opposed to representational or figurative art) "challenges some of the widely held beliefs and values of our time,"[17] thereby scaffolding the processes of attention, observation, interpretation, and facility with ambiguity that can allow physicians to grasp and navigate complex situations.

In 2012, Doukas et al. established the Project to Rebalance and Integrate Medical Education (PRIME),[18] convening an expert panel on how art, ethics, history, and literature should be integrated into medical education. They drew a direct link to professionalism, proposing that medical education in ethics and the humanities cultivates professional conduct in physicians by supporting skills in visual observation, textual reading and interpretation, oral reasoning, and writing, which in turn support critical thinking, privileging of multiple perspectives, eliciting and interpreting patients' stories, reasoning, and normative judgment, all important aspects of professionalism. They pointed out that such teaching has "an essential role to play in equipping medical students and residents with the tools to critically appraise the goals that the profession of medicine ought to pursue, ways the physician-patient relationship should be improved, and how the medical profession should understand and manage its complex relationship with society."[(p337)]

These ideas were elaborated over the next decade by the work of Arno Kumagai and the 2014 publication of *Health Humanities Reader* by Tess Jones, Delese Wear, and Les Friedman.[19] In 2015, the Health Humanities Consortium[20] was founded to promote health humanities scholarship, education, and practices.

In 2016, Haidet et al.[21] developed a conceptual model to support the design and evaluation of arts-based education, in which engagement with the arts leads to the construction of "new meanings," defined as self-awareness, openness to alternate perspectives, and the ability to cope with ambiguity. These qualities, in turn, translate into increased empathy and skills in communication and observation, ultimately improving clinical practice and professionalism.

The National Academies of Sciences, Engineering, and Medicine[22] as well as the AAMC,[23] have both strongly encouraged integration of the arts and humanities into curricula at all levels of medical education.

In the last decade, terminology has shifted from "medical humanities" to "health humanities" in order to include the broad range of professionals who care for patients and account for outside contributions to health and well-being that do not fall squarely in the field of medicine.[24] To be consistent, we use the term health humanities from this point forward.

Defining and Developing Professionalism—The Role of the Humanities

Vignette 5.1

What Is Professional Attire?

The older male physician wears a shirt and tie and a white coat. The younger physician, a female, is wearing what appears to be a white T-shirt, jeans, and a white coat. Who is more professional?

The older physician's shirt is a bit worn around the collar, the tie is knotted awkwardly, his white coat bears the stains of pen marks around the pocket and coffee stains. The young physician's white T-shirt is impeccably white, the jeans expensive and pressed, her white coat tailored and buttoned to perfection. Who is more professional?

The older physician's hair is combed, but he needs a haircut and a shave. The young physician bears facial piercings—brow, nose, and multiple earrings. Who is more professional?

Professionalism can be difficult to define. Some might describe it as being polite, punctual, and well dressed, while others might define it as prioritizing the patient's well-being above all else, even food or sleep. Others might say it means possessing an aura of wisdom or skill. Who should decide which is correct? The patient? The doctor? Society? The answer is not straightforward. This is because professionalism is a social construct, and like all social constructs, it is defined and judged in comparison with the established attitudes and behaviors of the group[25]—in this case, two groups: (1) doctors and the societies that govern and describe expectations and (2) patients, who provide feedback in various ways, including via social media, hospital-based surveys, and op-eds. Doctors also hold themselves to their own personal standards, based in part on their worldview and life experiences.

These forces and expectations can be—and often are—opposed to one another. The need to be safe, accurate, fast, empathic, and generate income are rarely all achievable at once.

As Herald Sox wrote in "Medical Professionalism in the New Millennium: A Physician Charter": "Forces that are largely beyond our control have brought us to circumstances that require a restatement of professional responsibility."[26(p115)]

Engagement with the humanities provides essential space for the individual to question established norms, adapt, and transform themselves—and sometimes their field—over the course of their career.

Consider the medical humanities as a parallel line that runs alongside the trajectory of our careers as physicians. In the short term, engagement with the arts and humanities helps us to think creatively so that we can be flexible and think on our feet when conflicts and tensions arise. It can allow us to hold two conflicting truths together—say, the need to "look like a doctor" and the concern that the white coat may symbolize superiority or patriarchy in a way that is uncomfortable for some patients[27]—and ask the question: "What does a doctor look like?" One can follow this idea further out, asking: "How has the image of a doctor changed over time? How should it change?" Dr. Thomas Stone, in Verghese's *Cutting for Stone*,[28] is well put together, admired for his economy of movement and calm under duress. But he has a sexual encounter with a nurse and abandons the children that result from this union. The humanities allows for close examination of such a character and the forces and values that shape their behavior. In addition, the lack of female physicians as characters in literature prior to the debut of female authors such as Perri Klass[29] and Ann Pachett[30] can also be understood as contributing to modern conceptions of "how a doctor looks."

In the long term, engagement with the arts and humanities can prepare us to negotiate the rapidly changing landscape of our work, as private equity,[31,32] the electronic medical record,[33,34] the pressures to garner attention and positive reviews on social media,[35,36] and the emergence of new and deadly pathogens[37] challenge our practice. We can use stories, poetry, and the visual arts to help identify and reinforce notions about what we are—and are not—willing to do, what we are called to do in our work, and how we can continue to move through our careers, negotiating our relationship with a continually shifting landscape.

In Toni Morrison's *Beloved*, Sixo and Schoolteacher debate the meaning of "stealing," and when Schoolteacher exacts a punishment, the narrator comments: "Definitions belong to the definers."[(p190)] It is important to reflect on this concept. In continual conversation with the arts and humanities, we ourselves can and should decide how we best embody professionalism when we move through clinical spaces.

Narrative-Based Skills: Hearing, Seeing, and Empathy

It is a given that doctors as professionals are meant to be good listeners, careful observers, empathic, and self-reflective. But how can we impart and support these characteristics?

Hearing

Careful listening is a key aspect of professionalism. But it is well known that physicians interrupt their patients after an average of eleven seconds.[38] The reasons for this include time pressure, financial pressure, burnout, and compassion fatigue. The clock is ticking, and the bottom line counts.

But it is important to try. As Rita Charon has written: "From the beginning of symptoms to the completion of treatment, illness has to be told—first, through symptoms . . . then to family or friends, and then to professionals, who repeat it among themselves."[39(p343)]

Vignette 5.2

The Importance of Telling and Listening

A three-year-old girl is brought to the emergency department by her parents because of poor oral intake for three days. She has had no fever, vomiting, or diarrhea. She continually declines food and leaves the table early. The attending spends a few minutes in the room, listening to the history while she performs a quick exam, which is normal. "It is probably normal toddler behavior," she says, as toddlers are known to be picky eaters. "She will eat when she's hungry." But the resident obtains more history: The parents had a premature infant that just passed away after a two-week neonatal intensive care unit stay. There have been many friends and relatives in the home, with mourning, crying, and displays of grief. The resident makes the decision to spend ten extra minutes with the family. She sits down, asks about their experience, and looks at their photographs of the baby as they share the story of the last two weeks. While the resident listens to them, the child life specialist brings the three-year-old to play with toys and eat a meal.

Professionalism is easy to define when it is found to be significantly lacking, that is, when physicians are rude, use insensitive language, or do not show up for scheduled obligations. It is more difficult to apprehend when the failure is nuanced. In the vignette above, the attending fails in a small but important way: She does not perceive that there is more to the story and fails to listen. This may be attributed to the many issues that compete for her time and attention, but the outcome remains the same. The root cause of the family's presentation to the emergency room has not been addressed; the professional obligation is unfulfilled.

The arts and humanities, particularly narrative medicine, provide an ample framework for receiving patient stories. They allow us to think through the components of story: what is left out, what assumptions are made, and how the order of events can influence our understanding.[40]

The humanities also provides direct examples of how one might listen deeply to a patient. For example, in Isabelle Allende's *The House of the Spirits*, a skillfully crafted scene shows Nana and Severo commiserating over the death of his child, Rosa, and illustrates the anatomy of a moment of deep listening, which takes place across wide gaps in social status, ethnicity, and gender. "Nana remained standing, her crossed arms holding her shawl against her chest. Severo pointed to the sofa and she approached him shyly. She sat down beside him. It was the first time she had been this close to her employer since she had lived in his house. Severo . . . buried his head in his hands, tearing his hair and murmuring a strange litany between his teeth. Nana, who was sitting stiffly on the edge of her seat, relaxed when she saw him cry. She stretched out her rough, chapped hand."[41(pp.28-29)] In this brief passage, we see an invitation to connect, a listener who *sits down* beside a bereft father, and the taking of a hand despite the many differences that might discourage this act.

Seeing

Close observation is one of the most important clinical skills at our disposal. It is a necessary component of clinical competence and quality of care, which are among the top qualities listed in "Medical Professionalism in the New Millennium: A Physician Charter."[42] Recognizing physical signs and changes in clinical status are key, as are observations about dynamics during the clinical encounter (i.e., whether our patient is anxious, in pain, mistrustful, or feels psychologically unsafe).

The arts and humanities can help us to hone our skills in observation, as well as consider its importance, and inspire curiosity, which impels our close observation.

How can this be achieved? Doukas and colleagues[43] propose that the study of art history can train students in "slow looking," by demonstrating the process of turning one's full visual attention to the single object in front of them. Much like Ocean Vuong relates in his novel *On Earth We're Briefly Gorgeous*,[44] looking closely can fundamentally change one's relationship to the object of their gaze, whether that object is a painting or a person. Work done with surgical residents[45] and medical students[46,47] has supported this idea.

Skills in observation are often invisible to new medical trainees because they are only tested when visual diagnosis techniques are addressed. To focus attention on the concept of close observation, one can use examples such as Luke Fildes's *The Doctor*, painted in 1887. The painting depicts four figures: a doctor, a sick child, and presumably a mother and father. The doctor sits beside the child in deep thought, his gaze singularly trained on her. One could ask: "What do you notice about the doctor's body language?" "What is it like to observe a patient so closely?" and "What are the obstacles to close observation in our daily clinical practice?" The same can be done with choreographer Jamar Roberts' piece, *Ode*, composed for the Alvin Ailey American Dance Theater in 2019 as a tribute to victims of gun violence. One could ask: "What do the dancer's bodies tell us about their history?" "What do you think they feel?"

Beyond pure observation, engagement with the visual arts can support different *ways of knowing* for medical trainees. In other words, such engagement may support the "knack for problem-solving, for seeing things from multiple perspectives at the same time, for maneuvering through and synthesizing complex ideas," so that they might contribute to "larger dialogues about medicine, science, politics, the law, and beyond."[48(p10)] These qualities, in turn, allow for applications of beneficence and justice that can serve the aims of professionalism.

Empathy

Empathy is perhaps the most important cornerstone of professionalism, yet in many ways it is the scarcest resource, constantly threatened by the stressors inherent to our work.

Empathy allows us to imagine other lives, recognize the humanity of every patient, and connect across difference to provide the best possible care. When we are surprised, frustrated, or otherwise knocked off balance by a patient or colleague, empathy allows us to respond with openness and flexibility. It also plays an important role in mitigating implicit bias.

Our patients inhabit worlds—both internal and external—that are distinct from our own. They may live with fear, mental illness, or chronic pain; they may have different socioeconomic, racial, ethnic, and religious backgrounds, immigration status, or abilities. Kidd and Castano showed that reading literary fiction (fiction that uses phonological, grammatical, and semantic stylistic devices) affects theory of mind processes by compelling the reader to engage in "mind reading" and character construction.[49] Other authors have had similar findings.[50,51,52]

What is it like to parent in poverty? What is it like to live with a seizure disorder? To be chronically ill, or dying? We can explore these experiences in work by novelists Toni Morrison,[53] Paul Harding,[54] John Green,[55] and many others.

While nobody can live all possible life experiences, many have been described in detail by poets and artists. Poets such as Audre Lord[56] and Camille Dungy[57] have painted life in the context of racism, persecution, and violence. Poets Laura Hershey,[58] Molly McCully Brown, and Susannah Nevison,[59] among others, have written about living with disability. Poets Yiyun Lee ("Immigrant Blues"), John Olivares Espinoza ("Spanish as Experienced by a Native Speaker"), and Zohra Saed ("Neptune Avenue"), among other artists, have captured life as immigrants to the United States. There is a wealth of artistic work about deeply personal topics from suicide[60,61,62,63] to wrestling with one's physicality[64,65] and sexuality.[66,67,68]

Conversely, through the arts and humanities we are reminded of feelings and experiences that are common to all humans—moments of mourning and moments of joy. For example, consider Joy Harjo's poem, "Perhaps the World Ends Here,"[69] which opens: "The world begins at a kitchen table. No matter what, we must eat to live," or Mary Oliver's "Wild Geese,"[70] which reads: "Whoever you are, no matter how lonely, /the world offers itself to your imagination,/ calls to you like the wild geese, harsh and exciting—/ over and over announcing your place/ in the family of things." Poetry and the arts often invoke universal human emotions that highlight the ways in which all people are connected.

Kidd and Castano[71] wrote: "The capacity to identify and understand others' subjective states is one of the most stunning products of human evolution."(p377) The arts and humanities bring us closer to this understanding, in turn deepening our capacity for professionalism.

Tolerance of Ambiguity

Vignette 5.3

An Uncertain Moment

A 45-year-old woman is referred to the emergency room because a routine complete blood count showed 70,000 white blood cells. Her partner wants to know if a definitive diagnosis can be made from this blood work and what next steps will be. The attending physician responds that more tests will need to be done, and as more information becomes available, it will be easier to respond in more detail. The partner shakes her head and says: "Basically, you know nothing." The physician searches for words, wondering what the most professional response might be. How does he turn this moment of ambiguity and uncertainty into a boon for professionalism?

Ambiguity and uncertainty are often perceived as negative states of being; the words "I don't know" are often taken as a failure of professional competence. However, there are many instances in both medicine and life where the answer cannot be known or a problem is too complex to make immediate conclusions or predictions. The arts and humanities can help shift our understanding of ambiguity from professional anathema to thought-provoking medium, an invitation to think deeply and speak honestly with the patient about the limits of our knowledge and abilities. Facility and comfort with ambiguity, then, are critical components of medical professionalism.

In terms of prognosis, uncertainty provokes understandable anxiety for patients and families. Many physicians, acting on the dual impulses—both rooted in the concept of professionalism—to alleviate anxiety and to have the answer, will struggle to respond to such questions or respond prematurely. This impulse likely contributes to the high rate of overestimation of survival for terminally ill patients.[72] However, as poet and physician Laura Kolbe has observed: "A physician's purpose is not perfect certainty, but the relief of suffering."[73] With this understanding, the physician can turn their focus from concern about the correct answer, to acknowledging uncertainty and providing support concretely by helping to normalize the uncertainty, address the patient's emotions, and help manage the effects of the uncertainty on their ability to live as well as possible in the current moment.[74] This process, as described by writer and physician Jay Baruch, represents "neither a lazy shrug nor permission to lower the intellectual bar, but a clarion call for a different type of rigor in medicine."[75(p42)]

Nowhere is there greater comfort with uncertainty than in the field of the arts and humanities. It is no surprise, therefore, that this discipline can be used in medical education to support skills in professionalism. Literature, film, and artwork can all be used to foster discussions about ambiguity and uncertainty, and reflective writing can be a valuable addition to this process.

Uncertainty and ambiguity, left unaddressed in the classroom, also can interfere with medical problem-solving and lifelong learning. Twenty-first-century medical education tends to separate subjects into disparate blocks of information. And, while this helps break down the enormous body of medical knowledge into more manageable pieces, this somewhat fragmented approach to medical education also sets the stage for anxiety and frustration during the clinical years. This is because the clinical environment is full of information that is difficult to fit together when using the reductionist approach to medicine. Moreover, it is rife with dissonance, such as conflicting recommendations from consulting services, discrepancies between a patient's presentation and the textbook's description of their presumed illness, and conflicting but equally valid priorities between family members.

Liou et al. have described the process of navigating such murky circumstances as "playing in the gutter."[76] In comic books, the gutter is the empty space between two panels of the story. The reader must actively engage with the gutters—imagining what has happened in that blank space—to explain the progression of the story from one frame to the next. Liou's group compares navigating this "messy, indeterminate zone" to navigating the analogous gutters of our professional work: the ambiguous spaces, observing that an understanding of the creative process can help transform the gutters from barriers to opportunities. Other authors have also postulated that creative processes drive learning by prompting students to consider connections between disparate facts and events.[77]

Openness to uncertainty is allied to professionalism in another way: It may help reduce medical errors. This is because discomfort with uncertainty may lead to ignoring information that doesn't fit neatly into a favored diagnosis or oversimplifying a complicated case. Comfort with ambiguity might allow the physician to greet the messy details with openness, rather than arriving at a premature resolution.[78] As Kolbe writes: "Our patients will tell us things that we cannot yet interpret, sending us to new questions, new shadings in the interrogative mood."[79(p75)]

Poet Mark Doty has proposed that uncertainty has dimensions that can support and enhance creative work. He writes: "In any process of inquiry, our uncertainty is our ally . . . "[80(p76)] Further, "it's that work—the work of uncovering, questioning . . . which makes the difference between a slight poem and a poem of substance." Perhaps the same could be said about difficult discussions with patients.

Ultimately, naming and exploring ambiguity and uncertainty are part of being honest to ourselves, our patients, and society. If we are not honest, we are in many ways "playing doctor," wearing a costume to portray a character. True professionalism lies in dealing squarely with the unknown and using it as a conduit toward professionalism.

Social Justice

Vignette 5.4

Race and Medicine

A senior attending is mentoring a fellow on a research project about the amount of pain medication received by emergency department patients with sickle cell crisis. The fellow decides to collect data on patient race as a predictor of their outcome of interest. The senior attending asks them to articulate why they believe that race might predict the amount of pain medication received. The fellow replies, "I've heard that pain thresholds vary between cultures."

Social Narratives

The American Society of Bioethics and Humanities has written: "Racism and racial injustice must be specifically recognized, combatted, and rejected as a matter of professionalism."[81] Justice, together with beneficence and autonomy, is a fundamental component of medicine's contract with society. In the vignette above, this principle is compromised by the fellow's socialization into a historic narrative that affects not only the doctor-patient relationship, but also the actual process of research design and data interpretation. The fellow might be correct in expecting the results to differ between racial and ethnic groups, but not because of variation in pain threshold—rather, because of *differential treatment based on race*. Historic narratives about aspects of race (e.g., vulnerability to pain) affect not only patient care, but also the design and interpretation of clinical research. Facility with the humanities is therefore critically important to physicians as a community of research scientists and educators. First, familiarity with US history allows, in this case, an understanding of the deep racist roots that underlie historic narratives about racial differences in pain threshold.[82] Second, familiarity with story facilitates an understanding of the power of "master narratives" (i.e., widely accepted stories about specific [usually minoritized] groups that persist despite clear evidence to the contrary).[83,84,85] Third, it creates physical and cognitive space for counterstorytelling, or stories that are generally neglected by mainstream representations.[86,87,88] The concept of counterstorytelling allows us to consider alternate hypotheses when patient outcomes differ by race. Rather than fall back on stereotypes about pain thresholds, the fellow might consider that the pain of Black patients is often undertreated and met with suspicion.[89,90] This matter is further complicated by the fact that there is no truly objective measure of pain; it can only be expressed through story,[91] which might be heard through the lens of implicit bias.

There are many examples of historic narratives about race being perpetuated over time and incorporated into scientific papers; these papers are then synthesized into clinical guidelines and reference value norms, creating disparate care for racial and ethnic minorities.[92,93,94] The arts and humanities provide a perfect scaffold to address social justice in our work, as they support conversations about critical thinking, United States and world history, and racialized narratives as arising from the dominant group. In fact, it has been proposed that artists be included on scientific research teams, as a way to incorporate different bodies of knowledge and invite different ways of problem-solving.[95] When we become aware of dominant and marginalized accounts of race, ethnicity, and other forms of difference, we can enter into patient care and clinical research that is more effectively aligned with principles of justice and, ultimately, professionalism.

Word Choice

Should physicians call one another "Doctor" or use first names? Should patients be called by the vocatives sir, miss, and sweetie? From descriptors like noncompliant, to labels such as *child with sickler cell disease or frequent flyer*, to first-person and antiracist language, attention to word choice is integral to enacting professionalism.[96] When we get the language wrong, our words are potential barriers to the vital connections we aspire to forge with our patients and colleagues.

Moreover, the words we choose are laden with signals about our conceptions of self and others; these signals in turn can shape clinical care, team cohesion, educational efforts, and patient trust, all of which relate to professionalism.

But in a clinical environment, with many competing tasks and urgencies, there is often inadequate time to consider the language we use. The arts and humanities remind us of the lexical baggage[97] attached to words, that is, the layers of meaning that words can assume based on life experience and worldview. Ferdinand Saussure, in his course on general linguistics,[98] described language as a system of signs (i.e., words) to which the listener responds in a predictable way. Signs are accompanied by "the signified" meaning, a mental concept. This concept is based on life experience and worldview and can differ greatly between individuals. Because of this, communication can be fraught with microaggressions and misunderstandings that are not intentional, but rather the result of word choice.

The arts and humanities support thinking deeply about language. For example, in Baldwin's novel *Giovanni's Room*,[99] the narrator speaks at length about the word "American," saying "When Giovanni wanted me to know that he was displeased with me, he said I was a *vrai American*. Conversely, when delighted, he said that I was not an American at all; and on both occasions he was striking, deep in me, a nerve which did not throb in him."[(p85)] Thinking deeply about how each character understands the word "American" can inspire thinking about the complexity and nuance of word choice. Reading poetry similarly allows for deep consideration of word meaning and allows for the understanding that meaning is subjective and contextual.

Most important, mutually respectful conversations about word choice and the nuances of what is being signified to the listener are critically important. Open and respectful conversation between colleagues, or between physicians and patients, is a hallmark of a professional environment. The way we speak to and about one another is a primary driver of what will happen in the clinical space.

Antiracism and Implicit Bias

As Maxine Hong Kingston wrote: "We're all under the same sky and walk the same earth; we're alive together during the same moment."[100(p171)] This emphasis on the universal is one of the most important qualities of the arts and humanities. Engagement with the arts and humanities often enhances the learner's understanding of personhood, the experience of being alive and living in a body that is vulnerable to illness and pain, which can in turn inform the way in which they relate to and understand their patients, translating into a respectful, open-minded, and professional approach.

The health humanities as a platform for antiracism education is an emerging and important branch of inquiry. Rita Charon writes: "Practice of narrative medicine requires attention to the processes of the teller/listener contract, the power hierarchies in place, the text and sub-text, and the rhetorical, linguistic, and metaphorical uses of race."[(p162)] Because of its emphasis on sociocultural critique and attention to inequitable systems, it can catalyze advocacy to address inequality.[101,102,103] Finally, it lends itself to understanding the perspectives of others,[104,105] humanization of the other,[106] and exploration of implicit bias.[107,108]

Both Charon[109] and Balhara[110] invoke the concept of the *third thing*[111,112] as a strength of the arts and humanities for studying a topic as rife with tension as antiracism. The third object—typically a poem, prose, visual image, or film—is a neutral "meeting ground" that can be discussed without making reference to immediate individuals or surroundings. This distance from the material being discussed can provide a feeling of psychological safety for participants and may allow for more open conversation. Charon writes: "We need messy spaces . . . that will make this possible as a learning, unlearning, and relearning space where fear is not the retort of first instance."[(p165)]

Finally, the pedagogy of the humanities lends itself to constructing neutral and nonhierarchical spaces for group discussion and models the very skills—careful listening, openness to multiple perspectives, and the valuing of diverse voices—that are being taught.[113]

Modes of Integration

How should the arts and humanities be integrated into the medical school curriculum? Several frameworks have been suggested.[114,115,116] Feasibility and scope depend on institutional and individual factors, for example, available resources and local expertise regarding the arts and humanities. Guiding principles include the following:

1. Frame proposals for humanities-based professionalism education to align with institutional goals and missions.

2. Work collaboratively. Nurture relationships with artists and thinkers from diverse fields at the institutional and community levels. Actively seek out those who are fluent in critical thinking and embrace problems as fundamental to professional modes of being.
3. Elevate and integrate voices that exemplify diverse worldviews, including race, ethnicity, and religion; gender and sexuality; immigration experience, ability, age, and region.
4. Include voices from the community. We can learn about professionalism through everyday interactions with the people around us, including patients, colleagues, trainees, friends, family, and people we do not know. Our clinic, or office, is an active classroom for continually learning and engaging with professionalism.
5. As a humanities educator, read broadly and deeply. Engage with visual art, film, and other forms of creativity as often as possible, and discuss with others. What do you see and feel? What do they see and feel? How are you the same? Different?
6. Create safe, respectful spaces for dialogue and allow for various interpretations and opinions. Avoid prescriptive discussions that move toward the "right answer"; embrace the messiness and uncertainty of discourse about professionalism. This is a unique function of the arts and humanities in medical spaces and should be used to the fullest.
7. Do not allow individual or institutional limitations to become barriers. Ideally, formal health humanities studies would be integrated into the medical school and continuing education curriculum. Practically, however, this is not the reality at many sites. It is okay to work with what you have, following the principles listed above. "One-off" sessions, while not ideal, may catalyze important conversations and spark important questions or insights about professional identity.
8. There is the potential for the humanities to move us to new ways of looking at ourselves and the world. This can make learners uncomfortable. Under the best of circumstances, this is a productive discomfort. Gia Merlo wrote: "Professional identity formation is not a matter of memorization and regurgitation: it requires receptivity, a spirit of anticipation, and an openness to change."[117(p8)]

One cannot discuss professionalism in the current day without acknowledging the many conflicting demands that challenge and problematize our notions of professionalism. Therefore, in teaching professionalism, we are primarily dialoguing about it, without prescribed answers. The arts and humanities allow us to acknowledge this position and reflect on the constantly evolving notion of professionalism while considering deeply who we are and why we have come to this place.

While certain classic texts are often used to support discussion about professionalism, there is no set curriculum. The body of available work is constantly growing and changing; new concepts and ways of thinking emerge. In tandem, the field of medicine, with its vulnerability to social and natural forces, also continues to change, challenging physicians daily to redefine their relationship to their field, their patients, and their work. Several useful databases for selecting material are listed in Table 5.1.

Despite the many conflicting forces that work on patients and physicians, their constancy as central characters does not change. Neither does their humanity nor their need for respect, safety, and professional care. This is, perhaps, the only constant in a continually evolving landscape.

Table 5.1 Professionalism: Selected Resources in the Arts and Humanities

Name	URL	Description
Sharetools.org	https://www.sharetools.org/	A resource for health professions educators to integrate humanities-based, antiracism education
Humanities at the Bedside	https://www.acep.org/education/humanities-at-the-bedside/	A health humanities curriculum resource generated by the ACEP Medical Humanities Section
Litmed	https://medhum.med.nyu.edu/	A searchable collection of literature, fine art, visual art, and performing art annotations created as a dynamic, comprehensive resource for scholars, educators, students, patients, and others interested in medical humanities
Poetry Foundation	https://www.poetryfoundation.org/	A searchable database designed to raise poetry to a more visible and influential position in culture
The Bellevue Literary Review	https://blreview.org/	An online literary magazine exploring humanity and the human experience
The Intima	https://www.theintima.org/	An online journal of narrative medicine

References

1. Monaghan P. *The Encyclopedia of Celtic Mythology and Folklore.* Infobase Publishing; 2004:296–297.
2. Estés CP. *Women Who Run With the Wolves: Myths and Stories of the Wild Woman Archetype.* Ballantine Books; 1992.
3. Fenki HI. Simchong: the blind man's daughter. Sejong Cultural Society. Accessed May 19, 2022. https://www.sejongculturalsociety.org/writing/current/tales/shimchong.php
4. Snow CP. Two cultures. *Science.* 1959;130(3373):419. doi:10.1126/science.130.3373.419
5. Sarton G, Siegel F. Seventy-first critical bibliography of the history and philosophy of science and of the history of civilization (to October 1947). *Isis.* 1948;39(1/2):70–139.
6. Kollmer Horton ME. The orphan child: humanities in modern medical education. *Philos Ethics Humanit Med.* 2019;14(1):1. doi:10.1186/s13010-018-0067-y
7. Hunter K. *Doctors' Stories: The Narrative Structure of Medical Knowledge.* Princeton University Press; 1991. https://doi.org/10.2307/j.ctv10vm1vd.
8. Charon R. At the membranes of care: stories in narrative medicine. *Acad Med.* 2012;87(3):342–347. doi:10.1097/ACM.0b013e3182446fbb
9. Arntfield SL, Slesar K, Dickson J, Charon R. Narrative medicine as a means of training medical students toward residency competencies. *Patient Educ Couns.* 2013;91(3):280–286. doi:10.1016/j.pec.2013.01.014
10. Association of American Medical Colleges Medical School Objectives Project. *Learning Objectives for Medical Student Education: Guidelines for Medical Schools.* Association of American Medical Colleges 1998.
11. American Society for Bioethics + Humanities. About. Accessed May 31, 2022. https://asbh.org/about/american-society-bioethics-humanities

12. Squier SM, Hawkins AH. Medical Humanities and Cultural Studies: Lessons Learned From an NEH Institute. *J Med Humanit.* 2004;25(4):243–253. doi:10.1007/s10912-004-4831-1

13. Hawkins AH. Epiphanic knowledge and medicine. *Camb Q Healthc Eth.* 2005;14(1):40–46. doi:10.1017/s096318010505005x

14. Shapiro J, Coulehan J, Wear D, Montello M. Medical humanities and their discontents: definitions, critiques, and implications. *Acad Med.* 2009;84(2):192–198. doi:10.1097/ACM.0b013e3181938bca

15. Dolev JC, Friedlaender LK, Braverman IM. Use of fine art to enhance visual diagnostic skills. *JAMA.* 2001;286(9):1020–1021. doi:10.1001/jama.286.9.1019

16. Bardes CL, Gillers D, Herman AE. Learning to look: developing clinical observational skills at an art museum. *Med Educ.* 2001;35(12):1157–1161. doi:10.1046/j.1365-2923.2001.01088.x

17. Schaff PB, Isken S, Tager RM. From contemporary art to core clinical skills: observation, interpretation, and meaning-making in a complex environment. *Acad Med.* 2011;86(10):1272–1276. doi:10.1097/ACM.0b013e31822c161d

18. Doukas DJ, McCullough LB, Wear S. Perspective: medical education in medical ethics and humanities as the foundation for developing medical professionalism. *Acad Med.* 2012;87(3):334–341. doi:10.1097/ACM.0b013e318244728c

19. Jones T, Wear D, Friedman LD. *Health Humanities Reader.* Rutgers University Press; 2014. https://www.degruyter.com/isbn/9780813562483

20. Health Humanities Consortium. About. Accessed May 31, 2022. https://healthhumanitiesconsortium.com/about/

21. Haidet P, Jarecke J, Adams NE, et al. A guiding framework to maximise the power of the arts in medical education: a systematic review and metasynthesis. *Med Educ.* 2016;50(3):320–331. doi:10.1111/medu.12925

22. National Academies of Sciences, Engineering, and Medicine *The Integration of the Humanities and Arts With Sciences, Engineering, and Medicine in HigherEducation: Branches From the Same Tree.* National Academies Press; 2018. https://doi.org/10.17226/24988

23. Howley L, Gaufberg E, King B. *The Fundamental Role of the Arts and Humanities in Medical Education.* AAMC; 2020.

24. Jones T, Blackie M, Garden R, Wear D. The Almost Right Word: The Move From Medical to Health Humanities. *Acad Med.* 2017 Jul;92(7):932–935. doi:10.1097/ACM.0000000000001518. PMID: 28657553

25. Goldberg JL. Humanism or professionalism? The white coat ceremony and medical education. *Acad Med.* 2008;83(8):715–722 doi:10.1097/ACM.0b013e31817eba30

26. ABIM Foundation, ACP-ASIM Foundation, European Federation of Internal Medicine. Medical professionalism in the new millennium: a physician charter. *J Am Coll Surg.* 2003;196(1):115–118. doi:10.1016/s1072-7515(02)01617-4

27. Cochran A, Upchurch GR. Has the physician's white coat seen its day? *JAMA Netw Open.* 2021;4(7):e2119881. doi:10.1001/jamanetworkopen.2021.19881

28. Verghese A. *Cutting for Stone.* Knopf; 2009.

29. Klass P. *Love and Modern Medicine.* Mariner; 2001.

30. Patchett A. *State of Wonder.* Harper; 2011.

31. Boddapati V, Danford NC, Lopez CD, Levine WN, Lehman RA, Lenke LG. Recent trends in private equity acquisition of orthopaedic practices in the United States. *J Am Acad Orthop Surg.* 2022;30(8):e664–e672. doi:10.5435/JAAOS-D-21-00783

32. Luh JY, Hansen ER, Liston S. Private equity and health care delivery. *JAMA.* 2021;326(24):2534. doi:10.1001/jama.2021.20431

33. Bodenheimer T, Sinsky C. From triple to quadruple aim: care of the patient requires care of the provider. *Ann Fam Med.* 2014;12:573–576. https://www.annfammed.org/content/12/6/573. https://doi.org/10.1370/afm.1713

34. Friedberg MW, Chen PG, Van Busum KR, et al. Factors affecting physician professional satisfaction and their implications for patient care, health systems, and health policy. *Rand Health Q.* 2014;3:1 https://www.ncbi.nlm.nih.gov/pmc/articles/PMC5051918/.

35. Damodar D, Donnally CJ 3rd, McCormick JR, et al. How wait-times, social media, and surgeon demographics influence online reviews on leading review websites for joint replacement surgeons. *J Clin Orthop Trauma.* 2019;10(4):761–767. doi:10.1016/j.jcot.2019.01.021

36. Sanati-Mehrizy P, Margulies I, Sayegh F, Ingargiola M, Taub P. The "realself effect." *Ann Plast Surg.* 2020;85(4):352–357. doi:10.1097/SAP.0000000000002245

37. Shapiro J, McDonald TB. Supporting clinicians during Covid-19 and beyond—learning from past failures and envisioning new strategies. *N Engl J Med.* 2020;383:e142. https://www.nejm.org/doi/10.1056/NEJMp2024834. https://doi.org/10.1056/NEJMp2024834

38. Phillips KA, Ospina NS, Montori VM. Physicians interrupting patients. *J Gen Intern Med.* 2019;34(10):1965. doi:10.1007/s11606-019-05247-5

39. Charon R. At the membranes of care: stories in narrative medicine. *Acad Med.* 2012;87(3):342–347. doi:10.1097/ACM.0b013e3182446fbb

40. Charon R. Chapter 1: accounts of self: exploring rationality through literature. In: *The Principles and Practice of Narrative Medicine.* Oxford University Press; 2017:15–34.

41. Allende I. 1982. *The House of the Spirits.* Alfred A. Knopf; 1982.

42. ABIM Foundation, ACP-ASIM Foundation, European Federation of Internal Medicine. Medical professionalism in the new millennium: a physician charter. *J Am Coll Surg.* 2003;196(1):115–118. doi:10.1016/s1072-7515(02)01617-4

43. Doukas DJ, McCullough LB, Wear S. Perspective: medical education in medical ethics and humanities as the foundation for developing medical professionalism. *Acad Med.* 2012;87(3):334–341. doi:10.1097/ACM.0b013e318244728c

44. Vuong, O. *On Earth We're Briefly Gorgeous.* New York: Penguin Press, 2019.

45. Kirkland KB, Craig SR. Exploring the surgical gaze through literature and art. *JAMA.* 2018;319(15):1532–1534. doi:10.1001/jama.2018.0396

46. Katz JT. Formal art observation training improves medical students' visual diagnostic skills. *J Gen Intern Med.* 2008;23:991–997.

47. Shapiro J, Rucker L, Beck J. Training the clinical eye and mind: using the arts to develop medical students' observational and pattern recognition skills. *Med Educ.* 2006;40(3): 263–268.

48. Auerbach K, Baruch M. Beyond comfort zones: an experiment in medical and art education. *J Learn Arts.* 2012;8(1).

49. Kidd DC, Castano E. Reading literary fiction improves theory of mind. *Science.* 2013;342(6156):377–380. doi:10.1126/science.1239918.

50. Djikic M, Oatley K, Moldoveanu M. Reading other minds: effects of literature on empathy. *Scientific Study of Literature.* 2013;3:28–47. .doi:10.1075/ssol.3.1.06dji

51. Bal PM, Veltkamp M. How does fiction reading influence empathy? An experimental investigation on the role of emotional transportation. *PLoS One.* 2013;8:e55341. doi:10.1371/journal.pone.0055341

52. Miall D, Kuiken D. Foregrounding, defamiliarization, and affect: response to literary stories. *Poetics.* 1994;22, 389–407. doi:10.1016/0304-422X(94)00011-5
53. Morrison T. *The Bluest Eye.* Holt, Rinehart and Winston; 1970.
54. Harding P. *Tinkers.* Bellevue Literary Press; 2009.
55. Green J. *The Fault in Our Stars.* Dutton Books; 2012.
56. Lorde A. *From a Land Where Other People Live.* Broadside Press; 1973.
57. Dungy C. *Suck on the Marrow.* Red Hen Press; 2010.
58. Day M, Herd M. *Laura Hershey: On the Life and Work of an American Master.* Pleiades Press; 2019.
59. McCully Brown M, Nevison S. *In the Field Between Us.* Persea Books; 2020.
60. Jackson D. "Bobolink." *Poem-a-Day*; 2021. https://poets.org/poem/bobolink
61. Wieners J. The Suicide. In: Wieners J. *Selected Poems, 1958–1984.* 1986Black Sparrow Books; 1986..
62. Baraka A. Preface to a Twenty Volume Suicide Note. In: Baraka A. *SOS: Poems, 1961–2013.* Grove/Atlantic; 2015.
63. Sanchez EL. Six Months After Contemplating Suicide. *Poetry Magazine.* 2015.
64. Rogers S. *Fat Girl Forms.* Saturnalia Books; 2021:20.
65. Zighelboim S. *The Fat Sonnets.* Argos Books; 2018.
66. Eugenides J. *Middlesex.* Picador; 2002.
67. Bennett B. *The Vanishing Half.* Penguin; 2020.
68. greathouse ta. *Wound From the Mouth of a Wound.* Milkweed; 2020.
69. Harjo J. Perhaps the world ends here. In: Harjo J. *The Woman Who Fell From the Sky* W. W. Norton & Company; 1994.
70. Oliver M. Wild geese. In: Oliver M. *Dream Work.* Atlantic Monthly Press; 1986:14.
71. Kidd DC, Castano E. Reading literary fiction improves theory of mind. *Science.* 2013;342(6156):377–380. doi:10.1126/science.1239918.
72. Christakis NA, Lamont EB. Extent and determinants of error in doctors' prognoses in terminally ill patients: prospective cohort study. *BMJ.* 2000;320:469–472.
73. Kolbe L. How COVID-19 changed medicine. *Yale Rev.* 2022;110(2). Accessed May 27, 2022. https://yalereview.org/article/covid-doctor-uncertainty-kolbe
74. Smith AK, White DB, Arnold RM. Uncertainty—the other side of prognosis. *N Engl J Med.* 2013;368(26):2448–2450. doi:10.1056/NEJMp1303295
75. Baruch J. Doctors as makers. *Acad Med.* 2017;92(1):40–44.
76. Liou KT, Jamorabo DS, Dollase RH, Dumenco L, Schiffman FJ, Baruch JM. Playing in the "gutter": cultivating creativity in medical education and practice. *Acad Med.* 2016;91(3):322–327. doi:10.1097/ACM.0000000000001018
77. Marshall J. Connecting art, learning, and creativity: a case for curriculum integration. *Stud Art Educ.* 2005;46:227–241.
78. Seaburn DB, Morse D, McDaniel SH, Beckman H, Silberman J, Epstein R. Physician responses to ambiguous patient symptoms. *J Gen Intern Med.* 2005;20(6):525–530. doi:10.1111/j.1525-1497.2005.0093.x
79. Kolbe L. How COVID-19 changed medicine. *Yale Rev.* 2022:110(2). Accessed May 27, 2022. https://yalereview.org/article/covid-doctor-uncertainty-kolbe

80. Doty M. In: Slager D, ed. *Views From the Loft: A Portable Writer's Workshop.* Milkweed Editions; 2010:75–82.

81. American Society for Bioethics + Humanities. ASBH Statement on Racial Injustice and Professionalism in Bioethics and Health Humanities. Accessed May 31, 2022. https://asbh.org/asbh-statement-on-racial-injustice-and-professionalism#:~:text=For%20professionals%20working%20in%20bioethics,injustice%20in%20their%20professional%20arenas

82. Washington HA. *Medical Apartheid.* Anchor Books; 2006.

83. Foucault M. *The Archeology of Knowledge.* Pantheon; 1972.

84. Hammack PL, Toolis EE. Putting the social into personal identity: the master narrative as root metaphor for psychological and developmental science. Commentary on McLean and Syed. *Hum Dev.* 2016;*58*(6):350–364. https://doi.org/10.1159/000446054

85. Braddock K, Dillard JP. Meta-analytic evidence for the persuasive effect of narratives on beliefs, attitudes, intentions, and behaviors. *Commun Monogr.* 2016;*83*(4):446–467.

86. Bamberg M, Andrews M, eds. *Considering Counternarratives: Narrating, Resisting, Making Sense.* John Benjamins; 2004.

87. Braddock K, Horgan J. Towards a guide for constructing and disseminating counternarratives to reduce support for terrorism. *Stud Confl Terror.* 2016;39(5), 381–404. https://doi.org/10.1080/1057610X.2015.1116277

88. Solórzano DG, Yosso TJ. Critical race methodology: counter-storytelling as an analytical framework for education research. *Qual Inq.* 2002;8(1):23–44. doi:10.1177/107780040200800103

89. Goyal MK, Johnson TJ, Chamberlain JM, et al; Pediatric Emergency Care Applied Research Network (PECARN). Racial and ethnic differences in emergency department pain management of children with fractures. *Pediatrics.* 2020;145(5):e20193370. doi:10.1542/peds.2019-3370

90. Johnson TJ, Weaver MD, Borrero S, et al. Association of race and ethnicity with management of abdominal pain in the emergency department. *Pediatrics.* 2013;132(4):e851–e858. doi:10.1542/peds.2012-3127

91. Baruch J, Springs S. Opioids and pain in the emergency department: a narrative crisis. *Med Humanit.* 2018;44(3):213–216. doi:10.1136/medhum-2017-011429

92. Braun L. *Breathing Race Into the Machine: The Surprising Career of the Spirometer From Plantation to Genetics.* University of Minnesota Press; 2014.

93. Kowalsky RH, Rondini AC, Platt SL. The case for removing race from the American Academy of Pediatrics Clinical Practice Guideline for Urinary Tract Infection in Infants and Young Children With Fever. *JAMA Pediatr.* 2020;174(3):229–230. doi:10.1001/jamapediatrics.2019.5242

94. Vyas DA, Eisenstein LG, Jones DS. Hidden in plain sight—reconsidering the use of race correction in clinical algorithms. *N Engl J Med.* 2020;383(9):874–882. doi:10.1056/NEJMms2004740

95. Springs S, Baruch J. Artists on the research team: an interdisciplinary approach to team science, research rigor, and creative dialogue. *Health Promot Pract.* 2021;22(1 suppl):83S–90S. doi:10.1177/1524839921996301

96. Taneja S, Kuriakose T, Vinci RJ. The weight of our words: how medical communication perpetuates bias. *Pediatrics.* 2022;149(3):e2021054296. doi:10.1542/peds.2021-054296

97. Sally McConnell-Ginet. *Words Matter: Meaning and Power.* Cambridge University Press; 2020:26.

98. Saussure F de, Bally C, Sechehaye A. *Course in General Linguistics.* McGraw-Hill; 1966.

99. Baldwin J. *Giovanni's Room.* Delta Trade Paperbacks; 2000.

100. Kingston MH. *The Woman Warrior: Memoirs of a Girlhood Among Ghosts.* Vintage, 2010.

101. Dennhardt S, Apramian T, Lingard L, Torabi N, Arntfield S. Rethinking research in the medical humanities: a scoping review and narrative synthesis of quantitative outcome studies. *Med Educ.* 2016;50(3):285–299. doi:10.1111/medu.12812

102. Moniz T, Golafshani M, Gaspar CM, et al. The prism model: advancing a theory of practice for arts and humanities in medical education. *Perspect Med Educ.* 2021;10(4):207–214. doi:10.1007/s40037-021-00661-0

103. Balhara KS, Ehmann MR, Irvin N. Antiracism in health professions education through the lens of the health humanities. *Anesthesiol Clin.* 2022;40:287–299.

104. Charon R, Trautmann Banks J, Connelly JE, et al. Literature and medicine: contributions to clinical practice. *Ann Intern Med.* 1995;122:599–606.

105. Hurwitz B, Charon R. A narrative future for health care. *Lancet.* 2013;381:1886–1997.

106. Murphy-Shigematsu S. Teaching cross-cultural competence through narrative. *Fam Med.* 2009;41(9):622–624.

107. Ross PT, Lypson ML. Using artistic-narrative to stimulate reflection on physician bias. *Teach Learn Med.* 2006;2014(4):344–349.

108. Balhara KS, Ehmann MR, Irvin N. Antiracism in health professions education through the lens of the health humanities. *Anesthesiol Clin.* 2022;40:287–299.

109. Charon R, Irvine C, Ngozi Oforlea A, Rivera Colon E, Smalletz C, Spiegel M. Racial justice in medicine: narrative practices toward equity. *Narrative.* 2021; 29(2):160–177. Project MUSE. doi:10.1353/nar.2021.0008

110. Balhara KS, Ehmann MR, Irvin N. Antiracism in health professions education through the lens of the health humanities. *Anesthesiol Clin.* 2022;40:287–299.

111. Gaufberg E, Batalden M. The third thing in medical education. *Clin Teach.* 2007;4(2):78–81.

112. Ogden T. The analytic third: implications for psychoanalytic theory and technique. *Psychoanal Q.* 2004;73(1)):167–195.

113. hooks b. Transformative pedagogy and multiculturalism. In: Perry T, Fraser JW, eds. *Teaching in the Multicultural Classroom.* Routledge; 1998:91–98.

114. Shapiro J, Coulehan J, Wear D, Montello M. Medical humanities and their discontents: definitions, critiques, and implications. *Acad Med.* 2009;84(2):192–198. doi:10.1097/ACM.0b013e3181938bca

115. Doukas DJ, McCullough LB, Wear S. Perspective: medical education in medical ethics and humanities as the foundation for developing medical professionalism. *Acad. Med* 2012;87(3):334–341. doi:10.1097/ACM.0b013e318244728c

116. Haidet P, Jarecke J, Adams NE, et al. A guiding framework to maximise the power of the arts in medical education: a systematic review and metasynthesis. *Med Educ.* 2016;50(3):320–331. doi:10.1111/medu.12925

117. Merlo G. *Principles of Medical Professionalism.* Oxford; 2021.

6

Professionalism of Solidarity and the Social Contract

Marco Antonio de Carvalho Filho, Renato Soleiman Franco, and Edison Iglesias de Oliveira Vidal

Key Points

- The social contract metaphor may be insufficient to address the evolving dynamics between the medical profession and society.
- Combining concepts from critical pedagogy (liberation, critical consciousness, full citizenship, education for change, and dialogue) with cultural humility proposes a "professionalism of solidarity."
- Situated learning, critical consciousness, and liberation expand the social contract metaphor to promote social justice.
- Acknowledging the complexity of modern medical practice is crucial, and a professionalism of solidarity empowers patients and fights injustice.
- Administrative evil and the Lucifer effect explain why fixed organizational structures may resist a professionalism of solidarity.
- The future envisions a medical community embracing complexity while promoting social justice.

Introduction

In the last 20 years, the social contract metaphor has shed light on the relationship between the medical profession and society.[1] In the first part of this chapter, we explore how this metaphor is helpful in understanding and conceptualizing the different levels of this complex relationship (individual, organizational, and public levels). However, we also discuss the limitations of this metaphor to capture the ever-evolving nature of this relationship. In a global world marked by profound economic inequality, deeply influenced by the wonders of scientific and social developments, there is no one contract capable of covering all the nuances of the complex interactions between healthcare providers and the societies they serve. Prescriptive professionalism falls short in front of such complexity. Currently, reaching professional "phronesis" (practical wisdom) demands the ability to apply the core values of the profession, such as beneficence and social justice, to uncertain, complex, and ambiguous situations, keeping patients' best interests in mind while creating space for patients' autonomy to flourish in the context of dialogical interactions, in which power is shared and used to liberate and not to oppress.[2]

In the second part of this chapter, we build on the concepts of situated learning, critical consciousness, liberation, and education for change as suggested by the movement called "critical pedagogy," started by the Brazilian educationalist Paulo Freire to devise a "professionalism of solidarity."[2–4]

Finally, in the third part, we discuss how the concept of cultural humility,[5] together with a professionalism of solidarity, may expand and democratize the current professionalism discourse to include patients' voices and needs and promote social justice. We also alert how the Lucifer effect (i.e., the social dynamics of power influencing ordinary people into engaging in behaviors that impart suffering on others) may explain why fixed organizational structures may offer resistance to such professionalism.

The Social Contract Metaphor

More than 300 years after the definition of the social contract, discussions about its application are still alive in ethics, politics, and history. The philosophers Thomas Hobbes, John Locke, and Jean-Jacques Rousseau defined the social contract as the codes, norms, and customs, including implicit and explicit rules, that guide the relationship between the individual and the State.[6] In the context of medical education, the social contract has been used as a metaphor to explore, problematize, and explain the relationship between the medical profession and society. For example, in this relationship, society expects doctors' respect, integrity, competence, and the promotion of individual and community well-being. The medical profession, in turn, expects autonomy, self-regulation, trust, financial reward, and social recognition through the public appreciation of their work and adequate working conditions.[1,7]

Presenting the social contract to medical students inserts the relationship between doctors and patients in a sociocultural perspective, built throughout history and influenced by the cultural, economic, and political context.[8] Reflecting on the social contract allows students to understand the concessions, privileges, expectations, and obligations related to the practice of medicine. This reflection expands the understanding of the doctor-patient relationship and health care while allowing for a more in-depth discussion about medical professionalism.[9] In the social contract context, nurturing medical professionalism must contemplate fostering moral values that transcend time to honor society's expectations.

However, considering the contract as a set of behaviors, expectations, and obligations in a prescriptive and static relationship between medicine and society is a simplification that does not correspond to the expectations and requirements of today's medicine.[10]

As an evolution, Hafferty and Castellani proposed a model to understand and study medical professionalism, comprehending micro, meso, and macro dimensions.[11] These dimensions interact and influence each other. In the micro dimension, professionalism comprises each doctor's work—their clinical practice while caring for patients and their families. In the meso dimension, professionalism focuses on the professional relationships within the social structures surrounding the medical profession. In the macro dimension, professionalism presents itself as a social movement with political, ideological, economic, commercial, corporate, and cultural facets.[11]

This multidimensional perspective of professionalism incorporates the complexity of modern medical practice by understanding that the medical profession is influenced and modulated by diverse social forces in a dynamic and evolutionary balance. Thus, the relationship between medicine and society would involve a complex system integrating aspects of professional and personal relationships between

- doctors and patients/family members;
- doctors and the general community;
- doctors, society, and culture;
- doctors among themselves;
- doctors and other professionals; and
- doctors and institutions (medical schools, state jurisdictions and actors, industries, and healthcare plans).

Suppose medical educators and professionals do not embrace this complexity. In that case, the profession risks losing its protagonist role, becoming a gear in an engine without knowing where it is going and why.

Can we have a critical perspective on personal, professional, institutional, and societal interests, behaviors, values, and ambitions?[12] The answer to this question is not simple, requires much debate, and may not have just one answer. We think that the movement known as critical pedagogy can contribute to this debate.

Critical Pedagogy and Professionalism

"Professionalism Happens In the World" —The Risk of Idealization

One of the first insights of Paulo Freire when alphabetizing adults in rural areas of the northeast of Brazil, was that education happens "in the world"—it is situated in a social, political, economic, and cultural context.[3,4] Acknowledging the social dimension of learning is not denying its neurobiological roots; it expands them. Paulo Freire also stressed that learning is born from the interaction between the learner and the world, which means it is actively constructed and contextualized. Why is this idea relevant for professionalism education and practice?

Professionalism also happens in the world.[13] However, professionalism education often happens in idealized contexts that fail to represent the complexity, uncertainty, and ambiguity of real-life scenarios. In several medical schools, the professionalism learning track starts already in the preclinical training, with bioethical discussions and paper-based clinical cases, which intend to reproduce the reality of the clinical practice. In general, these learning experiences follow the simple-to-complex approach adopted by the other disciplines in the health profession curriculum. This approach modulates complexity, aiming to optimize learning. In addition, the emotional aspects of the simulated problems are often suppressed, following the mistaken assumption that good decision-making demands emotional detachment.[9]

It is known that, when learning complex skills, students benefit from starting with simple problems, which may optimize students' limited work-memory capacity and facilitate the initial construction of cognitive representations (schemas) of the problems at hand.[14] After mastering the basics, teachers may progressively increase problems' complexity and variety to develop further students' cognitive schemas. Although this simple-to-complex approach seems to function well in developing practical and cognitive skills, it may represent a risk when teaching professionalism. Also, teachers unfamiliar with the reality of practice may underestimate the cognitive load and emotional labor related to handling professionalism dilemmas.[15]

Consequently, when educators simplify professionalism dilemmas to create simple-to-solve problems, students may understand that distinguishing right from wrong is easy and always possible, and those different perspectives can certainly be aligned. Students may consider that decision-making is like a multiple-choice question—there is an undoubtedly best answer to be marked and scored.

The other risk educators take when simplifying professionalism dilemmas is creating an idealized view of reality. Students may end up idealizing themselves, the patients, their colleagues, and the clinical environment, creating a wonderland where everything functions according to clear rules and regulations. When students transition to actual practice and finally understand how messy the clinical environment may be, how difficult it is to make wise decisions, and how imperfect people are, they experience a clash that may lead to identity dissonance, emotional detachment, and cynicism.[15]

We believe that introducing students as soon as possible to the reality of practice under the guidance of a skillful supervisor is the best way to teach professionalism. The simple-to-complex approach may happen in a different dimension. Instead of modulating the complexity of the problems, educators may modulate (1) the level of participation (from observation to peripheral participation, then to full participation, and, finally, to taking a leading role) and (2) the frequency of exposure (from once a month/week until everyday practice). This prevents idealization and allows students to reflect on real professional dilemmas, moving professionalism education away from a prescriptive stance to becoming participatory and engaged. This participatory approach will facilitate the development of a "critically conscious" professionalism.

Developing Critical Consciousness as a Step Toward Social Justice

Supervisors should stimulate students to take a critical, reflective stance, when exposed to real professional dilemmas. Freire believed that the educational process should shed light on the diverse forces acting on the individuals shaping their identity and modulating their behavior. These forces are often implicit, and when they limit individuals' development or freedom, they become oppressive and dehumanizing. In this context, Freire considered education a process of "liberation"; in his words: "Liberation is a praxis: the action and reflection of men and women upon their world in order to transform it." [4(p79)]

To reach liberation, health professionals need to develop a critical consciousness. Critical consciousness is a "reflection for action" process that, as Freire conceptualized, is marked by the testing of one's findings and by openness to revision; by the attempt to avoid distortion when perceiving problems and to avoid preconceived notions when analyzing them; by refusing to transfer responsibility; by rejecting passive positions; by soundness of argumentation; by the practice of dialogue rather than polemics; by receptivity to the new for reasons beyond mere novelty and by the good sense not to reject the old just because it is old—by accepting what is valid in both old and new. [3]

In professionalism education, liberation should encompass the personal, organizational, and social dimensions of professional practice. At a personal level, the liberation will demand the professionals in training to understand how their social trajectories influenced the way they see the world, the patients, and their profession. To become autonomous thinkers, they need to reflect on how their views on the world align (or not) with the future they want to construct for themselves within their professional and personal contexts. To reach liberation, students' reflections need to be followed by concrete actions. For instance, one may realize that being a white male from an upper social class may lead to implicit bias and a certain lack of awareness of the challenges faced by vulnerable social groups. In a liberation process, becoming aware means adopting an antiracist instance and an active approach to connect with the vulnerable, welcome their empowerment, and join the fight for social justice.

At an organizational level, the liberation process will stimulate the health professional to question the power imbalance that still marks interprofessional collaboration, the rarity of shared decision-making and patient centeredness, the structural racism, the gender imbalance in teams, and the lack of awareness of the LGBTQ+ community needs. This expanded comprehension will come with the need to engage in changing the health professional culture into one capable of embracing diversity as an asset, inclusion as a necessity, and compassion as its driving force.

At the social level, the liberation process makes explicit the connection between healthcare and society, which means that changing one should lead to the change of the other. For instance, this connection demands the creation of dialogical opportunities such as the empowerment of patients' associations, the inclusion of community representatives in the organization and planning of healthcare initiatives, and the empowerment of patients as active agents in the training of health professionals. This connection also makes health professionals responsible for joining in the efforts to increase marginalized groups' access to the system. Healthcare professionals pervaded by the spirit of liberation understand that their responsibility goes beyond caring for individuals to embody caring for the community they serve. For Freire, the educational process is never neutral; it always has a political dimension.[4,16] Without social justice, the work of a health professional is never complete.

The Professionalism of Solidarity

This lack of completeness should not be perceived as a burden but as an opportunity to connect with the world and transform it. The base of critical pedagogy is the connection between two people learning from each other. This connection is one based on dialogue and love. According to Freire: "Love is at the same time the foundation of dialogue and dialogue itself. . . . If I do not love the world—if I do not love life—if I do not love people—I cannot enter into dialogue." [16(p89)] Love is essential in dialogical relationships to allow the one who listens to step back from their prejudices and preconceived ideas to experience the world as perceived by the other. This listening attitude is not a passive one. It is a continuous process of co-constructing ideas to be enacted in the world. It has a purpose, meaning, and direction. It is a continuous process of reassuring our humanity and our connections with each other. It is an act of solidarity. We see the other, feel affected by this otherness, and become curious, alert, and ready to connect and take action when necessary.[4,16,17]

A professionalism of solidarity is born out of our connection with patients. We care about them, and they care about us, as in a symbiotic relationship. Different patients will need different relationships, and any prescribed behavior will be insufficient to cover the complexity of these relationships. This does not mean that boundaries are needless; this means that boundaries will depend on the nature of the relationship, on patients' and professionals' needs, and on what kind of dialogue is necessary to respect and empower patients to become protagonists of their own healthcare trajectories. As Freire believed in developing full citizenship (a status of full and autonomous participation in society),[4] we believe in full "patientship" (a status of full and autonomous participation in the therapeutic plan and healthcare system).

This connection with patients nurtures an attitude of mutual respect and shared understanding at the multiprofessional team level, which transforms "power over" into "power within" the team, canalized to foster mutual support and prioritize patients' needs over egoic battles. At the organizational level, this connection leads to a fight for equity, demanding cultural change. Microaggressions, structural racism, sexist stances, and moral harassment do not have space in a professionalism of solidarity. In this context, the unacceptable professional behavior is not the one that goes against the rules but the one that updates or changes the rules preventing human beings from becoming free individuals, agents of their own lives. The professionalism of solidarity is one of nonconformity.

At the societal level, this connection drives toward inclusion. Diversity becomes an opportunity to expand one's consciousness to understand different ways of professing similar values—an opportunity to open dialogues about different but legitimate ways of being in the world. A professionalism of solidarity does not accept that people with diverse, nonmajority cultural or ethnic backgrounds may have a different healthcare trajectory with unexpected adverse outcomes and experiences.[2]

This openness to dialogue does not mean that any behavior is acceptable. It means that the discussion about what is acceptable should be based on reaching common ground, defining what is precious about being human, and rescuing humanism from oppression. When conflict arises, complexity should be embraced, the values explicitly pondered, the context acknowledged, and the patient respected. Conflicts should be perceived as opportunities to deepen the understanding of the situation at hand through an open and democratic dialogue. This open dialogue needs cultural humility to strive.

Cultural Humility

Mr. AZ, an 85-year-old Black Brazilian man with advanced dementia, is admitted to the hospital because of recurrent aspiration pneumonia, whose first episode had occurred three months previously. The medical resident explains to his wife and two daughters that aspiration pneumonia is a common complication of advanced dementia, and that it results from impaired swallowing related to the progressive decline of brain functions that is typical of that condition. The resident also tells Mr. AZ's family that in such cases, the healthcare team recommends comfort feeding, that is, to carefully hand feed the patient with a focus on his comfort instead of achieving standard amounts of nutritional intake through a percutaneous endoscopic gastrostomy (PEG) tube. His wife and daughters are suspicious that the hospital is trying to deny appropriate care to Mr. AZ to decrease costs, and they express deep concern regarding the perspective of not giving Mr. AZ enough food. They insist that he must be fed by a PEG tube if he cannot eat safely without developing new pneumonia. The resident becomes increasingly frustrated as she believes that feeding the patient through a PEG tube would go against current best-practice guidelines for dementia care, represent a source of suffering to the patient, and be unethical.

This case portrays a situation of conflict between the healthcare team and the patient's family regarding what constitutes the best therapeutic approach for the patient and what is ethically appropriate. Situations such as this are a significant source of distress to patients' families and healthcare professionals and will often fuel distrust among those parties. The lack of a shared understanding of the clinical situation summed to a perceived moral misalignment set doctors and patients aside, hampering trust and creating suspicion. Considering Shapiro's wise definition of professionalism as "any intent, action or words that foster trustworthy relationships," [18(p169)] we would like to argue that cultural humility represents a critical ability that can help to bond doctors and patients and create trust.

Cultural humility is a concept developed in 1998 by Tervalon and Murray-García[5] to denote a lifelong process that requires humility for healthcare professionals (1) to engage in self-reflection and self-critique; (2) to bring into check the power imbalances that exist in the patient-professional encounters; and (3) to develop and maintain a respectful and nonpaternalistic partnership with communities on behalf of individuals. It was further conceptualized by Hook et al.[19] as the ability to maintain an other-oriented interpersonal stance characterized by a respectful openness to understand the patients' perspectives. Notably, cultural humility differs substantially from the often-misunderstood notion of "cultural competency" as equivalent to memorizing lists of specific cultural features of different ethnic groups, which often leads to unhelpful stereotyping of individuals belonging to those groups. In a certain sense, cultural humility is an antidote to the "culture of no culture" that is common in healthcare and lies at the heart of the conflict described in the case vignette.[20] However, before we delve into that argument, it will be useful to review the concept of culture.

Culture

Culture may be defined as a multidimensional and adaptive system that generates a social structure for a given population group providing its members with a set of expectations, beliefs, and means to achieve a sense of identity, safety, and meaning for life.[21] It is the lens through which each human being sees, makes sense of, and interacts with the world. Hence, culture significantly influences how people relate to the healthcare system, interpret verbal and nonverbal communication cues, make decisions, and deal with different illnesses. Importantly, every individual also belongs to multiple subcultures. For example, besides being a Brazilian, Mr. AZ has a particular gender and racial identity (i.e., Black male) and belongs to certain socioeconomic, linguistic, and religious groups, among several other groups (e.g., family, profession, and neighborhood). Ultimately, there are so many intersecting dimensions shaping an individual's (cultural) perception of the world that healthcare professionals must avoid stereotyping/making strong assumptions about issues such as patients' preferences of care or communication based on a single aspect of their cultural background (e.g., their ethnicity).

Culture of No Culture

Now back to the culture of no culture argument. The problem at the heart of the conflict described in the case vignette probably does not lie in the resident not knowing that the patient's family culture is influencing their request for the placement of a PEG tube. In cases such as that of Mr. AZ, commonly, a major root cause of the conflict between patients' families and physicians lies in the doctor's difficulty in understanding that their view of reality is not reality itself, but only a perception that was framed not only by the medical culture where they were educated and within which they practice, but also by other components of their cultural identity (e.g., ethnicity, gender, social class).[20,22] Indeed, the learning of medicine and other healthcare professions goes beyond acquiring factual technical knowledge and involves being immersed in a new culture. The problem is that healthcare professionals often have difficulty differentiating which components of their understanding of a given situation derive from technical facts (e.g., that PEG tubes are not better in extending the lives of people with advanced dementia than careful hand feeding by mouth[23,24]), from those that are shaped primarily by their culture (e.g., the meaning of suffering). Whenever healthcare professionals are not able to make that distinction, they cannot help but naturalize their own views/culture as the standard by which the patients' and their families' cultures must be judged. In those situations, healthcare professionals usually engage in communication processes where they believe it is their duty to persuade patients/families to adhere to the professionals' predefined plan. When patients/families resist, the conflict is often labeled/misdiagnosed as a form of denial, and conversations may often stall and impart suffering to all parties involved. Perhaps one of the reasons that those conversations stall is that, in the first place, they were never real conversations with two sides listening to each other. We argue that it is almost impossible to truly listen to someone else when we are so convinced that ours is the only possible correct way to address a particular problem that we believe our job is just to sway that person in favor of our predefined solution.

Most important, we contend that we can only be truly open to the ideas and views of someone else when we consider that person as having true value. Indeed, in sharp contrast to humility, arrogance stems from the belief that we are superior to others (i.e., that others have less value than we do). Interestingly, the concept of dignity in healthcare has been linked to how people perceive themselves as reflected through the eyes of the other.[25] Therefore, we reason that the necessary openness to the views of patients and their families that is embodied by cultural humility is an essential component of dignity-conserving care.[26]

In the same way that we can only see our own eyes through their reflection in a mirror or picture, we need humility to take a step back and start questioning through self-reflection and self-critique the extent to which our own beliefs and cultural identities are shaping our judgments toward our patients, their families, and communities. This questioning leads to reflecting on and acting on our prejudices and implicit biases, helping to build transparent and trustful relationships with patients and colleagues. We need humility to acknowledge that our views may be wrong, that our knowledge is imperfect, and that real-life situations are way more complex than textbooks.

Interestingly, Paulo Freire argued that one of the essential elements that make us humans is our ability to recognize our own incompleteness, our own unfinishedness.[16] He argued that it is through the recognition that humans are able to engage in learning and education that they may grow less incomplete, step by step. By acknowledging our unfinishedness and imperfections as a central component of our own humanity, we not only become less insecure about ourselves, but also more open to revisiting our own beliefs and learning from the perspectives of others. That understanding is completely aligned with the principles of cultural humility. It has been argued that cultural humility, more than a concept, is a framework that contributes to achieving the goal of partnering with individuals and populations with a sense of equity and respect: a framework that can be used to build mutual trust relationships and understand the root causes of suffering.[27] This is why we believe that cultural humility is central for a professionalism of solidarity worthy of its name. However, discussions around cultural humility are often restricted to the scope of the behavior of individuals. An intrinsic limitation of that approach is that it falls short of confronting major contextual elements that undermine the practice of a professionalism of solidarity. In the next section, we address that issue.

Professionalism, Administrative Evil, and the Lucifer Effect

A 20-year-old male, AM, with severe intellectual developmental disorder is cared for by his mother, who assists him in all his basic activities of daily living, including feeding, mobility, and toileting. He has limited speech and engages in self-injurious behavior when under stress. Around six months into the COVID-19 pandemic, he was brought to an emergency department due to respiratory symptoms and mildly decreased peripheral oxygen saturation ($SpO_2 \approx 91\%$). When the diagnosis of COVID-19 was confirmed, the attending physician explained to his mother that AM would be hospitalized and kept isolated following the hospital's standard procedures. His mother became immediately very distressed and argued that if her son were kept isolated from her in an empty room for the duration of his hospitalization, this would cause him so much suffering that it would equal torture. The attending responded that this was a standard procedure for all patients with COVID-19, which avoids the dissemination of SARS-CoV-2 (severe acute respiratory syndrome coronavirus 2) in the hospital, and that there was nothing that he could do to change that rule. He tried to explain that if AM would become agitated that he would be sedated. However, his mother, a former nurse who had quit the profession to care for her son, correctly counterargued that if she were allowed to be by his side, there would be no need to sedate him, and that sedating him could contribute to the worsening of his health status. In her despair, she threatened to take him home instead of allowing him to be hospitalized in an isolation room.

The case above describes a situation that is compatible with the definition of *administrative evil*, a term coined by Adams and Balfour in 1998 to denote a masked form of evil whereby ordinary people inflict pain and suffering on others but do so in the course of performing their organizational roles seemingly appropriately.[28] Many would easily claim that the physician, in that case, cannot be blamed for just following orders. Nevertheless, by so doing, they would be missing several relevant issues, as follows: First, although institutional protocols are often developed considering the average patient and may include the most appropriate decisions for the majority of the population, they may be insufficient to address significant issues related to the needs of specific vulnerable groups, as exemplified by those with severe disabilities. It is critical to consider that organizational protocols, like every human endeavor, are prone to imperfections and may require improvements and revisions. They should not be static and are not the ultimate representation of the greater good bestowed on organizations by omniscient heavenly beings. They are dynamic expressions of administrative decisions that change over time according to the balance of power and relative importance of competing values within institutions. Second, a simple examination of the bigger picture of how hospitals have dealt with the COVID-19 pandemic would show that children hospitalized due to that infection outside of intensive care units were not separated from their parents during their hospital stay because it was evident that keeping those children with their parents was necessary for their physical and mental well-being. Since adults with severe mental disability are often more dependent on their caregivers than many children are on their parents, and the suffering inflicted on them by such forced isolation may be even more pronounced, it is hard to justify different policies for children and adults with such conditions. Last, from the healthcare professionals' perspective, it is usually much easier to deny responsibility by claiming they were just following superior orders than to question the morality of administrative guidelines within highly hierarchically structured healthcare organizations.

As explained by Adam and Balfour, administrative evil is often difficult to identify and results directly from the culture of technical rationality, which is fairly strong in the field of healthcare.[28] We call particular attention to four enablers of administrative evil. First, language plays a pivotal role. The use of euphemisms and technical terms provides emotional distancing and prevents us from making the connection between our actions and moral categories such as good and evil, right and wrong. For example, during the Holocaust, the term "final solution" was used as a code word for killing, and "resettlement" was used to make the evacuation of an entire community to forced labor sound socially appropriate. Second, the representation of individuals as "bad people" or "not normal" leads to their dehumanization, which decreases the possibility of empathizing with and caring for them. The dehumanization of others may be marked, as in the Rwandan genocide of 1994, when the Tutsi minority was described in mainstream Rwandan radio stations as "cockroaches" or "snakes,"[29] or more subtly, for example, when healthcare professionals label certain patients as "multiple-complaint users."[30] Third, humans function in a mental autopilot characterized by automatic and learned behaviors during considerable portions of our daily lives.[31] That mechanism is essential for providing efficiency to many of our actions by sparing us from overthinking about actions and behaviors in familiar tasks, such as when driving home after work. Of course, the human brain also can develop adaptive responses to environmental changes by engaging other brain areas, such as the prefrontal cortex, outside the so-called default mode network responsible for those automatic behaviors. The problem is that, because administrative evil is usually masked within situations that we take for granted, we often fail to recognize the need to reconsider standard learned behavior of following organizational rules even when those rules harm others. Critical thinking over automatic behaviors is probably most challenging when working in time-pressured environments, such as in emergency departments and primary care. Fourth, hubris, as represented by a sense of inflated pride or superiority toward others, often contributes to our inability to turn off our automatic behaviors and question the morality or correctness of our actions.

Previously in this chapter, we argued that professionalism happens in the world, and that the teaching of professionalism should take place in real-life settings. A direct corollary of such an understanding is that the very environment where educational and clinical interactions take place influences the practice and learning of professionalism/unprofessionalism. By environment, we mean much more than the spatial characteristics of where those interactions take place. We mean both the explicit and implicit organizational and cultural rules that convey subtle yet powerful messages regarding what is valued and what is acceptable or not within healthcare institutions. Indeed, much of the literature about the all-too-common phenomenon of empathy decline and rising cynicism that happens along the process of medical education traces its origins to problems related to the hidden curriculum of healthcare organizations.[32,33] Declining empathy and rising cynicism have hugely negative implications regarding any form of professionalism defined as an endeavor aimed at building trustworthy relationships.

Social psychology experiments conducted in the 1960s and 1970s, such as Stanley Milgran's studies on obedience and authority[34] and Philip Zimbardo's Stanford prison experiment, have established how situational forces related to the social dynamics of power may influence ordinary people into engaging in behaviors that impart suffering on others, which was coined "the Lucifer Effect"[35]

We argue that developing a professionalism of solidarity should be rooted in both individual and organizational practices. Those practices involve, for example, promoting the principles of cultural humility as central components of interactions among people in healthcare; stimulating critical thinking about our own actions and organizational rules; allowing time to think through the possible unwanted consequences of individual decisions and administrative policies; promoting a diverse and safe work environment where different views are treated with respect; encouraging admission of individual and organizational mistakes as the first step in their mitigation; and discouraging ethical transgressions such as lying, cheating, and bullying through effective institutional policies.

Conclusion

We are hopeful that, in the next decades, we will witness the medical community embracing the complexity of the medical practice while developing a critical consciousness capable of igniting a continuous cycle of reflection and action toward promoting social justice. This critical consciousness, the base of a professionalism of solidarity, may inspire our community to empower patients; fight against injustice; promote diversity, equity, and inclusion; embrace interprofessional collaboration; and change cowardly structures of power. This new professionalism is only possible if we engage in a dialogical and democratic relationship with ourselves, our patients, and the communities we serve. The professionalism of solidarity is one of connection and love.

References

1. Cruess RL, Cruess SR. Professionalism, communities of practice, and medicine's social contract. *J Am Board Family Med.* 2020;33(suppl):S50–S56.
2. Razack S, de Carvalho Filho MA, Merlo G, Agbor-Baiyee W, de Groot J, Reynolds PP. Privilege, social justice and the goals of medicine: towards a critically conscious professionalism of solidarity. *Perspect Med Educ.* 2022;11(2):67–69.
3. Freire P. *Education for Critical Consciousness.* Vol 1. Bloomsbury Publishing; 1973:168.
4. Freire P. *Pedagogy of the Oppressed.* Bloomsbury Publishing USA; 2018:232.

5. Tervalon M, Murray-Garcia J. Cultural humility versus cultural competence: a critical distinction in defining physician training outcomes in multicultural education. *J Health Care Poor Underserved.* 1998;9(2):117–125.
6. Veitch S, Christodoulidis E, Goldoni M. *Jurisprudence: Themes and Concepts.* Routledge: Abingdon, Oxon; 2018:350.
7. Duracinsky M, Marcellin F, Cousin L, et al. Social and professional recognition are key determinants of quality of life at work among night-shift healthcare workers in Paris public hospitals (AP-HP ALADDIN COVID-19 survey). *PloS One.* 2022;17(4):e0265724.
8. Cruess RL, Cruess SR. Expectations and obligations: professionalism and medicine's social contract with society. *Perspect Biol Med.* 2008;51(4):579–598.
9. Prasad S, Alwan F, Evert J, Todd T, Lenhoff F. How the social contract can frame international electives. *AMA J Ethics.* 2019;21(9):742–748.
10. Manca A, Gormley GJ, Johnston JL, Hart ND. Honoring medicine's social contract: a scoping review of critical consciousness in medical education. *Acad Med.* 2020;95(6):958–967.
11. Hafferty FW, Castellani B. The increasing complexities of professionalism. *Acad Med.* 2010;85(2):288–301.
12. Rockich-Winston N, Taylor TR, Richards JA, White D, Wyatt TR. "All patients are not treated as equal": extending medicine's social contract to Black/African American communities. *Teach Learn Med.* 2021;34(3):238–245.
13. Roberts LW. High road, low road: professionalism, trust, and medical education. *Acad Med.* 2020;95(6):817–818.
14. Szulewski A, Howes D, van Merriënboer JJ, Sweller J. From theory to practice: the application of cognitive load theory to the practice of medicine. *Acad Med.* 2020;96(1):24–30.
15. Ribeiro DL, Costa M, Helmich E, Jaarsma D, de Carvalho-Filho MA. "I found myself a despicable being!": medical students face disturbing moral dilemmas. *Med Educ.* 2021;55(7):857–871.
16. Freire P. *Pedagogy of Freedom: Ethics, Democracy, and Civic Courage.* Rowman & Littlefield Publishers; 2000:176.
17. Freire P, Ara AM. *Pedagogy of the Heart.* Bloomsbury Publishing USA; 1998.
18. Shapiro J, Whittemore A, Tsen LC. Instituting a culture of professionalism: the establishment of a center for professionalism and peer support. *Jt Comm J Qual Patient Saf.* 2014;40(4):168–177.
19. Hook JN, Davis DE, Owen J, Worthington EL, Utsey SO. Cultural humility: measuring openness to culturally diverse clients. *J Couns Psychol Adv.* 2013;60(3):353–366.
20. Taylor JS. Confronting "culture" in medicine's "culture of no culture." *Acad Med.* 2003;78(6):555–559.
21. Cain CL, Surbone A, Elk R, Kagawa-Singer M. Culture and palliative care: preferences, communication, meaning, and mutual decision making. *J Pain Symptom Manage.* 2018;55(5):1408–1419.
22. Goold SD, Williams B, Arnold RM. Conflicts regarding decisions to limit treatment: a differential diagnosis. *JAMA.* 2000;283(7):909–914.
23. Davies N, Barrado-Martín Y, Vickerstaff V, et al. Enteral tube feeding for people with severe dementia. *Cochrane Database Syst Rev.* 2021;(8).
24. American Geriatrics Society Ethics Committee and Clinical Practice and Models of Care Committee. American Geriatrics Society feeding tubes in advanced dementia position statement. *J Am Geriatr Soc.* 2014;62(8):1590–1593.

25. Chochinov HM. Dignity and the eye of the beholder. *J Clin Oncol.* 2004;22(7):1336–1340.
26. Chochinov HM, Tataryn D, Clinch JJ, Dudgeon D. Will to live in the terminally ill. *Lancet.* 1999;354(9181):816–819.
27. Chavez V. Cultural humility: people, principles & practices. 2022. Accessed March 6, 2022. http://www.ces4health.info/find-products/view-product.aspx?code=XT4NJRJP
28. Adams GB, Balfour DL. *Unmasking Administrative Evil.* Routledge; 2014.
29. Ndahiro K. In Rwanda, we know all about dehumanizing language. *The Atlantic.* 2019. Accessed March 06, 2022. https://www.theatlantic.com/ideas/archive/2019/04/rwanda-shows-how-hateful-speech-leads-violence/587041/
30. Vescovi RGL, Souza LGS, Avellar LZ. Multiple complaints users: social representations built by the primary health care doctors. *Psicol Estud.* 2015.
31. Vatansever D, Menon DK, Stamatakis EA. Default mode contributions to automated information processing. *Proc Natl Acad Sci U S A.* 2017;114(48):12821–12826.
32. Neumann M, Edelhäuser F, Tauschel D, et al. Empathy decline and its reasons: a systematic review of studies with medical students and residents. *Acad Med.* 2011;86(8):996–1009. doi:10.1097/ACM.0b013e318221e615
33. Billings ME, Lazarus ME, Wenrich M, Curtis JR, Engelberg RA. The effect of the hidden curriculum on resident burnout and cynicism. *J Grad Med Educ.* 2011;3(4):503–510.
34. Milgram S. The dilemma of obedience. *Phi Delta Kappan.* 1974;55(9):603–606.
35. Zimbardo P. *The Lucifer Effect: How Good People Turn Evil.* Random House; 2011.

7

A Philosopher's Perspective

Aspirational Professionalism

David Ozar

Key Points

- While physicians begin to develop a sense of professionalism during medical school, the process of becoming and being a professional is a continual self-formation process that is lifelong.
- Professionalism education programs during undergraduate and graduate medical education should be structured to help learners become proficient in the skills necessary to engage in lifelong self-formation of their professionalism.
- Physicians need to develop an awareness and appreciation of the potential threats to professionalism that may affect them in independent practice, including those resulting from being fully responsible and accountable for a patient's care, different types of work environments and relationships, and commercial interests.

Introduction

Talk of professionalism can occur in many different contexts. Persons working in occupations not ordinarily considered professions or doing tasks not associated with the practice of a profession can nevertheless be described meaningfully as acting professionally. Sometimes this only means that this is how the person earns their living. But references to professionalism are more often used evaluatively to commend a person's technical proficiency or to commend how they relate to others while doing their work. In other words, they are being commended for acting "like a professional." That is, the most basic meaning of professionalism concerns how members of a profession are expected to act. It is widely accepted in our society (and in many other societies) that, when a person is admitted to a profession, the person takes on a set of additional obligations by doing so. Professionalism in this context points to the contents of this commitment to the society at large and to the other members of the profession that is made by every member of a profession. Professionalism in this context also implies, though it is not stressed as frequently, that the members of a profession commit themselves to making such changes in their lives as are necessary to dependably act in accord with these additional obligations and also commit themselves to assisting one another as colleagues in achieving this. It is these two meanings of professionalism that is the focus of this chapter.

Given this understanding of professionalism, it is clear that the professional formation of a physician is a long-term activity. While it begins in earnest in medical school during undergraduate medical education (UME) (assuming appropriate baselines through the medical school admissions process) and presumably continuing during graduate medical education (GME) programs, such as residencies and fellowships, a physician's professional formation does not end when the years of formal training are completed. It not only needs to continue, but also needs to increasingly become a self-directed process, a process of self-formation that is in fact a career-long, lifelong one. But for this to happen dependably and for it to be a dependable outcome of medical training rather than being the exception, effective education in the skills of self-formation, on which such long-term growth depends, needs to be a primary goal of and explicit focus of professionalism education in every medical school and every formal training program thereafter. This essay considers what a practicing physician's efforts at effective self-formation might look like in the years after formal medical training is done. But first we need to ask what medical schools, and then internship, residency, and postgraduate programs, need to do to contribute effectively to their students' lifelong medical professionalism by enhancing their skills in self-formation.

The professional formation of a physician necessarily attends to two different realms of physicians' professional life and practice. One focuses on the distinctive expertise of the medical profession by which physicians benefit the health of the individual patients and the public whom they serve. The goal of medical training and professionalism in this realm is, simply put, sufficient technical proficiency for the physician to practice independently. The other realm of medical professionalism concerns ethical values and conduct, the attitudes, relational skills, and habits that guide not only the physician's technical decisions, but also and especially the physician's relationships with those whom the physician serves and those who work with the physician in serving them. The appropriate educational outcomes and competencies for training medical students effectively in technical proficiency have been widely studied and are not discussed further here. But in the realm of ethical values and conduct, that is, medical professionalism, it is less clear how to effectively foster appropriate growth.

Professional Identity Formation

A large literature has grown up in search of clear answers to this concern about professional formation and in recent years has drawn valuably on the work of psychologists building on Erikson's theory of ego identity formation. Two of the leading contributors to medical education from this tradition, Cruess and Cruess, summarize this work:

> An extensive literature in developmental psychology illuminates how individuals develop a personal identity, and during the past decade, this scholarship has served as the basis of original and creative work examining the nature of physicians' professional identities and the factors that influence their emergence. . . . Conceptually, professional identity formation must be congruent with the processes through which human beings develop a personal identity. Psychological theories propose that individuals proceed through life continuously organizing their experiences into a meaningful whole that incorporates their personal, private, public, and professional "selves." As they pass through each stage, from infancy to childhood, adolescence, and beyond,

individuals gain experience and become capable of constructing an increasingly complex persona.[1] (p718)

This picture of physicians' growth as persons, including their growth in medical professionalism, has contributed a great deal to the understanding of professional formation in the medical schools and beyond. But it needs a conception of professionalism that explicitly incorporates its developmental perspective as aspirational professionalism does, and its practitioners, those guiding medical students and new physicians in their identity formation, need to incorporate into their pedagogies and learning outcomes mastery of the specific skills on which effective self-formation depends.

Aspirational Professionalism

The central thesis of this chapter is that professionalism formation in UME and GME must focus much more explicitly on the fact that professional formation is a long-term process and therefore that the most important educational outcomes of professional formation efforts during the training years are that the learners understand this fact and grow in proficiency in the skills of self-formation on which long-term success in professional self-formation depends. If this is the goal of professionalism education in UME and GME, then what picture of medical professionalism itself should these programs be communicating?

One picture of medical professionalism is as an "ideal" in the sense of the *complete* fulfillment of every positive aspect of conduct that the medical profession offers to individuals and to the community. In addition to the highest possible level of clinical skill in the service of individual patients and the public health, it includes ideal affective characteristics in relationships with patients, surrogates, families, and more, and in relationships with other professionals and coworkers, and in addition invariably correct ethical understanding and conduct in all matters.

Realistically, of course, such a condition is unachievable by actual human beings. Humans advance toward such an ideal only incrementally, and they invariably experience shortfalls in the process. Therefore, ideal professionalism is not a useful concept for physicians' professionalism education. Useful details about the contents of medical professionalism can certainly be found in medicine's professional societies' codes of medical ethics, in the scholarly literature on medical ethics, and also in the literature recounting the lives and qualities of admirable physicians. But even mastering such information is not itself sufficient for professional formation. More importantly, it would be very possible to interpret such resources as describing an unattainable ideal rather than being instrumental for developmental growth. What then is needed to guide learners in the kind of day-to-day effort required to make progress in professionalism is something "less ideal."

One of the problems with ideals is that they have no developmental component, no room for partial achievement, and no room for learning from shortfalls about what doing better looks like and then being motivated to reach for it rather than doubting it is too ideal to be reachable.

A further problem with ideals is that they are necessarily impersonal rather than articulated from within the lives and practice of actual, fallible physicians who are nevertheless genuinely admirable in important ways. Although cases in the medical ethics literature that are narrated in the first person can be an exception, abstractions alone, that is, abstractions that are not connected to some relevant person's motivation and effort, are frequently ineffective in changing an adult's, especially a young adult's, conduct.[a]

Therefore, the concept of professionalism that should guide educators in medical professionalism is what will here be called "aspirational professionalism." Its content, stated abstractly, is the values, attitudes, relational skills, and habits that are characteristic of admirable members of the medical profession. But for effective developmentally focused professional formation, the learners must encounter this concept, not as an abstract set of ideals, but as lived and practiced, that is, as the values, attitudes, relational skills, and habits of actual physicians rather than some abstract notion of an ideal physician. How this might look in practice is the focus of the next section.

Professional Formation in UME

Few students entering medical school will have personally experienced, much less carefully reflected on, the process of long-term self-formation that produces exemplary professionals, and few will have established the habits of self-reflection that make such growth possible. Therefore, for a medical school's professional formation program to be consistent with aspirational professionalism, the program should aim at cognitive and affective learning objectives that focus on this goal. The medical students need to acquire a clear understanding (cognitive) of aspirational professionalism and of what is needed to grow in it. But they also need to be guided to value (affective) aspirational professionalism and therefore also to value the kinds of reflection and effort that are the essential means to it.[b]

The Admission Process

The formation of aspirational professionalism specific to medicine begins during UME. But to make this possible, the admissions process needs to produce a group of learners who have made commitments to a social group that they have actively striven to fulfill and that are not only commitments to the applicant's own goals in spite of the intense competition characteristic of undergraduate premed experience. The prospective medical student may not have reflected carefully on the kind of commitments that the members of the medical profession make to the larger society.[c] But there needs to be evidence that he or she understands and has acted on commitments to a social group in order to benefit the group and ideally the larger society as well. The absence of such experiences in an applicant's background should raise serious questions about whether this person is capable of growing in medical professionalism during the medical school years.

[a] Another possible description of professionalism might be called "minimalist professionalism" because it focuses on the most obvious and basic standards of the medicine's ethics. It is what is ordinarily intended when conduct that falls short of these standards is declared *unprofessional*. An obvious example would be violating a patient's privacy by publicly sharing personal information about the patient without the patient's knowledge or consent. But this way of understanding medical professionalism asks far too little of trainees to be a focus or goal of professionalism education.[2]

[b] These cognitive and affective learning outcomes are described more fully in a white paper.[3]

[c] See "Professions and Professional Ethics" by David Ozar.[4]

Cognitive Learning Outcomes

There are three necessary cognitive learning outcomes. The first is understanding what is meant by aspirational professionalism. Otherwise, it is very likely that incoming UME students will think the goal is "ideal" professionalism and view professionalism as something that their medical training will automatically produce or, in more realistic moments, worry that they have no idea how to achieve it.

Second, cognitive learning needs to include the concrete contents of medical professionalism (i.e., the specific kinds of values, attitudes, relational skills, and habits that are characteristic of admirable members of the medical profession). Passive learning of the names and descriptions of these characteristics may help the students know what to look for, but most important is that they become able to identify specific instances of these characteristics as lived values, consistent attitudes, effective relational skills, and more of the physicians they actually encounter and in first- and third-person accounts of physician practice. Only when students are attentive to these characteristics as they are lived (and on their absence when they are missing) can they begin to imitate them. In addition to reading, discussing, and reflecting on first- and third-person accounts of physicians' practice, they will need honest, modest story sharing by ordinary good practitioners, including candid sharing of their shortfalls and their learning from these shortfalls.

In this connection, the students will definitely learn more effectively if they can process what they are learning in smaller groups where personal reflection and give-and-take conversation are possible rather than for a hundred students in a stacked lecture hall. As more fully examined in the chapters of the next section, small-group discussions, led by practicing physicians trained in facilitating open discussion or led by the students themselves, are the best means for drawing out and prompting reflection on what the students are observing.

The third cognitive learning outcome at the UME level is that the students first understand and appreciate that self-formation in professionalism involves a teachable skill set, and that, second, they learn what these skills are so they can begin to become proficient in developing them. The transition from learning about professionalism to professionalism becoming a matter of self-formation will only occur once this learning outcome is achieved. This skill set involves:

Self-assessment: the ability to earnestly reflect on one's behavior in relation to professionalism expectations.

Self-commendation: when one has acted professionally, recognition that one has done so and a commitment to act similarly in similar circumstances.

Self-correction: when one has acted unprofessionally, recognition of the behavior as unprofessional.and a commitment to modify one's behaviors toward avoiding similar future unprofessional acts.

Experience tells us that these skills are most easily learned by being practiced daily—ideally making time for them at the end of each day— not only to contribute effectively to the learner's growth in medical professionalism, but also to facilitate habituation of the skills themselves. Here, as above, there will be a place for didactic teaching, but more importantly students will need to be prompted to practice these skills and for educators to assess their contributions to the student's own growth. In addition, as above, students

Box 7.1 Cognitive Learning Objectives in Medical School Toward Aspirational Professionalism

By the completion of medical school training, learners should:

Know the differences between "Aspirational Professionalism" and "Ideal Professionalism."

Be able to identify "concrete" elements of medical professionalism in practice, or identify when there is an absence of these of these elements in practice:

- Values
- Attitudes
- Relational Skills
- Habits

Know and be able to utilize tools of continued self-formation post medical training, including:

- Self-assessment
- Self-commendation
- Self-criticism
- Self-correction

will need to be prompted and ideally provided with opportunities to share in small groups their experiences of self-assessment, self-commendation, and self-correction.

Affective Learning Outcomes

The corresponding affective learning outcomes concern students learning to value aspirational professionalism and the values, attitudes, relational skills, and habits of admirable physicians as these are lived. It has been known at least since Aristotle that the best way to guide a human to adopt new values and new ways of living is by directing their attention to characteristics they admire in others and prompting them to begin to imitate them. Most new medical students have encountered physicians whom they admire, and some of them will have known or worked with physicians concretely enough that the desire to become like them is motivationally effective. To build on this, the personal encounters with thoughtful, articulate physicians already described and the use of small-group discussions to facilitate careful reflection on what the students are observing will be the best ways to facilitate the students' growth in valuing these things.

It might be objected that students are quite capable of dissembling, of observing what is presented but not valuing it, and of saying what they know faculty want to hear. Ideally the admission process has made the presence of such students less likely. But if such resistance is encountered, unless the shortfall is severe enough to justify dismissal, any corrective actions employed by faculty must be explicitly from the perspective of aspirational professionalism. For valuing of the characteristics of admirable physicians to the point of striving to imitate them cannot be manufactured by coercion. It is only if a community of faculty, administrators, staff, and older students are genuinely committed to forming the school's newest students in aspirational professionalism and striving to live their own lives and to treat one another accordingly that the younger students will be motivated to value and begin to deliberately imitate the characteristics of admirable physicians.

Therefore, not only the professionalism education program, but also the school's institutional culture must uniformly indicate a clear commitment to forming the students in aspirational rather than ideal (much less minimal) professionalism.[1] The students will not dependably learn to value medical professionalism understood aspirationally unless it is the students' experience that, for every shortfall, even for conduct that falls short of the most obvious and basic standards of medicine's ethics, the responses of faculty, administrators, and staff to these shortfalls is consistent with aspirational professionalism. That is, they must experience this as an experience to be remembered and learned from, an indicator not merely that growth is needed, but also that growth is possible.[d]

The Didactic Versus Clinical Years

In this connection, faculty assessments of a student's progress in the technical content of medical expertise should also be expressed as much as possible from the point of view of aspirational professionalism and thus of developmental growth. The teaching of the technical subjects that dominates medical education in the didactic years can easily communicate a "yes or no" motivational message to the students: The message can easily be: "If you don't learn the relevant facts or if you don't learn how the procedure is done correctly, you may diagnose incorrectly or actually harm the patient, possibly hastening their death." It will take special effort, therefore, to structure how teaching and grading are done in technical fields so that, to the extent it is possible, even the technical subjects are being taught from the perspective of aspirational professionalism.

During the clinical years, even technical subjects are taught primarily by means of observation and imitation, that is, the same structure by which learning happens in the affective realm, and the strategies for forming students in medical professionalism recommended above and the small-group discussions described above should continue to be used during the clinical years where direct observation of practicing physicians is so prominent. Ideally, the clinical faculty in the various hospitals where the students rotate should be informed of the explicitly aspirational focus of the medical school's professional formation efforts and encouraged to work with the students accordingly.

GME Programs

By the time medical students are approaching residency or fellowship training, they will have had to make important life decisions about what kind of medicine they will practice and where. Many of them also will have had other life decisions to make by this time, and the same is even truer for postgrad programs. Some of these decisions may have focused their self-formation narrowly on technical expertise in spite of the medical school's efforts at professional formation. But most young physicians in GME programs have begun to

[d] The title of one of Charles Bosk's studies in the sociology of medicine is most apt in this connection.[5]

function as the principal actors in determining what kind of medical professionals they will become and have begun to employ the skills of self-assessment, self-commendation, and self-correction when needed at least in regard to their technical goals.

Regarding professional formation, if a GME program determines that its young physicians have not yet fulfilled the cognitive and affective learning objectives prescribed above for medical schools, its commitment to professionalism education would require it to establish those learning objectives as its own and devise educational programs to work toward them. In any case, every GME program should be prepared to assess its applicants accordingly. If these learning objectives have been achieved during medical school, then what the GME program needs to do to further the professional formation of its trainees is simpler. All that should be needed is for opportunity and appropriate prompting to be provided so that these young physicians can engage in small groups, either led by appropriate faculty or learner led, to continue the sharing their reflections on what they are observing about medical professionalism in the hospitals' practicing physicians and what they are learning from doing their own self-assessments. For if the above learning objectives have been achieved, the young doctors in these programs will not only be familiar with such conversations but also have learned to value them for the sake of their own and their colleagues' professional growth.

For the medical student, the most important challenge to the time and effort needed to achieve the learning objectives identified above is the immense amount of technical material to be mastered at the risk of missing a crucial fact or causal connection in a patient's presentation or botching an important procedure, not to mention failing a test or disappointing a faculty teacher or mentor, even if such shortfalls are in fact responded to in aspirational terms. In GME programs, however, the stakes are higher because it is actual patients that may be harmed by one's shortfall in expertise or suffer in other ways from one's failure to relate effectively, not to mention negative reports by teachers or mentors and potentially a dimmer future as a result, even if these shortfalls are responded to in aspirational terms. All throughout the training years, even when there is strong aspirational support in the institution's leadership and culture, the pressure to master medicine's constantly growing technical expertise will work to drain away the time and effort that is also needed to grow professionally. The learner needs be deliberately sensitive to this conflict of worthy goals and make it a practice to not shortchange his or her growth in medical professionalism as a result.

In addition, even during medical school, but especially during GME training, physicians will face many other challenges unrelated to mastering medical expertise and growing in medical professionalism. Mounting debt, relationship challenges, potential life commitments, as well as one's own and other's illnesses and deaths of dear ones, all can conflict with the time and effort needed to maintain one's professional growth. It is therefore important in each instance that, in addition to their individual efforts at self-formation in professionalism, there are both personal and institutional support systems that help prioritize young physicians' growth in professionalism along with their other important goals.

Self-Formation in Medical Practice and Some Barriers

Many of the questions that a practicing physician asks when acting professionally in any given situation will be worded in terms of "oughts" and "shoulds." But a central theme of this chapter is that answering such questions correctly depends first on asking: "What kind of physician am I?" and "What do I need to focus on to become the kind of physician I am striving to be?" So if the professionalism formation efforts during the training years have achieved their cognitive and affective goals, many of the should and ought questions that arise in daily practice will be easily answered, and the number of such questions that need to be explicitly addressed will gradually diminish as acting in ways consistent with medical professionalism becomes increasingly the focus of well-formed habits. Such a physician understands what growing in professionalism means and what skills are needed to do so successfully, as well as the kinds of time and effort that need to be culled from a busy life to do it.

If the professionalism formation efforts during the training years have not achieved their cognitive and affective goals, either because they were resisted by the physician-in-training or because of deficiencies in the professionalism education programs themselves, a physician committed to growing in professionalism has a lot of extra work to do. The cognitive and affective goals of professionalism education, and the specific learning outcomes described above, will need to become personal goals for such a physician, in addition to managing all the burdens and challenges of the daily practice of medicine and responding to the commitments and challenges the physician has outside the office. But if growing in professionalism is the physician's goal, there is no other way. This is why it is so important that UME and GME programs do not leave their learners to figure out professional self-formation later on their own.

Still, even the physician who has been well formed in professional growth during the training years will face new kinds of challenges to acting professionally when he or she enters daily practice as a fully trained, certified, and licensed physician. Few new physicians enter independent practice without an awareness, perhaps even the shock, of the burden of now being the fully responsible party for the diagnoses they make, the therapies they prescribe, and the procedures they perform. This burden includes legal responsibility as well, but for a physician committed to growing in professionalism, it is more often the burden of being fully responsible for changes in the patient's health and life that is felt most strongly. As the young physician responds to these feelings, it is the aspirational understanding of medical professionalism rather than the ideal understanding that yields the most appropriate understanding of what is going on, and is likely to be the most consoling as well.

A second important change when a physician's training years end is that the challenge of establishing an effective relationship with every patient is now fully this physician's responsibility. The care provided to patients during the training years is obviously better if it includes relating to patients respectfully but if the focus is on medical effectiveness, the trainee's role as a relator to patients is typically secondary. But when the training years are over, it is the new physician's relationship skills that every patient now depends on to receive respectful and effective care. Especially challenging patients, distrustful patients, uncertain family members, self-focused surrogates, and patients who see themselves as entitled cannot be "handed off" when you are the physician in charge. These challenges are even greater for physicians who rotate on and off service as hospitalists or as specialists at the request of an attending, where one must get to know one's patients very quickly to establish an effective and respectful relationship and where continuity of care depends on careful reports to the attending or on careful handoffs from the previous and to the next hospitalist in the rotation. Growing in these responsibilities and in the relational skills that are needed among caregivers is essential to a physician's growth as a professional and is, as above, best achieved by the physician who has an aspirational rather than ideal understanding of medical professionalism.

A third set of challenges that will become part of the new physician's life when the training years end concerns the commercial for-profit marketplace whose values and structures are so different from the service orientation of most dealings with patients during the training years. There are a number of different environments in which a new physician might practice. But every one of them is affected by the values and priorities of the commercial marketplace that challenge and can sometimes directly conflict with the values and priorities of medical professionalism.

For example, some new physicians join existing office-based practices and, depending on the new physician's status in the practice, as an employee or as the equivalent of a "junior partner," and the needs of the practice as a commercial enterprise will undoubtedly impact how he or she cares for patients. The same is true of those who become hospitalists or who join a hospital or system's large multispecialty group practice, even though the commercial decisions having the widest impact (whether it is a not-for-profit or a for-profit entity) will ordinarily be made by persons far removed from the physician's interactions with patients. The same is also true, though the structures may be different, for physicians who focus on public health, research, public service, or organizations committed to servicing the underserved. Healthcare in our society is much too closely joined to the commercial for-profit marketplace for a physician to think that serving one's patients professionally will not be challenged by the commercial marketplace's values and priorities.

The first requirement of medical professionalism regarding this challenge is to avoid overlooking it or ignoring it, but rather to examine the ways commercial concerns influence decisions that impact patient care directly or by their impact on physicians and other caregivers. Some of these impacts will be as obvious as inadequate staffing and time pressures that interfere with effective communication with patients and other caregivers. Others may be much subtler. But growing in professionalism first requires awareness of these challenges. A useful question to be asking is: "What would the public or my own patients think of my or my institution's commitment to medical professionalism if they looked carefully at the ways the values and priorities of the commercial market impact how my or this institution's patients are cared for?"

The second requirement would be action to address any shortfalls in medical professionalism caused by the impact of the commercial marketplace on patient care. What a new physician can do to lessen the negative impacts of the commercial marketplace will often seem very modest; but time in practice and increasing authority within the physician's institution can create opportunities for influencing institutional change. What is important in the meantime, and then as years in practice increase, is that one's commitment to medical professionalism does not permit either one's concern about the adverse impacts of the commercial marketplace on patient care or one's commitment to work for relevant change to become dulled. Continual awareness of shortfalls, including things that cannot be changed quickly, and a continual commitment to work to change them whenever and insofar as it is possible, is, after all, a central component of aspirational professionalism.

Many physicians in practice today are indeed admirable professionals, and the characteristics and skills that they have grown into admirable habits are indeed worthy of imitation by their younger colleagues and the students who are lucky enough to encounter them. But whatever actual training they received in professional formation was almost

Box 7.2 "Self-Formation" in Medical Practice

Challenges and barriers to medical professionalism in independent practice include:

Being responsible and accountable for developing effective patient-physician relationships.
Being responsible and accountable for the care provided to patients.
Being legally responsibility for care provided to patients.
Having to balance commercial interests.

certainly based on an ideal understanding of professionalism despite its inadequacies as a basis for professionalism education. What this chapter has argued is that the efforts of UME and GME programs to form their students in medical professionalism should instead be grounded in aspirational professionalism.

References

1. Cruess RL, Cruess SR, Boudreau JD, Snell L, Steinert Y. A schematic representation of the professional identity formation and socialization of medical students and residents: a guide for medical educators. *Acad Med.* 2015;90(6):718–725. doi:10.1097/ACM.0000000000000700
2. Brody H, Doukas D. Professionalism: a framework to guide medical education. *Med Educ.* 2014;48:980–987.
3. APHC Taskforce on Professionalism. White paper: defining medical professionalism. Academy for Professionalism in Health Care. May 2015; rev. March 1, 2019. https://doi.org/10.13140/RG.2.2.11070.29763. Accessed June 11, 2024.
4. Ozar DT. Professions and professional ethics. In; Jennings B, ed. *Encyclopedia of Bioethics,* Vol 5, 4th ed. Thomson/Gale; 2014:2526–2537.
5. Bosk C. *Forgive and Remember: Managing Medical Failure.* University of Chicago Press; 1979.

PART A: EPILOGUE

MEDICINE IN TWO WAYS

Thomas S. Inui

Making rounds in the US Public Health Service (USPHS) Indian Health Hospital in Albuquerque, New Mexico, was both familiar and exotically unfamiliar at the same time. Located just a parking lot and one ramp away from the University of New Mexico referral hospital and Cancer Center, the Indian Health Service (IHS) hospital was a small inpatient facility (thirty beds) with outpatient clinics for adults and children that operated five days a week, a clinical lab for basic hematology and chemistries, and a radiology suite. I had just finished my year as chief resident in internal medicine at Johns Hopkins Hospital. Dr. A. McGehee Harvey told me he selected me and a peer, Steve Achuff, for this role because "We were good at change." Fortunately, he was right. Over that special year, I coped with the unexpected loss of total vision in one eye (an episode of optic neuritis that largely resolved in several months but left me with scotomata and a lifetime worry about multiple sclerosis), surviving the rigors of fifteen-hour days in the hospital seeing patients and teaching, with every other Sunday off for rest. I turned in my whites to the Hopkins Hospital laundry, hopped into our VW 412 and motored west from Baltimore, through St. Louis, and down Route 66 to Santa Fe, New Mexico, then Albuquerque. Daily inpatient rounds and consultant visits to the seven southern Pueblos and Southwest Polytechnique Institute IHS clinic sites we served seemed like a role and a pace I could master. The southwest weather was sunny, and I had one of the best offices I ever occupied, a former four-bed bedroom with a wall of windows overlooking parking lots and the northern end of the Sandia Mountains.

There were some adjustments to be made medically. There were no Black patients in the hospital, no patients with sickle cell disease, and no patients with heroin complications. We admitted a patient with fever and a bubo, who had been camping close to a prairie dog colony (plague?). Alcoholism and its complications were evident, type 2 diabetes was practically a normal physiologic state, but there was virtually no ischemic heart or peripheral vascular disease. I got called to the adult outpatient clinic by an excited physician's assistant the first time a patient with chest pain and a classic electrocardiogram for an acute inferior myocardial infarction showed up. The patient had driven himself in from 40 miles away in a pickup truck. "Doc, I've never seen this on an EKG! What is it?" asked the PA. On the wards, there was a mix of Pueblo and Navajo patients. There was a mix of short-stay admissions in need of diagnosis and management of acute conditions and patients with longer, even indeterminate-length stays. The former patients were hospitalized for such conditions as regulating their diabetes regimens, pneumonia, and cellulitis treatment. The long-stay patients had cancer requiring radiotherapy or chronic renal failure requiring hemodialysis. They were in Albuquerque because there were no dialysis centers or radiotherapy units on the eastern Big Navajo reservation. Some of the oldest patients and most of the Navajo spoke little or no English. This made communication on ordinary matters a challenge. I rounded daily with one of the other doctors, the floor nurse, and our hospital social worker, Vi. She was truly bicultural and had been drafted during World War II by the army to serve as a "code talker," baffling the Japanese listening to US armed forces radio transmissions in the South Pacific by simply speaking straight Navajo. "No other language like it in the world, and none of the Japanese had ever studied it at places like Harvard!" said Vi.

On rounds, Vi handled or passed along to us many questions from curious patients and their families. The following are examples:

> What are these doctors doing when they walk around and study the charts that hang on our beds? What secret things are nurses writing about us on these charts? Why do they stand here and talk to one another? They don't even talk right. They interrupt one another and don't wait—after one of them talks—to see that first one has finished talking before saying something themselves. How come they tell us that they have medicines to treat us, but they never bring that medicine? Instead, one of these other people, the ladies, brings pills to us or hangs a bag of water on this pole. What are they doing with the blood they take from us and what do they do with it if there is some left over? Why do they keep talking about bad things that could happen to me? Don't they know that talking about these bad things actually makes them happen? Why do they keep sending me next door to the big hospital? Don't they know that hospital used to belong to us and we gave it away to the White People in return for free medical care forever. It turned out 'forever' was less than 10 years. Now they make us pay to go there.

Vi had her hands full of questions on rounds.

One patient admitted to our wards was particularly challenging on all fronts. She was an elderly Navajo woman who was febrile and only minimally responsive. Her chest x-ray showed evidence of possible active pulmonary tuberculosis, and her cerebrospinal fluid had elevated protein and some round cells. We thought she might have tuberculosis meningitis and tried to communicate the seriousness of her condition to her family, several of whom had accompanied her to the hospital. The family seemed to understand a good deal of what we were saying, but were adamant that she would not be sent next door to the big hospital or would stay in the Indian Hospital. They seemed to be about to take her away, back to their summer lean-to on the Rez. "Haven't people died here?" they asked. "Yes, but if we treat your mother with strong medicines, she doesn't have to die." I said with Vi's consecutive translation. "If she isn't eating, then she needs medicines put into her blood as well as in her mouth." We went around and around and finally (with Vi's help) we got it. If dineh (the Navajo people) die inside, their spirits are trapped and are angry. They make the sick even sicker and any others inside can also die. "Haven't many people died here?" To leave their mother in this "house of dead spirits" was to condemn her to certain death. What now?

> "Well," we said, "Now we think we understand some of your worries. How about this: this hospital has an outside deck area off the hallway on the second floor. We usually don't have any patients out there, but if we wheeled a bed out there with some other stuff we use to give medicines, the nurses could come out there to treat her. It's cold at night, but this time of year there's no rain and not too much wind. You could take blankets out there to keep her warm. No fires, please! We could provide water and

food if she'll eat. You can bring chairs or we can loan some to you so a family member can sit with her. What do you think?"

And we stood in silence waiting for them to speak [pause, pause . . .], just as they had listened to us in silence until they knew we had finished speaking. "We think we understand your worries," they said. "But how long will she have to say here?" [Pause, pause. . . .] "Maybe four weeks, maybe the whole moon." [Pause, pause. . . .] "That's a long time. If she needs to have a sing, can a blessing way be done here?" [Pause, pause. . . .] "If you want to do this, we will try to make space out there to do it." [Pause, pause. . . .] OK? OK . . . OK. . . .

Thanks, Vi. Medicine in two ways.

After reading this story, try using an exegesis method to explore its content.

1. Who in this story can I see as myself?
2. From the point of view of whomever you have chosen, what do you bring to the situation that makes these events possible?
3. Who else in this story (or its organizational or cultural context) influences this story?
4. Where/what in this story is "the good," the value, the virtue, the "North Star" or the principle we might seek to preserve?
5. What, then, ought I do?

PART B

UNDERSTANDING AND EDUCATING FOR MEDICAL PROFESSIONALISM ALONG THE CONTINUUM OF PHYSICIAN PRACTICE

8
Faculty Development for Professionalism

Marin Gillis and Judy Bolstad

Key Points

- Most clinical educators have little or no formal education on medical professionalism and are therefore unprepared to teach, assess, and role-model the lessons taught in the preclinical curriculum.
- Clinical educators are highly influential for inculcating, assessing, and role-modeling professionalism.
- Clinical educators need faculty development toward developing professional identities as educators.

Clinical Educators Need Development in Professionalism

It should be uncontroversial to say that educators should only be entrusted to teach when they possess the knowledge and skills to do so. When it comes to teaching professionalism, however, medical education has a problem: Those who have a great impact on students' professional identity formation, clinical educators, have not been adequately prepared to teach, assess, or role-model professionalism. This is not to say that these educators are necessarily unprofessional. Rather, it is to acknowledge that professionalism in medical education has been understood and taught differently over the years, and that current practicing physicians need explicit training to be the most effective clinical educators for our next generation of physicians.

Medical practice is a multifaceted and demanding enterprise that requires individual practitioners to apply scientific knowledge to support the health and address the suffering of individual patients, who have their own preferences, values, and agency. This is performed while working within complex systems of healthcare payment and delivery and social structures that are not inclusive, diverse, or equitable. For a significant number of physicians, the practice of medicine also involves teaching medical students and residents. The educator role of medical practitioners has been documented since the Hippocratic oath: Oath takers swear to respect and support their own teachers and to share medical knowledge with others who want to learn.[1,2] One needs to keep in mind what the practice of medicine entails to understand what it means to be a medical professional, and since the practice has been defined, medicine has included the directive to educate the next generation and thereby sustain the practice.

Teaching students how to be physicians is not exhausted by imparting bioscientific content, and the so-called art of medicine cannot be instilled only through role-modeling because the art, which has always seemed to refer to anything else that was not biomedical science, now includes evidence-based content in a wide number of subject areas. The human body is complex, and to manage this complexity, medical practice is divided into specialties. Moreover, advancing patient and population health and easing suffering are also too complicated for a single profession (medicine) and indeed, a single sector (healthcare). Reforms in medical education aspire to include instruction in relevant nonbiomedical sciences through a well-thought-out curriculum developed and delivered by teams of educators that include clinicians as well as professors and other experts in fields like education, humanities, social and behavioral sciences, public health, law, policy, business, and data science. Together they develop educational interventions to prepare students to practice medicine in contemporary healthcare settings that recognize health equity as a mission. This is a different medical education than most practicing clinicians received. More than 50% of physicians practicing in 2020 would have graduate medical school before professionalism and ethics were included in the formal curriculum.[3]

Medical education is a perennial pursuit for the practitioner. Lifelong learning is a professional obligation because of bioscientific knowledge's exponential growth,[4] research progress in areas that bolster the medical mission, the so-called art of medicine, and for the medical educator, curricular evolution in academic medicine. Preparing medical students to be lifelong learners themselves and developing effective continuing medical education systems is a professional obligation of medicine.

Toward a Better Professionalism Education

Historically, professionalism was inculcated through role-modeling, recitation of oaths, and solitary contemplation, but was not part of the formal (unhidden) medical school curriculum. In 1997, Cruess and Cruess argued that this resulted in a state of affairs where: "Most doctors do not fully understand the obligations they must fulfill to satisfy public expectations and maintain professional status."[5(p1674)] The Cruesses argued that physicians should learn the "origins and nature" of their obligations as professionals and that professionalism concepts should be formally addressed and assessed in the curriculum.[5] Significantly, this movement in education revealed that professionalism, like the rest of medical school curricula, requires an understanding of concepts, practice applying the concepts, and ultimately opportunities for the trainee to operationalize them in various aspects of medical practice; these include, but are not limited to, the underlying values and goals of medical practice, the virtues of the practitioner, and the relationship between professionals and society.[6,7] The argument for explicitly teaching medical professionalism, not just the expected behaviors of medical professionals, was that if medical students are taught their professional obligations, virtues, and values early, they would become internalized so that students could employ them when they started training in the clinical setting.

Professionalism instruction was accordingly introduced in the foundational years of medical school. These science-dense, mostly preclinical, years have not proven ideal for acceptance and appreciation of professionalism by students. The comparatively small amount of curricular time and space on examinations reveals to students that it has little relevance or value. While Step One of the US Medical Licensing Examination includes professionalism, ethics, and law, often the multiple-choice questions on professionalism are exhausted by legal topics like third-party permission for treatment, impaired physicians, and reporting guidelines. Of course, these topics are essential to professional medical practice, but they do not capture the often complicated and nuanced aspects of practice that require, in addition to content knowledge, skill development to deal with ambiguity that includes improving students' moral discernment and imagination, critical and creative thinking, and moral courage.

Professionalism topics are often absent from the clinical curriculum, and when they are present, they are usually taught by foundational year faculty who guide students through thinking about situations they have encountered rather than ensuring that clinical preceptors themselves integrate and discuss aspects of professionalism explicitly as part of clinical training.

Further, students who were taught professionalism in foundational coursework perceived their lessons to be corrupted or optional in clinical settings when they witnessed physicians practicing in ways that seemed inconsistent with their professionalism lessons.[8,9] It may be the case that what students interpreted as unprofessional was acceptable practice, but learners and teachers lacked a shared professionalism vocabulary with which to explore deeper or unspoken aspects of the situation that warranted the clinician's actions.

In the wake of the concern over the erosion of professionalism lessons in the clinical years, there has been an explicit shift in thinking about inculcating professionalism in students from teaching professionalism to supporting students as they develop their own professional identities.[10] Professional identity formation is described as "a representation of self, achieved in stages over time during which the characteristics, values, and norms of the medical profession are internalized, resulting in an individual thinking, acting, and feeling like a physician."[11(p1447)] Proponents note: "The acquisition of a professional identity by physicians is not a new phenomenon. Although the term was not used until recently, it has represented a foundational element of medical education for centuries, having been characterized in the past by words such as 'character' or possessing the right 'characteristics.'"[10(p647)]

This shift to "developing professional identity" as a learning objective puts the onus on the learners who seek to join medicine's community of practice and recognizes that "only the learner can determine who they wish to become."[10(p645)] Issues that raise professionalism concerns are often psychologically and morally distressing and may have cascading effects if not addressed.[12] Students' inexperience can amplify their sensitivity to professionalism issues because they lack a nuanced appreciation of the larger medical systems. A shared language and understanding of professionalism are important for students and clinical educators to cope with and learn from these situations when they arise. Guided and structured introspection activities are an important tool in the communities of practice model, with introspection guided by clinicians being particularly valuable.[13]

Communities of practice is a pedagogy to foster medical student professional identity formation.[10] It involves a recognition that medical practice is inherently a collegial endeavor and has its own structure as a learning community.[10(p644)] Acquiring a professional identity is part of fully joining the community. It is recommended that educational activities be directed at fostering students' self-images as members of the community who follow the norms and internalize the values of the medical profession. Proponents of this shift argue that the change in focus will make teaching professionalism more effective and efficient.[10] However, when educational attention is on the learners rather than teachers, the importance of role-modeling on professional identity formation may be unintentionally neglected. We believe that this shift in thinking rightly recognizes that practicing physicians already have a professional identity, but it does so without scrutinizing when and how those identities were formed.

To serve as sufficient role models, clinical educators need to exemplify the professional virtues and values academic medicine seeks to instill in students. This is a concordance measure to ensure that the lessons they instill are what the medical students, as future professionals, need to learn to address the health needs of patients and to practice in line with the values and goals of contemporary medicine.

Scholarship on teaching professionalism consistently shows that role modeling and experiential learning make a significant impact on what students internalize about their professional responsibilities.[10,14] Most clinical physicians were trained before 2000 and likely were not formally trained in professionalism. Indeed, today there are approximately more than 75,000 practicing physicians nationwide who graduated from medical school before 1976, more than a decade prior to formal inclusion of professionalism in the curriculum.[3] These most experienced physicians, who are more likely to be in clinical and administrative leadership positions, are the products of education that was less inclusive than today of female, minority, and students with disabilities and where hazing and other questionable rites of passage were present. As medical education becomes more inclusive, the number of reports of sexism, racism, and ableism in medical education increase and are higher than those from students in other disciplines documented by the National Academies of Sciences, Engineering, and Medicine.[15,16]

This is not to argue that all older physicians are sexist, racist, or ableist or that younger physicians lack these unconscious attitudes. Older physicians were, however, educated in a system where racism, sexism, and ableism were not universally excluded. When instituting curricular reforms aimed at significant change in medical practice, it is not enough to change the education of current students who will be sent out to practice with, be mentored by, and report to older, experienced, and highly valuable senior physicians. Curriculum designers must consider how currently practicing physicians were educated and what their professional identities entail and take deliberate action to ensure that they are prepared to instantiate, instill, and assess students based on professional values.

In a commentary addressing the many reports outlining vital changes needed to ensure the functioning of the academic health center (AHC), Davis and colleagues warn of the "lack of preparedness for clinical, educational, and even research changes on the part of nearly all faculty substantially limits any lasting reform."[17(p1079)] There is an assumption in reform proposals that faculty will "acquire new competencies and adopt new roles automatically or with minimal training or feedback."[17(p1079)] Davis and colleagues refer to this oversight as "a large 'elephant in the room' in the house of academic medicine."[17(p1079)]

The elephant in the room with professionalism education reform is that the clinical educators, on whom so much of medical education depends, are not supported as educators. The inclusion of professionalism in the preclinical medical curriculum, paired with the clinical faculty's level of facility with current literature on teaching professionalism—including terminology, underlying concepts, values, and principles—has led to a phenomenon where the formal professionalism lessons were almost expected to trickle up to clinical educators and out to the greater community of medical practice. Clinician educators are both clinicians and educators, and they can be considered professionals in each domain. Continuing medical education requirements for licensure and certification ensure that clinicians meet the professional obligation to keep up with advancing medical knowledge. Clinician educators must also be supported and developed as educators on advancements in the science of teaching and learning and on professionalism curriculum through programs of continuing professional development.

Clinical Faculty in the Academy

We have located a significant challenge in professionalism education that emerges from considerations of the importance of clinical educators in medical education. In this section we elaborate the organizational or systems issues that exacerbate this challenge toward finding a remedy to it. By looking at the spaces where medical education takes place and the years that learners spend there, the importance and influence of clinical educators in the delivery of undergraduate and graduate medical education becomes clear. In the United States and Canada, medical school is usually four years long, with the first two years traditionally dedicated to learning basic science material and the last two years dedicated to applying that basic science knowledge on various clinical rotations. This approach has changed somewhat over the past twenty years, but regardless of whether learning durations are described in term of years, periods, blocks, or phases, most curricula remain adaptations of the "two-and-two" model.[18]

Clinical education follows an apprenticeship approach as medicine is a practice that involves the application of knowledge, demonstration of skills, and operationalization of social values in a healthcare setting. The pedagogies used to teach clinical applications include cases, simulations, shadowing physicians, and peer-teaching opportunities. The adage, "see one, do one, teach one," attributed to the founder of the Johns Hopkins surgery residency, William Stewart Halstead,[19] summarizes this apprenticeship approach: First directly observe a task being performed, engage in hands-on practical experience by performing the task oneself under watchful eyes, and eventually show someone else how to perform the task. Learning through immersion in the future work environment allows learners to become progressively trustworthy at performing a task first with help toward mastery to practice autonomously. Of course, medical education has evolved with evidence-based active learning methodologies and high-tech simulations, but clinical pedagogy remains pretty much in line with the signature adage.

According to the American Hospital Association, there are over 1,000 teaching hospitals in the United States. Referred to as AHCs, these institutions train more than 75% of residents (graduate medicine education) and may include medical schools or be closely associated with medical schools (undergraduate medical education).[20] Nontraditional "community-based" medical schools are not integrated into an AHC system, but they also rely on clinical educators who work in hospitals as well as private clinical spaces in the medical school's geographic area.[21]

Clinical faculty are the backbone of medical education. These faculty are physicians who have appointments to occasionally teach, but for whom patient care remains a primary duty. Usually unpaid, they are sometimes referred to as voluntary-track faculty; they are appointed to medical schools with titles such as clinical instructor, clinical assistant, clinical associate, and clinical full professor; this is a parallel track to those physicians, PhDs, and others, whose primary appointments are in medical schools as professional educators. It may also be referred to as a courtesy appointment, recognizing their contribution to the education mission. Through their appointment, they are officially acknowledged as affiliated with the medical academy, the institution that creates and assesses evidence-based medical practice and admission to the practice. Clinical faculty are often given a medical school email address, usually only used to log into online course grade books, access to the medical school library, which they usually do not need if they already have access to robust hospital library services, and they may use their academic title professionally, under condition that the appointment remains up to date.

Often, promotion for clinician faculty is a matter of the number of years at a rank; usually it is five years before one is advanced, but it is not uncommon to find physicians who hold an assistant clinical professor rank for more than a decade. Advancement of clinical faculty does not follow traditional academic promotion that sees increasing responsibility and evidence of excellence as teachers, as knowledge generators, and as leaders directing and advancing the education, research, or clinical missions of academic medicine. The great need for clinical placements prompts the recruitment of clinicians to teach more than a clinician's passion for education and desire to be developed as a medical academician. For present purposes, it is worth noting that this educational necessity makes it difficult to standardize student experiences across clinical sites and relies heavily on the professionalism of the volunteer faculty to fuel excellence in role modeling.

Recognizing that hospital-based practicing physicians are vital to the education of future physicians, the American Medical Association (AMA) recently published concerns and guidance towards safeguarding the education mission of medicine, threatened in the wake of a strained and broken healthcare system due to the COVID-19 pandemic.[22] Already aware of structural social and economic challenges in academic medicine that make a great impact on medicine's social contract with society, something noted by the National Medical Association since its inception in 1895, the AMA's message is important, relevant, and powerful. If hospitals are beyond capacity, the educational mission of medicine will flounder, and if it is not revitalized, the future of medicine is at risk. The AMA guidance brings to the forefront systemic gaps in academic medicine that at once are dependent on clinician educators and at the same time do little to support them in their efforts. It is worth offering this section in full:

> Historically, key activities to support medical education are not sufficiently valued or protected by organizations; The medical education system lacks educational surge capacity; Medical educators function at the intersections of systems. Each educational program interacts with associated health system(s), accreditors and licensure systems that are also in flux. This places constraints on the educator's influence and creates tension; Career development among educators is languishing as they strive to meet the many challenges presented by recent disruptions; Well-being efforts appropriately focus on learners and on health care providers; however specific programming to support the unique needs of educators—and the diversity of needs among educators—is commonly neglected. [22(p2)]

The mechanism available to physician educators in clinical settings to support education and enhance lifelong learning is continuing medical education (CME). CME is a sanctioned professional obligation for (some) state licensure, hospital credentialing, and board certification.[23] There are several reasons for the ineffectiveness of hospital CME as the first, if not only, line of dissemination of new clinical knowledge and development of clinicians as medical educators.

First, CME usually appears in the form of one-time only, lecture-based topical sessions. Sessions are not part of an integrated learning curriculum, and improvement metrics are rarely recorded or tracked (e.g., whether after a CME intervention on clinical teaching effectiveness there were differences in learner outcomes). Second, CME content is offered to align with one's medical specialty, imparting important new clinical and procedural knowledge, but it is rarely designed to address systems issues or develop reflective knowledge, clinical educator skills, or other topics all physicians need to know.[24] Third, CME in AHCs is underresourced and usually run by administrators (directors and coordinators), whose main task is to ensure all accreditation requirements are met for the activities. Those who run CME are not usually educators, let alone medical academicians, which brings up a fourth issue. CME and medical school faculty development programs are usually isolated from one another, in both the academic health center and the community-based versions of medical education. Last, even though practitioners are eligible to take CME through their specialty organizations or at other national venues like conferences, which would well deliver more substantial development of clinical teaching and learning, time and expense of attendance are common barriers for busy clinicians.[25] To be sure, CME efforts are important and necessary to meet accreditation requirements, but they are piecemeal. While they may address discrete specialty gaps, they are systemically ineffectual at promoting, supporting, and instilling professionalism, which includes a commitment to teaching and learning and educational best practices.

A solution to the continuing education challenges is to align CME with the faculty development enjoyed by physician educators in academic medicine. Either under the auspices of an Office of Continuing Professional Development or a robust Office of Faculty Development in the medical school or university, programming should mirror professional academic faculty development. Development designed for university professors is easily adapted to advance physicians to deliver a medical curriculum that sees as its goal producing good physicians. This model structures programming and training around the different roles of faculty across their career life span: as a new faculty, advancing from assistant to associate professor, advancing from an associate to full professor, and as an emeritus faculty. It includes professional and personal development, instructor development, and organizational development.[26]

We propose that advancement of medical faculty should include professional development toward the ends of both professionalism as a medical provider and as an academic. Being an academic is different from being a physician, and success as an academic is not the same as success as a physician. It should also include personal development toward gaining adequate knowledge and skills aimed toward an authentic relationship with the values of education, for example, collegiality and academic honesty. Becoming a good academic involves, for example, self-assessment and reflection, time management, knowing when to ask for mentors and coaches, implicit bias training, and how to ethically self-promote. Instructor development should include programming to develop all competencies and skills related to courses, curriculum, and student success, including curriculum design, active learning pedagogies (e.g., case-based learning, real-time feedback, one-minute precepting) and the science of learning. Clinical educators need to learn nonbiomedical content from those who have expertise in the fields as part of their educator development, for example, science of learning and health equity. Last, programming for organizational development offers a structural lens to improve educational practices toward building systems that will be efficient and effective in supporting educators and students so that the teaching/learning process will thrive. It prepares faculty to be academic leaders by disseminating the trends that affect teaching and learning internally and externally beyond the medical school and the university to academic health centers, academic medicine organizations, accreditation bodies, and relevant state and national government offices. The overall goal is that through faculty development efforts, clinical educators will discover the importance of reflective practice oriented toward the goals and values of medicine and be empowered to take ownership of their various roles as clinicians, as researchers, as educators, and as academic leaders.

It is imperative that this robust faculty or professional development of clinical educators, as educators, is designed to be developmental because clinical faculty, like regular faculty, are at different stages in their academic careers. Advancement and promotion of clinical faculty should mirror that of regular faculty. A competency-focused curriculum with lessons delivered in self-contained smaller modules that are directly relevant to education roles is best because clinical educators are practicing physicians whose time is in vital demand. Content ought to be current and designed by experts who are themselves knowledge-producers because clinical educators need evidence-based material from several different disciplines whose research methodologies they may be unfamiliar with and therefore cannot self-assess, for example, those of the humanities, social sciences, education, public health, and law; and they require expert feedback and assessment that is useful and tracked with metrics. Online just-in-time technologies (JITT) and micro-credentialing are promising tools to consider for clinical educator faculty development and/or continuing professional education.[27,28]

Conclusion

Clinical faculty will become empowered to occupy the role of professional educator with robust development. Regular academic medicine faculty development, including advancement toward promotion, can be replicated for clinical faculty through collaboration between offices of faculty affairs at the medical school and university, continuing medical education, continuing professional development, medical education on the university and hospital campuses, and joint libraries and instructional design/information technology. Professional identity formation activities for medical students can be reproduced for clinicians toward including "being an academic" as part of their professional identity. There are learning technologies and pedagogies that can accommodate this, like JITT and communities of practice. Content should be provided by medical schools and their affiliated universities, thereby lessening the distance between the medical academy and professional medical practice, which in turn may promise space for future collaborations. Further, connecting the difficulties of modern medical practice with the deep values of the profession can have an immunizing effect against physician burnout.[29]

Of course in the end, one is called on as a medical professional to "declare ('profess') what the public and individual patients can expect regarding shared competency standards and ethical values and to implement trustworthy means to ensure that all medical professionals live up to these promises." [30(p2)] Understanding the values of the profession, the relationship between physicians and society, and internalizing those values is critical to empower physicians to practice with maximal competence and be effective educators. Attending to the faculty development aspect of medical education for professionalism will be fruitful, not only for medical students as they learn and become good physicians, but also for the clinical educators themselves, who may have developed their own professional identity at a time when healthcare systems were simpler and when racism, sexism, and ableism, for example, were acceptable, or at least tolerated, aspects of medical education. To be sure, not all clinical educators will be interested in or amendable to faculty development of this sort, and the need for clinical educators will require many schools to continue using these underdeveloped faculty. However, evidence suggests that clinical educators are often eager for, and highly interested in, developing clinical teaching skills.[31,32]

Practitioners may bristle at the notion that they need more training in professionalism because it may feel like an assault on their character. Yet it is important to remember that the values of medicine are not so easily applied, especially when medical knowledge and techniques are growing rapidly, and medical systems become increasingly complex. The values of the medical profession may overlap or reinforce each other, but they can also conflict and pull apart in complicated ways that do not always yield clear answers. Recall that medical knowledge and skill unmoored from professional values is risky and has led to practitioner involvement in unethical human subject experimentation, facilitation of torture, eugenics, and limiting or revoking personal liberties. Further, the profession is autonomous and has a monopoly because society empowers, entrusts, and protects physicians to cure, palliate, rehabilitate, and prevent disease and suffering as well as create, manage, and continually assess the process of admitting and educating new trainees. Physicians swear to practice according to the same set of humanitarian values, including the primacy of the patient welfare, respect for patient autonomy and persons, and promotion of social justice; these promises take a professional lifetime of learning.

References

1. Hippocrates. The Hippocratic oath. North M, trans. National Library of Medicine; 2002. Last updated February 7, 2012. Accessed May 31, 2022. https://www.nlm.nih.gov/hmd/greek/greek_oath.html
2. Lasagna L. The Hippocratic oath: modern version. 1964. Accessed May 31, 2022. https://www.pbs.org/wgbh/nova/doctors/oath_modern.html
3. Young A, Chaudhry HJ, Pei X, Arnhart K, Dugan M, Simons KB. FSMB census of licensed physicians in the United States, 2020. *J Med Regul.* 2021;107(2):57–64.
4. Densen P. Challenges and opportunities facing medical education. *Trans Am Clin Climatol Assoc.* 2011;122:48–58.
5. Cruess SR, Cruess RL. Professionalism must be taught. *BMJ.* 1997;315(7123):1674–1677.
6. American Board of Internal Medicine. Project Professionalism. 2001. https://www.scribd.com/document/442593155/project-professionalism-pdf
7. Inui TS. A flag in the wind: educating for professionalism in medicine. AAMC. February 2003. https://med.fsu.edu/sites/default/files/userFiles/file/professinalism.pdf

8. O'Doherty D, Culhane A, O'Doherty J, et al. Medical students and clinical placements—a qualitative study of the continuum of professional identity formation. *Educ Prim Care.* 2021;32(4):202–210. doi:10.1080/14739879.2021.1879684
9. Parsons AS, Kon RH, Plews-Ogan M, Gusic ME. You can have both: coaching to promote clinical competency and professional identity formation. *Perspect Med Educ.* 2021;10(1):57–63. doi:10.1007/s40037-020-00612-1
10. Cruess SR, Cruess RL, Steinert Y. Supporting the development of a professional identity: general principles. *Med Teach.* 2019;41(6):641–649. doi:10.1080/0142159X.2018.1536260
11. Cruess RL, Cruess SR, Boudreau JD, Snell L, Steinert Y. Reframing medical education to support professional identity formation. *Acad Med.* 2014;89(11):1446–1451. doi:10.1097/ACM.0000000000000427
12. Epstein EG, Hamric AB. Moral distress, moral residue, and the crescendo effect. *J Clin Ethics.* 2009;20(4):330–342.
13. Mann K, Gordon J, MacLeod A. Reflection and reflective practice in health professions education: a systematic review. *Adv Health Sci Educ Theory Pract.* 2009;14(4):595–621. doi:10.1007/s10459-007-9090-2
14. Monrouxe L. Theoretical insights into the nature and nurture of professional identities. In: Cruess RL, Cruess SR, Steinert Y, eds. *Teaching Medical Professionalism: Supporting the Development of a Professional Identity.* 2nd ed. Cambridge University Press; 2016:37–54.
15. Hill KA, Samuels EA, Gross CP, et al. Assessment of the prevalence of medical student mistreatment by sex, race/ethnicity, and sexual orientation. *JAMA Intern Med.* 2020;180(5):653. doi:10.1001/jamainternmed.2020.0030
16. National Academies of Sciences, Engineering, and Medicine. *Sexual Harassment of Women: Climate, Culture, and Consequences in Academic Sciences, Engineering, and Medicine* (Johnson PA, Widnall SE, Benya FF, eds.). National Academies Press; 2018:24994. doi:10.17226/24994
17. Davis DA, Rayburn WF, Smith GA. Continuing professional development for faculty: an elephant in the house of academic medicine or the key to future success? *Acad Med.* 2017;92(8):1078–1081. doi:10.1097/ACM.0000000000001777
18. Duffy TP. The Flexner Report—100 years later. *Yale J Biol Med.* 2011;84(3):269–276.
19. Osborne MP. William Stewart Halsted: his life and contributions to surgery. *Lancet Oncol.* 2007;8(3):256–265. doi:10.1016/S1470-2045(07)70076-1
20. American Hospital Association (AHA). AHA Certification Center. Accessed May 30, 2022. https://www.aha.org/career-resources/certification-center
21. Association of American Medical Colleges (AAMC). AAMC Data Snapshot. April 2024. Accessed June 6, 2024. https://www.aamc.org/media/75561/download?attachment
22. American Medical Association (AMA). Protecting the education mission during sustained disruption: organizational steps to support medical educators. 2022. Accessed May 29, 2022. https://www.ama-assn.org/system/files/protecting-education-mission.pdf
23. Davis N, Davis D, Bloch R. Continuing medical education: AMEE education guide no 35. *Med Teach.* 2008;30(7):652–666. doi:10.1080/01421590802108323
24. Lucey C, Souba W. Perspective: the problem with the problem of professionalism. *Acad Med.* 2010;85(6):1018–1024. doi:10.1097/ACM.0b013e3181dbe51f
25. O'Brien Pott M, Blanshan AS, Huneke KM, Baasch Thomas BL, Cook DA. Barriers to identifying and obtaining CME: a national survey of physicians, nurse practitioners and physician assistants. *BMC Med Educ.* 2021;21(1):168. doi:10.1186/s12909-021-02595-x

26. Gillespie KH. *A Guide to Faculty Development.* 2nd ed. Jossey-Bass; 2010.

27. Lok P, Beyene K, Awaisu A, Woods D, Kheir N. Microcredentials training in pharmacy practice and education: an exploratory study of its viability and pharmacists' professional needs. *BMC Med Educ.* 2022;22(1):332. doi:10.1186/s12909-022-03341-7

28. Yilmaz Y, Lal S, Tong XC, et al. Technology-enhanced faculty development: future trends and possibilities for health sciences education. *Med Sci Educ.* 2020;30(4):1787–1796. doi:10.1007/s40670-020-01100-1

29. Merlo G. *Principles of Medical Professionalism.* Oxford University Press; 2021. doi:10.1093/med/9780197506226.001.0001

30. Hafferty F, Papadakis M, Sullivan W, Wynia M. ABMS Definition of Professionalism (Short Form). ABMS.org. January 18, 2012.

31. Steinert Y, Mann K, Anderson B, et al. A systematic review of faculty development initiatives designed to enhance teaching effectiveness: a 10-year update: BEME Guide No. 40. *Med Teach.* 2016;38(8):769–786. doi:10.1080/0142159X.2016.1181851

32. Trainor A, Richards JB. Training medical educators to teach: bridging the gap between perception and reality. *Isr J Health Policy Res.* 2021;10(1):75. doi:10.1186/s13584-021-00509-2

9

Discrimination, Bias, and Their Effects on Professionalism Standards for Underrepresented Groups

Vanika Chawla and Amy Alexander

Key Points

- This chapter explores unique considerations of the applications of professionalism for underrepresented in medicine groups, including first-generation physicians, international medical graduates, LGBTQ+ physicians, physicians with disabilities, Asian medical trainees and physicians, and racial and ethnic minorities, including Black, Latinx, and Native American medical students and physicians.
- We explore how constructs of professionalism are often applied inequitably in a way that disadvantages underrepresented groups, and bias and discrimination toward certain groups can often be guised as "professionalism" issues.
- We advocate for our profession to move toward a culture that can celebrate and embrace differences and diversity.

Who Is Underrepresented in Medicine?

As of March 2004, the Association of American Medical Colleges (AAMC) defined those who are underrepresented in medicine as: "Those racial and ethnic populations that are underrepresented in the medical profession relative to their numbers in the general population." Before this new definition, the AAMC used the term "underrepresented minority," which consisted of Blacks, Mexican Americans, Native Americans (American Indians, Alaska Natives, and Native Hawaiians), and mainland Puerto Ricans. The new definition shifts from a fixed group of racial and ethnic groups to an evolving and more dynamic definition that is reflective of changing demographics of society and specific local regions.[1] The National Instituted of Health offers a broader definition for those who are underrepresented in the scientific workforce. In addition to individuals in racial and ethnic groups that are underrepresented, they also include individuals with disabilities, individuals from disadvantaged backgrounds, and women.[2] It is important to note, however, that the concept of representation alone may not account for other processes of marginalization. For example, while Asian physicians are not underrepresented in medicine in general, there is a disparity in their representation in leadership positions.

For this chapter, we have used a broad definition of those who are underrepresented in medicine.

Despite efforts to increase diversity, medical school faculty continue to be predominantly white (63.9%) and male (58.6%), especially in leadership positions and at higher ranks, such as at the level of professor.[3] While the representation of women and Asian men has increased in medicine, the percentages of medical students and physicians from Black, Hispanic, and other racial and ethnic groups that are underrepresented in medicine are significantly below the percentages of these groups in the national census.[4] Although Black, Latinx, and Native American physicians comprise approximately one-third of the US population, they only account for 9% of practicing physicians, and this rate has not changed in a meaningful way over the last few decades.[5,6] There is also a "leaky pipeline" at varying stages of medicine (medical school admissions, residency, faculty promotions) that results in a lack of diversity in medicine. Unfortunately, those who are underrepresented in medicine are less likely to be promoted,[7] and they receive lower compensation than their white male counterparts.[8] There are additive stressors for those with intersectional identities. Recent data from the Accreditation Council for Graduate Medical Education also shows that underrepresented trainees are dismissed from training programs at higher rates.[9,10] Thus, unfortunately, the physician workforce and leadership do not reflect the diversity of the patient population they serve, thereby negatively impacting patient care. Research shows that patients prefer physicians who are concordant with their race/ethnicity.[11] Physician diversity is associated with improved access and better quality care for underserved populations.[12]

The Stanford Medicine Leadership Education in Advancing Diversity (LEAD) Program is a 10-month longitudinal leadership program for residents and fellows (scholars) across Graduate Medical Education to develop leadership and scholarship skills in addressing issues related to diversity, equity, and inclusion (DEI); to produce leaders in academic medicine dedicated to DEI; and to improve the culture of medicine. The program includes the development of an educational workshop on a DEI topic of the scholars choosing, which is presented at the Annual Diversity & Inclusion Forum. A former LEAD group presented their workshop, Dismantling Professionalism (Fisk et al., 2022), and encouraged the audience to identify, acknowledge, and challenge bias in notions of professionalism that disadvantages marginalized groups.[13] This workshop has inspired this book chapter. Those who are underrepresented in medicine experience constructs of professionalism differently, and this chapter explores special considerations for these groups. Specifically, we explore special considerations for gender and sexual minorities, first-generation physicians, international medical graduates, racial and ethnic minorities and Asian medical students, residents, and physicians. However, we acknowledge that this list and the subsections may not capture the experiences of all who are underrepresented in medicine and instead serves as a collection of examples and considerations that could inspire one to make necessary changes within one's own workplace and training context.

Underrepresented in Medicine and Professionalism

In 2019, the *Journal of Vascular Surgery* published an article that involved a study of social media behavior among young surgeons: "Prevalence of Unprofessional Social

Media Content Among Young Vascular Surgeons."[14] Three male researchers created social media accounts to search and evaluate publicly identifiable social media accounts of vascular surgery trainees. Based on criteria they had set, they labeled content as "unprofessional," and this included "holding or consuming alcohol" and "inappropriate attire" such as swimwear. Ultimately, the article was retracted in response to the outcry on social media by the medical community. The authors issued an apology and acknowledged that the definitions of professionalism in this article were "entrenched with conscious and unconscious bias."[15] While the construct of professionalism was developed as a set of ethical-, behavioral-, value-, and competency-based standards, professionalism and its associated aspects were developed when the workplace was based on a white-dominant culture. Bias in current notions of professionalism or narrow applications of the definition of professionalism may inadvertently represent the "white majority view" and implicitly disadvantage those who do not fit this mold.[16]

A study examined how professionalism is experienced in diverse healthcare and learning environments using a qualitative survey in a large university health network. In this survey of over 3,000 respondents, several key themes emerged that highlighted how underrepresented populations experience professionalism differently.[17]

Those who are underrepresented in medicine had increased criticism over their actions and what was considered "professional." The study describes narratives from participants, "There are some examples, but they are subtle yet apparent. One thing I have noticed is that . . . residents of color seem to get criticized for things that the majority do not, even if they do the same things. There is this microscope that is applied to them which . . . is subtle, yet present."[17(p9)] This can range from scrutiny over dress, speech, accents, work styles, and so forth. "Every time the [minority group] resident came late to rounds, even if he/she was accompanying a patient to a test, it was documented in writing. It didn't matter if White residents came later to rounds or conferences; their lateness was never documented."[17(p8)]

The standards of professionalism were not applied equitably. Even though Underrepresented in Medicine (URM) trainees were under greater scrutiny under the guise of professionalism when it came to their own actions, on the contrary, they experienced a greater violation of professional boundaries from others in the workplace, ranging from microaggressions to overt harassment and discrimination.[17] This phenomenon disproportionately impacted women and gender and sexual and racial/ethnic minorities.[17] A representative quotation that illustrates this example is as follows: "The physician grabbed my right forearm and pulled it towards the patient. The physician asked the patient 'does it [the patient's color of diarrhea] look like her arm or is it lighter?' . . . The physician chuckled and said 'your skin is the perfect color for this job.' "[17] Thus, a double standard exists whereby the inequitable application of professionalism holds URM groups to a different standard when it comes to their own behaviors, yet they are subjected to greater discrimination and harassment by others in the workplace.

Further, respondents felt that notions of professionalism were not inclusive. URM trainees felt pressured to assimilate into their environments, and this often meant conforming to "white norms" and concealing their identities, including aspects of culture and religion due to fear that these were not "professional."[17] For example, " Many internationals compromise personal dignity and values so they don't get kicked out, but ultimately it only promotes intolerance and behavior aimed at silencing their voices and opinions rather than making them feel included and welcome."[17(p10)] Participants were left with the choice of either staying and compromising their sense of self and identity or leaving the environment. The study also noted these biases manifesting in professional disciplinary actions. "I was called into a standard/probation meeting on a Muslim learner. . . . [I]t was commented on the case that the individual 'would not even eat our foods' as a reason to question their academic performance . . . as 'the learner only ate halal foods.' "[17(p10)] If medical professionalism is applied through unequal standards it can, as a result, be "weaponized" against marginalized groups and applied in a way that penalizes those who do not fit group norms through disciplinary actions.[17] This pressure to conform also counteracts efforts for diversity and may "silence" voices due to fear of the backlash of "unprofessionalism."[17] Dr. Duaa AbdelHameid shares in a narrative piece in the *New England Journal of Medicine*: "Professionalism is refraining from discussing race at work for fear of being labeled an 'angry Black woman.' "[18] Bias in notions of professionalism can also contribute to significant pressures for URM trainees to be "perfect" at all times and overcompensation for fear of repercussions otherwise and to feel that they belong: "You just want to make sure that what you're doing is top-notch, because you know for others, they may use your mistakes and then kind of pair that with your race."[19(p7)]

These biases in notions of professionalism can impact professional identity formation. Professional identity formation is a complex transformational process by which one's identity evolves into a future professional self and one learns to "think, act, and feel" like a physician.[20] Recent literature has emerged noting that URM trainees face unique challenges in professional identity formation, including "stereotype threat," which is a phenomenon by which people may perform poorly due to fear of conforming to negative stereotypes of their identity groups.[21] "Minority tax" is also noted to be an additional stressor and barrier to optimal professional identity formation. Minority tax refers to learners being taxed with additional work, such as being burdened with having to "fix" all problems related to DEI, taking on additional care for patients of their identity group, and being tasked as an expert or ambassador for their group.[21] This may contribute to a sense of "othering" and gives the message that those who are URM do not belong or fit the mold of what it means to be a physician, and this serves to hinder the process of identity formation.[21] Further an immense pressure to be perfect, as well as fear that aspect of one's personal identity is not considered professional can impact the integration of one's personal and professional identity, which is a necessary process in professional identity formation.

Microaggressions are unfortunately another common experience of those who are underrepresented in medicine and are also postulated to impact professional identity formation.[21] The term *microaggression* was initially coined in 1970 by Harvard psychiatrist Chester Pierce and refers to the minor yet damaging humiliations and indignities experienced specifically by Black Americans. They are described as "subtle, stunning, often automatic, and non-verbal exchanges which are 'put downs.'"[22] Sue et al. describe microaggressions as "brief and commonplace daily verbal, behavioral, or environmental indignities, whether intentional or unintentional, that communicate hostile, derogatory, or negative slights and insults that potentially have harmful or unpleasant psychological impact on the target person or group."[23] Microaggressions can occur against any marginalized group and are often a manifestation of bias. The experience of microaggression is alarmingly common and frequent among trainees. A study found that 60% of respondents experienced at least one microaggression per week, and 33.9% reported one microaggression daily. Gender (64.4%), race/ethnicity (60.5%), and age (40.9%) were the most commonly reported reasons for experiencing a microaggression.[24]

People With Disabilities

One study examined the prevalence of US practicing physicians with disabilities. It estimated an overall disability prevalence of 3.1%, with chronic health conditions being the most common disability followed by mobility and psychological disabilities. Among physicians with disabilities, approximately 17% identified as other underrepresented groups.[25] There were 2.7% of medical students who reported a disability in 2016, and this number increased to 4.6% in 2019.[26] Physicians with disabilities are subjected to high rates of discrimination. A study found that physicians with disabilities had a significantly higher likelihood of experiencing every type of mistreatment from both patients and coworkers.[27] A narrative by Maïté Van Hentenryck, who is a medical student with a disability reflects: "I thought medical school would be different: people would understand my history, yet not define me by it. But in modern medicine, people with disabilities are our patients, not our colleagues."[28] Hentenryck shares extensive barriers for applicants with disabilities to enter medical school.[28] Hentenryck adds that trainees often have to "fight for needed accommodations" once matriculated.[28] Nearly one-fifth of the US population has a disability.[29] Physicians with a disability can provide better care for patients and can empathize better with those with disabilities and can serve as models for their peers and facilitate greater learning and awareness of disabilities.[26] Meeks et al. note barriers that physicians with disabilities face, including those related to access to accommodations, policies and procedures, the physical environment, and lack of support.[26] Physicians with disabilities feel that they need to perform better than their peers to be accepted, have to advocate to receive basic services, struggle with stigma, and receive messages that they do not belong.[26] Furthermore, the professional competencies of a physician are often determined from the view of ableism. Anecdotally, trainees have reported their disabilities as being viewed by programs as the trainee's performance problems, rather than viewing them as something for the program to accommodate. Programs instead should create environments where all trainees can succeed and thrive. Meeks et al. encourage the medical body to critically think about what counts as "qualified," or in other words professionally competent.[26]

Gender and Sexual Minorities

A systematic review and meta-analysis evaluated data from over 30,000 trainees globally (both medical students and residents), and the results showed that there were high rates of discrimination and harassment.[30] Over half of the trainees reported experiencing discrimination and harassment. The most commonly reported form of harassment included verbal, and the most commonly reported form of discrimination was due to race or gender. Female trainees were at the highest risk.[30] While the proportion of medical students graduating who are female has increased, and women now constitute over half of the national medical study body, discrimination and disparity still persist.[4] Women physicians are paid less, are less likely to be promoted, and are underrepresented in leadership positions.[31–33] They also experience high rates of discrimination and harassment. For example, 30% of women in medicine report experiencing sexual harassment, compared to 4% of men.[34] Further, physicians who are pregnant and have children face additional challenges, including gendered job expectations, limitations in opportunities for advancement, lack of support during pregnancy and the postpartum period, and lack of support with work and life balance.[35] One participant in a qualitative study on maternal discriminatory experiences notes that they were: "Told that taking maternity leave was a bother to everyone and that I can't just 'keep going on vacation for 6 weeks.'" Another shares: "As a resident pumping for my 3 month old child (after coming back to work 4 weeks postpartum) I was told by my associate program director that my 'personal life was interfering with my ability to perform my work responsibilities' because of taking breaks to pump every 4–6 hours. Despite the fact that I was pumping in a public workspace surrounded by attendings, residents, medical students, and occasionally consultants from other services so as not to miss any important clinical work or decisions rather than pump in private."[35] It is also an important consideration to expand parental leave policies to encompass diverse and unique family structures, including those who may not be able to biologically carry a child and to accommodate varying types of methods of conceiving.

Lesbian, Gay, Bisexual, Transgender, Queer/Questioning, Intersex, Asexual, Two spirit (LGBTQIA2S+) residents report high rates of discrimination, including being harassed by colleagues and patients, witnessing disparaging care toward LGBTQIA2S+ patients, being denied referrals, and being socially ostracized by their peers in medicine.[36] As a result, they experienced higher levels of depression and anxiety than their heterosexual counterparts, associated with lower perceived belonging.[37] Approximately 1% of graduating medical students identified as transgender or gender expansive (e.g., nonbinary, genderqueer, agender).[38] Transgender and gender-expansive physicians report high rates of discrimination, including transphobia and being misgendered and witnessing discriminatory care toward patients. As a result, many experience emotional distress, fear for their physical and psychological safety in the workplace, and feel that they need to hide or conceal parts of their identity.[39] In a report by the British Medical Association, only 43% of LGBTQIA2S+ physicians felt comfortable disclosing their sexual orientation at the workplace, and only 34% felt comfortable disclosing their gender identity.[40] A "rigid gender binary paradigm" and structural and institutional factors are contributory.[39] A participant in a qualitative study on the experiences of transgender and gender-expansive physicians shares: "I found it very difficult to weigh my what I felt to be my duty to speak up against injustice with my desire to remain safe. . . . There's a lot of power differential. . . . I was very much afraid that not only would there be professional repercussions, but also there might be personal repercussions if I was then sort of suspected as being aligned with the community."[39] Political factors need to be considered as well, and physicians who identify as gender and sexual minorities may face discrimination from their patients and communities depending on the context of where they live and practice, and they may require additional support and consideration. Rather than offer support and make work environments more inclusive, professionalism can be utilized as a means to disparage and penalize physicians for aspects related to their identity.

Asian Trainees and Physicians

While the percentage of Asian medical students in the United States has grown twelvefold since the 1970s to a high of 24% in 2022, of which over 50% are women, Asian physicians are less likely to occupy leadership positions compared to white counterparts.[41,42] Further, Asian trainees are often stereotyped as a group, to their detriment. Asian trainees and physicians are often stereotyped by the "model minority myth," which implies that Asians are hardworking and highly educated and objectively successful.[43] This serves to invalidate and downplay any lived experiences of racism or discrimination and can also create a divide among different racial groups.[43] Further, the Asian population is no monolith; however, several subpopulations are often grouped under one category, which neglects to capture the significant diversity and differences in this group.[43] The term *Asian American* constitutes over 20 different ethnic groups, all with distinct identities, histories, and experiences.[44] Further, Asian trainees endure microaggressions, implicit biases, exoticization, and educational profiling as "passive" and "quiet," and they also hit a "bamboo ceiling" without opportunities to progress in academic medicine.[44,45] They are stereotyped as being "shy" and "quiet," and assumptions may be made that they are not interested in leadership opportunities.[43] Asian trainees are more likely to experience medical student mistreatment.[46] Even when controlling for factors such as Step 1 scores, research productivity, leadership, and community service, Asian medical students were less frequently selected for induction into Alpha Omega Alpha society compared with white students, likely reflecting a selection bias. During clerkships, Asian medical students were less likely to receive positive comments compared with white students and more likely to receive lower clerkship grades.[47,48] These findings suggest bias and discrimination on the part of evaluators when evaluating Asian medical trainee performance and professionalism. There is a long history of anti-Asian discrimination in the United States, described in concepts that include "yellow peril," a racist color metaphor that depicts people in East and Southeast Asia as an existential threat to the Western world; the "perpetual foreigner," a racist, xenophobic form of nativism in which naturalized and even native-born citizens are perceived by some members of the majority as foreign because they belong to a minority ethnic or racial group; "the model minority myth," where Asian Americans are stereotyped as studious, successful, smart—a model minority who excels in education and accomplishes the "American dream," yet ignores the reality of systemic racism and creates racial divisions; and the "invisible Asian," the expectation that Asians will be quiet, not cause problems, stay "in line," not complain, and will not hold leadership positions and essentially stay quiet and nonthreatening as a group.[49–52] In addition, the COVID-19 pandemic has led to a rapid rise in hate incidents targeting people of Asian descent since early 2020. Over 10,000 incidents were reported during the first 18 months of the COVID-19 pandemic.[53] Anti-Asian racism and harassment have been directed against Asian medical trainees and Asian physicians alike. Intersectional challenges additionally compound the above problems for Asian women and Asian sexual minorities.

First Generation in Medicine

First-generation medical students are the first in their families to attend medical school, while first-generation college students are the first in their families to attend college. These are distinct populations that may overlap. First-generation students, both college and medical, come from different backgrounds and may differ in terms of racial/ethnic, immigration, and socioeconomic factors; however, they are more likely to come from minority backgrounds, have financial disadvantages, and be non-US citizens compared to non–first-generation students.[54] This adds to the challenges they experience as being the first in their families to navigate college and medical school with less guidance and experience. Family misunderstandings and additional family burdens and responsibilities, lack of professional networks, and psychological challenges such as confusion, guilt, and imposter syndrome are possible challenges they may face.[55] First-generation medical students may also be more self-reliant, and they may experience stigma related to asking for assistance and support. Studies of first-generation college students show higher rates of academic and financial distress and higher work hours, coupled with lower levels of support and self-care.[54,56] In medical school and residency, this may result in academic and training challenges or performance issues that are mistaken as "professionalism issues" rather than a broader complex problem for a system that does not provide specific support to first-generation trainees.

International Medical Graduates

International medicine graduates (IMGs) are defined as individuals who completed their primary medical degree from a medical school outside of the United States.[57] Twenty-five percent of licensed US doctors are IMGs, and this number has been and continues to grow. The largest number of licensed IMGs have graduated from schools in India, followed by the Caribbean.[58] IMGs may or may not be US citizens, and the definition relates to the primary country of training rather than the citizenship of the physician. However, nearly 80% of IMGs are not US born.[59] Studies show that some IMGs had better outcomes than their US-trained counterparts.[60] IMGs play an important role in the workforce and in providing care in underserved areas and in primary care.[59]

IMGs must overcome significant barriers to transition to the United States. This includes challenges with writing several examinations, including the Step 1, 2, and 3 exams.[61] They encounter much less certainty when it comes to matching compared to graduates of US medical schools.[61] This may lead to significant delays in matching or not obtaining the specialty of choice. They also need to navigate immigration challenges such as receiving visas. Once in the United States as a physician, they are not only navigating the process of immigration but also simultaneously need to start the process of residency.[61]

In addition to the baseline challenges that are present with the transition point from medical school to residency, IMGs need to adapt to the complexities of a new healthcare system and familiarize themselves with new cultural nuances, standards of "professionalism," and communication skills.[61] They encounter microaggression, bias, and a lack of support groups and mentorship,[61] and they may face isolation and insensitivity in the workplace.[59] They are less likely to obtain academic positions.[61] One family physician from the Middle East notes his transition to a US residency program and describes this process as turbulent: "They related it all to incompetence.... Some of us were even called antisocial.... [I think] it's all cultural. We were all from different countries.... Sometimes people ... that's just their way of talking and you would think that they're either being rude or either they're screaming at you or they are mad or, you know?"[59]

A study in the United Kingdom showed that those who have received their medical qualifications outside the United Kingdom and Black and minority ethnic groups were more likely to have formal disciplinary investigations for concerns about fitness to practice. White physicians trained in the United Kingdom were least likely to be reported for disciplinary investigations.[16] IMG doctors noted that these disciplinary investigations and sanctions were harsher than those issued to white doctors for similar actions.[16]

In a study in Australia, IMGs were more likely than Australian medical graduates to receive complaints from medical boards and adverse disciplinary findings.[62] IMGs face similar challenges as other underrepresented medicine groups and are subject to similar bias in notions of professionalism. Residency programs need to consider the specific training needs and provide support to IMGs during their training and beyond. While it is important to support the transition of the IMGs to the US culture and medical systems to provide quality and safe patient care, it is also important that their personal identity and culture are not compromised, and that the unique and diverse attributes, strengths, and skills they bring and experiences they have are valued. Further, professional standards must be applied equitably and be based on objective criteria rather than differences in dress, speech, culture, and so forth.

Underrepresented Racial/Ethnic Groups

Many of the studies discussed in this chapter have focused on racial and ethnic minorities. A qualitative study of Black, Latinx, and Native American resident physicians found that their experience of training is different from nonminority counterparts, ascribed to additional challenges such as microaggressions and bias, minority tax, and challenges negotiating professional and personal identity.[19] Residents felt they needed to choose between their work and personal identity due to the perception that their personal identity was not accepted at their workplace and the implication that aspects of their racial and ethnic identities "lack professionalism," such as hair, speech, body language, clothing, food. In a piece, "Is this hair professional enough," Bizimungu shares: "At the start of clerkship, however, I had qualms about whether my short Afro hair would be deemed professional enough for a clinical setting. On several occasions when I was mistaken for a nurse, an orderly or a janitor, I asked myself if—on top of my visibly Black skin—my hairstyle did not fit with society's image of a doctor-to-be."[63]

An additional consideration is physicians with names that do not sound white. One resident recounted a common experience, "'Oh, wow, that last name is different. How do I say it? Where is that from? Is English your first language? Where are you from?' They would not just accept Texas."[19(p4)] An individual's name is a big part of their identity. A study by Greene et al. shows that some patients exhibited a preference for physicians with a name that implied they were white and male, regardless of quality scores compared to non–white-sounding names.[64] Thus, URM physicians with non–white-sounding names may experience discrimination from their colleagues and patients even before the actual encounter or interaction, simply based on their name. Anecdotally, physicians with non–white-sounding names also describe that often patients and colleagues and those in leadership are not able to pronounce or remember their names. Could this impact opportunities for promotions by leadership, or opportunities for patients to leave positive comments about their physician? Research shows that people with non–white-sounding names find it more difficult to get responses to their job applications, despite having the same credentials.[65] Intersectionality is a concept that refers to the "multiple social forces, social identities, and ideological instruments through which power and disadvantage are expressed and legitimized."[66] Those with intersectional identities have exacerbated challenges.

Negative Consequences

Research consistently shows that diversity can help organizations improve both patient care quality and financial results.[67] We know that ultimately diverse healthcare providers are best for patient care. Unfortunately, there continues to be a lack of diversity in medicine and bias, discrimination, and lack of adequate support contribute to this. Academic culture is based on cultural norms that exclude underrepresented groups, and this contributes to mental health challenges.[68] The prevalence of depressive symptoms or depression among resident physicians is 28.8% and increased over time in training, based on a systematic review and meta-analysis involving 17,560 resident physicians.[69] A recent meta-analysis showed high rates of burnout among trainees (50%).[70] Burnout is more prevalent among physicians versus the general US population, and residents are more likely to exhibit symptoms of depression than population control samples.[71]

Conclusion

This chapter has covered how constructs of professionalism are often applied inequitably in a way that disadvantages underrepresented groups. This chapter explores how bias and discrimination toward certain groups can often be guised as "professionalism" issues. We have explored literature, and narrative experiences of underrepresented groups, including racial and ethnic minorities, Asian medical trainees, sexual and gender minorities, physicians with disabilities, and first-generation and international medical graduates and have explored unique considerations for each of these groups and how they may be impacted by notions of professionalism. We reiterate that this list is not exhaustive and does not capture the experiences of all those who are underrepresented in medicine. In their 2022 on *Dismantling Professionalism,* Fisk et al. urge us to dismantle institutional systems and policies that advantage some learners and disadvantage others and instead create environments that are supportive and inclusive.[13] They advocate for a definition of professionalism that encourages individuality rather than conformity and decolonizes professionalism.[13] We urge readers to reflect on their own institutions and contexts and reflect on how professionalism standards are applied at your own institution and the bias that may exist in your contexts. A formal curriculum and training on professional identity formation can help. Mentorship is crucial for those who are underrepresented in medicine and can help ameliorate challenges related to optimal professional identity formation.[13,21] However, this onus should not fall on URM physicians, and non-URM physicians should receive training in mentoring URM students.[13] Ongoing efforts for allyship, activism, and resources for those who do this work are imperative.[13] Professionalism standards must be continually examined and updated in a way that represents all voices, including those that are typically marginalized or silenced.[13] Identifying, addressing, and eradicating bias in notions of professionalism standards is imperative in order to operationalize a construct of professionalism that is equitable.[13] Osseo-Arre et al. advocate for a definition of professionalism that focuses on "the fair/respectful treatment of patients and colleagues regardless of position or personal characteristics, such as gender identity, sexual orientation, and race/ethnicity."[19] As a profession we must reflect on what it means to be professional in a way that moves us toward a culture that can celebrate and embrace differences and diversity.

Acknowledgments

We would like to acknowledge Drs. Cameron Alec Fisk, Diana Marlene Pena, Stephanie Harman, Travis Lee Reece-Nguyen, Lauren Elizabeth Rivkin, Tiffany Chambers, Kristen Meiling Ng, and Chiazotam Nkemdilim Ekekezie, and members of the Stanford LEAD group who developed and presented the workshop entitled "Dismantling Professionalism", which has inspired this chapter and content.

References

1. Association of American Medical Colleges. Underrepresented in Medicine Definition. Accessed March 1, 2023. https://www.aamc.org/what-we-do/equity-diversity-inclusion/underrepresented-in-medicine
2. National Institutes of Health. Populations underrepresented in the extramural scientific workforce. Accessed March 1, 2023. https://extramural-diversity.nih.gov/diversity-matters/get-the-facts#:~:text=Underrepresented%20groups%20include%20individuals%20from,from%20disadvantaged%20backgrounds%2C%20and%20women
3. Ogunyemi D. *Affinity Groups: Unique Populations.* Unique Populations. https://www.aamc.org/professional-development/affinity-groups/gfa/unique-populations
4. Morris DB, Gruppuso PA, McGee HA, Murillo AL, Grover A, Adashi EY. Diversity of the national medical student body—four decades of inequities. *N Engl J Med.* 2021;384(17):1661–1668. doi:10.1056/NEJMsr2028487
5. *Section II: Current Status of the US Physician Workforce.* Association of American Medical Colleges (AAMC). 2014. https://aamcdiversityfactsandfigures.org/section-ii-current-status-of-us-physician-workforce/. Accessed March 1, 2023.
6. Deville C, Hwang WT, Burgos R, Chapman CH, Both S, Thomas CR. Diversity in graduate medical education in the United States by race, ethnicity, and sex, 2012. *JAMA Intern Med.* 2015;175(10):1706. doi:10.1001/jamainternmed.2015.4324
7. Nunez-Smith M, Ciarleglio MM, Sandoval-Schaefer T, et al. Institutional variation in the promotion of racial/ethnic minority faculty at US medical schools. *Am J Public Health.* 2012;102(5):852–858. doi:10.2105/AJPH.2011.300552
8. Ly DP, Seabury SA, Jena AB. Differences in incomes of physicians in the United States by race and sex: observational study. *BMJ.* Published online 2016;353:i2923. doi:10.1136/bmj.i2923
9. Vela MB, Chin MH, Peek ME. Keeping our promise—supporting trainees from groups that are underrepresented in medicine. *N Engl J Med.* 2021;385(6):487–489. doi:10.1056/NEJMp2105270
10. *The Program Directors' Guide to the Common Program Requirements (Residency).* Accreditation Council for Graduate Medical Education (ACGME); 2020:376.
11. Takeshita J, Wang S, Loren AW, et al. Association of racial/ethnic and gender concordance between patients and physicians with patient experience ratings. *JAMA Netw Open.* 2020;3(11):e2024583. doi:10.1001/jamanetworkopen.2020.24583
12. Marrast L, Zallman L, Woolhandler S. Minority physicians' role in the care of underserved patients: diversifying the physician workforce may be key in addressing health disparities. *JAMA Intern Med.* 2014;174(2):289–291.

13. Fisk A, Pena D, Ng K, et al. Dismantling professionalism. Presented at: Stanford Medicine 5th Annual Diversity and Inclusion Forum; June 2022; Stanford University, Stanford, CA.
14. Hardouin S, Cheng TW, Mitchell EL, et al. RETRACTED: prevalence of unprofessional social media content among young vascular surgeons. *J Vasc Surg.* 2020;72(2):667–671. doi:10.1016/j.jvs.2019.10.069
15. Hardouin S, Cheng T, Mitchell EL, et al. Reply. *J Vasc Surg.* 2020;72(5):1830. doi:10.1016/j.jvs.2020.08.020
16. Dave A, Bhatti N, Grover J, et al. Does a narrow definition of medical professionalism lead to systemic bias and differential outcomes?: A narrative commentary. *Sushruta.* 2021;14(1):1–12. doi:10.38192/14.1.13
17. Alexis DA, Kearney MD, Williams JC, Xu C, Higginbotham EJ, Aysola J. Assessment of perceptions of professionalism among faculty, trainees, staff, and students in a large university-based health system. *JAMA Netw Open.* 2020;3(11):e2021452. doi:10.1001/jamanetworkopen.2020.21452
18. AbdelHameid D. Professionalism 101 for Black physicians. *N Engl J Med.* 2020;383(5):e34. doi:10.1056/NEJMpv2022773
19. Osseo-Asare A, Balasuriya L, Huot SJ, et al. Minority resident physicians' views on the role of race/ethnicity in their training experiences in the workplace. *JAMA Netw Open.* 2018;1(5):e182723. doi:10.1001/jamanetworkopen.2018.2723
20. American Association of Colleges of Pharmacy. Professional identity formation. Accessed March 1, 2023. https://www.aacp.org/article/professional-identity-formation#:~:text=Professional%20identity%20formation%20is%20a,feeling%20like%20pharmacists%20upon%20graduation
21. Trevino R, Poitevien P. Professional identity formation for underrepresented in medicine learners. *Curr Probl Pediatr Adolesc Health Care.* 2021;51(10):101091. doi:10.1016/j.cppeds.2021.101091
22. Pierce CM, Carew JV, Pierce-Gonzalez D, Wills D. An experiment in racism: TV commercials. *Educ Urban Soc.* 1977;10(1):61–87.
23. Sue DW, Capodilupo CM, Torino GC, et al. Racial microaggressions in everyday life: implications for clinical practice. *Am Psychol.* 2007;62(4):271–286. doi:10.1037/0003-066X.62.4.271
24. Anderson N, Lett E, Asabor EN, et al. The association of microaggressions with depressive symptoms and institutional satisfaction among a national cohort of medical students. *J Gen Intern Med.* 2022;37(2):298–307. doi:10.1007/s11606-021-06786-6
25. Nouri Z, Dill MJ, Conrad SS, Moreland CJ, Meeks LM. Estimated prevalence of US physicians with disabilities. *JAMA Netw Open.* 2021;4(3):e211254. doi:10.1001/jamanetworkopen.2021.1254
26. Meeks LM, Herzer K, Jain NR. Removing barriers and facilitating access: increasing the number of physicians with disabilities. *Acad Med.* 2018;93(4):540–543. doi:10.1097/ACM.0000000000002112
27. Meeks LM, Conrad SS, Nouri Z, Moreland CJ, Hu X, Dill MJ. Patient and coworker mistreatment of physicians with disabilities: study examines mistreatment of physicians with disabilities. *Health Aff.* 2022;41(10):1396–1402. doi:10.1377/hlthaff.2022.00502
28. Van Hentenryck M. Growing Pains. *JAMA.* 2020;324(8):745–746. doi:10.1001/jama.2020.13442.

29. *25th Anniversary of Americans With Disabilities Act: July 26.* United States Census Bureau; 2015. Accessed March 1, 2023. https://www.census.gov/newsroom/facts-for-features/2015/cb15-ff10.html

30. Fnais N, Soobiah C, Chen MH, et al. Harassment and discrimination in medical training: a systematic review and meta-analysis. *Acad Med.* 2014;89(5):817–827. doi:10.1097/ACM.0000000000000200

31. Whaley CM, Koo T, Arora VM, Ganguli I, Gross N, Jena AB. Female physicians earn an estimated $2 million less than male physicians over a simulated 40-year career: study examines estimated career gap in pay between female physicians and male physicians. *Health Aff.* 2021;40(12):1856–1864. doi:10.1377/hlthaff.2021.00461

32. Richter KP, Clark L, Wick JA, et al. Women physicians and promotion in academic medicine. *N Engl J Med.* 2020;383(22):2148–2157. doi:10.1056/NEJMsa1916935

33. Reed DA, Enders F, Lindor R, McClees M, Lindor KD. Gender differences in academic productivity and leadership appointments of physicians throughout academic careers. *Acad Med.* 2011;86(1):43–47. doi:10.1097/ACM.0b013e3181ff9ff2

34. Jagsi R, Griffith KA, Jones R, Perumalswami CR, Ubel P, Stewart A. Sexual harassment and discrimination experiences of academic medical faculty. *JAMA.* 2016;315(19):2120. doi:10.1001/jama.2016.2188

35. Halley M, Rustagi A, Torres J, et al. Physician mothers' experience of workplace discrimination: a qualitative analysis. *BMJ.* 2018;363(4926). doi:10.1136/bmj.k4926

36. Dimant OE, Cook TE, Greene RE, Radix AE. Experiences of transgender and gender nonbinary medical students and physicians. *Transgend Health.* 2019;4(1):209–216. doi:10.1089/trgh.2019.0021

37. Wang K, Burke SE, Przedworski JM, et al. A comparison of depression and anxiety symptoms between sexual minority and heterosexual medical residents: a report from the Medical Trainee CHANGE Study. *LGBT Health.* 2020;7(6):332–339. doi:10.1089/lgbt.2020.0027

38. Tanmoy Das L. We need more transgender and gender nonbinary doctors. Accessed March 15, 2023. https://www.aamc.org/news-insights/we-need-more-transgender-and-gender-nonbinary-doctors

39. Westafer LM, Freiermuth CE, Lall MD, Muder SJ, Ragone EL, Jarman AF. Experiences of transgender and gender expansive physicians. *JAMA Netw Open.* 2022;5(6):e2219791. doi:10.1001/jamanetworkopen.2022.19791

40. *Sexual Orientation and Gender Identity in the Medical Profession.* British Medical Association; 2022:70. https://www.bma.org.uk/media/6340/bma-sogi-report-2-nov-2022.pdf

41. *Table B-3: Total U.S. MD-Granting Medical School Enrollment by Race/Ethnicity (Alone) and Gender, 2018–2019 through 2022–2023.* Association of American Medical Colleges (AAMC). 2023. Accessed March 1, 2023. https://www.aamc.org/media/6116/download

42. Morris-Wiseman LF, Cañez C, Romero Arenas MA, Hsu CH, Nfonsam VN. Race, gender, and international medical graduates: leadership trends in academic surgical societies. *J Surg Res.* 2022;270:430–436. doi:10.1016/j.jss.2021.09.043

43. Liu CZ, Wang E, Nguyen D, Sun MD, Jumreornvong O. The model minority myth, data aggregation, and the role of medical schools in combating anti-Asian sentiment. *Acad Med.* 2022;97(6):797–803. doi:10.1097/ACM.0000000000004639

44. Ahn DJ, Garg N, Naik AG, et al. Where do I fit in? A perspective on challenges faced by Asian American medical students. *Health Equity.* 2021;5(1):324–328. doi:10.1089/heq.2020.0158

45. Hyun J. *Breaking the Bamboo Ceiling*. HarperCollins; 2009.

46. Hill KA, Samuels EA, Gross CP, et al. Assessment of the prevalence of medical student mistreatment by sex, race/ethnicity, and sexual orientation. *JAMA Intern Med*. 2020;180(5):653. doi:10.1001/jamainternmed.2020.0030

47. Lee KB, Vaishnavi SN, Lau SKM, Andriole DA, Jeffe DB. Cultural competency in medical education: demographic differences associated with medical student communication styles and clinical clerkship feedback. *J Natl Med Assoc*. 2009;101(2):116–126. doi:10.1016/S0027-9684(15)30823-3

48. Lee KB, Vaishnavi SN, Lau SKM, Andriole DA, Jeffe DB. "Making the grade:" noncognitive predictors of medical students' clinical clerkship grades. *J Natl Med Assoc*. 2007;99(10):1138–1150.

49. Odijie M. The fear of "yellow peril" and the emergence of European federalist movement. *Int Hist Rev*. 2018;40(2):358–375. doi:10.1080/07075332.2017.1329751

50. Sefa Dei G, Hilowle S. *Cartographies of Race and Social Difference*. Springer; 2018.

51. Debunking the model minority myth. Accessed March 29, 2023. https://pacificasiamuseum.usc.edu/exhibitions/online-exhibitions/debunking-the-model-minority-myth/

52. Shih K, Chang J. The invisible costs of the model minority myth on Asian American families. September 27, 2021. Accessed March 29, 2023. https://www.ncfr.org/ncfr-report/fall-2021/invisible-costs-model-minority-myth-asian-american- families

53. Yellow Horse A, Jeung R, Matriano R. Stop AAPI Hate National Report. 2020:19. Accessed March 29, 2023. https://stopaapihate.org/national-report-through-december-31-2021/

54. Romero R, Miotto K, Casillas A, Sanford J. Understanding the experiences of first-generation medical students: implications for a diverse physician workforce. *Acad Psychiatry*. 2020;44(4):467–470. doi:10.1007/s40596-020-01235-8

55. Gallegos A, Gordon LK, Moreno G, et al. Visibility & support for first generation college graduates in medicine. *Med Educ Online*. 2022;27(1):2011605. doi:10.1080/10872981.2021.2011605

56. House LA, Neal C, Kolb J. Supporting the mental health needs of first generation college students. *J College Stud Psychother*. 2020;34(2):157–167. doi:10.1080/87568225.2019.1578940

57. American Academy of Family Physicians. Residency application requirements for international medical graduates. Accessed March 2, 2023. https://www.aafp.org/students-residents/medical-students/become-a-resident/applying-to-residency/international-medical-graduates.html

58. American Medical Association. How IMGs have changed the face of American medicine. October 19, 2021. https://www.ama-assn.org/education/international-medical-education/how-imgs-have-changed-face-american- medicine. Accessed March 1, 2023.

59. Chen PGC, Curry LA, Bernheim SM, Berg D, Gozu A, Nunez-Smith M. Professional challenges of non-U.S.-born international medical graduates and recommendations for support during residency training. *Acad Med*. 2011;86(11):1383–1388. doi:10.1097/ACM.0b013e31823035e1

60. Tsugawa Y, Jena AB, Orav EJ, Jha AK. Quality of care delivered by general internists in US hospitals who graduated from foreign versus US medical schools: observational study. *BMJ*. 2017;356:j273. doi:10.1136/bmj.j273

61. Zaidi Z, Dewan M, Norcini J. International medical graduates: promoting equity and belonging. *Acad Med*. 2020;95(12S):S82–S87. doi:10.1097/ACM.0000000000003694

62. Elkin K, Spittal MJ, Studdert DM. Risks of complaints and adverse disciplinary findings against international medical graduates in Victoria and Western Australia. *Med J Aust.* 2012;197(8):448–452. doi:10.5694/mja12.10632

63. Bizimungu S. Is this hair professional enough? *CMAJ.* 2021;193(7):E254–E255. doi:10.1503/cmaj.201871

64. Greene J, Hibbard JH, Sacks RM. Does the race/ethnicity or gender of a physician's name impact patient selection of the physician? *J Natl Med Assoc.* 2018;110(3):206–211. doi:10.1016/j.jnma.2017.05.010

65. Bertrand M, Mullainiathan S. *Are Emily and Greg More Employable Than Lakisha and Jamal? A Field Experiment on Labor Market Discrimination.* National Bureau of Economic Research; 2003:40.

66. Crenshaw K. *On Intersectionality: Essential Writings.* New Press; 2017.

67. Gomez LE, Bernet P. Diversity improves performance and outcomes. *J Natl Med Assoc.* 2019;111(4):383–392. doi:10.1016/j.jnma.2019.01.006

68. Asai DJ. Race Matters. *Cell.* 2020;181(4):754–757. doi:10.1016/j.cell.2020.03.044

69. Rotenstein LS, Ramos MA, Torre M, et al. Prevalence of depression, depressive symptoms, and suicidal ideation among medical students: a systematic review and meta-analysis. *JAMA.* 2016;316(21):2214. doi:10.1001/jama.2016.17324

70. Zhou AY, Panagioti M, Esmail A, Agius R, Van Tongeren M, Bower P. Factors associated with burnout and stress in trainee physicians: a systematic review and meta-analysis. *JAMA Netw Open.* 2020;3(8):e2013761. doi:10.1001/jamanetworkopen.2020.13761

71. Dyrbye L, Shanafelt T. A narrative review on burnout experienced by medical students and residents. *Med Educ.* 2016;50(1):132–149. doi:10.1111/medu.12927

10

Assessment of Professionalism

A Manageable Challenge

Elizabeth Krajic Kachur

Key Points

- Clear definitions are the first step for developing professionalism assessment strategies.
- Effective professionalism assessment approaches must address knowledge, skills, attitudes/values and behaviors.
- Professionalism is a multifactorial competency and requires multiple assessment and remediation tools throughout the continuum of medical education.

The Mandate for Assessing Professionalism

In the past, the importance of professionalism was implied in oaths and laws. However, over the last few decades it has become a "Core Competency" for healthcare providers. For example, in 1999 the Accreditation Council for Graduate Medical Education (ACGME) institutionalized it as a key component of every medical training program.[1] Other healthcare professions made it a similar explicit standard for their trainees and practitioners.[2] This has implications for teaching as well as for learner assessment.

Given the current educational mandates, there is an urgency to develop valid, reliable, feasible, and fair assessment instruments. Without quality data, it is difficult to assign learners to effective remediation or even prevent them from graduating even if they are unfit for advancing or clinical practice. Single documented lapses, even if severe, are often not enough to put a stop to someone's career, as we could see in cases such as Michael Swango, who was caught falsifying charts but was not prevented from graduating from Southern Illinois University Medical School in 1982. He then went on to murder up to 60 patients under his care.[3] While Swango can be considered an outlier, patients, other healthcare providers, and society are affected by unprofessional behaviors to a high enough degree to warrant major efforts in intervention and prevention.

There have been various efforts to compile lists of available assessment tools.[4,5,6,7,8] New tools are emerging continuously.[9,10,11] This chapter provides a framework to assist educational programs with creating a comprehensive and fair assessment plan.

The Need for Clarity in Definition and Scope

Although assessment is critical for every educational endeavor, it is a loaded word for many and can come in many formats, as detailed in Table 10.1. Is it *for* learning (i.e., formative) or is it *of* learning, to make promotion decisions (i.e., summative)? Is it valid (i.e., does it measure what it is supposed to measure) and reliable (i.e., would a repetition of the assessment lead to the same result)? Does it treat all learners in an equitable fashion or will it introduce biases towards specific groups (e.g., gender, race). In other words, is it fair?

Every learner evaluation needs to start with clear definitions: What are we assessing? Without such certainty, every tool will be inadequate to achieve fair and equitable results. There must be some agreement about what is right and what is wrong while acknowledging that there is a large "gray" or borderline area that deserves equal attention. Looking at the concept of professionalism more closely, one can see that it has undergone major paradigm shifts, as highlighted in 2019 by Wamsley and Thompson.[12] We have moved from viewing professionalism as a character trait to a personal capacity, from rules, roles, and models to skill development, and from assumption to assessment. Lapses are no longer viewed as flaws but as deficiency, and institutional responses have changed their focus from disciplining and removal to coaching and prevention. Similar to the way we look at medical mistakes, professionalism lapses are now seen through a systems lens. All these shifts have major implications for producing, selecting, and applying effective assessment tools throughout the continuum of health professions education.

Changes in definition can occur rapidly, in step with societal transformations. For example, the 2005 Physician Charter developed by the American Board of Internal Medicine (ABIM)[13] does not mention "wellness and self-care" as one of the core values all physicians should adhere to. However, a recent book, *Principles of Medical Professionalism*, devoted several chapters to this topic.[14] There are also social justice implications. For example, some people consider the term *professionalism* itself to have racist undertones. They argue that it mainly focuses on dress code and appearance, which may be slanted toward prevailing standards in specific racial, gender, and generational groups.

Professionalism is also context specific, as Mintz et al. (three medical students) pointed out.[15] Being late to a session could appear unprofessional to the teacher who is running the class. However, if the reason is due to a patient requiring further attention, delaying departure from the clinical site would be the professionally appropriate action to take. Understandably, learners are very concerned that they are evaluated fairly, and that an uninformed assessment could harm their reputation.

Clearly, professionalism is a term that is fraught with emotions. The differences in definition can be traced back to cultural (institutional or national), generational, or profession-specific factors. Changes in technology (e.g., e-professionalism), therapeutics, and care delivery further influence the values and standards of each healthcare profession. Complicating the matter further is the potential compartmentalization of professional demeanor. For example, someone can act very properly toward peers, but act differently when in multiprofessional settings. Consequently, valid assessments require a holistic approach that uses a multitude of sources and tools. Many educators argue for a "programmatic assessment," described in Table 10.1 as best practice.

Table 10.1 Assessment Types and Terms Commonly Used in Health Professions Education

Diagnostic assessment	To identify gaps; can be used to inform a curriculum (e.g., a pretest) or to make admission decisions.
Formative assessment	*For* learning: requires a major emphasis on providing effective feedback to stimulate and guide further learning.
Summative assessment	*Of* learning: performed at the end of a course or program to make promotion decisions (e.g., Entrustable Professional Activities [EPAs]).
Standardized tests	All test takers respond to the same written or performance-based challenge and are assessed against uniform standards.
Performance-based assessment	Requires learners to demonstrate applied knowledge, skills, and attitudes while being observed.
Work-based assessment	Requires learners to demonstrate behaviors that imply knowledge, skills, and attitudes in an everyday work setting.
Progress testing	At routine intervals, the same assessment is given to all training levels to identify improvement and growth over time (e.g., according to Milestone expectations).
Sequential testing	Starting out with a limited screening test, one identifies individuals who clearly demonstrate the sought-after competencies. Those who do not or are borderline undergo further testing until a performance level can be determined with confidence.
Programmatic assessment	A system of assessments that is built into the curriculum and produces frequent quantitative and/or qualitative feedback loops to learners and programs.

Systematic Approaches to Professionalism Assessment

In 1990 George Miller introduced the "Miller's pyramid," which illustrates four levels of assessment: Knows, Knows How, Shows How, and Does.[16] In 2016 Cruess et al. highlighted the importance of professional identity formation by adding a fifth evaluation dimension,[17] as illustrated in Figure 10.1.

With so many competency levels at play, it becomes quite clear that no single tool can offer an adequate professionalism assessment. Table 10.2 provides an overview of Miller's pyramid regarding the type of competencies targeted, opportunities, and challenges, as well as some sample assessment formats that fall into these categories. All can be used for pre/posttesting to evaluate educational interventions, and all can be administered in person or online. Of course, it will be easier to create an online multiple-choice quiz (MCQ) than to implement a virtual Objective Structured Clinical Exam (OSCE). However, the latter will be able to assess a broader range of competencies regardless of administration mode.

Level 1: Know

As illustrated in Table 10.1, knowledge is at the very basis of every competence. At that level it is the ability to restate and identify "facts." MCQs are a useful tool to ascertain whether someone knows specific information and concepts. Bloom's Taxonomy of Educational Objectives with its more recent update[18] can help to make such type of

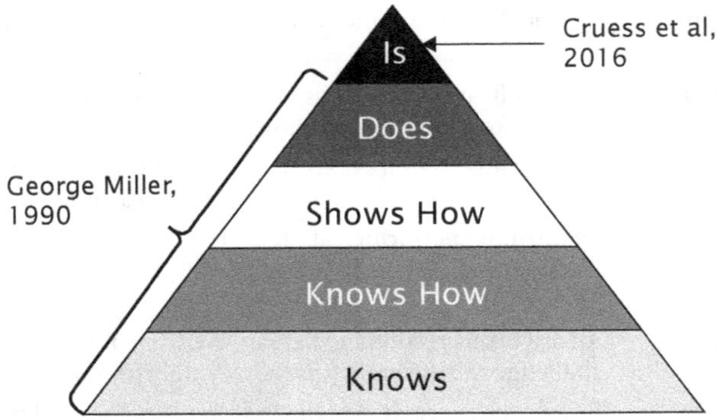

Figure 10.1 Miller's pyramid, adjusted for Professionalism.

questions go beyond mere recall. Table 10.2 provides more suggestions for how MCQs can assist with assessing professionalism.

While knowledge is a very basic competence, knowing ethical rules and laws is important. They can be a precursor of professional behavior. For example, it is worthwhile to ensure that learners know all the confidentiality laws if we want them to be able to apply them in a simulated or clinical setting.

Level 2: Knows How

One step up on the pyramid is "Knows How." This level addresses the learner's ability to select appropriate behaviors when given a specific scenario. Situational judgment tests (SJTs) are designed to do just that. They have become popular in business and other people-oriented professions as selection strategy because they are easy to administer, and they have been researched extensively. The latter included predictive studies that were able to show at least a modest ability to identify individuals who are at risk for subsequent disciplinary actions.[19]

The Association of American Medical Colleges (AAMC) has been working on such type assessments for a while,[20] and, in 2021, they launched the PREview™ Exam.[11] It covers the following domains: Service Orientation, Social Skills, Cultural Competence, Teamwork, Ethical Responsibility to Self and Others, Resilience and Adaptability, Reliability and Dependability, and Capacity for Improvement. In this computerized test, examinees are presented with medical school–related scenarios, and they can select from several response options. Scoring is based on how well each option corresponds with the choices made by medical education experts. The fact that this standardized test was developed in collaboration with medical schools makes it especially suitable for those type of admission decisions.

There are other SJTs that target social intelligence and professionalism more generically. Casper (Altos Company) has been producing them for a while longer than the AAMC and has recently expanded their assessments to fifteen word- or video-based scenarios. The response options similarly include text and video responses. All are subsequently evaluated by trained raters. Their new product focuses on the transition to graduate medical education and includes an SJT for application to residency programs.[21]

Table 10.2 Assessment Options Based on the Adapted Miller's Pyramid

Level	Competence Type	Assessment Formats	Opportunities	Limitations
1. Knows	K	Multiple Choice Questions (e.g., FERPA/HIPPA Quiz[18])	• Review of professional and legal standards • Easy to develop and easy to score • Results can be norm- or criterion referenced • Can be administered online	• Main focus is on recall
2. Knows How	K, A	Vignettes/Case-based questions with behavioral options or short-answer responses (e.g., Situational Judgment Test[11]) AAMC	• Ability to select answers based on knowledge and values • Correct answer can be based on expert consensus • Vignettes can be tailored to learner's context	• Social desirability can obscure true values
3. Shows How	K, S, A	Observation-based assessments of behavior (e.g., Objective Structured Clinical Exam – OSCE[10]) Walker-Descartes	• Can determine what someone is able to do in simulated or work-based setting • Skills cannot be faked so easily • With stimulus standardization and rater training observational assessments can become more reliable	• Performance under pressure may not be representative of actual behaviors, they could be worse or better • The test stimulus could lack uniformity for all learners (e.g., variations in standardized patient case portrayal) • Ratings can be biased
4. Does	K, S, A, B	Performance data collection under real life conditions (e.g., 360 Degree Evaluations[19])	• Based on actual behaviors and their outcomes • Multi-source evaluations by faculty, teams, peers, patients over an extended time period • Unannounced standardized patients can assess performance under actual work conditions	• Inadequate data collection (e.g., lack of patient feedback) • Departmental dynamics (e.g., hierarchy) can prevent honest assessments or reporting • Ratings can be biased
5. Is	A	Portfolio with reflections or essays with prompts (e.g., Professional Identity Essay[9]) Kalet	• Attempts to capture true/lived values • Can be aligned with developmental stages • Easy to set up • Artificial intelligence can facilitate scoring	• Difficult to analyze and interpret

K = Knowledge, S = Skills, A = Attitudes/Values, B = Behavior.

Level 3: Shows How

The third level toward the top of the pyramid is called "Shows How." It more directly assesses what someone is actually able to do, albeit under test conditions. It is a step up because it requires the demonstration of skills that can occur in a simulated environment or an actual clinical setting through direct observation with standardized rating forms.

The OSCEs are a multistation formative or summative assessment in which scenarios, learner tasks, rating forms, and timing are fully standardized. Since 1975,[22] these types of assessments have been used worldwide, even for national exams. Some such programs use professionalism as a performance dimension that is being assessed in all stations. Other OSCEs include specific stations that address professionalism-related tasks. Dealing with a medical mistake is a very frequently used scenario, but there are many others, such as confronting a colleague about unprofessional behaviors, staying professional while dealing with a biased patient, or changing gears when realizing that a colleague is impaired and cannot perform as expected. Some programs have developed OSCEs that are entirely devoted to professionalism.[23] But, even if such stations are just embedded in a more general formative OSCE, they can have a long-lasting effect on learners.[24,25]

Many non-OSCE simulations involve teamwork, and they also can provide excellent opportunities to evaluate interprofessional behaviors by including standardized team members. Another example is a procedural simulation with a mannequin that results in a negative outcome that the learner then has to communicate to a standardized family member. Through simulation, one can recreate real-life events that are important, but too difficult to capture for professionalism assessments.

Mini Clinical Evaluation Exercises (Mini CEXs) have become a very popular work-based assessment. Following the same principles of sampling performance when observing learners in clinical settings, Cruess et al. introduced the Professionalism–Mini Evaluation Exercise (P-MEX) in 2006.[26] Since then, the instrument has been translated and examined in several countries, and it is promoted by the ACGME. Various studies have been performed to address the validity and reliability of the original instrument. While there is some debate about individual items, the four domains remain constant: Doctor-Patient Relationship Skills, Reflective Skills, Time Management, and Interprofessional Relationship Skills. Although a shorter list than the above described AAMC PREview[11] domains, the categories definitely overlap.

Level 4: Does

The fourth level focuses on the "Does," how competencies are practiced in the daily work environment, without direct observation. Professionalism lapses are not uncommon; most people will admit that no one is immune to them, and theories have been developed to explain how they come about.[27] Of course, lapses range in severity and persistence, but they do require common standards and agreement about the behavioral manifestations. Due to the diversity of definitions described above, multiple perspectives are needed to provide a reliable and fair assessment.

Some institutions have developed critical incident reporting systems to document professionalism issues.[28] They vary in terms of format, such as the level of detail, anonymity of reporter, processing strategies, and consequences. Typically, such reports trigger remediation efforts, and a significant number of them can result in dismissal. To implement such a system, there needs to be a clear understanding about the various types and levels of transgression. It is only fair to the learners that such "measurements" are publicized widely among all involved. One critique about using this tool is that it often only focuses on negative behavior (i.e., lapses) and does not provide opportunities to give credit for outstanding professionalism performance.

Multisource feedback, also referred to as 360-degree evaluations, can be more successful in capturing negative and positive professional behaviors.[19] They incorporate multiple perspectives, which provides a more comprehensive assessment by expanding the observation opportunities exponentially. In addition to supervisors, 360-degree assessments also collect evaluations from peers (at, above, and below the learner's level of training), other healthcare providers (e.g., nurses), and patients and/or families. Each evaluator type can be influenced by factors such as institutional hierarchies, generational and cultural differences, or dependencies for grading or patient care. However, incorporating multiple perspectives can help balance out some of the biases that can creep into performance evaluations. Typically, learners are also asked to provide a self-assessment, which can later be compared to the assessments by others. Although such types of assessment are difficult to implement (especially collecting meaningful data from patients and families), the wider the circle, the better the chance for capturing the true level of professionalism.

To address the challenges of collecting multiple assessments for each learner, the ACGME recently installed an online system to elicit, collect, and analyze evaluations that are personalized for each learner.[29] The Teamwork Effectiveness Assessment Module (TEAM) consists of the following steps: (1) The resident or fellow completes a self-assessment. (2) The program identifies interprofessional healthcare providers he or she worked with during a rotation. These providers are contacted via email to provide ratings and feedback about the learner's performance. (3) The data are collected from the designated team members, and ratings as well as comments are compiled in a report. (4) Based on the report the learner creates a plan for improvement or for building on the identified strengths, which is discussed with the program director or advisor. Evaluator comments add more specificity to the ratings and further illuminate what behaviors to keep and what to change.

Unannounced standardized patients provide unique opportunities to merge the benefits of standardization with the benefits of assessing competencies in a natural context.[30] The scenario and case are kept constant, standardized patients are rehearsed, rating forms are uniform and trained for, but the examinee is not aware of being observed in their clinical environment. Thus, this evaluation strategy has a good chance to create a valid assessment result. For ethical reasons examinees are informed that they will receive a visit from such a "secret shopper," but they don't know when and research has shown that the detection rate is generally low.[31]

Level 5: Is

The top of the pyramid represents professionalism identity formation, often abbreviated as PIF.[32] It takes a developmental approach and is similar to Milestones. Staging professional developments is complex and requires a theoretical framework that postulates how professionals develop their identity over the course of their training or maybe even beyond that, their careers. There is also a need for clearly specified and accurate measurements and well-trained raters. Of course, progress on the professionalism trajectory can also be tracked by some of the previously discussed evaluation tools that are not necessarily tied to a developmental scheme.

Reflections are considered a preferred pathway to gain insight into a person's values and level of maturity. They have even been linked with professionalism lapses,[33] which makes them especially useful. Portfolios that require reflective comments are often considered a go-to assessment tool to demonstrate professional growth. The Professional Identity Essay (PIE) operates on a similar principle. Examinees are given a series of prompts to choose from (e.g., What will the profession expect from you? What would be the worst thing for you if you failed to live up to the expectations of your patients?). The resulting essay is then analyzed by a trained and blinded rater using a rubric that is keyed into a theoretical development model. Research has demonstrated improvement over preclerkship training. [9] Similar strategies have been applied to assess professionalism growth during the COVID-19 pandemic[34] and posed questions such as: "What have you done to adapt to this situation?" to Indonesian students at various levels of undergraduate medical education. Using qualitative research tools for analysis, they could demonstrate different levels of professional maturity.

Triangulating Data to Arrive at Justifiable Judgments

Calling someone out for being unprofessional is difficult. Many people will avoid communicating such judgments for fear of damaging the relationship or potential legal repercussions (e.g., a defamation lawsuit). Since there is no single "perfect" assessment, we need to apply multiple tools, multiple times for a better chance to approximate the truth about someone's level of professionalism. Only when bringing all the data together can a clear picture emerge.

Beyond the issue of "fairness," one also must ask whether the problem is really a professionalism issue. All tools previously described have a significant link to communication skills: verbal, nonverbal, or written. Separating these two competencies can be difficult, maybe sometimes even impossible. Language fluency and cultural differences can also be a major contributor to behavior that may just appear to be caused by a lack of professionalism.[35] Other factors to consider are bias, law, contextual factors (e.g., a provocative patient), personal problems, and mental health issues. When reaching the Does level, one must also consider the institutional culture, the hidden curriculum, and role modeling that can facilitate or prohibit professional behavior and lead to wrong assumptions about someone's identity formation. For example, in a study of medicine clerkship student entries into a professionalism journal, the number of stories related to role models interacting respectfully with patients were primarily positive, whereas the interactions with colleagues recorded were entirely negative.[36] As Rougas et al. highlight, one can't underestimate the power of role models, and educators need to have some robust understanding of learners' experience before judging their behavior.[37]

Summary

Clearly, healthcare educators are taking the need for teaching and assessing professionalism very seriously. By making it a core competency, a new urgency to find quality assessment tools has emerged. Unfortunately, this is a complex undertaking, and there are no easy fixes. In addition to coming up with effective assessment tools, there are also many logistical concerns. It is reassuring that organizations like the ACGME or AAMC as well as industry-based companies are developing programs to address administrative needs. Organizations like the Academy for Professionalism in Healthcare (APHC) can advance our definition and understanding of the competency itself and help with disseminating tools and strategies for its assessment.

In 2013, Goldie identified the assessment of professionalism as an "evolving field,"[38] and we are clearly still far from having conquered the intricacies of making professionalism-related judgments. More strategies and research will be needed to develop best practices and robust systems that can adjust to the changes in our definitions and cultural contexts. One thing is very clear: We cannot rely on a single sample of professional or unprofessional behavior to make a definitive judgment. A complex and multifactorial competency like professionalism requires the thoughtful selection, administration, analysis, and interpretation of multiple assessment tools to allow for meaningful and timely remediation or to provide justification and documentation for withholding promotions, which would have been very important in the case of Michael Swango, where a lack of taking action had such disastrous results.[3]

References

1. Exploring the ACME Core Competencies: Professionalism. Accessed March 25, 2023. https://knowledgeplus.nejm.org/blog/acgme-core-competencies-professionalism/
2. Cao H, Song Y, Wu Y, et al. What is nursing professionalism? A concept analysis. *BMC Nurs.* 2023;22:34. https://doi.org/10.1186/s12912-022-01161-0
3. Stewart JB. *Blind Eye: How the Medical Establishment Let a Doctor Get Away With Murder.* Simon & Schuster; 1999.
4. Wilkinson TJ, Wade WB, Knock LD, Aiyer MK. A blueprint to assess professionalism: results of a systematic review. *Acad Med.* 2009;84(5):551–558.
5. Rider EA., Nowotny N, Smith MA. Assessing professionalism: a review of the literature. *J Gen Intern Med.* 2007;22(5):670–674.
6. Klemenc-Ketiš Z, Vrecko H. Measuring medical professionalism: a systematic review of instruments and their measurement properties. *J Educ Eval Health Prof.* 2015;12:39.
7. Li H, Ding N, Zhang Y, Liu Y, Wen D. Assessing medical professionalism: a systematic review of instruments and their measurement properties. *PLoS One* 2017;12(5):e0177321. https://doi.org/10.1371/journal.pone.0177321
8. Tay KT, Ng S, Hee JM, Chia EWY, et al. Assessing professionalism in medicine—a scoping review of assessment tools from 1990 to 2018. *J Med Educ Curric Dev.* 2020;7:2382120520955159. doi:10.1177/2382120520955159
9. Kalet A, Buckvar-Keltz L, Monson V, et al. Professional identity formation in medical school: one measure reflects changes during pre-clerkship training [version 1]. *MedEdPublish.* 2018;7:41. https://doi.org/10.15694/mep.2018.0000041.1
10. Walker-Descartes I, Kachur E, Altshuler L, Beckett O, Johnson Z. Addressing sexual harassment allegations with a colleague: a challenging OSCE station. *J Grad Med Educ.* 2020;12(3):352–353. doi:10.4300/JGME-D-19-00836.1
11. AAMC PREview™ Professional Readiness Exam. Accessed March 25,2023. https://students-residents.aamc.org/aamc-preview/aamc-preview-professional-readiness-exam

12. Wamsley M, Thompson V. Debriefing a professionalism lapse. Accessed March 25, 2023. https://meded21.ucsf.edu/sites/g/files/tkssra796/f/wysiwyg/W15%20Professionalism.pdf)
13. American Board of Internal Medicine (ABIM). Medical professionalism in the new millennium: a physician charter. https://abimfoundation.org/wp-content/uploads/2015/12/Medical-Professionalism-in-the-New-Millenium-A-Physician-Charter.pdf
14. Merlo G. *Principles of Medical Professionalism.* Oxford University Press, 2021
15. Mintz R, Pierson L, Miller DG. Rethinking professionalism assessment in medical education. *Ann Intern Med.* 2022;175(7):1030–1031. https://doi.org/10.7326/M22-0488
16. Miller GE. The assessment of clinical skills/competence/performance. *Acad Med.* 1990;65:S63–S67. doi:10.1097/00001888-199009000-00045
17. Cruess RL, Cruess SR, Steinert Y. Amending Miller's pyramid to include professional identity formation. *Acad Med.* 2016;91(2):180–185. doi:10.1097/ACM.0000000000000913
18. Anderson LW, Krathwohl DR, Bloom BS. *A Taxonomy for Learning, Teaching, and Assessing: A Revision of Bloom's Taxonomy of Educational Objectives.* Longman; 2001.
19. Tiffin PA, Sanger E, Smith DT, Troughton A, Paton LW. Situational judgement test performance and subsequent misconduct in medical students. *Med Educ.* 2022;56(7):754–763. doi:10.1111/medu.14801
20. AAMC PREview Professional Readiness Exam Research. Accessed March 25, 2023. https://www.aamc.org/services/admissions-lifecycle/aamc-preview-professional-readiness-exam-research
21. Dou T. Casper is changing for 2022–23. 2022, February 15. https://takealtus.com/2022/02/casper-is-changing-for-2022-23
22. Harden RM, Stevenson M, Downie WW, Wilson GM. Assessment of clinical competence using objective structured examination. *Br Med J.* 1975;1(5955):447–451. doi:10.1136/bmj.1.5955.447
23. Hochberg MS, Kalet A, Zabar S, Kachur E, Gillespie C, Berman RS. Can professionalism be taught? Encouraging evidence. *Am J Surg.* 2010;199(1):86–93. doi:10.1016/j.amjsurg.2009.10.002
24. Aeder L, Altshuler L, Kachur E, Langenau E. Fostering an atmosphere of professionalism in a residency program: Learning how to address the unprofessional behavior of colleagues through OSCEs. *Mededportal.* 2012;8(4):9168. https://www.mededportal.org/doi/10.15766/mep_2374-8265.9168
25. Aeder L, Altshuler L, Kachur E, Walker-Descartes I. Empowering trainees to promote professionalism. *Clin Teach.* 2018;15(4):304–308. doi:10.1111/tct.12680
26. Cruess R, McIlroy JH, Cruess S, Ginsburg S, Steinert Y. The Professionalism Mini-evaluation Exercise: a preliminary investigation. *Acad Med.* 2006;81(10 suppl):S74–S78. doi:10.1097/00001888-200610001-00019
27. Chang HJ, Lee YM, Lee YH, Kwon HJ. Causes of resident lapses in professional conduct during the training: a qualitative study on the perspectives of residents. *Med Teach.* 2017;39(3):278–284. doi:10.1080/0142159X.2017.1270432
28. Rademacher R, Simpson D, Marcdante K. Critical incidents as a technique for teaching professionalism. *Med Teach.* 2010;32(3):244–249. doi:10.3109/01421590903197001
29. Accreditation Council for Graduate Medical Education (ACGME). Teamwork Effectiveness Assessment Module. Accessed March 28, 2023. https://dl.acgme.org/learn/course/team-website-instructions/team-instructions/team-guide-for-users

30. Taormina DP, Zuckerman JD, Karia R, Zabar S, Egol KA, Phillips DP. Clinical skills and professionalism: assessing orthopaedic residents with unannounced standardized patients. *J Surg Educ.* 2018;75(2):427–433. doi:10.1016/j.jsurg.2017.08.001

31. Franz CE, Epstein R, Miller KN, et al. Caught in the act? Prevalence, predictors, and consequences of physician detection of unannounced standardized patients. *Health Serv Res.* 2006;41(6):2290–2302. doi:10.1111/j.1475-6773.2006.00560.x

32. Teo KJH, Teo MYK, Pisupati A, et al. Assessing professional identity formation (PIF) amongst medical students in oncology and palliative medicine postings: a SEBA guided scoping review. *BMC Palliat Care.* 2022;21:200. https://doi.org/10.1186/s12904-022-01090-4

33. Hoffman LA, Shew RL, Vu TR, Brokaw JJ, Frankel RM. Is reflective ability associated with professionalism lapses during medical School? *Acad Med.* 2016;91(6):853–857. doi:10.1097/ACM.0000000000001094

34. Findyartini A, Anggraeni D, Husin JM, Greviana N. Exploring medical students' professional identity formation through written reflections during the COVID-19 pandemic. *J Public Health Res.* 2020;9(suppl 1):1918. doi:10.4081/jphr.2020.1918

35. Hodges B, Paul R, Ginsburg S, Ottawa Consensus Group Members. Assessment of professionalism: from where have we come—to where are we going? An update from the Ottawa Consensus Group on the assessment of professionalism. *Med Teach.* 2019;41(3):249–255. doi:10.1080/0142159X.2018.1543862

36. Karnieli-Miller O, Vu TR, Holtman MC, Clyman SG, Inui TS. Medical students' professionalism narratives: a window on the informal and hidden curriculum. *Acad Med.* 2010;85(1):124–133. doi:10.1097/ACM.0b013e3181c42896. Erratum in: Acad Med. 2011;86(1):29.

37. Rougas S, Gentilesco B, Green E, Flores L. Twelve tips for addressing medical student and resident physician lapses in professionalism. *Med Teach.* 2015;37(10):901–907. doi:10.3109/0142159X.2014.1001730

38 .Goldie J. Assessment of professionalism: a consolidation of current thinking. *Med Teach.* 2013;35(2):e952–e956. doi:10.3109/0142159X.2012.714888

11
Assessing Professional Identity Formation
Mission Impossible?

Suzanne Goh, Shiva Sarraf-Yazdi, and Lalit Kumar Radha Krishna

Key Points

- Professional identity formation (PIF) is conceptually different from professionalism. PIF is the activity through which professionalism is attained, and it has multiple different assessment strategies.
- Core elements of PIF assessment include that it is individualized, multidimensional, longitudinal, flexible and accessible, institutionally supported, and regarded as valuable to learners.
- Reflective portfolios are a key component to teaching PIF and developing professionalism among medical professionals.

Introduction

Professional identity formation (PIF) has been considered the backbone,[1] the highest purpose and the "principal objective"[2(p1450)] of medical education. While implied as a goal of medical education, attending to PIF has not always been explicit.

Flexner,[3] in his 1910 report on medical education, identified a failure to focus on PIF as one of the four key deficits in medical education. In 1957, Merton rang that gong again when he laid out the expectations of medical schools to provide students with a professional identity that enables them to "think, act and feel like a physician."[4(p7)] Yet, it is perhaps the 2010 Carnegie Foundation call for reform in medical education related to explicitly cultivating the formation of professional identity[5] that has significantly focused efforts to support PIF along the medical education continuum.

Assessment of such an ethereal construct as identity formation is understandably complex and challenging. In this chapter, we focus on PIF and consider the strategies and approaches to its assessment. Notwithstanding that this may potentially be a fool's errand, the aim is to provide literature-backed direction, rather than instruction, for those seeking an approach to assessing PIF.

A Précis of Professional Identity Formation

Myriad affordances and hindrances, from an individual's existing values, norms, and expectations to those at institutional and societal levels, come to shape one's professional identity. For example, factors that influence students' PIF in medical school run the gamut from the formal curriculum to the co-curricular space and the learning environment. Curricular efforts are primarily focused on ethics and professionalism education, reflective practice, medical humanities, and various experiences involving real and standardized patients.[6,7] In the co-curricular arena, platforms typically include opportunities for community service and professional socialization.[7] Approaches aimed at shaping the culture and environment involve mentoring and role-modeling initiatives, symbolic socialization events (e.g., white coat ceremony, donor memorial service), and acknowledging the informal and hidden curriculum.[6]

However, the use of intentional, focused, and guided reflective practice remains the sine qua non for effective support of PIF.[6,8] This is not surprising when considering that identity formation is an internal process that is invisible, intangible, fluid, unceasing, nonlinear, and individualized, while also encompassing the professional community's values and practices and social context.

Given its complex nature, it is also unsurprising that there is no single, gold standard, evidence-based method of assessing PIF. As stated by Cruess et al. about PIF assessment: "A single standard as an educational objective is not only impossible, it is undesirable."[9(p183)] In the absence of a holy grail of valid, reliable, and feasible assessment methods to do just that, how then do we ensure that medical students and trainees are on track as they strive to developmentally "think, act, and feel like a physician"?[4(p7)]

The Power of PIF

Over the last two decades, efforts to understand PIF through underlying theories and models have grown significantly, but why is attending to PIF important?

There is growing evidence to suggest that effective PIF can support physician well-being and resilience.[10,11] Toubassi et al. have postulated that curricular strategies to support learners' PIF improves their well-being.[12] While not preventive, such an approach may attenuate the negative effects of encountering challenges, enable individuals "to realize and value the significance of their efforts" that they come to consider as "worthwhile and justifiable," and to "potentially even celebrate, their purpose as physicians."[12(p307)]

The consequences of poor PIF are too significant to ignore. Diminished physician well-being can lead to erosion of empathy, substandard patient care, and increased frequency of medical errors.[13–15] Dissonance between one's personal and professional identities and expectations can lead to unethical behavior, professional misconduct, poor well-being and burnout, leaving the profession, and even suicide,[16–22] all of which are on the rise and suggested to be "observable manifestations of poor PIF."[23(p247)]

With the urgency and spotlight on the well-being of healthcare professionals globally brought on by the COVID-19 pandemic, there is a rising tide of recognition that something needs to be done, done well, and done now. In response to this, the National Academy of Medicine launched the National Plan for Health Workforce Well-Being in the United States in October 2022 "to drive collective action to strengthen health workforce well-being and restore the health of the nation."[24] Other countries have also developed resources and support services aimed at promoting the well-being of health professionals.[25–27] However, beyond supporting those in crisis, it behooves medical educators to collectively pay heed to this groundswell of attention on healthcare professionals' well-being and to actively cultivate PIF in the effort to develop resilient practitioners. This necessitates systems-level and organization-directed strategies.[28]

Professional Identity Formation Versus Professionalism

When attempting to identify an assessment strategy for PIF, a question often surfaces of where professionalism ends and PIF starts. Intrinsically and inextricably linked, just as an artist cannot be separated from their art, Moseley et al. described PIF as "an internal, perceptional process of development," while "professionalism is the outward display of professional behaviors."[29] Professionalism in medicine is committing to the medical profession and expectations demanded of physicians, which requires adoption of a shared belief system. As the person internalizes and assimilates professional traits into intrinsic characteristics and observable actions, they become more committed and further demonstrate professional behavior. In the process, an evolving integrated personal and professional identity is formed and reformed. On the other hand, identifying as a member of the profession and striving to form an identity consistent with those members through socialization necessitates that the professions' values and behaviors be upheld and demonstrated. Upholding the profession's expectations and embodying its roles and responsibilities foster the forming of professional identity. PIF is thus "a necessary foundation for professionalism,"[30(pe603)] while learning professionalism is a means to help learners and practitioners shape their professional identity.[9]

These distinct, albeit related, constructs are often conflated and used interchangeably, as are their overlapping assessment strategies. As interlinked as these concepts are, however, one should not be subsumed within the other. In Figure 11.1, we use examples to draw distinctions between PIF and professionalism and suggest potential outcomes depending on permutations with and without each construct.

		Professionalism	
		+	–
Professional Identity Formation	+	Deepening commitment Professional fulfillment	Safe practice, poor bedside manner (e.g., television personality "Dr House")
	–	Dissonance Disillusionment	Unsafe practice Attrition

Figure 11.1 Potential permutations of professionalism and PIF resulting in different outcomes.

There are four different permutations to consider when it comes to professionalism and PIF:

1. Those who have both positive PIF and professionalism: These individuals conduct themselves professionally because professionalism is an essential part of their identity. They possess a strong sense of professional values and beliefs that guides their behavior.
2. Those who have PIF but lack professionalism: This group may have developed a sense of professional identity, but they struggle to adhere to professional standards and conduct themselves appropriately. Their behavior may not align with the expectations of their field, indicating a gap between their identity and their actions. Dr. House from the popular medical drama TV series is a clear example of a doctor who has a sense of PIF but exhibits poor professionalism. Despite his exceptional diagnostic skills and dedication to medicine that point to a level of PIF, he typically ignored protocols, behaved rudely toward others, and crossed ethical boundaries, demonstrating poor professionalism.
3. Those who demonstrate professionalism but lack well-formed PIF: These individuals are capable of behaving professionally and meeting the standards of their profession, but they may not have developed a deep-rooted professional identity. They may follow the rules and expectations out of external pressures or fear of consequences rather than a genuine internal commitment and may struggle to do so when circumstances prove challenging or potentially disadvantageous.
4. Those who lack both PIF and professionalism: This category includes individuals who neither possess a well-formed professional identity nor exhibit professional behavior. They are considered unsafe and unreliable in their professional practice and should not be allowed to continue in their field.

Failing to appreciate the differences could lead, for example, to primarily assessing externally observed behaviors, independent of a person's values and beliefs that drive their way of "being." That said, assessing the latter poses a formidable challenge. Indeed, assessing PIF separately from professionalism is problematic—perhaps even questionable.

PIF Theoretical and Conceptual Models

Before discussing assessment strategies, an overview of the underlying theories and conceptual models may help inform the development of more effective and meaningful PIF assessment strategies, which can in turn help to support the development of the learners.

There has been an abundance of PIF theories in the last two decades, spanning the individualist to the social-cultural and contextual spectrum.[31,32] These provide a framework for understanding how professional identity evolves over time. By identifying key domains, stages, or processes of PIF, these theories and models can guide the development of assessment approaches aligned with the complexity and multidimensionality of PIF. While a comprehensive presentation and discussion of all the theories is beyond the scope of this chapter, a summary is shown in Table 11.1.

Table 11.1 Select PIF Theories and Conceptual Models

Theory/Model	Authors	Premise
Kegan's Stages of PIF "Orders of Consciousness"[38]	Kegan, 1982	Proposes that individuals progress through five stages of development as they grow and mature in their professional roles. These stages include the Impulsive Self, Socialized Self, Self-Authoring Self, Self-Transforming Self, and Self-Transcending Self. Each stage involves a greater level of self-awareness, autonomy, and complexity in one's thinking and behavior.
Reflective practice model[42]	Schön, 1983	This model suggests that professional identity is formed through ongoing critical reflection and self-evaluation of one's professional practice.
Social cognitive career theory[44]	Lent et al., 1994	This model emphasizes the role of social and contextual factors when forming a professional identity, including the influence of mentors, peers, and organizational culture.
Socialization theory[33]	Hafferty, 2000	Suggests that medical professionals are socialized into their roles through a process of observation and imitation. According to this theory, medical students learn what it means to be a doctor by observing and emulating the behaviors and attitudes of their colleagues.
Narrative theory[35]	Charon, 2001	Suggests that PIF is related to the stories that medical professionals tell about themselves and their experiences. By creating a coherent narrative that connects their experiences and actions, medical professionals can construct a professional identity that is meaningful and coherent.
Communities of practice model[41]	Wenger, 2007	This model posits that professional identity is developed through participating in the activities of a community in which a common set of professional practices and values are shared.
Self-authorship model[43]	Baxter Magolda, 2009	This model proposes that professional identity is developed through a process of self-authorship, which involves developing an integrated and coherent sense of self grounded in personal values and beliefs.
The Ring Theory of Personhood[36]	Krishna & Alsuwaigh, 2015	Conceptualizes personhood as a series of concentric rings, with the central ring representing the individual's core identity. As an individual moves outward through the rings, they encounter experiences and socialization factors that influence their identity formation. This theory emphasizes that personal and professional identities are interconnected and integrated.
The Onion Model of PIF[37]	Barnhoorn, 2016	The onion metaphor suggests that PIF is a dynamic, layered, and multi-dimensional process that involves the interaction of multiple identity components, rather than a linear, hierarchical progression. Barnhoorn identifies six layers: individuality, community, institutional culture, personal values, role conception, and profession-specific skills and knowledge. These layers are interconnected and interact with one another, shaping the individual's professional identity as they progress through their career.

(continued)

Table 11.1 Continued

Theory/Model	Authors	Premise
The PIF Model by Cruess et al.[9]	Cruess et al., 2016	This model involves four stages: anticipatory, professional identity formation, consolidation, and continuing professional identity formation. These represent a process of ongoing development and evolution of a healthcare professional's identity and sense of belonging to the profession.
Cognitive development theory[34]	Durning et al., 2016	Suggests that PIF is related to cognitive development. As medical professionals progress through their training, they develop more complex cognitive structures that allow them to integrate and make sense of their experiences.
The Integrated Model[40]	Haidet et al., 2016	This model emphasizes the importance of three key domains in PIF: personal, social, and cultural. Personal domain refers to an individual's internal self-concept, social domain entails interactions with others in the profession, and cultural domain refers to the larger societal context of medicine.
The Dual Processing Model[39]	Helmich et al., 2018	Proposes that professional identity is formed through two processes: socialization and self-construction. Socialization is the process by which students adopt the norms and values of the medical profession, while self-construction involves integrating personal experiences and beliefs into the professional identity.

Many current theories of PIF have shifted focus on the introduction, integration, and expression of the desired values, beliefs, and principles required by the organization, society, and profession to a more expansive idea of PIF. Guided by recent studies, new models of PIF pay due consideration to the context-sensitive, personalized, longitudinal nature of this "transformative journey through which one integrates the knowledge, skills, values, and behaviors of a competent, humanistic physician with one's own unique identity and core values."[2, 5(p762)] This holistic, multidimensional perspective has ramifications on assessments of PIF.

Parameters for Assessing PIF

Given the all-encompassing nature of PIF, clearly identifying and demonstrating what constitutes "success" is no easy task. Adding to the challenge, as society and healthcare evolve, it is inevitable that new medical competencies and aspects of professional expectations and identities emerge, such as with the advent of telemedicine, electronic medical records,[45] and even the evolution of the professional dress code.

Any assessment of PIF should thus account for the individual's experiences within the social context of the professional setting. The messiness of the construct itself reinforces the need for a multiprong assessment approach. There is growing evidence that PIF assessment should have the following characteristics and parameters[46]:

1. Be individualized and personalized.[9,47]
2. Be multisourced (including self, faculty, patients, peers)[7,48] and multidimensional[49]; employ multiple and mixed methods[29,48]; and be context dependent[50] to allow a holistic sampling that more accurately represents the person.
3. Be longitudinal and conducted at multiple time points including key transitions.[3,7,29,51,52] This allows capturing the developing professional identity and recognizing and responding to any support needs in a timely manner.
4. Be accessible[53] and sufficiently flexible.[54–58] This would improve feasibility and learner ownership and buy-in, contributing to authenticity.
5. Have institutional support and oversight.[59] Viewing PIF assessment as an individual construct puts the onus on the individual to "be" the good doctor without due attention to the wider context, such as hidden curricula or institutional cultures. The logistical complexity of multifaceted PIF assessments further render it unfeasible without support and oversight by the host organization. The institution should, for example, ensure faculty training and development to enable effective feedback and fair assessment.[60] Program evaluations, as well as providing timely support for learners,[46] should be driven by the host organization.
6. Be regarded as valuable by the learners.[60] They are more likely to engage meaningfully with the process and the feedback they receive when they buy-in to the value of the assessments, thus supporting PIF.

PIF and Miller's Pyramid

Miller's pyramid has long been used to guide decisions on assessment and program evaluation strategies in medical education. When considering professionalism, Hafferty posed the question about whether the focus should be on "what one is rather than what one does."[61(p54)] Cruess et al. championed the intentional shift in emphasis from "doing" to "being" with PIF and amended Miller's pyramid to better account for PIF by proposing a fifth and apex level, "Is," to describe one who "consistently demonstrates the attitudes, values, and behaviors expected of one who has come to think, act, and feel like a physician."[9(p181)]

While Cruess's fifth level is intended to reflect PIF holistically, assessing PIF can target each of the lower levels to capture the various components that contribute to PIF, including professionalism. In Table 11.2, we show examples of assessment objectives for professionalism and PIF, suggesting how these may manifest in a medical student who is not yet a full-fledged professional. In crafting a PIF assessment strategy, the objectives would focus more on affective components such as commitment and belonging to the medical community.

If we assert that "doing" alone cannot ultimately define having effectively formed one's professional identity, then learners lacking the level of expertise to act like a physician can still demonstrate "thinking and feeling" like one, all the while doing what is developmentally appropriate. In this case, to reflect the continuum within which PIF progresses, rather than a distinct arrival into Is, we explicitly recognize a process of "becoming" when transitioning from doing (e.g., in medical school and early training years) to "being" (e.g., in later periods of training and in clinical practice).

Table 11.2 Examples of Assessment Objectives for Professionalism and PIF

Miller's Pyramid Stage	Professionalism Objectives	Examples of How It May Manifest in an Early Medical Student	PIF Objective	Examples of How It May Manifest in an Early Medical Student
Knows	Identify key elements of professional behavior	The student can articulate key elements of professional behavior, such as accountability, honesty, and ethical conduct, and can demonstrate an understanding of how these elements relate to the practice of medicine.	Identify personal values and beliefs that align with the medical profession	The student can identify their personal values and beliefs and reflect on how they align with the values of the medical profession.
Knows How	Demonstrate ethical decision-making in clinical scenarios	The student can explain the steps involved in ethical decision-making, such as identifying the ethical dilemma, gathering information, and considering alternative courses of action.	Begin to articulate how personal values and beliefs may inform ethical decision-making	The student can demonstrate some understanding of ethical principles and their application to clinical scenarios and can begin to reflect on how their personal values and beliefs may inform their ethical decision-making.
Shows How	Consistently exhibit professional behavior in all aspects of medical education	The student can consistently exhibit professional behavior in all aspects of medical education (e.g., attending all required classes, meeting assignment deadlines, and collaborating respectfully with peers).	Reflect on how exposure to clinical settings has impacted their view of the medical profession	The student can reflect on their experiences in clinical settings and can identify specific instances in which these experiences have impacted their views of the medical profession and their own professional identity.
Does	Demonstrate professional behaviors and attitudes in all aspects of patient care	The student can demonstrate professionalism by arriving on time to clinical rotations, dressing appropriately, being respectful and courteous to patients and colleagues, and completing all expected learning requirements on time.	Assess and reflect on personal and professional growth in relation to professional identity formation	The student can reflect on their experiences in medical school thus far and can identify specific instances in which they have grown both personally and professionally, as well as how these experiences have impacted their development of a professional identity.

Table 11.2 Continued

Miller's Pyramid Stage		Professionalism Objectives	Examples of How It May Manifest in an Early Medical Student	PIF Objective	Examples of How It May Manifest in an Early Medical Student
Is	Becoming	At the level of "Is", professionalism becomes integrated into the developing professional identity. Begin to integrate personal and professional values into a developing professional identity			The student can be a role model for professionalism by demonstrating ethical and compassionate behavior, integrity, and by treating others with respect and dignity. They can link this with their developing professional identity grounded in personal and professional values and can identify areas for growth.
	Being	Integrate personal and professional values into a cohesive professional identity that guides practice			The student can embrace professional behavior as a core component of medical practice into their personal and professional values, believing in the importance of this behavior for building trust and rapport with patients, collaborating effectively in teams, and maintaining a professional reputation.

PIF Assessment Tools

There are a multitude of methods and tools aimed at assessing elements of PIF, yet none wholly effective on its own. Tools commonly utilized to assess PIF are summarized in Table 11.3. These include reflective writing (with or without prompts), surveys, inventories, questionnaires, and guided feedback. Many existing tools for assessing PIF emphasize character traits and attributes, professional conduct, foundational knowledge of ethical and professionalism principles, moral reasoning, communication skills, and show of empathy.[46] In a recent critical review of PIF interventions in medical education, Mount et al. demonstrated that the key ingredient to most, if not all, PIF-related

Table 11.3 Approaches and Tools for Assessing PIF

Assessment Approaches and Tools for PIF	
Reflection-Based (With and Without Facilitated Discussions)	
Guided feedback62	Focuses on providing personalized, appropriate, specific, and timely feedback on a clinician's developing critical thinking skills and competencies over their learning trajectory. It helps clinicians generalize specific interactions to their wider practice, supports confronting challenging experiences, explores and validates emotional responses, fosters courage and tolerance of uncertainty, and builds resilience. It challenges the clinician to advance to the next competency level.
Structured activity: "A Learning Experience" (ALE)63	To elicit and examine the description and depth of reflections
Brown's Guide/ BEGAN tool (the Brown Educational Guide to the Analysis of Narrative)64	To guide faculty to provide concise, individualized feedback on a piece of reflective writing, integrating quotations from the narratives with pertinent faculty comments, personal experiences, elements of close reading and reflection, inviting questions
Reflection Evaluation for Enhanced Competences Tool Rubric (REFLECT)65	To facilitate multidimensional analysis of writing spectrum, presence, description of conflict, attending to emotions and meaning making to appraise "reflection-on-action" processes
Thematic scoring ("to map and grade the reflection themes") and Reflection score65	To quantitatively evaluate the number of themes identified in reflective writing, used in conjunction with the REFLECT rubric
Self-Reflection and Insight Scale (SRIS)66	To determine the individual's readiness for self-regulated behavior change by determining their motives and clarity of insight (self-administered, 20-item closed questionnaire)
Groningen Reflection Ability Scale (GRAS)67	To appraise a clinician's self-reflection, empathetic reflection, and reflective communication
Reflective ability rubric68	To assess an individual's level of reflective ability in essays written around a specific prompt or topic
Reflection-in-Learning Scale (RLS)69	Assesses conscious engagement, meaningfulness, self-confidence, depth and self-efficacy in the process of self-regulated learning
Self-assessments	Based on personal reflection
Moral reasoning assessments	Based on personal reflection
Professional identity essay (PIE)70	To determine the developmental level of PIF and promote in-depth reflections
Mentor-facilitated conversations71	To facilitate frank discussions and reflections on patient encounters facilitating professional growth and humanism
Surveys, Scales, Inventories, or Questionnaires	
Stage-specific attribute scales (SASs) (1)72	To assess the maturation and socialization of the individual's PIF
Developing Scale73	To assess an individual's self-control as a professional, awareness of being a doctor, reflection as a medical doctor, their execution of social responsibility and the external and internal self-harmonization (developed with SAS)

Table 11.3 Continued

Assessment Approaches and Tools for PIF	
Physician professional identity survey74	To gauge a physician's identity integration or identification with various groups (a pictorial format survey)
Identity integration (IdIn) survey49	To measure the fusion of personal and professional identity (a pictorial measure used with the Physician Professional Identity (PPI)
Professional Self-Identity Questionnaire (PSIQ)75	To measure professional identity in 9 domains: teamwork, communication, conducting assessment, cultural awareness, ethical awareness, using records, dealing with emergencies, reflection, and teaching (multifaceted tool)
Professional Identity Questionnaire (PIQ)76	To identify the extent of an individual's social identification with the medical profession
Observation Based	
Observation of clinical performance	To directly observe work-based performance, including mini-Clinical Evaluation Exercise, Professionalism Mini-evaluation exercise, multisource feedback, and patient opinions

interventions is reflection.[8] Accordingly, a majority of PIF assessment tools target reflective work.

Given the complexities of PIF, one way to capture its features into one strategy is through the use of a reflective portfolio[77] in which to collate "evidence that through critical reflection on its contents demonstrate achievement as well as personal and professional development."[77, 78(p1)]

Reflective Portfolios

Millman et al. in 1990 instigated the idea[79] of incorporating portfolios in higher education to assess tasks in authentic settings.[80] Adopted along the medical education continuum, several forms and functions have been attributed to portfolios. Holmboe et al. described portfolios as "collections of work, evaluations, and products of the learner over time"[81(p710)] and elaborated further on how a portfolio is not "a single evaluation 'tool' but represents a framework and process for collecting, analysing, and documenting the successful acquisition of the general competencies."[81(p710)] Driessen described a framework that allocates three main functions to a portfolio: learning, assessment, and personal development.[82] Carraccio recommended that a portfolio system of assessment should feature: "(1) interaction between the learner and a mentor, each playing an active role, (2) multiple assessment methods including reflection and self-assessment that when aggregated, contribute to a comprehensive assessment of the learner, and (3) a longitudinal perspective that demonstrates growth over time."[83(p38)] Pandya et al. described a reflective portfolio as "a collection of evidence that attests to achievement as well as personal and professional development through critical analysis and self-reflection."[84(p78)]

In systematic reviews of effectiveness of portfolios in health professions education, implementing portfolios is found to support learning and assessment of competencies, including critical thinking, reflective ability, personal and professional development, communication skills, and empathy.[57,80,85,86] Other beneficial effects include improved learner knowledge, self-awareness, reflective engagement, independent learning, integration of theory with practice, and improved relationships with—and feedback from—instructors.[85,87] The portfolio has been specifically identified as a method to enable students to uncover aspects of the hidden curriculum as they reflect on their developing professional identities.[86]

As is the case with all assessments, "authenticity" is vital to the validity of a reflective portfolio; authenticity refers to the extent to which the outcomes measured represent appropriate, meaningful, significant and worthwhile forms of human accomplishments.[88]

Friedman Ben David et al. described portfolios as ideal for assessing the professional development of the medical learner over time and through different stages, being personalized to the learner, offering possibilities for formative and summative assessment, with contributions of quantitative as well as qualitative data.[80] They also suggested strategies for improving standardization and authenticity and hence reliability and validity.

Beck Dallaghan et al. described several challenges of using portfolios, which may be related to people, processes, and technology.[59] People involved, including medical school administrators, clinical supervisors, portfolio coaches, and medical students themselves, may have different concerns and barriers to buy-in for developing a portfolio program. The process itself, such as how data are accessed and reviewed, can also pose challenges, and technology issues related to using an electronic platform must also be considered. Clarity of purpose and a well-designed process can help address these challenges and ensure the success of a medical student portfolio program.

Thus, adding to the above-mentioned parameters for PIF assessment, other components, and parameters to consider for a reflective portfolio could include

1. Personal reflection along with guided feedback by trained faculty, mentors, and/or supervisors on experiences, ethical issues, and disorienting dilemmas.[47,63,77,89,90]
2. Contents that are selected by the learner.[80,91] This can enhance personal ownership, support self-directed learning, promote deeper levels of reflection, and develop metacognitive skills.[63] Allowing the learner to take control of the reflective process can more authentically represent their learning and development.
3. Clear structures, goals, and guidelines for learners *and* assessors, ensuring broad sampling of learners' tasks, work-related activities,[80] and other relevant content.
4. Rigorous faculty (mentors and assessors) training, feedback, and standardization processes to minimize decision inconsistencies.[80]
5. Manageability of portfolios, which has been cited as a critical factor in maintaining learner motivation.[85,92,93]

Driessen et al. also suggested that integrating portfolios with other curricular elements is advantageous, while including a summative assessment component can help to maintain the validity of portfolio assessment amid competition from other summative evaluations.[57]

Conclusion

Identity formation is by its nature (involving an individual's identity) a complex, evolving phenomenon, while within the medical profession, forming a professional identity is rooted in socialization. Assessing PIF on an individual level alone is thus a limited and limiting endeavor. Be it portfolio or any other assessment tool and technique, as Messick concluded: "Interpretation of such teaching and learning consequences as reflective of test validity (or invalidity) assumes that all other aspects of the educational system are working well or are controlled. Thus, in practice the issue is not just the systemic validity of the tests but rather the validity of the system as a whole for improving teaching and learning."[94(p16)]

That there is no perfect way of assessing PIF does not mean it cannot be assessed or that it is not worth the effort to assess, as the consequences of poorly formed professional identity can leave long-lasting, negative effects on individual, institutional, and societal levels.

Attaining and assessing PIF remain complex endeavors—both ideologically and logistically. Yet they are clearly worthwhile pursuits, and the proverbial journey of a thousand miles must begin with a single step.

References

1. Cooke M, Irby D, O'Brien B. *Educating Physicians: A Call for Reform of Medical School and Residency*. Jossey-Bass Publisher; 2010.
2. Cruess RL, Cruess SR, Boudreau JD, Snell L, Steinert Y. Reframing medical education to support professional identity formation. *Acad Med*. 2014;89(11):1446–1451.
3. Flexner A. *Medical Education in the United States and Canada*. Science and Health Publications; 1910.
4. Merton RK. *Some Preliminaries to a Sociology of Medical Education*. The Student-Physician: Introductory Studies in the Sociology of Medical Education. Harvard University Press; 1957.
5. Irby D, Cooke M, O'Brien B. Calls for reform of medical education by the Carnegie Foundation for the advancement of teaching: 1910 and 2010. *Acad Med*. 2010;85(2):220–227.
6. Sarraf-Yazdi S, Teo YN, How AEH, et al. A scoping review of professional identity formation in undergraduate medical education. *J Gen Intern Med*. 2021;36(11):3511–3521.
7. Holden MD, Buck E, Luk J, et al. Professional identity formation: creating a longitudinal framework through TIME (Transformation in Medical Education). *Acad Med*. 2015;90(6):761–767. doi:10.1097/acm.0000000000000719
8. Mount G, Kahlke R, Melton J, Varpio L. A critical review of professional identity formation interventions in medical education. *Acad Med*. 2022;97(11S):S96–S106.
9. Cruess RL, Cruess SR, Steinert Y. Amending Miller's pyramid to include professional identity formation. *Acad Med*. 2016;91(2):180–185.
10. Chandran L, Luli R, Strano-Paul L, Post S. Developing "a way of being": deliberate approaches to professional identity formation in medical education. *Acad Psychiatry*. 2019;43(5):521–527.
11. Cullum R, Shaughnessy A, Mayat N, Brown M. Identity in lockdown: supporting primary care professional identity development in the COVID-19 generation. *Educ Prim Care*. 2020;31(4):200–204.
12. Toubassi D, Schenker C, Roberts M, Forte M. Professional identity formation: linking meaning to well-being. *Adv Health Sci Educ Theory Pract*. 2022;28(1):305–318. Advance online publication:1–14.

13. Dewa C, Loong D, Bonato S, Thanh N, Jacobs P. How does burnout affect physician productivity? A systematic literature review. *BMC Health Serv Res.* 2014;14:325.
14. Shanafelt T, Bradley K, Wipf J, Back A. Burnout and self-reported patient care in an internal medicine residency program. *Ann Intern Med.* 2002;136:358–367.
15. West C, Huschka M, Novotny P. Association of perceived medical errors with resident distress and empathy: a prospective longitudinal study. *JAMA.* 2006;296(9):1071–1078.
16. Papadakis M, Hodgson C, Teherani A, Kohatsu N. Unprofessional behavior in medical school is associated with subsequent disciplinary action by a state medical board. *Acad Med.* 2004;79(3):244–249.
17. Kow CS, Teo YH, Teo YN, et al. A systematic scoping review of ethical issues in mentoring in medical schools. *BMC Med Educ.* 2020;20(1):246.
18. Dzau V, Kirch D, Nasca T. To care is human—collectively confronting the clinician-burnout crisis. *N Engl J Med.* 2018;378:312–314.
19. Wright A, Katz I. Beyond burnout—redesigning care to restore meaning and sanity for physicians. *N Engl J Med.* 2018;378(5):309–311.
20. Lee FQH, Chua WJ, Cheong CWS, et al. A systematic scoping review of ethical issues in mentoring in surgery. *J Med Educ Curric Dev.* 2019;6:2382120519888915. doi:10.1177/2382120519888915
21. Reis SP, Wald HS. Contemplating medicine during the Third Reich: scaffolding professional identity formation for medical students. *Acad Med.* 2015;90(6):770–773. doi:10.1097/ACM.0000000000000716
22. Sabanciogullari S, Dogan S. Relationship between job satisfaction, professional identity and intention to leave the profession among nurses in Turkey. *J Nurs Manag.* 2015;23(8):1076–1085.
23. Holden M, Buck E, Clark M, Szauter K, Trumble J. Professional identity formation in medical education: the convergence of multiple domains. *HEC Forum.* 2012;24(4):245–255. doi:10.1007/s10730-012-9197-6
24. National Academy of Medicine. Dzau V, Kirch D, Murthy V, Nasca T, eds. *National Plan for Health Workforce Well-Being.* National Academies Press; 2022.
25. Cordis EC. Improving quality and safety in the hospital: the link between organisational culture, burnout, and quality of care. https://cordis.europa.eu/article/id/91388-preventing-physician-burnout
26. General Medical Council. Wellbeing resources for doctors. https://www.gmc-uk.org/news/news-archive/wellbeing-resources-for-doctors
27. Limb M. Covid-19: Doctors' wellbeing must be "critical priority" after pandemic mistakes, says BMA. *BMJ Open.* 2022;377:o1284.
28. Ngamaba KH, Panagioti M, Armitage CJ. How strongly related are health status and subjective well-being? Systematic review and meta-analysis. *Eur J Public Health.* 2017;27(5):879–885. doi:10.1093/eurpub/ckx081
29. Moseley L, McConnell L, Garza K, Ford C. Exploring the evolution of professional identity formation in health professions education. *New Dir Teach Learn.* 2021;2021(168):11–27.
30. Crossley J, Vivekananda-Schmidt P. The development and evaluation of a Professional Self Identity Questionnaire to measure evolving professional self-identity in health and social care students. *Med Teach.* 2009;31(12):e603–e607.
31. Smith B, Sparkes A. Contrasting perspectives on narrating selves and identities: an invitation to dialogue. *Qual Res.* 2008;8(1):5–35.

32. Monrouxe L, Rees C. Theoretical perspectives on identity: researching identities in healthcare education. In: Cleland J, Durning SJ, eds. *Researching Medical Education.* Wiley Blackwell; 2015:129–140.

33. Hafferty F. Beyond curriculum reform: confronting medicine's hidden curriculum. *Acad Med* 2000;75(6):549–556.

34. Durning S, Artino A, Boulet J, Dorrance K, van der Vleuten CLS. The implications of three major learning theories for simulation-based assessment of clinical competence: a review and synthesis. *Acad Med.* 2016;91(6):865–871.

35. Charon R. Narrative medicine: a model for empathy, reflection, profession, and trust. *JAMA.* 2001;285(15):1897–1902.

36. Krishna L, Alsuwaigh R. Understanding the fluid nature of personhood—the ring theory of personhood. *Bioethics.* 2015;29(3):171–181.

37. Barnhoorn P. Professional identity formation: onions rather than pyramids. *Acad Med.* 2016;91(3):291.

38. Kegan R. *The Evolving Self: Problem and Process in Human Development.* Harvard University Press; 1982.

39. Helmich E, Bolhuis S, Laan R, Koopmans R, Grol R. Toward a shared understanding of competence in medicine: a systematic review of the concept of competence. *Med Educ.* 2018;52(11):1109–1122.

40. Haidet P, Stein H, Kelly P, Levine R, Koenig T. The role of the humanities in medical education: a survey of medical students, residents, and deans at 25 US medical schools. *Acad Med.* 2016;91(7):978–985.

41. Wenger E. Communities of practice, a brief introduction. *Sci Investig Rep.* 2007:17–22 .

42. Schön D. *The Reflective Practitioner: How Professionals Think in Action.* Basic Books; 1983.

43. Baxter Magolda MB. Developing Self-Authorship in Graduate School. The Experience of Being in Graduate School: An Exploration. In Anderson MS, ed. *New Directions for Higher Education.* Jossey-Bass; 1998;101:41–54.

44. Lent R, Brown S, Hackett G. Toward a unifying social cognitive theory of career and academic interest, choice, and performance. *J Vocat Behav.* 1994;45(1):79–122.

45. Kenny N, Shelton W. Lost virtue: professional character development in medical education. *Adv Bioeth.* 2006;10:xi–xvii.

46. Teo KJH, Teo MYK, Pisupati A, et al. Assessing professional identity formation (PIF) amongst medical students in oncology and palliative medicine postings: a SEBA guided scoping review. *BMC Palliative Care.* 2022;21(1):200.

47. Tay K, Ng S, Hee J, et al. Assessing professionalism in medicine—a scoping review of assessment tools from 1990 to 2018. *J Med Educ Curricr Dev.* 2020;7:1–9.

48. Irby DM, Hamstra SJ. Parting the clouds: three professionalism frameworks in medical education. *Acad Med.* 2016;91(12):1606–1611.

49. Buck E, West C, Graham L, Frye A, Teal C. Challenges to assessing professional identity in medical students: a tale of two measures. *Med Educ Online.* 2019;24(1):1–5.

50. Mak-van der Vossen M, Peerdeman S, van Mook W, Croiset G, Kusurkar R. Assessing professional behaviour: overcoming teachers' reluctance to fail students. *BMC Res Notes.* 2014;7:368. doi:10.1186/1756-0500-7-368

51. Kalet A, Buckvar-Keltz L, Harnik V, et al. Measuring professional identity formation early in medical school. *Med Teach.* 2017;39(3):255–261.

52. Aagaard E, Moscoso L. Practical implications of compassionate off-ramps for medical students. *Acad Med.* 2019;94(5):619–622.

53. Ten Cate O, Graafmans L, Posthumus I, Welink L, van Dijk M. The EPA-based Utrecht undergraduate clinical curriculum: Development and implementation. *Med Teach.* 2018;40(5):506–513. doi:10.1080/0142159X.2018.1435856

54. ten Cate O. AM last page: what entrustable professional activities add to a competency-based curriculum. *Acad Med.* 2014;89(4):691.

55. Carraccio C, Englander R, Gilhooly J, et al. Building a framework of entrustable professional activities, supported by competencies and milestones, to bridge the educational continuum. *Acad Med.* 2017;92(3):324–330.

56. ten Cate O, Taylor D. The recommended description of an entrustable professional activity: AMEE Guide No. 140. *Med Teach.* 2021;43(10):1106–1114.

57. Driessen E, Tartwijk J, van der Vleuten C, Wass V. Portfolios in medical education: why do they meet with mixed success? A systematic review. *Med Educ.* 2007;41:1224–1233.

58. Davis M, Ponnamperuma G. Portfolio assessment. *J Vet Med Educ.* 2005 32(3):279–284.

59. Beck Dallaghan G, Coplit L, Cutrer W, Crow S. Medical student portfolios: their value and what you need for successful implementation. *Acad Med.* 2020;95(9):1457.

60. Brainard AH, Brislen HC. Viewpoint: learning professionalism: a view from the trenches. *Acad Med.* 2007;82(11):1010–1014. doi:10.1097/01.ACM.0000285343.95826.94

61. Hafferty F. Professionalism and the socialization of medical students. In: Cruess RL, Cruess SR, Steinert Y, eds. *Teaching Medical Professionalism.* Cambridge University Press; 2016:54–68.

62. Wald H, Davis S, Reis S, Monroe A, Borkan J. Reflecting on reflections: enhancement of medical education curriculum with structured field notes and guided feedback. *Acad Med.* 2009;84(7):830–837.

63. Mann K, Gordon J, MacLeod A. Reflection and reflective practice in health professions education: a systematic review. *Adv Health Sci Educ Theory Pract.* 2009;14(4):595–621.

64. Wald H, Reis S, Monroe A, Borkan J. The loss of my elderly patient: interactive reflective writing to support medical students' rites of passage. *Med Teach.* 2010;32(4):e178–e184.

65. Ament Giuliani Franco C, Franco R, Cecilio-Fernandes D, Severo M, Ferreira M, de Carvalho-Filho M. Added value of assessing medical students' reflective writings in communication skills training: a longitudinal study in four academic centres. *BMJ Open.* 2020;10(11):e038898.

66. Roberts C, Stark P. Readiness for self-directed change in professional behaviours: factorial validation of the Self-Reflection and Insight Scale. *Med Educ.* 2008;42(11):1054–1063.

67. Aukes L, Geertsma J, Cohen-Schotanus J, Zwierstra R, Slaets J. The development of a scale to measure personal reflection in medical practice and education. *Med Teach.* 2007;29(2/3):177–182.

68. O'Sullivan P, Aronson L, Chittenden E, Niehaus B, Learman L. Reflective Ability Rubric and user guide. *MedEdPORTAL.* 2010;6:8133.

69. Sobral D. Medical students' mindset for reflective learning: a revalidation study of the Reflection-in-Learning Scale. *Adv Health Sci Educ Theory Pract.* 2005;10(4):303–314.

70. Kalet A, Ark T, Monson V, et al. Does a measure of medical professional identity formation predict communication skills performance? *Patient Educ Couns.* 2021;104(12):3045–3052.

71. Olive K, Abercrombie C. Developing a physician's professional identity through medical education. *Am J Med Sci.* 2017;353(2):101–108.

72. Tagawa M. Scales to evaluate developmental stage and professional identity formation in medical students, residents, and experienced doctors. *BMC Med Educ.* 2020;20(1):40.

73. Tagawa M. Development of a scale to evaluate medical professional identity formation. *BMC Med Educ.* 2019;19(1):63.

74. van Mook WN, Muijtjens AM, Gorter SL, Zwaveling JH, Schuwirth LW, van der Vleuten CP. Web-assisted assessment of professional behaviour in problem-based learning: more feedback, yet no qualitative improvement? *Adv Health Sci Educ Theory Pract.* 2012;17(1):81–93. doi:10.1007/s10459-011-9297-0

75. Haruta J, Maeno T, Takayashiki A, Goto R, Ozone S, Maeno T. Validation of the professional self-identity questionnaire for medical students during clinical practice in Japan. *Int J Med Educ.* 2021;12:160–165.

76. Toben D, Mak-van der Vossen M, Wouters A, Kusurkar R. Validation of the professional identity questionnaire among medical students. *BMC Med Educ.* 2021;21(1):359.

77. Kalet AL, Sanger J, Chase J, et al. Promoting professionalism through an online professional development portfolio: successes, joys, and frustrations. *Acad Med.* 2007;82(11):1065–1072.

78. Plaza C, Draugalis J, Slack M, Skrepnek G, Sauer K. Use of reflective portfolios in health sciences education. *Am J Pharm Educ.* 2007;71(2):34.

79. Millman J, Bird T, Darling-Hammond L. The schoolteacher's portfolio: an essay on possibilities. In: Millman J, Darling-Hammond L, eds. *New Handbook of Teacher Evaluation: Assessing Elementary and Secondary School Teachers.* Sage Publications; 1990:241–255.

80. Friedman Ben David M, Davis M, Harden R, Howie P, Ker J, Pippard M. AMEE Medical Education Guide No. 24: portfolios as a method of student assessment. *Med Teach.* 2001;23(6):535–551.

81. Holmboe E, Rodak W, Mills G, McFarlane M, Schultz H. Outcomes-based evaluation in resident education: creating systems and structured portfolios. *Am J Med.* 2006;119(8):708–714.

82. Driessen E. *Educating the Self-Critical Doctor. Using a Portfolio to Stimulate and Assess Medical Students' Reflection.* Maastricht University; 2008.

83. Carraccio C. Portfolios in Medical Education. In: Schwartz A, ed. *Assessment in Graduate Medical Education: A Primer for Pediatric Program Directors.* Chapel Hill, NC: American Board of Pediatrics; 2011:37–45.

84. Pandya H, Slemming W, Saloojee H. Reflective portfolios support learning, personal growth and competency achievement in postgraduate public health education. *Afr J Health Prof Educ.* 2017;9(2):78–82.

85. Buckley S, Coleman J, Davison I, et al. The educational effects of portfolios on undergraduate student learning: a Best Evidence Medical Education (BEME) systematic review. BEME Guide No. 11. *Med Teach.* 2009;31(4):282–298.

86. Hall P, Byszewski A, Sutherland S, Stodel E. Developing a sustainable electronic portfolio (ePortfolio) program that fosters reflective practice and incorporates CanMEDS competencies into the undergraduate medical curriculum. *Acad Med.* 2012;87(6):744–751.

87. Driessen E, van der Vleuten C, van Tartwijk J, Vermunt J. The use of qualitative research criteria for portfolio assessment as an alternative to reliability evaluation: a case study. *Med Educ.* 2005;39:214–220.

88. Archbald D, Newmann F. *Beyond Standardized Testing: Assessing Authentic Academic Achievement in the Secondary School.* National Association of Secondary: School Principals and National Center on Effective Secondary Schools; 1988.

89. Humphrey H, Smith K, Reddy S, Scott D, Madara J, Arora V. Promoting an environment of professionalism: the University of Chicago "roadmap." *Acad Med.* 2007;82(11):1098–1107.

90. Steinert Y, Cruess RL, Cruess SR, Boudreau JD, Fuks A. Faculty development as an instrument of change: a case study on teaching professionalism. *Acad Med.* 2007;82(11):1057–1064.

91. Driessen E, Van Tartwijk J, Vermunt J, Van Der Vleuten C. Use of portfolios in early undergraduate medical training. *Med Teach.* 2003;25(1):18–23.

92. Gadbury-Amyot C, Kim J, Palm R, Mills G, Noble E, Overman P. Validity and reliability of portfolio assessment of competency in a baccalaureate dental hygiene program. *J Dent Educ.* 2003;67(9):991–1002.

93. Jenkins L, Mash B, Derese A. The national portfolio for postgraduate family medicine training in South Africa: a descriptive study of acceptability, educational impact, and usefulness for assessment. *BMC Med Educ.* 2013;13:101.

94. Messick S. The interplay of evidence and consequences in the validation of performance. *Assess Educ Research.* 1994;23(2):13–23.

12
Compassion and Professional Formation

Steven Rosenzweig

Key Points

- Compassion is the capacity to sustain empathy and be with suffering in ways that are open-hearted and comforting to both patient and physician.
- Distinguishing the vicarious pain of empathy from the positive affective qualities of compassion is a necessity for the professional formation of physicians.
- Virtue ethics, neuroscience, and early studies provide a framework for compassion training in medical education.

Suffering, Compassion, and the Mission of Medicine

A core mission of medicine is the alleviation of human suffering from illness, injury, and disability.[1] It is our primary ethical duty to provide care that is compassionate as well as competent.[2] At the bedside, this means turning toward and attending to our patient's suffering in ways that go beyond treating their disease. Every physician knows how challenging this is because of the enormity and intensity of suffering we encounter, its resistance to medical treatment alone, its overdetermination by social injury and traumatic life circumstances, and its inevitability as part of illness, aging, and dying.

This mission to relieve suffering is the subtext of medicine's social contract with patients and communities who turn to us for aid. Many, if not every one of us, feel called to the practice of medicine in order to alleviate suffering. The difficult truth is that engaging with patients' suffering often overwhelms our professional and personal resources. One of the most significant factors is that others' pain can cut too close to our own bones. We demand empathy from ourselves but are not trained to manage our own empathic distress. Our capacity to engage with our patients' suffering is further limited by work conditions that drive burnout, exacerbate vicarious trauma,[3] or disenfranchise our grief.[4]

Stakes are high. Whether intentionally or unintentionally, physicians too frequently engage with patients in ways that are emotionally distant or otherwise dismissive of their suffering. Patients reach out to us in their vulnerability, often to experience disconnection, rejection, isolation, or even emotional abandonment. As a result, patient suffering is compounded by feelings of rejection that lead to alienation and hopelessness.

We physicians are also harmed by these kinds of interactions that may be a source of moral distress and even moral injury.[5] Aware of our social contract and professional calling, our self-esteem and professional identity may sustain injury when we fail to provide compassionate care. We may maladaptively cope with feelings of deficiency through rationalization or denial, reinforcing behaviors that lead to dissatisfaction, burnout, or depression.

The central premise of this chapter is that the capacity to engage our patients' suffering is foundational to professionalism *and* there are successful ways to cultivate this capacity of compassion.

Professionalism and Professional Formation

Medicine's social contract with society is the bedrock of professionalism. We physicians are entrusted with the power and privilege to heal and not harm. Just being deemed as patient fiduciaries is not enough: Trustworthiness requires each physician to be capable of deserving and guarding every patient's trust. This is what is meant by professional formation: the development of our moral, cognitive, emotional, social, and spiritual capacities to fulfill our social contract.

An important example is made clear by examining the highly regarded physician charter,[6] widely regarded as a consensus formulation of medicine's social contract. Reading this document closely, we discover that the terms *compassion* and *caring* fail to appear even once. Mention of these essential, personal qualities of each physician's character are completely missing. The charter lays out core principles and commitments. Beyond these, physicians are also responsible for providing care as people who are compassionate, trustworthy, just, morally courageous, altruistic, and steadfast.

Compassion, Capacity, and Physician Formation

Compassion is widely understood as

> attunement to suffering characterized by caring, kindness and the motivating wish to ease that suffering.

Our professional, ethical mandate is not only to move toward suffering to alleviate it, but to cultivate our capacity to do so. Consider the surgeon fully supported by technical knowledge and instrumental skills—capacity—to do work that is otherwise inconceivable. Recognized as capacity, compassion can be understood as the necessary inner support to address suffering with sensitivity, kindness, and caring, even under conditions that are stressful, constraining, and potentially overwhelming.

This chapter examines the cultivation of our capacity as physicians to bring compassion to the bedside as a core component of professional formation. To do so, we employ the framework of virtue ethics, study compassion in its various aspects, examine the felt experience of compassion, and consider methods to support compassion cultivation.

Compassion Capacity as Virtue

Contemporary virtue ethics is highly relevant to professional formation and the development of a physician's compassion and other moral capacities.[7] Pellegrino and others championed the role of virtue in contemporary bioethics; virtue ethics plays an important role in current thinking about professionalism and professionalism education in medicine and healthcare.[8]

As discussed, fulfillment of medicine's social contract with society may be defined as adherence to ethical principles and duties that guide professional behavior.[6] The emergence of modern bioethics was particularly grounded in establishing fundamental principles such as autonomy and beneficence as the basis of ethical deliberation and action.[9]

By contrast, virtue ethics is concerned with what it means to be a good person who develops the character and proclivity to act morally. Virtues are those ideal moral qualities that form our character and shape our disposition toward ethical action. The virtuous physician has the capacity to apply ethical principles in the right way and for the right reason and to negotiate moral ambiguity when principles are in conflict.

The Aristotelian virtue of fortitude is a useful example that is highly relevant to clinical practice. Fortitude is not a decision-making principle. Rather, fortitude is a moral capacity, strengthened over time through self-regulation and self-discipline. It is demonstrated through steadfast service to a patient's welfare, despite mounting stressors, distractions, and excuses to cut corners in care.

Given the core mission of medicine is the relief of suffering, compassion is prima facie an essential physician virtue. All virtues are to be intentionally developed; we return to a discussion of how virtue is cultivated further in this chapter in the section on compassion training.

Compassion and Spirituality

In addition to the contemporary, secular understanding of virtue, it is important also to note the history of this idea in religious and spiritual teachings. In secular thinking, virtue is treated as an abstracted ideal. In spiritual traditions, the good originates in a realm of the transcendent and the sacred. Accordingly, the source of compassion lies beyond the individual person yet is realized and lived through that person. Examples include the naming of compassion as *fruit of the Holy Spirit* in Catholicism, *divine attribute* in Islam and Judaism, *divine abode* (brahmavihārā) in Buddhism, or *essence* in other spiritual paths. Physicians immersed in any of these traditions would view development of moral capacity within a wider, spiritual context.

Aspects of Compassion

Compassion is often described in terms of aspects that include

1. Cognitive: awareness of suffering
2. Affective: caring and attuned concern
3. Intentional: wish to relieve or ease suffering
4. Behavioral: stance and readiness to take action

Examining each aspect sheds additional light on what it means to cultivate compassion as a capacity to respond to suffering.

Cognitive Aspects: Awareness of Suffering. *Perspective taking* is required to recognize the suffering of others (cognitive empathy) and is only possible by overcoming mental filters and implicit biases that obscure or numb recognition of another's distress.

Personal insight is necessary for awareness of our own suffering so that we see through our psychological defenses of denial, minimization, and deflection. We must also recognize cruel self-judgments with which we shame ourselves for needing self-compassion.

Mindfulness means being fully present to our experience in the moment. Mindfulness includes awareness of not only thoughts, but also feelings. Attuning to suffering requires self-regulation of attention that may otherwise be deflected by anxiety, aversion, disgust, vulnerability, or other negative emotions. Conversely, we attune to compassion by paying attention to its naturally arising positive emotions. Mindfulness includes interoception, the awareness of body feelings and sensations. Feeling tight and contracted, we tend to disengage; mindfully relaxing the jaw, softening shoulders, and allowing diaphragms to move (belly breath) can support our presence and openness.

Affective Aspects: Caring and Attuned Concern. Much has been written in recent years about compassion and its associated *positive* affective experience. This is perhaps the most important point of distinction between empathy with someone's suffering and compassion for that suffering. As an experiment, you might pause briefly now, settle yourself for a few moments, then bring into your awareness someone who is dear to you—this could be a relative, a friend, a pet, really anyone for whom you have some affection. Knowing that life brings difficulties, allow a few moments to sense and feel your caring for them, your loving wish that they not suffer and have as much ease as possible. As we turn toward our experience of compassion, we may notice an arising of positive feelings and sensations of kindness, affection, tenderness, caring, and connection. The body may feel slightly softer, pleasantly warmer, or more spacious.

We recognize that *compassion is characterized by a positive, affective experience of kindness, caring, affection, and affiliation.* As we cultivate the capacity for compassion, we can bring greater attention to our positive feelings and stabilize them. Although aware of pain and suffering, we learn to feature, expand, and orient toward these naturally arising feelings of kindness, caring, and even love for a fellow human being. This positive, emotional climate is deeply supportive of the caregiver.

Intentional and Behavioral Aspects: Wish to Relieve Suffering and Readiness to Act. At the bedside, the wish to ease suffering and the sense of readiness and availability to afford that relief are deeply interconnected. They are the foundation of overt, compassionate actions. Both the wish and readiness to ease suffering are expressed to the patient through words, paralanguage, and nonverbal cues. A stance of compassion is itself an act of compassion, breaking a patient's sense of isolation in the meeting of human kindness, even when no additional treatments are possible at that time. This relates to the understanding of compassionate presence, as discussed in the next section.

Compassion and Interpersonal Resonance

We build the capacity to offer compassion even when there are no specific interventions that can be taken to ease pain or suffering. When you attune to suffering with mindfulness, detach as much as you can from distracting thoughts and allow the feelings of kindness, caring, concern, and human connection to pervade your inner climate, we are *being* compassionate. You communicate compassion spontaneously through facial microexpressions and body micromovements and consciously through language, prosody (voice rhythm and intonation), body posture, proxemics (appropriate physical closeness), supportive silence, and comforting gestures.

As you attune to your patient in this way, your patient attunes to your compassion. You feel and respond to each other's presence. The biological understanding of shared neural activations is relevant here. The term *mirror neurons* refers to certain networks that activate when observing another person, seemingly internally mirroring the other person's actions and even intentions.[10] Intersubjective neuronal sharing involving physician and patient mirror neurons seems to evoke patient neuroception of safety and comfort.[11] A sort of emotional contagion occurs.[12] There is a neurobiology of *we* (chapter 3, pp58-62.)[13]

Resonance means the "coupling of two autonomous entities into a functional whole."[13] Neuronal sharing would not only relate to my ability to empathize with my patient, but *also* support my patient to register my compassionate kindness, warmth, and caring. This resonance unfolds as a shared balm of comfort and connection between physician and patient.

Compassion Versus Empathy

Certain defining characteristics of compassion are made clearer when contrasted with those of empathy. Although a construct of empathy as perspective taking has gained popularity in medical education research, the clinical reality of empathy is multidimensional. Trailblazing humanistic psychotherapist Carl Rogers defined empathy as entering the world of the patient to register their emotions and meanings as if one were the other person but without losing the "as if" condition.[14] Empathy is both perspective taking *and* felt experience. Empathizing with a baby erupting in laughter, I am not simply understanding their point of view, I emotionally register their joy and delight. Empathy with pleasure is pleasurable.

Obviously in the clinical setting we focus on our ability to empathize with patients' suffering. We all know that empathy with distress is distressing; it hurts you to feel my pain. It is not surprising that neuroimaging of empathy pathways demonstrates activation of emotional pain centers of the anterior insula and the anterior medial cingulate cortex.[15] Empathizing may even increase sensitivity to one's own physical pain.[16] Hour after hour and day after day, empathizing with the suffering of our patients can become too much to tolerate; empathy tips over into empathic distress, leading to risks of burnout and vicarious trauma.

The experience of compassion is completely different. Kindled by empathic concern, compassion is the attunement and sensitivity toward suffering permeated with caring, kindness, connection, and warm wishes for the ease of that suffering. It is a *positive*, affective experience. A parent embraces their distressed child with loving feelings that envelop them both. Similar warm feelings of caring and connection ease the empathic suffering of a physician attending a patient in great distress. Rather than constricting with vicarious pain, that physician might bring attention to these warm, positive feelings and allow them to unfold even more in order to comfort and be comforted.

A medical student during her pediatric clerkship told the story of rounding daily on a toddler with staph scalded skin syndrome, an infection resulting in skin that looks and feels scalded or burned. The child stood sobbing on her bed each morning as necessary but painful dressing changes were performed. Witnessing this child's ordeal day after day, this empathic student became very distressed. One day the student moved to the child's side and offered her hand which the child hesitantly took, then squeezed throughout the procedure. The student reflected that moving in closer, taking that hand, and just being a compassionate presence not only seemed to comfort the child but also filled her with warm feelings of caring that eased her own empathic distress and sense of helplessness.

Neurobiological research has shown that compassion is associated with activation of not only empathy centers[17] but also neural networks of affiliation, love, and reward (orbitofrontal cortex, ventral striatum, and pregenual anterior cortex).[18] In the brain, compassion, love, and pleasure signal together. Compassion is its own reward, downregulating limbic stress axes and upregulating dopamine, vasopressin, endorphin, and nitrous oxide in key pathways.[19]. Put more humanistically: "If you want others to be happy, practice compassion. If you want to be happy, practice compassion."[20(pX)]

Compassion Increases Empathy

The positive, affective experience of compassion is not a bypass of empathy with suffering. Compassion practice appears to actually sensitize us to the suffering of others while supporting our capacity to be with suffering. Expert Tibetan monk meditators, in a tradition that is strongly grounded in compassion contemplation, demonstrate heightened physiologic response (pupil dilatation and activation of insula and cingulate cortex) to sounds of suffering compared to novice meditators.[21] Research subjects were randomized to a secular training in compassion-based cognitive therapy and assessed using the Reading the Mind in the Eyes Test and functional magnetic resonance imaging (fMRI) brain scanning. Compassion training was associated with increased activation of empathy neural pathways and greater empathic accuracy.[22]

Near Enemies of Compassion

It is helpful to reference a traditional, Buddhist set of practices for cultivating compassion and other virtues (*brahmavihārās*) of loving kindness, equanimity, and altruistic joy. Each virtue is understood to have its "far enemy" (opposite); sadism would be the opposite of compassion. In addition, each virtue has its "near enemy" (imposter), a negative quality that may be mistaken for the virtue. For example, a near enemy of equanimity is indifference.

Empathic distress can be viewed as a near enemy of compassion. As discussed, empathic distress is a vicarious suffering that can carry us away from the actual, positive affect and comfort of compassion. Ultimately, empathic distress leads to the emotional numbing or flooding that shut down compassion.

Pity is another near enemy of compassion. When I pity someone, I psychologically distance myself from them. There is a hierarchy of power as I look down on them from a position of privilege. They are adrift but I feel relief that I am on dry land. While the term *sympathy* has various usages and is sometimes used to imply empathy, in the literature on compassion, sympathy relates to pity. Sympathy means how your pain makes me feel bad in some way. It separates us. I comfort you to make me feel better. By contrast, the social bonding of compassion carries a sense of common humanity. There is comfort and support for us both in our caring relationality and shared humanity.

Equanimity Supports Compassion

Equanimity is a quality of mind characterized by imperturbability rooted in insight into the truth of things. Sir William of Osler described it as "coolness and presence of mind under all circumstances, calmness amid storm, clearness of judgment," a requirement for the practice of medicine.[23(p4)] In Buddhist virtue (*brahmavihārā)* practice, equanimity carries additional meanings of openness, spaciousness, and perceptual clarity. As already noted, equanimity is to be discriminated from its near enemy of indifference or apathy. Development of equanimity is a major benefit of mindfulness meditation practices that foster nonreactive, moment-to-moment awareness of the present moment.[24,25]

Equanimity supports compassion. There are times when the suffering we encounter is too much to bear, and we need to step back, gain some wider perspective, have more breathing room inside ourselves. We recognize not only our striving to fix and heal, but also our human limitations. Our inability to save the patient from their suffering is just the truth of things, not a failure, denial, or escape. We understand that life situations are determined by an infinite chain of conditions and circumstances. We allow our field of awareness to open more widely, become more relaxed and allowing of the truth, and gain more calm and clarity. After some time and when skillful to do so, we can reattune to our patient's need for compassion, offering a more spacious and grounded presence. Equanimity supports the compassion that holds the empathy. Compassion and equanimity cultivation are essentially interconnected.

A medical student shared his worry with me that he had lost his empathy. On rotation in the emergency department, he was drawn into a trauma resuscitation. This student was disturbed because he had not registered the emotions of the moribund patient. As we inquired together, he realized that he *had* experienced great calm, clarity, openness to present moment experience, and an ability to respond to needs and participate fully in the intense treatment efforts. He realized he was not disconnected, indifferent, or uncaring. His equanimity supported his caring about the patient and his care of the patient.

Self-Compassion

It is a common observation that most of us are less kind and caring toward ourselves than toward others. We've internalized cultural biases that confuse self-compassion with narcissism, self-indulgence, or self-pity. Our inner critic or inner judge is a psychic structure related to the superego that forms in early childhood; we experience it through internal messaging that is typically exacting, harsh, and even abusive.[26,27] Rather than functioning as a benevolent coach or loving advisor, the inner critic functions through shame, fear, guilt, and denigration. We punish ourselves for our own pain and human needs.

Historically, the culture of medicine amplified voice of the inner judge through unrealistic and harmful professional idealizations. Aspirational virtues of altruism and excellence were perverted into expectations of self-sacrifice and perfectionism. In this brutal

Box 12.1 "On-the-Spot" Self-Compassion Practice[30]

This practice incorporates mindfulness, kindness and common humanity. At any moment of my life I may notice my own distress: (1) I turn inwardly toward my suffering with caring, as I would turn toward the distress of a dear one; (2) I acknowledge my human desire to not suffer, (3) I wish for myself—*and all others who are suffering like me in this moment*—relief, comfort, greater ease, happiness. This can be coupled with the breath: Breathing-in I turn toward my human experience of suffering, breathing-out I offer kind and caring wishes to myself and all others who are suffering like me.

framework, a "real" doctor's personal needs and pain are failings that are to be ignored and suppressed.

In stark contrast, self-compassion is the sensitive attunement to one's own physical, emotional, social, or spiritual suffering with clarity and kindness. We suffer because we have universal human needs and limitations. Rather than viewing our own suffering as a deficiency or failing that separates us from others, self-compassion is decentering: We see how suffering arises from our human condition and connects us profoundly to all others.[28] Self-compassion promotes social bonding, altruism, empathic concern, and forgiveness.[29]

We've named two dimensions of self-compassion: kindness to self and common humanity. A third is mindfulness, the self-regulation of attention necessary to witness and be present to our own suffering, rather than simply being caught up in it or automatically reacting to it.[28] Thinking in terms of virtue, we can cultivate the same compassion disposition toward our own pain as toward the pain of others.

A brief, self-compassion practice is provided in Box 12.1.

Compassion Training

Virtue Cultivation. There is a general method for acquiring virtue. We begin by inquiring into the meaning of a virtue. We contemplate, analyze, explore, and discover its truth and depth. We identify its expression in others and allow ourselves to be inspired by and emulate our role models. We learn to recognize it in ourselves, bring attention to it, value it, cultivate it. Finally, we practice the virtue in the way we might practice any skill, honing through repetition. We develop a disposition toward any virtue by putting it into practice, again and again.

It is an ethical imperative to cultivate the virtue of compassion by

1. Aspiring to the virtue ideal. We remind ourselves of our mission as physicians and healers and our deep wish to relieve suffering.
2. Becoming students of the virtue. We inquire into the meaning of compassion, distinguish it from its near enemies of empathic distress and pity, understand more about its nature, process, and value.
3. Learning to recognize virtue in others and ourselves. We pay more attention to how others embody or express compassion in order to emulate them. At the same

time, we bring mindful attention to compassion as it arises in us, intentionally allowing compassion to unfold more fully.
4. Practicing in order to hone our capacity and disposition. We practice by allowing compassion to arise, intentionally kindling its positive feelings of kindness, caring, and connection; being mindful of interfering thoughts, emotions, and attitudes; and expressing compassion through our presence even when interventions are not available.
5. Developing, ultimately, a disposition toward the virtue, living out the virtue more and more completely over time. Compassion becomes more and more of a constant in our daily lives. Our capacity grows even more as we also feel supported, soothed, and comforted by kindness and caring for others. We are further enriched and enlivened through compassionate connection with others.

An Experimental Model. Results of one controlled study of compassion training are illustrative.[31] Researchers demonstrated that compassion training resulted in neuroplastic changes in the brain, activating areas previously established as associated with compassion neural networks. The study also showed how the practice of compassion toward suffering is associated with positive emotions.

All ninety-four female subjects were exposed to standardized video recordings of people suffering from injuries or natural disasters; these were interspersed with video segments of people in emotionally neutral situations. During these exposures, psychometric measures of empathy, positive affect, and negative affect were obtained and fMRI scanning performed.[32]

Subjects randomized to the intervention group participated in a six-hour compassion training that included a theoretical introduction explaining the features of compassion. Subjects were then guided through meditations that invoked and developed feelings of kindness and caring, initially directed toward loved ones. They were then taught to extend these feelings in a general way, first toward strangers and then toward all human beings. Members of this group were instructed to perform regular formal home practices and also practice informally in daily life. Controls received memory training and performed formal memory exercises at home. After the intervention, both groups were exposed to a second, similar set of video stimuli and postintervention measures were obtained.

In this experimental model, subjects who studied, rehearsed, and practiced compassion demonstrated neurobiological changes associated with activation of previously identified compassion networks associated with positive valuation, love, and affiliation. They experienced significantly greater positive emotions while exposed to distressing video material of human suffering. At the same time, they maintained their empathy and even seemed to have lowered their threshold for experiencing empathy. These changes were not seen in the control group.

Programmatic Compassion Training. Historically, methods for cultivating compassion have been an important part of religion-based, contemplative traditions. More recently, secular models of compassion training have been developed. Drawing from traditional practice as well as contemporary psychology, these approaches include cognitive-based compassion training,[33,34] compassion cultivation training,[35] compassion-focused therapy,[36] mindful self-compassion training,[37] and contemplative/emotion training.[38]

Compassion training is not new to the medical community. The Being with Dying Professional Training Program for Clinicians, created in 1972, may be the oldest secular compassion training program in the United States.[39] Other educational models that include core elements of compassion training that have been taught to medical students and physicians include Mindfulness-Based Stress Reduction,[40–44] and The Healer's Art elective for medical students.[45,46]

Common Elements of Compassion-Training. These various models of compassion-training share the following common elements:

Inquiry. Inquiry is a process of ongoing discovery, discernment, and broadening and deepening of insight. For example, the learner investigates the central question: "What is compassion?" in a way that is open ended and leads to growing insight and understanding. Using methods of self-inquiry, the learner employs self-observation and reflection to investigate their own responses to suffering and also their experiences of giving and receiving compassion.

Mindfulness and Self-Regulation of Moment-to-Moment Attention. As discussed, compassion responsiveness requires mindfulness: intentionally bringing attention to experience in the present moment without automatically reacting to the experience in some way. Mindfulness practice is associated with greater calm, empathy, and compassion.[24,43,44,47,48]

Expansion of Empathy. Research has shown how human beings are generally more empathic with members of their social in-group and are more likely to be unfeeling and dismissive toward suffering by the "other."[49,50] Inquiry and structured contemplative exercises are employed to expand the psychological boundaries of in-group affiliation in order to identify with human experience more universally.[51]

One such exercise that fosters realization of common humanity is the "just-like-me" practice.[52] In this practice, we regard a stranger while affirming a sequence of recognitions that include the following: This person has a body and a mind, just like me. This person has feelings, emotions, and thoughts, just like me. This person has, in his or her life, experienced physical and emotional pain and suffering, just like me. This person wishes to be free from pain and suffering, just like me.

Compassion Rehearsal and Practice. Through structured contemplation, the learner intentionally attunes to and develops the various experiential components of compassion, such as caring, kindness, affiliation, and the felt wish for the other's comfort, ease, and well-being. Box 12.2 provides a foundational form of this practice.

In more advanced practices those feelings of affection and caring can then be extended towards others, oneself, and even strangers. Using informal, "on-the-spot" practices[53], the learner "catches" opportunities as they spontaneously arise during the day to feature an experience of compassionate connection and caring.

Researchers have begun to examine the effects of compassion training by employing psychometric testing, examining biological markers, and studying neurobiological effects measured by functional brain imaging. Studies have reported positive changes in psychological well-being and emotional self-regulation, increased altruism and prosocial behavior, enhanced empathy, diminished empathic distress, and reduced markers of inflammation (interleukin 6, cortisol); associated pre-post changes on fMRI have been described.[22,31–34,54–56] This builds on findings already reported in the literature associating mindfulness-based interventions with outcomes of increased compassion, self-compassion, and empathy in physicians and medical students.[42–44]

Box 12.2 Guidance for Compassion Practice

Find a relatively quiet place where you won't be bothered for a few minutes and turn off your devices. Get comfortable in your seat and as much as possible allow yourself to relax a bit more, allowing your shoulders to drop or soften, opening your mouth slightly to unclench your jaw, settling into the support of your chair and the ground beneath your feet. You might take a few relaxed breaths, breathing in slowish through the nose, breathing out slower-ish through the mouth with a vocalized sigh or soft whistle . . .

Bring into your awareness someone for whom you have a natural sense of affection. A baby or pet is ideal for this practice. Sense their presence: This could be a visualization or a "feelingization", a felt imagination of them here with you right now, or you with them wherever that is. This felt imagination is something you do naturally when you think of them. As you do this, also notice positive feelings that arise, feelings of caring or love. Notice how these feelings are registered in the body through pleasant sensations arising in the throat or heart or belly or anywhere else. There may be warmth, tingling, softness, or other sensations. Take a few moments to be with these arising sensations and loving feelings . . .

Acknowledging that life brings difficulties to everyone, notice your wish that this being know as much ease and happiness in their life as is possible. Sense into this wish as it arises and is offered with an open heart. Sense into the caring, kindness, connection, and love of your caring wishes. Take a few more moments to explore and discover this terrain of compassion.

Conclusion

Compassion is the sensitive attunement to suffering characterized by caring, kindness, and the wish and motivation to ease that suffering. The experience, stance, and expression of compassion are comforting, supportive, and self-rewarding. Compassion is at the heart of the practice of medicine with its mission to relieve suffering. More than a guiding principle or duty of social contract, compassion is a capacity or virtue that persons who are physicians must intentionally cultivate.

A singular emphasis on teaching empathy in medical education has failed to adequately address the risks of empathic distress and generally ignores the essential difference between empathy and compassion. This is a failed enterprise given that the positive, affective, self-rewarding experience of compassion is essential for tolerating empathy. Compassion also plays an important part in increasing empathy.

It is time to feature the cultivation of compassion—capacity and virtue—as central to professional formation. Decades of collaborative work among psychologists, educators, neuroscientists, and contemplatives has laid a groundwork for compassion cultivation in medical training. These methods are rooted in the vast experience of traditional practices, appropriately transposed into secular trainings, buttressed by growing empirical evidence. They offer a path toward greater compassion for our patients and ourselves.

References

1. Cassel EJ. The nature of suffering and the goals of medicine. *N Engl J Med.* 1982;306(11):639–645. doi:10.1056/NEJM198203183061104
2. Parsa-Parsi RW. The International Code of Medical Ethics of the World Medical Association. *JAMA.* 2022;328(20):2018–2021. doi:10.1001/jama.2022.19697
3. Vohra S. A piece of my mind. Learning not to move forward. *JAMA.* 2014;312(21):2215–2216. doi:10.1001/jama.2014.12931
4. Lathrop D. Disenfranchised grief and physician burnout. *Ann Fam Med.* Jul 2017;15(4):375–378. doi:10.1370/afm.2074
5. Epstein EG, Hamric AB. Moral distress, moral residue, and the crescendo effect. *J Elin Ethics.* 2009;20(4):330–342.
6. ABIM Foundation, ACP-ASIM Foundation, European Federation of Internal Medicine. Medical professionalism in the new millennium: a physician charter. *Ann Intern Med.* 2002;136(3):243–246.
7. Pellegrino ED. Toward a virtue-based normative ethics for the health professions. *Kennedy Inst Ethics J.* 1995;5(3):253–277.
8. Doukas DJ, Ozar DT, Darragh M, de Groot JM, Carter BS, Stout N. Virtue and care ethics & humanism in medical education: a scoping review. *BMC Med Educ.* 2022;22(1):131. doi:10.1186/s12909-021-03051-6
9. Beauchamp T, Childress J. *Principles of Biomedical Ethics*: marking its fortieth anniversary. *Am J Bioeth.* 2019;19(11):9–12. doi:10.1080/15265161.2019.1665402
10. Lamm C, Majdandzic J. The role of shared neural activations, mirror neurons, and morality in empathy—a critical comment. *Neurosci Res.* 2015;90:15–24. doi:10.1016/j.neures.2014.10.008
11. Geller SM, Greenberg LS. *Therapeutic Presence: A Mindful Approach to Effective Therapy.* American Psychological Association; 2012:vi.
12. Herrando C, Constantinides E. Emotional contagion: a brief overview and future directions. *Front Psychol.* 2021;12:712606. doi:10.3389/fpsyg.2021.712606
13. Siegel DJ. *The Mindful Therapist a Clinician's Guide to Mindsight and Neural Integration.* Sound recording. W. W. Norton & Company: Brilliance Audio; 2011.
14. Rogers CR. *A Way of Being.* Houghton Mifflin; 1995:xviii.
15. Singer T, Seymour B, O'Doherty J, Kaube H, Dolan RJ, Frith CD. Empathy for pain involves the affective but not sensory components of pain. *Science.* 2004;303(5661):1157–1162. doi:10.1126/science.1093535
16. Loggia ML, Mogil JS, Bushnell MC. Empathy hurts: compassion for another increases both sensory and affective components of pain perception. *Pain.* 2008;136(1–2):168–176. doi:10.1016/j.pain.2007.07.017
17. Mathur V, Harada T, Lipke T, Chiao J. Neural basis of extraordinary empathy and altruistic motivation. *NeuroImage.* 2010;51(4):1468–1475.

18. Klimecki OM, Leiberg S, Ricard M, Singer T. Differential pattern of functional brain plasticity after compassion and empathy training. *Soc Cogn Affect Neurosci.* 2014;9:873–879. doi:10.1093/scan/nst060

19. Esch T, Stefano GB. The neurobiological link between compassion and love. *Med Sci Monit.* 2011;17(3):RA65–RA75. doi:10.12659/msm.881441

20. Bstan 'dzin rgya M, Cutler HC. *The Art of Happiness: A Handbook for Living.* Riverhead Books; 1998:x.

21. Lutz A, Brefczynski-Lewis J, Johnstone T, Davidson RJ. Regulation of the neural circuitry of emotion by compassion meditation: effects of meditative expertise. *PloS One.* 2008;3(3):e1897. doi:10.1371/journal.pone.0001897

22. Mascaro JS, Rilling JK, Tenzin Negi L, Raison CL. Compassion meditation enhances empathic accuracy and related neural activity. *Soc Cogn Affect Neurosci.* 2013;8(1):48–55. doi:10.1093/scan/nss095

23. Osler W. *Aequanimitas.* P. Blakiston's Son; 1905.

24. Lutz A, Slagter HA, Dunne JD, Davidson RJ. Attention regulation and monitoring in meditation. *Trends Cogn Sci.* 2008;12(4):163–169. doi:10.1016/j.tics.2008.01.005

25. Shapiro SL, Carlson LE, Astin JA, Freedman B. Mechanisms of mindfulness. *J Clin Psychol.* 2006;62(3):373–86. doi:10.1002/jclp.20237

26. Brown B. *Soul Without Shame: A Guide to Liberating Yourself From the Judge Within.* Shambhala; 1999:xxiv.

27. Harding C. *Dissecting the Superego: Moralities Under the Psychoanalytic Microscope.* Routledge, Taylor and Francis Group; 2019:xvi.

28. Neff KD. Self-compassion: theory, method, research, and intervention. *Annu Rev Psychol.* 2023;Jan 18(74):193–218. doi:10.1146/annurev-psych- 032420-031047

29. Germer CK, Neff KD. Self-compassion in clinical practice. *J Clin Psychol.* 2013;69(8):856–867. doi:10.1002/jclp.22021

30. Chödrön P. *Good Medicine.* Sounds True; 1999.

31. Klimecki OM, Leiberg S, Ricard M, Singer T. Differential pattern of functional brain plasticity after compassion and empathy training. *Soc Cogn Affect Neurosci.* 2013;9(6):873–879. doi:10.1093/scan/nst060

32. Klimecki OM, Leiberg S, Lamm C, Singer T. Functional neural plasticity and associated changes in positive affect after compassion training. *Cereb Cortex.* 2013;23(7):1552–1561. doi:10.1093/cercor/bhs142

33. Pace TW, Negi LT, Adame DD, et al. Effect of compassion meditation on neuroendocrine, innate immune and behavioral responses to psychosocial stress. *Psychoneuroendocrinology.* 2009;34(1):87–98. doi:10.1016/j.psyneuen.2008.08.011

34. Desbordes G, Negi LT, Pace TW, Wallace BA, Raison CL, Schwartz EL. Effects of mindful-attention and compassion meditation training on amygdala response to emotional stimuli in an ordinary, non-meditative state. *Front Hum Neurosci.* 2012;6:292. doi:10.3389/fnhum.2012.00292

35. Jazaieri H, McGonigal K, Jinpa T, Doty JR, Gross JJ, Goldin PR. A randomized controlled trial of compassion cultivation training: effects on mindfulness, affect, and emotion regulation. *Motiv Emot.* 2013;38(1):23–35. doi:10.1007/s11031-013-9368-z

36. Gilbert P. *Compassion Focused Therapy: Distinctive Features.* CBT Distinctive Features Series. Routledge; 2010:viii

37. Neff KD, Germer CK. A pilot study and randomized controlled trial of the mindful self-compassion program. *J Clin Psychol.* 2013;69(1):28–44. doi:10.1002/jclp.21923

38. Kemeny ME, Foltz C, Cavanagh JF, et al. Contemplative/emotion training reduces negative emotional behavior and promotes prosocial responses. *Emotion*. 2012;12(2):338–350. doi:10.1037/a0026118

39. Rushton CH, Sellers DE, Heller KS, Spring B, Dossey BM, Halifax J. Impact of a contemplative end-of-life training program: being with dying. *Palliat Support Care*. 2009;7(4):405–414. doi:10.1017/S1478951509990411

40. Kabat-Zinn J. *Full Catastrophe Living: Using the wisdom of Your Body and Mind to Face Stress, Pain, and Illness*. Paperback Reissue ed. Delta Trade Paperbacks; 2005:xxxiii.

41. Rosenzweig S, Reibel DK, Greeson JM, Brainard GC, Hojat M. Mindfulness-based stress reduction lowers psychological distress in medical students. *Teach Learn Med*. 2003;15(2):88–92. doi:10.1207/S15328015TLM1502_03

42. Erogul M, Singer G, McIntyre T, Stefanov DG. Abridged mindfulness intervention to support wellness in first-year medical students. *Teach Learn Med*. 2014;26(4):350–356. doi:10.1080/10401334.2014.945025

43. Krasner MS, Epstein RM, Beckman H, et al. Association of an educational program in mindful communication with burnout, empathy, and attitudes among primary care physicians. *JAMA*. 2009;302(12):1284–1293. doi:10.1001/jama.2009.1384

44. Fortney L, Luchterhand C, Zakletskaia L, Zgierska A, Rakel D. Abbreviated mindfulness intervention for job satisfaction, quality of life, and compassion in primary care clinicians: a pilot study. *Ann Fam Med*. 2013;11(5):412–420. doi:10.1370/afm.1511

45. Rabow MW, Wrubel J, Remen RN. Authentic community as an educational strategy for advancing professionalism: a national evaluation of the Healer's Art course. *J Gen Intern Med*. 2007;22(10):1422–1428. doi:10.1007/s11606-007-0274-5

46. Rabow MW, Evans CN, Remen RN. Professional formation and deformation: repression of personal values and qualities in medical education. *Fam Med*. 2013;45(1):13–18.

47. Kabat-Zinn J. Mindfulness-based interventions in context: past, present, and future. *Clin Psychol Sci Pract*. 2003;10:144–156. doi:10.1093/clipsy.bpg016

48. Hofmann SG, Sawyer AT, Witt AA, Oh D. The effect of mindfulness-based therapy on anxiety and depression: a meta-analytic review. *J Consult Clin Psychol*. 2010;78(2):169–183. doi:10.1037/a0018555

49. Xu X, Zuo X, Wang X, Han S. Do you feel my pain? Racial group membership modulates empathic neural responses. *J Neurosci*. 2009;29(26):8525–8529.

50. Bernhardt BC, Singer T. The neural basis of empathy. *Annu Rev Neurosci*. 2012;35:1–23. doi:10.1146/annurev-neuro-062111-150536

51. Hopkins J, Bstan 'dzin Rgya M. *A Truthful Heart: Buddhist Practices for Connecting With Others*. Snow Lion Publications; 2008.

52. Ram D, Bush M. *Walking Each Other Home: Conversations on Loving and Dying*. Sounds True; 2018:xxii.

53. Chödrön P, Oliver JD. *Living Beautifully With Uncertainty and Change*. Shambhala; 2012:ix.

54. Pace TW, Negi LT, Sivilli TI, et al. Innate immune, neuroendocrine and behavioral responses to psychosocial stress do not predict subsequent compassion meditation practice time. *Psychoneuroendocrinology*. 2010;35(2):310–315. doi:10.1016/j.psyneuen.2009.06.008

55. Weng HY, Fox AS, Shackman AJ, et al. Compassion training alters altruism and neural responses to suffering. *Psychol Sci*. 2013;24:1171–1180. doi:10.1177/0956797612469537

56. Mascaro JS, Kelley S, Darcher A, et al. Meditation buffers medical student compassion from the deleterious effects of depression. *J Posit Psych*. 2018;13(2):133–142. doi:10.1080/17439760.2016.1233348

13
Ecosystems of Professionalism
Moving From Student to Professional

Laura Edgar, Nathan R. Selden, and Timothy P. Brigham

Key Points

- Medical professionalism develops and matures over time; the ACGME created and implemented milestones to identify and track developmental expectations as medical residents progress through their residency training programs.
- Medical residency is the most prominent time in the development of medical professionalism, as this is the formal period in which a person wanting to be a physician transforms into a physician.
- Data collected and analyzed about residents' Milestones achievements shows that professional, ethical, accountable behavior grows during residency and is influenced by the culture of the clinical learning environment.

Introduction

Professionalism is a core component of the practice of medicine whether the clinician is a medical student, resident, fellow, or practicing physician. Indeed, the recognition of professionalism as a key component of medical practice extends to ancient times.[1] The clinician's career stage can impact the way in which professionalism is demonstrated and understood. To effectively identify and remediate problems, understanding this trajectory is essential. Professionalism is not binary: present or absent. As physicians progress through residency and fellowship training, they are evaluated using a set of developmental professionalism subcompetencies every six months.[2] These residency milestones data, collected by the Accreditation Council for Graduate Medical Education (ACGME), demonstrate that professionalism develops and matures over time in a fashion similar to traditional knowledge and technical skills.

Milestones

The Milestones developmental subcompetencies are a required component of each ACGME-accredited training program. The Milestones were developed as a mechanism to aid residents and fellows by providing an opportunity for transparency in learning and assessment, encouraging self-assessment and self-directed learning, and promoting self-directed feedback-seeking behaviors.[3] Derived in part from the Dreyfus model of skill acquisition, the Milestones include five progressive levels, each with a specific descriptive narrative: novice, advanced beginner, competent, proficient, and expert.[4] This model also works in harmony with the competency-based education and the path to mastery as there is no expected time for progression from one level to the next.[5,6] The Milestones use a stepwise process to document that journey. At each residency program, faculty members serving on a clinical competency committee (CCC) assign Milestone levels in each subcompetency a minimum of twice each year. The CCC compares the totality of assessments collected over the specified evaluation time to the individual Milestone subcompetency narratives to identify the appropriate Milestones level in each instance.[7] Some specialties have independently created milestone developmental sub- competency narratives suitable to assess medical students and another to assess physicians in the first stage of independent practice (e.g., "Society of Neurological Surgeons Recruitment Guidelines," 2022).[8,9] Indeed, the Milestones progressive developmental assessment rubric lends itself to a lifelong learning model that encompasses a path to mastery extending well beyond the formal training period.

In 2016, the ACGME brought together a diverse group of experts to create a set of professionalism milestones that could be used by every accredited specialty.[10,11] Reflecting a fundamental core of shared concepts and behaviors that comprise medical professionalism, these milestones allow minor edits by each specialty but assess the same competencies across the breadth of the field. The new professionalism milestones have been included and evaluated by specialties revising their initial Milestones sets since July 2018. This chapter focuses on three of those milestones: professional behavior, ethical principles, and accountability and conscientiousness (accountability), and delves into the individual professional growth that happens throughout the assessed transitions in each subcompetency.[12]

Professional Behavior

The medical historian Kenneth Ludmerer, MD, wrote in his second book, *Let Me Heal*, that "the greatest influence on professional identity formation takes place during residency."[13(pix)] It is in the crucible of the formal phases of medical education in which we participate with the learner in an almost alchemical process where a person who *wants* to *be* a physician is transformed into a physician. The process of identity formation described elsewhere in this book, at its best, involves the incorporation of certain core values and virtues central to the profession of medicine into the very fabric of their being. Professionalism is the manifestation of these values and virtues in the practice of medicine that signals to the patient and the public that the physician and the profession are worthy of their trust. The Royal College of Physicians London[14] describes professionalism as "a set of values, behaviors, and relationships that underpins the trust the public has in doctors."[14,15 (p8)] Thomas Nasca, MD, MACP, CEO (chief executive officer), and president of the ACGME, writes: "The observable professional and healer behaviors that are manifestations of underlying values and virtues of the profession are **the** basis of the social contract" (Nasca, 2018; emphasis mine).[16] These observable behaviors include demonstrating the following to patients, colleagues, and society:

- Compassion, integrity, and respect for others
- Responsiveness to patient needs that supersedes self-interest
- Respect for patient privacy and autonomy
- Accountability to patients, society, and the profession
- Respect and responsiveness to diverse patient populations[16]

The importance of demonstrating professional behavior to the practice of medicine cannot be underestimated. Without it, patient, colleague, and societal trust erode.

As described previously, the Milestones provide a developmental framework that provides scaffolding for assessment, evaluation, feedback, and developing a learning plan

Table 13.1 Professionalism 1: Professional Behavior

Professionalism 1: Professional Behavior				
Level 1	Level 2	Level 3	Level 4	Level 5
Demonstrates professional behavior in routine situations	Identifies potential triggers for professionalism lapses and accepts responsibility for one's own professionalism lapses	Demonstrates a pattern of professional behavior in complex or stressful situations	Recognizes situations that may trigger professionalism lapses and intervenes to prevent lapses in oneself and others	Coaches others when their behavior fails to meet professional expectations
Comments:				Not Yet Completed Level 1

Used with permission from the ACGME.

and collaborative working partnership with the learner. The Milestones for professional behavior provide an informal yet potent method to assess where this learner might be in their development (Table 13.1). Asking questions with empathy and openness can help create a safe space for dialogue to ascertain where this learner "is" on the developmental trajectory for professional behavior and what actionable feedback the faculty member can deliver to help them begin to progress to the next level and/or reinforce the progress they have already made. While the urge to ameliorate any demonstration of poor professional behavior as quickly as possible might cast an overwhelming shadow, it is wise to pause and see this as a moment to contribute to the professional growth and identity of a learner. Step 1 might be assessment: Where is this learner on the continuum of development in their journey of professionalism?

Kenneth Blanchard and Paul Hersey[17] have designed a four-dimensional model that might prove useful. Depending on where you have determined a learner to be in their professionalism journey and their level as a learner, you can "direct," "coach," "partner" with, or "delegate" to the learner. If the learner clearly knows something was wrong about an interaction they witnessed but is frozen by ignorance of what to do, or indecision, or fear, you might take a very direct approach and tell the learner what to do, what needs to happen next, their role in the plan and as you longitudinally work with them, what steps, with the department's support, they need to take in their own professional journey. If they are further along the developmental continuum, the faculty member might adopt more of a "coaching" role. A more "partnering" or "delegating" style might be appropriate if the learner demonstrates level 3 or 4 thinking, deciding on an appropriate action plan together.

Feedback and developing a learning plan are crucial. And remembering that diagnosing a learner in any situation does not provide the faculty member with enough data to determine whether the learner is a novice, advanced beginner, competent, or proficient (or expert for that matter) in professional behavior. A summative judgment like that depends on a constellation of multiple observations by multiple observers. The question is where is the learner in this situation and what needs do they have to grow and develop as a professional?

It is also crucial to note that when using the Professional Behavior milestone to assess, diagnose, and develop a learning plan for your learners that the Milestones should not be used simplistically and cavalierly. Growth and development in professional behavior is a complex and dynamic phenomenon that should not be conceived as a continuum that moves from someone who frequently has professionalism lapses, to someone who sometimes has them, to a super being who never has a professionalism lapse. Everyone has lapses, residents and faculty included. We are all human after all. There are a variety of factors that can trigger a lapse—from the personal (life concerns, fatigue, family issues, issues related to self-confidence, etc.) to the professional (learning the specialty, caring for patients, workload, etc.). The difference between a level 1 and a l evel 5 in professional behavior is in increasing one's ability to recognize things, issues, situations, and more that trigger unprofessional behavior, increasing one's ability to accept responsibility, and intervening when a lapse (in self or others) may be about to occur or has occurred. The journey of professional behavior is a lifelong one for your residents—it is not without potholes and stumbling blocks. But it can also be a journey of joy and deep meaning. It is a vital component of a physician's healing arsenal that contributes greatly to the trust between the physician and the patient and the profession and society and to the development of a deep and necessary therapeutic relationship with patients and families.

A word on one more thing: the importance of culture in this instance. A clinical learning environment is an ecosystem characterized by experiential learning. The learner is always learning, more likely from what they observe from role model behaviors than the words that are preached. Culture shapes behaviors in ways in which most people are not even aware.[18] If the environment is one in which hierarchy supersedes accountability, then *any* learner, however mature in their professional development, might be paralyzed by fear of retribution or make a decision that dealing with the poorly behaved individual is a risk not worth jeopardizing their professional, educational, and psychological safety. For the learner to grow and develop as a professional, an environment of department support and personal safety coupled with behavioral norms that reinforce professional behavior and redirect and remediate unprofessional behavior is imperative. Otherwise, the learner's development as a professional can be seriously impaired, and the lesson learned the opposite of what the learner, the profession, society, and patients need and deserve in order to develop trust and solidify the social contract.

Consider the following scenario: A resident meets with the program director to discuss a conversation that was overheard between a first-year resident and a chief resident. The chief resident said that they were disappointed in the first-year resident's performance and that they seemed to be falling behind their colleagues in their command of medical knowledge and clinical judg ment, and that they needed them to step their game up or they were going to put patients in danger and risk their place in the program. The chief then added that we have never had a (Black, Hispanic, woman, other?) resident in this program, and that they took a chance ranking the first-year resident because of all the "wokeness" going on around the country. The chief resident said that they were not really expecting much from someone like them but more than they were getting.

When thinking about this event, the chief resident did not display professional behavior and in the moment would be rated as "Not Yet Completed Level 1," which is often associated with a level for remediation.

The resident who brought this to the program director would be assessed as level 3 as they demonstrated professional behavior in a complex situation. Had this resident intervened in the conversation and attempted to deescalate the situation, they would have been a level 4. To then develop an ongoing coaching relationship with the chief resident to help them understand the problem and how to improve would have made this resident a level 5.

However, the Milestones are not intended to be a single measurement in time, and it would be necessary to review other assessments, including multisource feedback that would include a diverse population of assessors.

Ethical Principles

In the clinical environment, ethical actors such as clinicians must analyze a vast variety of practical ethical problems, make specific decisions, and act. Various ethical principles may simultaneously inform such analyses, decisions, and actions (Table 13.2). In modern Western medicine, the most commonly cited framework for medical ethical analysis and decision-making subsumes four equal principles: respect for patient autonomy, beneficence, nonmaleficence, and justice.[19,20]

- Respect for autonomy recognizes patients as independent rational agents with the right to make informed and voluntary decisions free of coercion or undue external influence.[21] For example, the principle of autonomy is cited as justification for the practices of informed consent, truth-telling, and confidentiality.[20]
- The principle of beneficence derives from the Hippocratic imperative to carry out only those actions that are of benefit to the patient. Beneficence incorporates the modern concept of patient centeredness, seen by many clinicians as the central duty of professionalism to put a patient's needs before one's own.
- The principle of nonmaleficence derives from the aphorism to "do no harm," commonly attributed to the Hippocratic corpus.[22] Nonmaleficence carries not only a duty of intention but also competence and reasonable care.[23]
- The principle of justice, in the context of medical ethics, includes a duty to treat patients equally without regard to status, wealth, or identity, as well as a duty to reasonably distribute medical care as a scarce resource.[21] Recent attention to the principle of justice in healthcare has been associated with an effort to improve the social determinants of health.[24]

Many dilemmas in medical ethics reflect a conflict between competing principles.[23] For example, a surgeon may feel compelled to transfuse a patient during an operation without their consent in order to carry out a safe and successful surgery and secure a cure for the patient's disease (beneficence), but feel bound to respect the patient's wishes and only administer care that has been agreed to (autonomy). While these and various other ethical systems may be heuristically useful, especially to early learners, they represent only one of many different ways to organize, assess, and implement ethical behavior

Table 13.2 Professionalism 2: Ethical Principles

Professionalism 2: Ethical Principles				
Level 1	Level 2	Level 3	Level 4	Level 5
Demonstrates knowledge of basic ethical principles	Applies basic principles to address straightforward ethical situations	Analyzes complex situations using ethical principles and identifies the need to seek help in addressing complex ethical situations	Analyzes complex situations and engages with appropriate resources for managing and addressing ethical dilemmas as needed	Identifies and seeks to address system-level factors that induce or exacerbate ethical problems or impede their resolution
Comments:				Not Yet Completed Level 1

Used with permission from the ACGME.

in clinical medicine.[25] In real practice, clinical ethics depends on a complex and nuanced set of personal and systemic influences.[26]

Standard medical ethics assumes that routine patient care is given with the sole interest of benefitting the patient's health in mind. In contrast, additional ethical duties apply to the conduct of medical care in the context of research. These additional duties stem from recognition of abuses of medical experimentation that both exploited and harmed research subjects, observed during research conducted by Nazi physicians in World War II and later by other physicians in other contexts, such as research conducted on the Tuskegee airmen in the United States without their knowledge or consent. Modern protections against medical research abuse arise from the Nuremberg Code and the US Belmont Report. Medical research, intended to advance knowledge with the hope of benefitting future patients, might only incidentally benefit the subjects of the research itself. The inherent conflict between the interests of the research subject and the researcher (with implications for the principles of autonomy, beneficence, and nonmaleficence) calls for additional protections as part of the informed consent procedure. This is especially true of research involving vulnerable persons, including prisoners, intellectually disabled persons, and children.

Ethics theories and principles may be taught to medical students and trainees both in concept and as part of case-based learning during medical practice.[27] In 2018, students from various health care professions at a US medical school reported limited exposure to formal medical ethics training but a high interest in participating in formal medical ethics curricula.[28] During clinical residencies, formal ethical training is significantly less frequent, but potentially beneficial to both residents and patients.[29] During practice, many medical professional organizations, such as the American Medical Association, embody ethical principles as part of their guidelines and/or requirements for membership and practice. For example, the AMA Principles of Medical Ethics draw on the above four core principles to enumerate nine more specific behaviors and responsibilities for its members.[30]

Consider the following scenarios: An orthopedics resident admits a patient with long-standing metastatic breast cancer and a thoracic vertebral body lesion causing spinal cord compression. After presenting the case over the telephone to her attending surgeon, she describes to the patient the nature and length of the operation, its inherent risks, the alternative of local radiation therapy, and the rationale for choosing surgery in her situation. While answering the questions about the operation, it becomes clear to the resident that her patient erroneously believes the operation will also contribute to a curative intent for her underlying disease. The resident is confused as to why the patient who has been under the active care of her oncologist and other surgeons for almost two years, with multiple recurrences, holds this view, and whether she has a duty to correct the misperception or simply to describe tomorrow's operation (level 2).

An obstetrics and gynecology resident scrubs with a senior attending on a laparotomy procedure to remove multiple large fibroids from the uterus of an otherwise healthy patient in her early 30s. As the operation proceeds, blood control from the uterine wall at the site of each fibroid excision is poor, and the overall blood loss mounts. Despite the anesthesiologist warning about a sagging blood pressure, the attending surgeon expresses a desire to push ahead and "finish the last few" but seems to have difficulty managing the already ongoing bleeding. The resident quietly and respectfully asks the circulating nurse to page another attending to come assist with the rest of the procedure (level 3).

A senior medicine resident on the ICU service is treating an elderly patient with multi system organ failure, who has no advanced directive in place. If elected, further treatment—in the best of circumstances—will require placement of tracheostomy and feeding tubes and an extended, perhaps permanent, stay in a skilled nursing facility. The patient's daughter insists that he would "want everything done," but his son insists that he would prefer "a natural death" at this point. The medicine resident summons his attending physician for additional advice and suggests to the attending that they call an ethics team consult (level 4).

Advanced learners and practitioners may reach levels of ethical competency beyond that deemed necessary for independent practice (i.e., level 5 competency according to the rubric of the ACGME Milestones). For example, level 5 competency might be reflected by a clinician who creates resources for teaching medical ethics to others, such as an ethics case-based rounds, or for supporting complex ethical decisions, such as an ethics team or review board.

Accountability and Conscientiousness

Accountability is typically identified as a personal characteristic, like internal motivation, and conscientiousness as a personality trait that reflects self-governance and mastery. Accountability is often defined as the act of justifying and taking (or not taking) responsibility for one's own actions.[31–34] A review of the literature demonstrates that conscientiousness, accountability, and commitment to duty are a core component of professionalism that should be mastered.[33–37]

Economic, political, and professional accountability are all important models within the practice of medicine.[37] In basic terms, economic accountability looks at the value for the service provided, resource utilization, and targeted diagnostics and treatment. Political accountability can be thought of as the relationship between physicians and insurers or governing bodies. Professional accountability, the focus of this section , is a commitment to lifelong learning, completion of patient care tasks, and ultimately, the care of patients as individuals.[37] And yet others consider four domains of health system accountability to include a social, political, organizational, and provider dimension.[34] However the construct of accountability is determined, it can be thought of as including three "complementary and synergistic" elements: accountable party, subject matter, and processes for accountability.[34,35] Conscientiousness is significantly related to accountability and as such was included in the subcompetency.[38,39]

Low levels of conscientiousness in medical students have been demonstrated to correlate with negative faculty assessments for professionalism; unprofessionalism in medical students may predict disciplinary action by state medical boards. [40,41] And Sanfey et al.[42] identified that 50% of concerns related to professionalism, and 50% of malpractice claim costs, are related to less than 15% of all physicians. In considering the impact of developmental learning as it is related to accountability and conscientiousness, the Milestones data will demonstrate this growth. The literature provides multiple examples of the problems and the best times to be identified.

As indicated, issues with accountability and conscientiousness begin in medical school. For residency programs, it is suggested that a critical review of their attitudes and behaviors be completed within the first six months of training.[42] Through multiple assessment methods and multiple assessors, a cause of the problem may be identified.

Once identified, a plan of action to improve can be determined. These actions should include continued feedback, coaching, and role playing.[3]

A survey conducted in 2007 showed that 68% of attending physicians (ages 50 –65) thought that recent resident graduates were less dedicated and hardworking than their cohort.[43] And yet, multiple studies demonstrate the importance of professionalism to students and residents, including high ratings for accountability and conscientiousness, with residents scoring the highest.[43–45] O'Flynn et al.[44] showed that these personal characteristics were more important for medical students and residents than they were for faculty.

The Milestones serve as an example of how learners develop in their levels of accountability and conscientiousness (Table 13.3). As with many physician-related tasks, it takes time to develop the skills to manage the individual tasks in routine and complex situations while demonstrating care and compassion.

Consider the following scenarios: A medical student is about to complete a four-week rotation with the inpatient medical team. During the final night shift there is only one urgent patient issue, two admissions, and the team is fully staffed. This student completes the shift with the final notes being made and sign out made to the resident. The student would certainly demonstrate a beginning level of accountability and conscientiousness in this routine situation (level 2). They may not yet have the professional experience or foresight to demonstrate higher levels.

A resident is completing their notes for a patient with a complex treatment plan in the medical record as part of the evening sign out. The next day they note that the patient had an adverse event overnight, and on reviewing the medical record identify that some key patient information was not included in the previous note. The resident takes responsibility for the error by professionally discussing the event with the attending and other residents and with the patient and family. At this point the resident is clearly competent in this subcompetency as they take responsibility in a complex situation (level 3). A student may not have noticed what they missed and would likely be unable to talk with the patient and family about the error.

An attending physician recognizes that an intern seems to be struggling to keep up with patients in the clinic and with the notes in the medical record. To better understand the problem, the attending spends more time observing the intern and offers

Table 13.3 Professionalism 3: Accountability/Conscientiousness

Professionalism 3: Accountability/Conscientiousness				
Level 1	Level 2	Level 3	Level 4	Level 5
Performs administrative tasks and patient care responsibilities, with prompting	Performs administrative tasks and patient care responsibilities in a timely manner in routine situations	Performs administrative tasks and patient care responsibilities in a timely manner in complex or stressful situations	Proactively implements strategies to ensure that the needs of patients, teams, and systems are met	Creates strategies to enhance other's ability to efficiently complete administrative tasks and patient care responsibilities
Comments:				Not Yet Completed Level 1

Used with permission from the ACGME.

suggestions for more efficiency. This proactive approach helps the team and the patients (level 5).

Milestones Data and Growth

The literature provides the evidence behind growth in these three areas of professionalism over time and training. ACGME collects the individual learners' Milestone achievement twice each year, as determined by the CCCs . Th ese data show that learners do grow over time. Box plots are used to demonstrate this point through aggregate data reported at the end of the 2021 –2022 academic year. Box 13.1 explains how the box plots are interpreted. Data are demonstrated for each academic cohort in the specialty. Th ese data are reported publicly each year through the Milestones National Report.[2]

Professional Behavior

The box plots for Professional Behavior from internal medicine, rheumatology (a subspecialty of internal medicine), and vascular surgery demonstrate growth over time (Figure 13.1). Internal medicine shows a higher starting point at the end of their first year in the program as compared to Ethical Principals. Rheumatology looks like the infectious disease box plot in the next example. Vascular surgery demonstrated varying levels over time. Although the aggregate is increasing, the minimums are moving up and down, with program year 2 learners lower than program year 1 and program year 5 learners lower than program year 4.

Ethical Principles

The box plots for Ethical Principles come from internal medicine, infectious disease (a subspecialty of internal medicine), and vascular surgery (Figure 13.2). The growth across each program year is easily recognized, with higher interquartile range and mean. Internal medicine and infectious disease minimums were lower the second year than the first. In vascular surgery, note that the maximum for program year 1 learners is higher than program year 2.

Accountability

Accountability demonstrates similar patterns of overall growth for internal medicine, rheumatology, and vascular surgery, with variable minimum values. In all three examples, program year 2 learners have the lowest minimum for accountability (Figure 13.3).

Although these box plots do demonstrate growth over time, it is recognized that there could be many factors that impact these scores, including transition from intern to resident, the number of assessments collected in both evaluation periods, the pandemic that disrupted healthcare and training, and others.

Box 13.1 Interpretation of Box Plots

The median Milestone level for each program year (listed at the bottom of the box plot) is represented by the horizontal line, bounded by the 25th and 75th rank of Milestone ratings, also known as the interquartile range (IQR). The mean rating is represented by the diamond but should be interpreted with caution given the Milestones are ordinal, not interval data. "Min" represents the lowest level and "Max" the highest level (the "whiskers"), excluding outliers (represented by the open circles) (Milestones Report)[2]

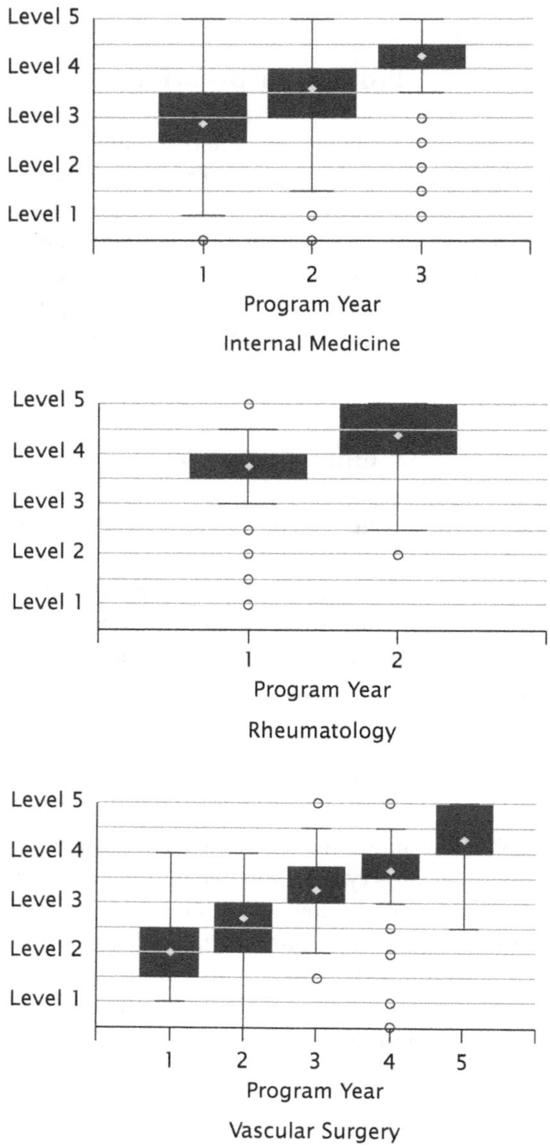

Figure 13.1 Box plots for professional behavior Milestone scores for internal medicine, infectious disease, and vascular surgery.

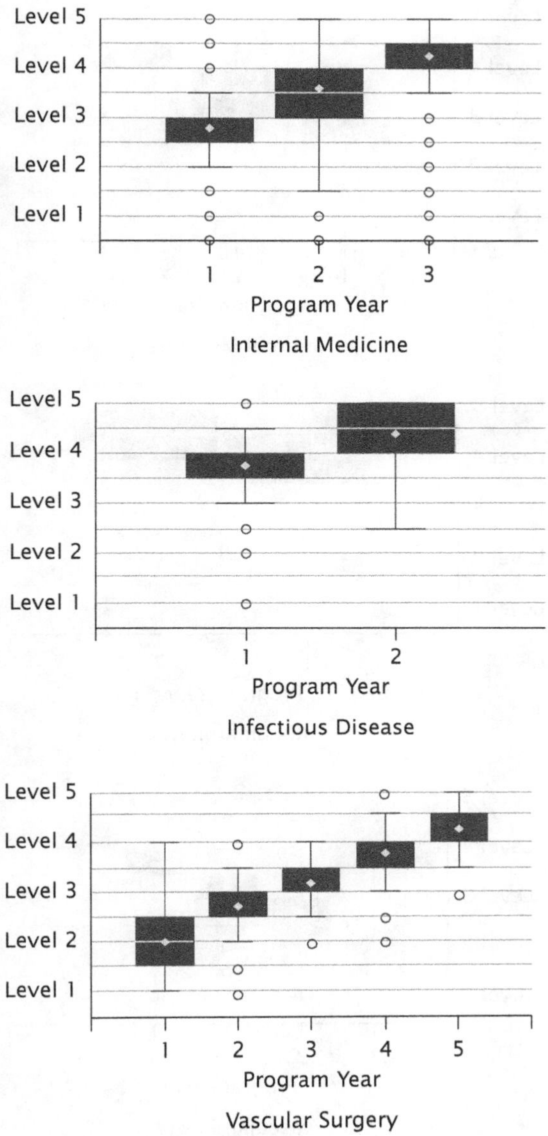

Figure 13.2 Box plots for ethical principles Milestone scores for internal medicine, infectious disease, and vascular surgery.

Conclusion

Medical professionalism is a complex and nuanced topic that presents challenges for both didactic and experiential learning. The ACGME Milestones represent a system of developmental checkpoints relevant to both knowledge and clinical proficiency as well as general competencies, including professionalism.[46,47] Predicting performance in technical versus general competency areas is difficult. For example, United States Medical Licensing Examination exams more closely correlate with early Milestone attainment in the technical competencies, while structured application interviews more

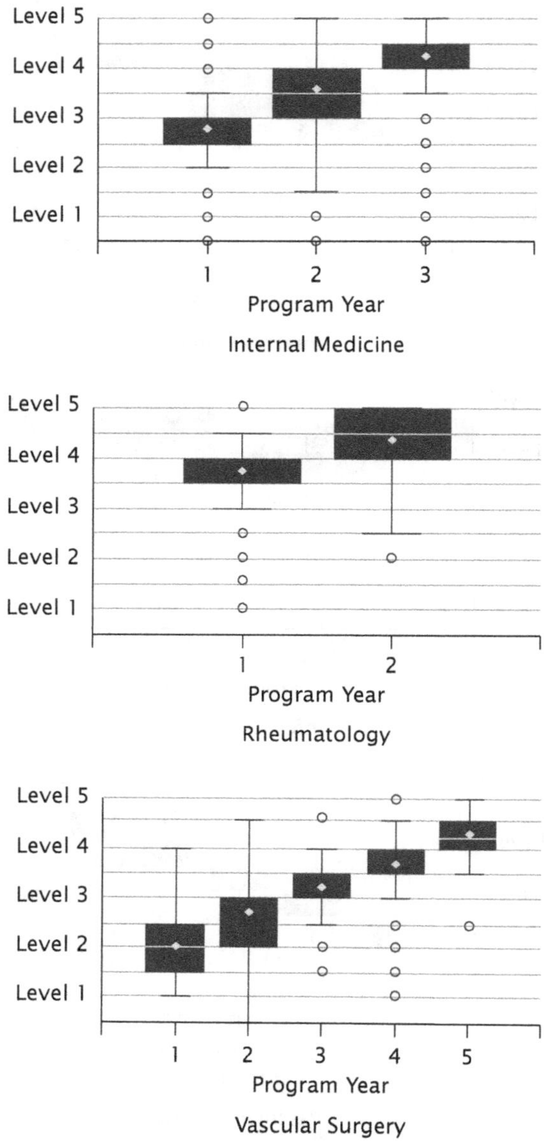

Figure 13.3 Box plots for accountability Milestone scores for internal medicine, rheumatology, and vascular surgery.

closely correlate with the general competencies, including interpersonal and communication skills as well as professionalism.[48]

This chapter considered progress in three subcompetencies of the ACGME Professionalism competency (ethical principles, professional behavior, and accountability) in part by using vignettes to illustrate the challenges posed by various clinical situations and the Milestone levels achieved, in a progressive fashion, by mastering them. As illustrated, early data from nationwide input of Milestone data in various specialties validates that this developmental assessment tool measures statistically defined aggregate progress across the training interval in both medical and surgical specialties. Within aggregate progress, however, there is hidden variability and even individual unevenness of progress. This variability exists, in part, because general competencies are much more susceptible than technical competencies to degradation over time, related to life and career stressors, burnout, and the relative accuracy of subsequent observations. Understanding and identifying individual variability is highly important to both career success and patient safety.

While clinical care delivery environments are changing at an accelerated pace in the wake of the COVID-19 pandemic, fundamental professionalism competencies remain necessary to achieve core aspects of effective and compassionate care in any and every clinical environment. In order to navigate change successfully, medicine must continuously evaluate and evolve the pedagogy of professionalism education, track its success in readying trainees for practice, and ensure the maintenance of professionalism principles and attributes as part of lifelong learning.

References

1. Nicholson N , Selden N R. *The Rhetoric of Medicine: Lessons on Professionalism from Ancient Greece.* Oxford University Press; 2019.
2. Edgar L, Hogan SO, Holmboe ES, et al. Milestones Report 2022. Acgme.org. October 2022. Accessed November 14, 2022. https://www.acgme.org/globalassets/pdfs/milestones/1160-ACGME-Milestones-Report-2022-R22.pdf
3. Edgar L, McLean S, Hogan SO, Hamstra S, Holmboe ES. The Milestones Guidebook version 2020. Acgme.org. 2020. Accessed September 3, 2022. https://www.acgme.org/globalassets/milestonesguidebook.pdf
4. Dreyfus SE, Dreyfus HL. *The Five Stage Model of the Mental Activities Involved in Directed Skill Acquisition.* University of California, Berkeley; 1980
5. Bloom B S, Baldwin T S, Hastings J T, Madaus G F. *Handbook on Formative and Summative Evaluation of Student Learning.* McGraw-Hill; 1971.
6. Van Melle EV, Frank JR, Holmboe ES, Dagnone D, Stockley D, Sherbino J. A core components framework for evaluating implementation of competency-based medical education programs. *Acad Med.* 2019;94(7):1002–1009. doi:10.1097/ACM.0000000000002743
7. Andolsek K, Padmore J, Hauer KE, Ekpenyong A, Edgar L, Holmboe ES. Clinical Competency Committees: A Guidebook for Programs. 3rd ed. January 2020. Accessed September 3, 2022. https://www.acgme.org/globalassets/acgmeclinicalcompetencycommitteeguidebook.pdf
8. The Society of Neurological Surgeons. Recruitment guidelines. Society of Neurological Surgeons .org. June 26, 2022. Accessed August 28, 2022. https://www.societyns.org/medical-students/external-medical-student-rotations.
9. Selden NR, Barbaro NM, Barrow DL, et al. Neurosurgery residency and fellowship education in the United States: 2 decades of system development by the One Neurosurgery Summit organizations. *J Neurosurg.* 2021;136(2):565–574. doi:10.3171/2020.10.JNS203125
10. Edgar L, Roberts S, Holmboe E. Milestones 2.0: a step forward. *J Grad Med Educ.* 2018;10(3):367–369. doi:10.4300/JGME-D-18-00372.1
11. Marco CA, Adams K, Leep Hunderford AN, et al. Refining the milestones for assessment of professionalism skills . Supplemental publication to Edgar L, Roberts S, Holmboe

E. Milestones 2.0: A Step Forward. *J Grad Med Educ.* 2018;10(3):367–369. https://meridian.allenpress.com/jgme/article-supplement/33604/pdf/jgme-10-03-37_s03/

12. Milestones 2.0 completed specialties and subspecialties and effective dates. Acgme.org. Published July 2022. Accessed September 3, 2022. https://www.acgme.org/Portals/0/PDFs/Milestones/Milestones2.0EffectiveDates.pdf.
13. Ludmer K. *Let Me Heal: The Opportunity to Preserve Excellence in American Medicine.* Oxford University Press. 2014.
14. Working Party of the Royal College of Physicians. Doctors in society. Medical professionalism in a changing world. *Clin Med (Lond).* 2005;5(6 suppl 1):S5–S40.
15. Halpern EJ, Spandorfer JM. Professionalism in radiology: ideals and challenges. *AJR Am J Roentgenol.* 2014;202(2):352–357. doi:10.2214/AJR.13.11342
16. Nasca TJ. President's address. Presented at: 2018 ACGME Annual Educational Conference; 2018; Orlando, Florida.
17. Hersey P , Blanchard K H. *Management of Organizational Behavior—Utilizing Human Resources.* Prentice Hall; 1972.
18. Wheelan SA. *The Handbook of Group Research and Practice.* Sage Publications; 2005. doi:10.4135/9781412990165
19. Beauchamp T, Childress J. *Principles of Biomedical Ethics.* 7th ed. Oxford University Press, 2013.
20. Varkey B. Principles of clinical ethics and their application to practice. *Med Princ Pract.* 2021;30(1):17–28. doi:10.1159/000509119
21. McCormick T R. Principles of bioethics. Department of Bioethics and Humanities, University of Washington ; 2018 ; accessed August 28, 2022. https://depts.washington.edu/bhdept/ethics-medicine/bioethics-topics/articles/principles-bioethics
22. Markel H. "I swear by Apollo"—on taking the Hippocratic oath. *N Engl J Med.* 2004;350(20):2026–2029. doi:10.1056/NEJMp048092
23. Taylor RM . Ethical principles and concepts in medicine In: Bernat J, Beresford RH, ed. *Handbook of Clinical Neurology.* Elsevier Science Publishing; 2013 :118:1–9.
24. O'Sullivan L, Aldasoro E, O'Brien Á, Nolan M, McGovern C, Carroll Á. Ethical values and principles to guide the fair allocation of resources in response to a pandemic: a rapid systematic review. *BMC Med Ethics.* 2022;23(1):70. doi:10.1186/s12910-022-00806-8
25. Hundert EM. A model for ethical problem solving in medicine, with practical applications. *Am J Psychiatry.* 1987;144(7):839–846. doi:10.1176/ajp.144.7.839
26. Madani M, Vedadhir A, Larijani B, Khazaei Z, Gharamaleki AF. Bridging the gap between ethical theory and practice in medicine: a constructivist grounded theory study. *Sci Eng Ethics.* 2020;26(4):2255–2275. doi:10.1007/s11948-020-00217-1
27. Langerman A, Cutrer WB, Yakes EA, Meador KG. Embedding ethics education in clinical clerkships by identifying clinical ethics competencies: the Vanderbilt experience. *HEC Forum.* 2020;32(2):163–174. doi:10.1007/s10730-020-09410-y
28. DeFoor MT, Chung Y, Zadinsky JK, Dowling J, Sams RW 2nd. An interprofessional cohort analysis of student interest in medical ethics education: a survey-based quantitative study. *BMC Med Ethics.* 2020;21(1):26. doi: 10.1186/s12910-020-00468-4
29. Helft PR, Eckles RE, Torbeck L. Ethics education in surgical residency programs: a review of the literature. *J Surg Educ.* 2009 ;66(1):35–42. doi: 10.1016/j.jsurg.2008.10.001

30. Principles of medical ethics. Ama-assn.org. 2016. Accessed August 28, 2022. https://www.ama-assn.org/about/publications-newsletters/ama-principles-medical-ethics

31. Kok AA, Plaisier I, Smit JH, Penninx BW. The impact of conscientiousness, mastery, and work circumstances on subsequent absenteeism in employees with and without affective disorders. *BMC Psychol.* 2017;5(1):10. doi:10.1186/s40359-017-0179-y

32. Roberts BW, Lejuez C, Krueger RF, Richards JM, Hill PL. What is conscientiousness and how can it be assessed? *Dev Psychol.* 2014;50(5):1315–1330. doi:10.1037/a0031109

33. Emanuel EJ, Emanuel LL. What is accountability in health care? *Ann Intern Med.* 1996;124(2):229–239. doi:10.7326/0003-4819-124-2-199601150-00007

34. Van Belle S, Mayhew SH. What can we learn on public accountability from non-health disciplines: a meta-narrative review. *BMJ Open.* 2016;6(7):e010425. doi:10.1136/bmjopen-2015-010425

35. Emanuel LL. A professional response to demands for accountability: practical recommendations regarding ethical aspects of patient care. Working Group on Accountability. *Ann Intern Med.* 1996;124(2):240–249. doi:10.7326/0003-4819-124-2-199601150-00008

36. Guraya SS, Guraya SY, Harkin DW, Ryan Á, Mat Nor MZB, Yusoff MSB. Medical Education e-Professionalism (MEeP) framework; from conception to development. *Med Educ Online.* 2021;26(1):1983926. doi:10.1080/10872981.2021.1983926

37. Gunderman RB, Streicher DA. Accountability in professionalism. *AJR Am J Roentgenol.* 2012 ;198(4):W344–346. doi: 10.2214/AJR.11.7767

38. Arthur W Jr, Graziano WG. The five-factor model, conscientiousness, and driving accident involvement. *J Pers.* 1996 ;64(3):593–618. doi: 10.1111/j.1467-6494.1996.tb00523.x

39. Drach-Zahavy A, Srulovici E. The personality profile of the accountable nurse and missed nursing care. *J Adv Nurs.* 2019;75(2):368–379. doi:10.1111/jan.13849

40. Papadakis MA, Teherani A, Banach MA, et al. Disciplinary action by medical boards and prior behavior in medical school. *N Engl J Med.* 2005;353(25):2673–2682. doi:10.1056/NEJMsa052596

41. Stern DT, Frohna AZ, Gruppen LD. The prediction of professional behaviour. *Med Educ.* 2005;39(1):75–82. doi:10.1111/j.1365-2929.2004.02035.x

42. Sanfey H, Darosa DA, Hickson GB, et al. Pursuing professional accountability: an evidence-based approach to addressing residents with behavioral problems. *Arch Surg.* 2012;147(7):642–647. doi:10.1001/archsurg.2012.832

43. Morreale MK, Balon R, Arfken CL. Survey of the importance of professional behaviors among medical students, residents, and attending physicians. *Acad Psychiatry.* 2011;35(3):191–195. doi:10.1176/appi.ap.35.3.191

44. O'Flynn S, Power S, Horgan M, O'Tuathaigh CM. Attitudes towards professionalism in graduate and non-graduate entrants to medical school. *Educ Health (Abingdon).* 2014;27(2):200–204. doi:10.4103/1357-6283.143770

45. Reed DA, Levine RB, Miller RG, et al. Effect of residency duty-hour limits: views of key clinical faculty. *Arch Intern Med.* 2007;167(14):1487–1492. doi:10.1001/archinte.167.14.1487

46. Conforti LN, Yaghmour NA, Hamstra SJ, et al. The effect and use of milestones in the assessment of neurological surgery residents and residency programs. *J Surg Educ.* 2018;75(1):147–155. doi:10.1016/j.jsurg.2017.06.001

47. Swing SR, Beeson MS, Carraccio C, et al. Educational milestone development in the first 7 specialties to enter the next accreditation system. *J Grad Med Educ.* 2013;5(1):98–106. doi:10.4300/JGME-05-01-33

48. Marcus-Blank B, Dahlke JA, Braman JP, et al. Predicting performance of first-year residents: correlations between structured interview, licensure exam, and competency scores in a multi-institutional study. *Acad Med.* 2019;94(3):378–387. doi:10.1097/ACM.0000000000002429

PART B: EPILOGUE

A WINDOW ON MY FUTURE

Thomas S. Inui

The first time I saw the linen room window was when I was being introduced to Osler 3 by my resident. I was about to start my third-year internal medicine clerkship at the Johns Hopkins Hospital, and the third-floor ward in the Osler building was to be my home floor for the next month.

"Welcome to Osler 3," said Mike, "I'm one of the two JARs [junior assistant residents] in charge of the team. You're here at a good time; our attending physician, Dr. C____, is terrific. He walk-rounds on all the patients, is an infectious disease guy, and is a former Osler chief resident. Work hard, know your patients, don't bullshit or brown-nose him, and you'll have a great rotation. By the way, he writes excellent recommendations for residencies. If you hope to stay here or go to another good place, there'd be no better person to ask for a letter."

The ward tour was more complex than I imagined. We were introduced to the charge nurse Amy, who was red-haired, somewhat intimidating, and younger than I thought she would be. My mother and godmother had been Hopkins nurses, so I listened closely to what she had to say about Cardex rounds (weekly nursing orders review), the importance of getting our work done with the patients before team bedside rounds involving her in the morning, and working with Sylvia, the Black ward clerk "who knows everything." Sylvia filled us in on the floor's diurnal rhythms—when to draw blood from patients, when food carts arrived, when visiting hours were, when nursing shifts changed, and where the forms were located for orders/referrals/informed consent for procedures and the like. Both Amy and Sylvia emphasized that "stealing leftover food" from patients' trays was a no-no and that sleeping in empty patient beds was forbidden. I began to think that long hours would be part of my rotation.

As the tour went on, there were other impressions. All the patients were Black and in four-person shared rooms, with yellow pull-aside curtains between beds and one chair at each bed. Mike said that the room across from the ward clerk and nursing station was where the sickest patients were put, so Sylvia and others could "keep an eye on them." Was this the intensive care unit (ICU)? There was a breezy "porch" bedroom at the end of the floor with multiple windows that admitted air and light. He said that patients with pneumonia in preantibiotic days took "winter cures" in this room, where they would be moved to breathe cold air, hoping to quell the inflammation and bacteria in their lungs. Now, it was a good room to put noisy patients who might keep everyone else awake at night, perhaps patients in restraints who couldn't move. Who were those patients I wondered, and who could keep an eye on them at the end of the hall? Why were there heavy security screens on all the windows, and how did the rest of the floor get breezes or other "air conditioning"? I saw radiators but felt no cool air moving. Where were the white patients?

The doctors' workroom was just off the nurses' station. "Sit at any desk," said Mike. "The other JAR and I usually sit at the end of the room over here, and the interns will sit next to us. Choose any other desk. Your coats can hang on these pegs, and your black bags can slide into the shelves down here. By the way, these little bottles here are Ritalin. Help yourself when you need it." Who dispenses this stuff? Why is it in sample bottles? "The clinical lab where you will do all the admission basic labs is right off the floor, next to the elevator, and the teaching room for professor's rounds is across the hall from the lab. The equipment for blood drawing on our patients is in the supply and linens closet. If you've got a stat lab or are paged to an arrest, don't take the elevator. Run the steps. The elevator is too slow without the ladies who run it in the daytime." Who are those ladies?

"Finally," said Mike, "here is the supply and linen room," as he led the way across the hall from the nursing station. It was a modest-size room with linens/towels/washcloths on shelving on the right, an inner door on the left, shelving on the wall beyond this door with wash basins, emesis basins, tubes for blood, needles, and tourniquets at the back. On the room's far wall there was a sizable window with a heavy-duty security screen visible. "This door is the staff bathroom. Don't enter without knocking, day or night. The nurses, nursing assistants, and ward clerks have first dibs on the toilet. You're welcome to use it if they are not in there. I want each of you to look out this window. It's important you know about this. See that roof below us? It's two stories down. On one occasion when our attending Dr. C____ was an intern, a patient of his with delirium tremens, who was wildly agitated by his hallucinations, jumped out of this window before anyone could restrain him. When Dr. C____ arrived and looked down, his patient was face down on the roof, not moving, and unresponsive. Dr. C____ didn't hesitate, he jumped out of the widow, dragged himself to his patient, tried to rouse him and, failing that, to resuscitate him. The patient had a broken neck and was dead. Dr. C____ had a broken leg. He was able to return to his duties with a cast and crutches the next day. After that incident, a security screen was installed in this window."

I began to know my place in the organization as well as some of my duties. It was both thrilling and sobering.

After reading this story, try using an exegesis method to explore its content.

1. Who in this story can I see as myself?
2. From the point of view of whomever you have chosen, what do you bring to the situation that makes these events possible?
3. Who else in this story (or its organizational or cultural context) influences this story?
4. Where/what in this story is "the good," the value, the virtue, the "North Star," or the principle we might seek to preserve?
5. What, then, ought I do?

PART C

PROFESSIONALISM IMPLEMENTATION IN CLINICAL PRACTICE

14

Lifestyle Medicine in Patient Care

Christopher P. Fagundes, Gia Merlo, and James M. Rippe

Key Points

- The biopsychosocial model assumes good health is determined by biological, psychological, and social factors that interact to promote health and disease.
- Lifestyle medicine is an evidence-based lifestyle therapeutic intervention—including a whole-food, plant-predominant eating pattern, regular physical activity, restorative sleep, stress management, avoidance of risky substances, and positive social connection—as a primary modality, delivered by clinicians trained and certified in this specialty, to prevent, treat and often reverse chronic disease.
- The behaviors, social connections, and emotions that characterize people's lives shape their quality of life and physical health.

Humans are living longer than ever before thanks to advances in modern medicine. Before 1900, acute infectious illnesses resulted in the most common causes of illness and death in the United States and other developed nations.[1] At the turn of the twentieth century, infectious diseases such as tuberculosis, influenza, and pneumonia were responsible for more than twice the number of deaths as heart disease, the number one cause of morbidity and mortality today. Indeed, chronic diseases such as heart disease, diabetes, stroke, and cancer are responsible for most deaths in the United States and other developed countries.[2] More than three-fourths of those over 65 have at least one chronic illness[3] or condition.[4] Collectively, chronic diseases comprise over 80% of annual healthcare costs in the United States.[3]

Unlike acute illnesses and disorders that can be understood and treated within a traditional biomedical framework, chronic diseases are developed, prevented, managed, and treated through a complex array of biological, psychological, and social influences.[4] Consider a recent report from the US Centers for Disease and Control Prevention asserting that eradicating smoking, physical inactivity, and poor diet would eliminate 40% of all cancers and 80% of heart disease, stroke, and type 2 diabetes in the United States; over one-third of deaths in the United States are attributed to these three health behaviors, along with alcohol abuse.[5] Accordingly, the promotion of lifestyle interventions that prevent and manage chronic diseases should be an international priority.

New Model of Health and Disease

The Second World War motivated the world's sovereign states to prioritize international cooperation as it became abundantly clear that the health and security of citizens in each country depended on the health and security of citizens in every other. Thus, a specialized agency of the United Nations named the World Health Organization (WHO) was formed for the purpose of "the attainment by all peoples of the highest possible level of Health."[6,7] In 1948, the chartered members of WHO defined health as "a complete state of physical, mental, and social well-being and not merely the absence of disease or infirmity."[7] Innovative and forward-looking at the time, it would take another half-century before medicine started to embrace a healthcare model that extended beyond a biomedical framework that exclusively relied on pharmacological and surgical interventions.

The biopsychosocial model assumes good health is determined by biological, psychological, and social factors that interact to promote health and disease.[8] Rather than viewing disease as an aberration needing medical intervention to *return to one's "normal"* state, the biopsychosocial model contends that good health can be worked for and attained by living a lifestyle characterized by good health behaviors and psychological health. The translational potential of this model requires that physicians and other medical professionals deliver *lifestyle interventions* to promote habits and practices to prevent and mitigate chronic diseases.[8]

Barriers to Progress

Most medical schools fail to cover basic information about the impact of nutrition, physical activity, stress, sleep, addiction, and close relationships on physical health. For example, less than one-third of medical schools provide the recommended 25 hours of nutrition science education.[9–11]When asked about their perceptions of clinical nutrition education after medical school, more than 70% of recent medical graduates reported insufficient training and knowledge. The lack of nutrition education is evident in a recent study examining fourth-year medical students' basic nutritional knowledge; fewer than 15% of those surveyed knew basic nutritional information, such as the recommended percentages for carbohydrates, protein, and fat in a daily diet.[9–11]Furthermore, the current economic model for healthcare delivery generally disincentives physicians from providing lifestyle interventions. Counseling patients on health behaviors and psychological health takes time and is not nearly as lucrative as administering medical procedures. While pharmaceutical companies spend billions on research and advertising, there is no immediate financial incentive for the industry to research, advertise, and train physicians on evidence-based lifestyle interventions.

Lifestyle Medicine: A Discipline and Philosophy

A relatively new discipline, lifestyle medicine "is an evidence-based lifestyle therapeutic intervention—including a whole-food, plant-predominant eating pattern, regular physical activity, restorative sleep, stress management, avoidance of risky substances

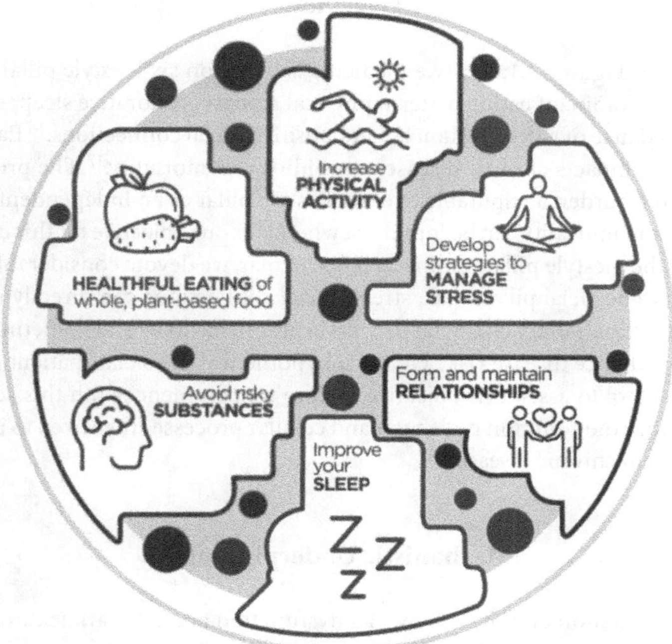

Figure 14.1 Six pillars of lifestyle medicine.

and positive social connection—as a primary modality, delivered by clinicians trained and certified in this specialty, to prevent, treat and often reverse chronic disease" (see Figure 14.1).[12] We have been deeply involved in lifestyle medicine from its inception. Indeed, one of the coauthors (JMR) named the field "lifestyle medicine" in the academic literature with the first edition of his eponymous 1999 textbook published.[13] This discipline provides a framework to produce the knowledge base necessary for physicians and other health practitioners to reduce the risk and impact of chronic diseases. Notably, a key aspect of this discipline is that physicians and other health professionals are encouraged to counsel patients on healthy eating, regular physical exercise, adequate sleep, stress management, avoiding drug and alcohol abuse, and the importance of high-quality social relationships.[14] Importantly, lifestyle medicine does not discount the importance of pharmacological and surgical interventions. Instead, it assumes good patient care requires counseling patients to engage in good health behaviors in unison with pharmacological and surgical interventions.[14]

Although physicians report being ill-prepared to deliver "lifestyle interventions," the demand for knowledge and training in this area has grown exponentially.[14] The need for training and research in lifestyle medicine was the impetus for the American College of Lifestyle Medicine (ACLM), founded in 2004.[15]This professional organization educates and advocates for lifestyle medicine "as a foundation of a transformed and sustainable healthcare system." They now offer certification in lifestyle medicine for physicians, specialists, and other professionals to show that one has the knowledge base necessary to prevent, treatment, and reverse chronic disease through evidence-based practices.[15]

Overview

As illustrated in Figure 14.1, lifestyle medicine is based on six lifestyle pillars: a whole-food, plant-predominant eating pattern; physical activity; restorative sleep; stress management; avoidance of risky substances; and positive social connections.[16] Each of these lifestyle pillars impacts chronic disease, morbidity, and mortality.[17] The proportion of disease-specific burden attributable to each lifestyle pillar as an independent risk factor of morbidity and mortality can be found elsewhere[18] as our objective for this chapter is to explore how the lifestyle pillars connect; in particular, we devote considerable attention to how the psychosocial pillars (i.e., stress, social connection) can directly impact and be impacted by the pillars characterized by health behavior—and sometimes interact to reduce or enhance disease risk. We use a hypothetical physician-patient scenario as an illustrative tool to assist this objective. Before we commence with this scenario, we briefly introduce the common molecular and cellular processes theorized to mediate the lifestyle pillars to chronic disease.

Mechanistic Underpinnings

Chronic inflammation and mitochondrial dysfunction are hallmark features of senescence and chronic disease.[19] *Inflammaging* is an emerging term in the literature characterizing the low-grade, chronic, systemic inflammation in aging that is an important indicator of morbidity and mortality.[20] There is a plethora of epidemiological evidence that a mild chronic inflammatory state is predictive of an aging phenotype.[20] Chronic inflammation is an essential biological mechanism that promotes declines in physical function leading to frailty and impaired functional activity. Persistent low-grade proinflammatory cytokine activity and mitochondrial dysfunction play a central role in risk and progression of cardiovascular disease (CVD), type II diabetes, several neurological diseases, rheumatoid arthritis, metabolic disorders, and some types of cancer regardless of the age of the individual.[21–23]A chronically overactive proinflammatory state promotes mitochondrial dysfunction, which stimulates indiscriminant amounts of reactive oxygen species (ROS); when oxidative damage is excessive, the risk for cellular senescence, premature aging, and chronic disease increases.[24–26]As a result of the cellular stress that ensues, cell-free mitochondrial DNA (mtDNA) induces proinflammatory cytokine activity, causing a feedback loop. Lifestyle medicine interventions have the potential to thwart this vicious cycle. There is strong evidence for the scientific premise that all six lifestyle pillars (Figure 14.2) can exacerbate and mitigate age-related increases in chronic inflammation (i.e., inflammaging) and associated mitochondrial dysfunction.[6,18]

Assessment and Implications of the Six Lifestyle Pillars

Consider the following example of how a physician trained in lifestyle medicine might interact with a 76-year-old patient named Jack, who has come in for an annual exam. Typical measurement assessments of height, weight, and vital signs are taken on Jack's arrival, and the first issue his physician notices when looking at Jack's chart is weight gain. Jack's body mass index (BMI) has increased from 24 to 31 over the last 12 months.

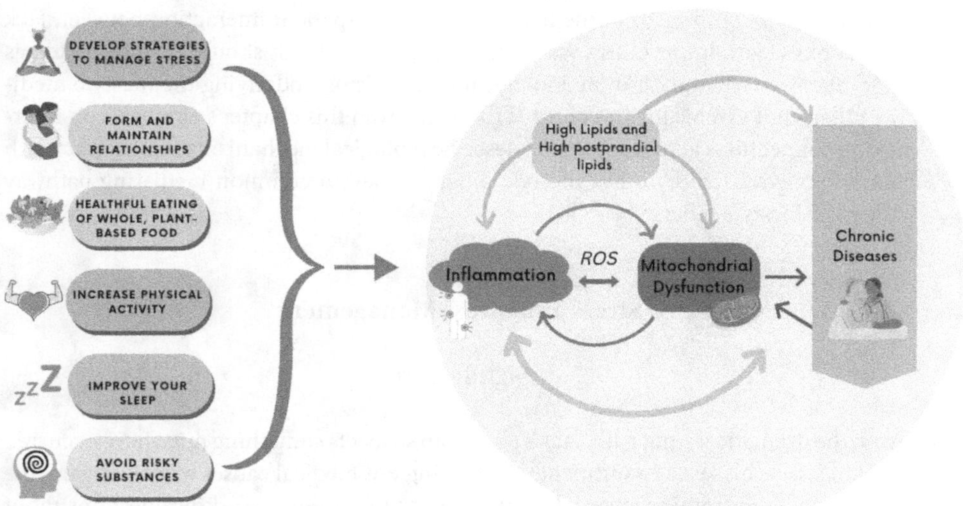

Figure 14.2 Six biobehavioral mechanisms linking lifestyle pillars to chronic disease.

With a BMI over 30, Jack is meeting the diagnosis of obesity; at this BMI, his risk for chronic disease and premature mortality is relatively high.[27–29]Obesity is a significant risk factor for chronic diseases and premature mortality; depending on the severity, obesity decreases life expectancy by 5–20 years.[30]

Obesity results from a complex interaction of biological, genetic, environmental, cultural, behavioral, and psychosocial factors influencing hunger, satiation, and body fat.[31] Approximately one-third of the global population is considered overweight or obese.[32]The rise in obesity has come at a high financial cost. Indeed, each person living in the United States who is obese cost the United States over $1,900 each year. Obesity and associated metabolic disturbances affect almost every physiological function and contribute to most chronic diseases. For those with a healthy weight, adipocytes store lipids and ensure metabolic processes remain in a state of homeostasis.[33]

It would be tempting for Jack's physician to articulate the health risks associated with obesity and explain that he needs to eat fewer calories and expend more energy. Yet, a physician trained in lifestyle medicine has learned that there is no evidence that a patient will lose weight after explaining how energy imbalance promotes obesity.[34] Furthermore, presenting data on the consequences of poor health behaviors only motivates behavior change under specific contexts and when delivered in particular ways.[34] When health messaging includes scare tactics for morbidity and mortality, motivation for positive health behavior change typically decreases.[35,36]

In our view, the pillars of lifestyle medicine should not be conceptualized as independent identities but as part of a dynamic system of interlocking factors contributing to health and well-being. Certain lifestyle medicine pillars have specific recommended guidelines generated by government health agencies and other governing bodies and organizations (e.g., the ACLM). Physicians trained in lifestyle medicine are encouraged to assess how their patient is doing in relationship to each pillar by taking lifestyle medicine vital signs. As we describe the significance, physiological processes, and health recommendations and guidelines associated with each pillar, we commence by illustrating the assessment component of the fictitious physician-patient interaction between Jack and his physician. Importantly, we want to emphasize that it should be interpreted as comprehensive when describing biological mechanisms underlying the lifestyle medicine pillar's links to health and chronic disease. Given this chapter's emphasis on interlocking connections across pillars, we describe biological mechanisms that interact with biomarkers governed by other lifestyle pillars or have a common mediating pathway with other lifestyle pillars.

Stress and Stress Management

Significance

Given the dramatic weight gain, Jack's physician suspects something must have occurred in his life since his last appointment. After ruling out medical causes of weight gain, the lifestyle medicine training material emphasizes the importance of asking questions about their patient's perceptions of stress and inquiring about recent life stressors, given their powerful impact on people's physiology, the risk for depression, and health behaviors.[37] Multiple studies have shown that those under chronic stress for a considerable period (e.g., dementia spousal caregivers) are at greater risk for morbidity and mortality than matched comparisons.[38,39] Both health behaviors and the physiological wear and tear on the body are thought to contribute to morbidity and mortality risk[40,41] jointly. Thus, the first lifestyle vital sign Jack's physician addresses is stress. In so doing, Jack explains that his wife of thirty years died six months ago. Although his grief symptoms have subsided, he has difficulty adjusting, and his lifestyle was quite unhealthy. Administration of the Hamilton depression rating scale indicates mild-to-moderate depression with a score of fifteen (which was clinically confirmed to be moderate depression), making it unlikely primary depressive illness is solely responsible for this dramatic weight change. Jack explains his symptoms of grief as manageable and does not consider himself depressed. However, he describes feelings of significant stress trying to address all the secondary stressors related to the loss (e.g., learning how to do household tasks his wife used to do, keeping track of various health-related issues; initiating social plans).[40–42]When evaluating the stress management vital sign in lifestyle medicine, it is critical the physician inquire about the patient's current approach to stress management.[43] Jack described a glass or two of wine as his primary tool to manage stress. However, he also mentions taking up smoking again. Using substances such as tobacco or alcohol is a common way for people to cope with negative emotions in times of stress, which is elaborated in more detail in the substance use section.

Mechanisms and Interactions With Other Pillars

When an event or stimuli is interpreted as stressful, the sympathetic–adrenal–medullary (SAM) system and the hypothalamic–pituitary–adrenal (HPA) axis are activated. As a result, the catecholamines norepinephrine and epinephrine are released in the periphery, resulting in increased heart rate and blood pressure and several other physiological alterations (e.g., eye dilation, digestive system decreases). Simultaneously, the hypothalamus releases corticotrophin-releasing factor (CRF), which facilitates the blood supply to the pituitary gland to stimulate adrenocorticotrophic hormone (ACTH). In turn, ACTH activates the adrenal cortex to produce cortisol, the type of glucocorticoid secreted in humans.

Although glucocorticoid activity is adaptive when released in the context of an acute stressor, chronic cortisol release can have adverse health consequences. First, glucocorticoids are immunosuppressive, which partially explains why those under chronic psychological stress are less likely to sustain a fourfold increase in antibody titers to the influenza vaccine, more likely to exhibit latent herpesvirus reactivation, and are more susceptible to the common cold.[44–50]One necessary and adaptive function is that cortisol serves to decrease inflammation. Yet, when people are under chronic stress, immune cells become desensitized to the anti-inflammatory effects of cortisol, leaving the system susceptible to prolonged levels of systemic inflammation when the body mounts a proinflammatory response.[19] Proinflammatory cytokine activity increases as a result of acute stress[46,47,49]; furthermore, chronic stress, loneliness, grief, and depression all prime the inflammatory stress response to mount an excessive and prolonged response when exposed to subsequent acute stressors.[47,51] Accordingly, the acute everyday hassles Jack experiences in his daily life likely put much more significant wear and tear on his body than they would at other times in his life.

Guidelines and Recommendations

Specific stress management guidelines are not as concrete as they are for some of the other lifestyle pillars; yet the field of lifestyle medicine encourages people to actively adopt techniques to manage their stress. Such practices include regularly participating in mind-body interventions such as yoga and tai chi.[52] Mindfulness-based stress management practices are also endorsed. Each of these has a strong evidence base for reducing psychological and physical health consequences of stress.[53] There is strong evidence that mind-body practices such as yoga even reduce people's level of chronic low-grade inflammation.[52] In addition to active stress management practices mind-body medicine approaches provide, some people under chronic stress may benefit from cognitive behavioral therapy to learn how to target dysfunctional and reframe dysfunctional thoughts that may be causing their stress; both in person and internet-based treatment have been shown to be highly efficacious to reduce symptoms of psychological stress and depression.[54,55]

Physical Activity

Significance

Next, Jack's physician asks about current physical activity levels, knowing that depression and stressful life events can thwart exercise routines.[56] Exercise lowers the risk for most chronic diseases.[57] People like Jack, who are under a great deal of psychological distress, report they lack the time, energy, and motivation to exercise when encouraged to do so for their mental and physical health.[58] Yet there is a large evidence base showing activity is highly efficacious in reducing and preventing symptoms of psychological stress and depression; this relationship appears to be linear.[59,60]

Table 14.1 Physical Activity Guidelines for Children, Adolescents, and Adults

Age Range	Frequency Duration	Type of Physical Activity
6–17 years	<60 min/day	Moderate- or vigorous-intensity aerobic, with some muscle strengthening
>18 years	<150 min/wk	<150 min/wk of either moderate- or vigorous-intensity aerobic or <75 min/week of mixed moderate- and high-intensity aerobic, preferably spread throughout the week; plus 2 days/wk of resistance training involving moderate to high intensities for all major muscle groups

In general, over 80% of adults do not meet the recommended requirements for physical activity (see Table 14.1 for definition by age).[61,62] Recent estimates suggest that the United States spends between $100 and $350 billion each year as a result of inactivity.[63] This amounts to over 10% of total US healthcare costs.[63] Physical activity is a significant risk factor for chronic disease in those over thirty.[62] Physical activity has a dose-response relationship with incident CVD, cardiovascular-related mortality, and all-cause mortality; those who meet current guidelines for moderate-to-vigorous physical activity reduce the risk of cardiovascular-related morbidity and mortality by over 75%.[64] Recent estimates suggest that 1.5% of all cancer in men and 4.5% in women can be attributed to physical inactivity.[65] Physical activity delays the onset of cognitive decline and some forms of dementia.[66]

Mechanisms

Physical activity can be best conceptualized mechanistically as a protective factor that reduces chronic disease risk.[62] Physical activity dramatically impacts various molecular and cellular processes associated with chronic disease.[67] The variability in heart rate mediated by the vagus nerve provides an index of parasympathetic function; stress and depression lower vagally mediated heart rate variability (HRV).[68–73]Low HRV is prognostic for CVD-related morbidity and mortality.[74–77]For example, after a myocardial infarction (MI) (i.e., heart attack), having lower vagally mediated HRV was a significant independent predictor of mortality.[78–80]In an older adult sample within the Framingham Heart Study (736 men and women with an average age of 72), having lower HRV was associated with higher all-cause mortality.[77] The mechanisms by which lower vagally mediated HRV boosts CVD risk, heart attack, and CVD-related mortality are multifactorial.[81] Because the vagus nerve innervates the heart's sinoatrial node (i.e., the heart's pacemaker), it can modulate rapid heart rate fluctuations to restore normal function. Low vagally mediated HRV is also inversely associated with hypertension, diabetes, and lower high-density lipoprotein (HDL), even after accounting for age, BMI, smoking, and alcohol consumption.[82–87]Via the cholinergic anti-inflammatory pathway, raising vagally mediated HRV through regular exercise can lower chronic low-grade inflammation.[88–90]Interventions that boost moderate activity have been shown to increase HRV, lower blood pressure, reduce insulin sensitivity, glucose, insulin sensitivity, low-density lipoprotein (LDL) cholesterol, and triglycerides (TGs).[67,91–96]

Physical Activity Recommendations

As can be seen in Table 14.1, the most recent exercise guidelines state that adults should do at least 150 minutes of moderate-intensity or 75 minutes a week of vigorous-intensity aerobic physical activity, or an equivalent combination of moderate- and vigorous-intensity aerobic activity.[97] In comparison, children and adolescents require 60 minutes a day of moderate or vigorous exercise. Those that do not meet physical activity requirements are at 10% greater risk of premature mortality compared with those that do.[63]

Example Interactions Across Lifestyle Pillars: Exercise and Stress

Not only does exercise promote physical health, but also it has a strong impact on mental health.[98] There is a well-established link between stress, depression, and physical activity. A meta-analysis of 49 prospective studies showed that those with moderate levels of fitness had a 23% greater risk of developing major depression than those with high levels of fitness. Furthermore, those who exhibited low levels of fitness had a 47% greater likelihood of developing depression than those with high levels of fitness.[99] Likewise, physical activity is also associated with lower levels of anxiety.[100]

Substance Use

Significance

Jack's physician knows Jack's risk of substance use increased after the death of his spouse. Furthermore, his risk for complicated grief increases among those who use substances while they grieve.[101,102] Substance use is a significant health problem, and avoiding addictive substances is a critical component of lifestyle medicine. Approximately 11% of the US population has a substance use disorder. Addiction is defined as the continued use of a drug despite negative consequences.[103]

Tobacco use is the leading preventable cause of death and disability in the United States,[1,2] with 30% of all cancers directly attributable to tobacco.[3,4] In addition, 5.6% of incident cancer cases in the United States are attributable to alcohol use; indeed, ethanol boosts acetaldehyde, promoting DNA damage.[65,104] Concerning other chronic diseases, tobacco and alcohol use are associated with arrhythmias, cardiac insufficiency, MI, chronic obstructive pulmonary disease, pulmonary hypertension, and diabetes.[105–109]

In addition to alcohol and tobacco use, prescription and illicit drug misuse is a major source of premature morbidity and mortality. Indeed, benzodiazepines, stimulants, and especially opioids have the potential for abuse.[110] The use of illicit drugs, such as heroin and cocaine, and abuse of prescription drugs (e.g., oxycodone) contribute to drug-related overdoses; except for the year, 2017, age-adjusted drug overdose rates have consistently increased every year since the turn of the century.[111] Addiction of many different types is a significant health problem. The array of substance types and specific psychological and physiological repercussions they produce prohibits us from parsimoniously describing specific biological mechanisms linking this lifestyle pillar to chronic disease.

Example Interactions With Other Pillars

Numerous conceptual models and robust empirical evidence underscore the interaction of emotion, context, and genetics in predicting addiction potential. The heritability of substance use disorders is about 0.5.[112–116]Stress and depression are among the most significant risk factors for substance abuse.[117] Troubled past and current relational experiences are also strong predictors of addiction risk.[118–122]Exercise has been shown to reduce the risk of addiction and promote addiction recovery. Given our discussion of vagally mediated HRV, we refer the reader to a series of well-controlled laboratory studies showing low vagally mediated HRV indexes and an inability to resist the temptation to drink alcohol among those recovering from an alcohol use disoder[69]; furthermore, a recent meta-analysis of several observational studies indicate a reliable link between low vagally mediated HRV and alcohol use disorder.[123]

Sleep

Assessment and Significance

Keeping with the pillars of lifestyle medicine, Jack's physician inquires about his sleep. Inadequate sleep and sleep disorders are vital risk factors for chronic disease and contribute to obesity. Given her background in lifestyle medicine, Jack's physician always asks her patients about sleep. Yet, she is particularly concerned about Jack's sleep, given he is grieving his spouse's death and experiencing considerable stress due to secondary stressors associated with the bereavement context. Indeed, insomnia occurs with greater frequency among those who are bereaved than those who are not.[124,125] More broadly, sleep represents a common complaint among those with a mental health diagnosis and a core feature and risk possible risk factor for stress-related disorders.[126,127] Sleep duration is an independent risk factor for cardiovascular-related morbidity and mortality; those who sleep less than 5 hours are at exceptionally high risk, as well as those who sleep over 10 hours daily.[128] In addition, sleep-disordered breathing and sleep apnea syndrome are particularly potent risk factors for CVD-related mortality and all-cause mortality.[128–130]In fact, disordered sleep is responsible for up to 40% of all CVD. Impaired sleep is also associated with the incidence and progression of obesity, cancer, and type 2 diabetes.[131–134]Mechanisms

Sleep is essential to good health; insufficient sleep dysregulates the autonomic nervous system, diurnal cortisol patterns, and the synthesis of proteins. [135,136] Multiple mechanisms underlie the link between sleep and chronic health conditions.[137] When circadian systems are dysregulated, adiposity is metabolically processed. Concerning CVD, poor sleep reduces HRV, raises blood pressure and heart rate, and leads to an overactive proinflammatory state.[133]

The mechanisms linking sleep to various forms of cancer are less established than those related to CVD, but it is a topic of active investigation. Night shift workers have a higher risk of breast cancer[138]; circadian disruption has been implicated as the most likely culprit for breast cancer risk and progression because clock genes and circadian dysregulation impact DNA damage repair, cellular apoptosis, survival, and even cell proliferation.[139] Persistent inflammation, a hallmark feature of inadequate sleep, can induce genetic instability and promote cell mutations.[140] In addition, inflammation promotes angiogenesis and metastasis.[140] Finally, poor sleep dysregulates cytokine production balance from Th1 to Th2 cytokines, leading to inadequate immune surveillance of abnormal cell mutations.[141] The impact of sleep disruption on cancer risk and progression appears to be greater among those also reporting high levels of psychological stress and depression.[142]

Recommendations

The recommended amount of sleep for optimal health changes across the life span. Humans need less sleep for good health as they age; infants need upward of 16 hours, while most adults need between 7 and 8 hours each day[143]; if adults sleep less than 6 hours daily, the risk of poor health and chronic disease increases.

Close Relationships

Significance (Loneliness and Social Isolation)

When Jack's physician inquiries about his social connections, Jack describes having difficulty attending social functions. Although his grief is still poignant, he describes overwhelming anxiety when asked to participate in social gatherings as his primary reason for avoiding these events. He worries people are inviting him out of pity. Because his wife was the extravert, he always quietly followed her lead at social events. Furthermore, he worries something may happen at a social event that triggers feelings of grief and lead to embarrassment. Because of this anxiety, he isolates himself more, increasing his anxiety and feelings of loneliness even more. This cycle is typical, especially among those with social anxiety. As someone trained in lifestyle medicine, Jack's physician knows the importance of helping her patients identify and overcome the barrier of fear to engage in healthy lifestyle choices by encouraging gradual exposure and instilling self-efficacy in her patient.[144–146]

There has been considerable research to show that objective social isolation and loneliness enhance the risk of poor quality of life and disease.[147–150]In light of the COVID-19 pandemic, loneliness has recently been highlighted as a major public health problem needing public health–type interventions.[151–153]Perceptions of social isolation are characterized by feelings of being unsafe, making one hypervigilant to stressors. In turn, perceptions of being socially isolated produce more negative social interactions. There is misperception that the internet makes people less lonely, while in fact the internet limits discussion of deeply personal issues.[154] They also make one remember previous negative interactions more negatively than they were, causing avoidance of future social interactions.[155] Across two other longitudinal studies, loneliness was a risk factor for developing pain, depression, and fatigue independent of standard risk factors.[67]

According to recent estimates of US adults over 45, one-third report being lonely.[156] Compared to those who report being less lonely or socially isolated, people who report being lonely have higher rates of dementia, CVD, and stroke.[147,157,158,159] They are also more likely to abuse substances.[160,161] Indeed, a meta-analysis of 148 different prospective studies showed that feeling socially connected is associated with a 50% risk reduction of premature mortality.[162] Furthermore, based on data from 3.4 million adults, loneliness, social isolation, and living alone were independent risk factors for early mortality; indeed, the relative risk of excess mortality was more significant due to being lonely and socially isolated than for having a BMI over 30.[163]

Mechanisms (Loneliness and Social Isolation)

In an 18-year study of 6,729 individuals from the National Health and Nutrition Examination Survey assessing social isolation and multiple markers of chronic inflammation, chronic inflammation mediated (explained) the link between social isolation and mortality.[149] In an experimental investigation of stress and loneliness in breast cancer survivors, lonelier posttreatment breast cancer survivors exhibited a more elevated and prolonged proinflammatory response to an acute experimental stressor.[64] Compared with those less lonely, adults who are more lonely exhibit greater latent herpesviruses cytomegalovirus and Epstein-Barr virus reactivation, an indicator of dysregulated cellular immunity; they also have shorter telomeres, an indicator of premature aging.[164]

Significance and Mechanisms (Marital Relationships and Health)

Marriage represents the most central relationship in most people's lives, and it is not surprising that the death of Jack's spouse poses a significant stressor. In addition to marital status, marital quality has a power impact on people's physical health; marital strife's harmful effects include increased risk and poorer outcomes for inflammation-related disorders, including depression, CVD, metabolic syndrome, and the onset of many forms of dementia, including Alzheimer disease.[165–168]Multiple research groups have shown that marital disagreements, characterized by high negativity rates, promote alterations in the autonomic, neuroendocrine, and immune systems, including elevated proinflammatory cytokine production.[169] Marital interaction studies have provided some of the best work demonstrating the importance of marital quality. Hostile marital interactions have significant negative physiological consequences. In one study in which couples engaged in a supportive discussion and a marital problem discussion across two separate sessions, the more hostile couples produced more of the proinflammatory cytokine interleukin 6 (IL-6) after the conflict discussion than the supportive discussion (113% vs. 45%). In contrast, less hostile couples' IL-6 production was similar after both discussions (70% vs. 65%).[170] Another study showed that couples who were more positively engaged with their marital partner during a laboratory-induced marital disagreement exhibited less IL-6 and tumor necrosis-alpha (TNF-α) over the next 24 hours after the disagreement.[171]

Example Interaction Across Pillars: Close Relationships and Diet

Close relationships and diet are intertwined. Evidence suggests that highly palatable, high-saturated-fat "fast-food-type" meals reduce loneliness by activating the same neuropathways that are triggered by feelings of belonging and security[172]; thus, individuals who experience loneliness may implicitly turn to high-saturated-fat meals to feel better. Interestingly, toxic marital relationships may synergistically interact with unhealthy fast-food-type meals to produce a more robust and sustained postprandial proinflammatory cytokine response. In one study, couples who exhibited problematic interpersonal behaviors (as indexed by coded facial expressions of hostility) during a standardized marital interaction assessment had higher postprandial levels of inflammation than those who exhibited low levels of hostility when they participated in a controlled feeding study within a laboratory environment.[173]

Diet

Research has consistently shown that people under chronic stress are more likely to have a diet consisting of "comfort foods" and fast-food-type meals high in sugars and saturated fats than a whole-food, plant-based diet prescribed to patients by physicians trained in lifestyle medicine.[174] Comfort foods and fast-food-type meals reflect a "western-style" diet, which is a term used in nutrition science to describe a high-saturated-fat diet consisting of high intakes of processed meat, red meat, butter, fried food, high-fat dairy products, and baked desserts. Because these food are highly caloric, if a person increased the frequency they ate this type of diet without altering their activity habits, weight gain would follow.[175–180]

In addition to the convenience fast-food-type meals provide, there are basic physiological processes that explain Jack's behavior. Specifically, people's food preferences shift when under chronic stress to desire high-caloric foods.[181] High-saturated-fat comfort foods appear to reduce feelings of sadness, independent of taste. Using a clever methodological approach, researchers injected either saline or fat directly into their participants' stomachs; then participants were exposed to sad images and music. Those who were in the "high-fat condition" (i.e., injected with fat) were 50% less impacted by the sad images and sad music than those in the control condition (i.e., injected with saline).[181] Accordingly, it is highly likely people condition themselves to turn to unhealthy foods in times of distress to reduce negative emotions.

Disease Implications, Risk Biomarkers, and Mechanisms

Those who follow a Western-style diet characterized by comfort foods and fast-food-type meals spend approximately 75% of their day in a postprandial state, which is associated with persistence substrates in circulation that have a significant health impact.[182] Those who follow a high saturated fat diet spend approximately 3/4ths of their day in a state of postprandial hyperlipidemia (i.e., a fed condition with elevated levels of fats, cholesterol, or TGs circulating in the blood).[183] TGs also provoke monocytes to produce proinflammatory cytokines. One study showed that postprandial hyperlipidemia led to a tenfold increase in the proinflammatory cytokine TNF-α within human aortic endothelial cells.[184]

Fasting and nonfasting TGs are strongly associated with MI, ischemic heart disease, cardiovascular events, and cardiovascular death. TGs and LDL cholesterol promote fatty buildup in the blood vessel wall, which narrows as a result. Through this process, elevated LDL and TGs play a significant role in atherosclerosis.[185,186] In addition to fasting levels, multiple studies have shown that postprandial lipid levels, especially TG levels (hypertriglyceridemia), predict CVD-related morbidity and mortality better than fasted levels.[187,188] In the Copenhagen City Heart Study, 7,587 women and 6,394 men were followed for approximately three decades; postprandial triglycerides were prognostic for future CVD events and premature mortality for both sexes.[189] In a study of 101 males

(61 with coronary heart disease and 40 without), postprandial TG levels predicted the presence of coronary artery disease better than fasting levels.[190]

Fasting triglycerides are also predictive of cognitive decline and incident Alzheimer disease and related dementia.[191–194]In a study of 202 older adults, those with elevated TGs had a twofold increased risk of cognitive impairment compared with those not at elevated risk.[195] A case-control study comparing those with mild cognitive impairment (MCI) to matched comparisons showed that TGs were higher in the MCI group.[196] A high-fat diet also promotes negative alterations in mitochondrial function,[197] which results in decreased oxidative respiration, decreased ATP production, and increased oxygen radical production; moreover, the morphology of mitochondria changes under high-fat overload, as shown by atypical morphology, loss of mitochondrial cristae, and shortened length.[198]

Poor diet carries enormous implications for diseases such as COVID-19. Individuals who were obese or had hypertension were three to four times as likely to be hospitalized or die from COVID-19.[199] Much of this can be attributed to poor diet. In addition, there is higher prevalence of both of these conditions in the Black and Hispanic populations in our country, which points to health equity issues. It is also worth noting that the recommendation to isolate during the COVID-19 pandemic probably caused changes in daily eating patterns and timing, which further exacerbated this problem.

Healthy Diet Recommendations

Lifestyle medicine advocates for a whole, primarily plant-based diet that includes fruits and vegetables, whole grains, seafood, legumes, and nuts. Importantly, the field of lifestyle medicine recommends a diet low in red and processed meats, sugary beverages, refined grains, and other sources of saturated and trans fats. These guidelines accord with diets recommended by US government health organizations, such as the Mediterranean diet and Dietary Approaches to Stop Hypertension (DASH) diet. They also reflect the current dietary guidelines for Americans. The *Dietary Guidelines for Americans* provides evidence-based guidelines for Americans at every stage. Most recently updated in 2020, it includes four overarching guidelines[200]:

1. Follow a healthy dietary pattern at every life stage.
2. Customize and enjoy nutrient-dense food and bereaving choices to reflect personal preferences, cultural traditions, and budgetary considerations.
3. Focus on meeting food group needs with nutrient-dense foods and beverages and stay within calorie limits.
4. Limit foods and beverages higher in added sugars, saturated fat, and sodium and limit alcoholic beverages.

Example Interactions Across Pillars: Diet and Stress

Postprandial TGs and proinflammatory cytokine production can be diminished by multiple lifestyle pillars, including exercise, sleep quality, and changes in dietary macronutrients to align with lifestyle medicine's recommendations. In addition, as we discuss in light of Jack's current context, psychological stress has a powerful impact on the postprandial response. Recall that Jack reports frequent psychological stress and moderate levels of depression, which is not surprising given he is in the first year of widowhood. An unhealthy diet may be more detrimental to him (by boosting risk health biomarkers higher and for more prolonged periods) than it would to someone not under this chronic stress. Frequent psychological stress may directly affect obesity, regardless of calories. Those who experienced a more significant number of prior-day stressors exhibited lower resting energy expenditure after eating a standardized high-saturated-fat meal than those who experienced fewer prior-day stressors. In this study, the difference converted into 104 kcal, which would mean a person under chronic stress with the same diet and activity levels would gain eleven extra pounds over a year.[201]

Frequent psychological stressors and the negative emotions they generate appear to potentiate the adverse repercussions of eating high-saturated-fat comfort foods because the postprandial (postmeal) response of lipids and proinflammatory cytokines are exaggerated when one experiences frequent stress. Psychological stress can promote lipidemia (high lipid content in the blood) by enhancing TG responses to a high-saturated-fat meal and inhibiting clearance.[202]

In one study, total triacylglycerol (TG) and very low-density lipoprotein (VLDL) TG areas under the curve were 50% or higher during a stressful condition than a control condition.[203]Increased postprandial changes were independent of baseline triacylglycerol levels.[203] In another study, acute stress also slowed TG clearance.[204] Compared to the nonstress condition, clearance of an exogenous fat load took 14% longer on average following a laboratory stressor.[204]

A different research group provided participants the same 4,186 kg meal consisting of bread, butter, ham, apple marmalade, and cottage cheese across two visits; in one visit, participants repeatedly engaged in a mental stressor designed to elicit a stress response. On the other visit, they completed a benign keyboard task. Postprandial VLDL and TGs were higher during the stress condition than the nonstress condition; furthermore, VLDL-cholesterol response, calculated as the area under the curve, was higher during the mental task than during the control sessions.[203] Fast-food-type meals high in saturated fat may prime immune cells to be more responsive to psychological stress and depression.[205,206]

In another study,[120,121] fifty-nine participants participated in a meal challenge study; after fasting for twelve hours, participants had a small intravenous catheter inserted on the day of the visit, and baseline samples were drawn, followed by a twenty- to thirty-minute adaptation period. Then they received a standardized high-saturated-fat meal; those with depression had a sharper increase. Likewise, in response to the meal, depressed women had 12% more elevated TGs than nondepressed women, and this effect persisted throughout the entire postmeal period.[201]

Evidence-Based Interventions as Cornerstone

A key component of lifestyle medicine is its focus on evidence-based interventions. It is well recognized among physicians and other health professionals that scientific knowledge must move from the basic sciences to clinical practice through rigorous phases of translational research.[207] Many medical professionals may be surprised that this same evidence-based approach is used when developing and implementing lifestyle interventions.[208] Commencing with basic science research, these interventions undertake rigorous clinical trials in the laboratory before being manualized and disseminated to health providers with the goal to produce highly potent and maximally implementable behavioral interventions that improve health and well-being. Not only must these interventions work, but also, as in pharmacological trials, mechanisms of change must be determined.[208]

When considering interventions to modify lifestyle factors, it is essential to consider the level of influence to target. Socioecological models of chronic disease posit that distal, intermediate, and proximal level factors impact chronic disease through biological and environmental interactions.[209] Distal factors include broad-based social conditions, policies, and institutional contexts. At this level of influence, interventions include changing rules, economic rewards, and institutional cultures.[209] For example, an intervention to promote lifestyle medicine at the distal level of influence could consist of creating a financial structure that reimburses for the time and energy it takes to implement successful lifestyle interventions.[210] One relatively low-cost intervention at the distal level of influence that has received support from public health advocates and policymakers is to make parks more accessible and safe for physical activity, especially in low-income communities,[211] targeting policy change to fund better lighting in gardens and walkways.

According to sociological models, people's social context (e.g., neighborhood context, local community norms, and habits) are considered "intermediate factors that influence chronic disease." Interventions that target these intermediate factors are often tailored for specific communities. One well-known example of a successful lifestyle intervention targeting intermediate factors addressed the high risk of CVD in non-Hispanic African American men living in urban areas within the United States.[212–214]Given the role hypertension plays in CVD, researchers sought to address the high rates of hypertension that were identified among non-Hispanic Black men by encouraging frequent blood pressure monitoring and healthy lifestyle behaviors. Toward this end, they did basic science research to determine the best place to intervene to change behavior at the community level. They identified barbershops as an ideal setting to implement lifestyle interventions because the barbershops are accessible, trusted, and frequently visited among non-Hispanic Black men living in urban environments. Initial intervention work employed community health workers to work with Black barbers to evaluate their patrons' blood pressure. In addition to regular blood pressure monitoring, numerous lifestyle interventions have been successfully implemented in collaboration with barbershop owners[212–214]to encourage good health behaviors to reduce risk. Other interventions that have been successfully implemented at this level of influence include group-based walking interventions that simultaneously promote social support for rural women.[215]

Proximal level of influence

In 2010, a diverse group of physicians developed a set of core competencies that physicians should know to have the skills and knowledge base necessary to provide lifestyle interventions. In 2015, the ACLM and the American College of Preventive Medicine worked together to develop a lifestyle medicine training program and lifestyle medicine certification process.[14,216,217] Updated in 2022, there are now eighty-eight competencies that fall within ten broad categories: general introduction to lifestyle medicine; role of practitioner's personal health and community outreach; nutrition science, assessment, and prescription; physical activity sciences, assessment, and prescription; sleep health science and interventions; treating tobacco use disorder and managing toxic exposures; clinical processes; fundamentals of behavior change; emotional and mental health assessment and interventions; and role of social connectedness and positive psychology.[218] Importantly, except for the section on practitioner's personal health and community advocacy, each section was developed so that physicians have the clinical knowledge and skills necessary to prescribe lifestyle interventions; accordingly, the content is designed to intervene at the proximal level of influence.[218]

Evidence-Based Intervention Skills and Approaches

A plethora of available manualized evidence-based treatment protocols have been shown to be efficacious in improving dietary choices, inactivity, substance abuse, disordered sleep, social connectedness, and levels of psychological stress. Most of these protocols target a single lifestyle factor and provide content and delivery instructions for the practitioner to follow to elicit long-term change. Typically, these manuals require the practitioner to meet with the patient multiple times in a predetermined time frame. For example, if we consider the fictitious provider-patient interaction, if Jack's physician wanted to focus solely on a single lifestyle pillar and meet with him multiple times over several weeks or months, she would be able to identify numerous evidence-based protocols.[219,220] These protocols would all have undergone rigorous clinical trials and were shown to be highly efficacious.[221] Even if Jack's physician had the time and compensation model necessary to deliver this type of intervention, it would be highly unlikely that she would be able to identify an evidence-based manual that explicitly addresses Jack's combination of lifestyle factors as many treatment manuals focus on a single health behavior or disorder.[218]

Transdiagnostic Approach

Transdiagnostic intervention approaches that address multiple health behaviors and social and affective processes using the same underlying treatment principles are well suited for lifestyle medicine practitioners.[222] These interventions target a common process or mechanism using the same intervention tools or approach when treating a range of maladaptive behaviors and clinical disorders (e.g., eating disorders, sleep disorders).[223,224] Transdiagnostic intervention approaches have both practical and functional utility for physicians that incorporate lifestyle medicine approaches into their practices.[225] A transdiagnostic intervention approaches better addresses heterogeneity than singularly focused interventions while also allowing for greater treatment flexibility when considering how a patient's relationship with one lifestyle pillar impacts their relationship with another pillar and vice versa.[222] By providing a common set of tools that can be implemented over variable lengths of time, this approach allows physicians to adopt an evidence-based approach to lifestyle interventions with the necessary flexibility to modify and tailor based on their patient needs, time constraints, and financial model.[222] In addition to the flexibility transdiagnostic intervention approaches provide, having one intervention approach that addresses multiple different lifestyle factors, transdiagnostic interventions also reduce the number of training protocols a lifestyle practitioner must master to provide evidence-based treatments.[226]

After assessing Jack's experiences and behavioral patterns since the death of his spouse, it has become abundantly clear to Jack's physician he is struggling with each pillar of lifestyle medicine. It is not practical for Jack's physician to provide or prescribe a different evidence-based intervention protocol to address each pillar. Even if Jack were receptive to such a time-intensive plan, there is evidence to suggest that targeting multiple health behaviors and social-psychological difficulties simultaneously may be more efficacious than targeting them separately.[227] Thus, Jack's physician has Jack engage in a series of online trainings and readings on the acceptance and commitment approach to mindfulness after explaining its basic principles and providing him handouts.[227] This transdiagnostic approach is one of many evidence-based approaches that have been shown to address multiple lifestyle pillars with the same tools.[228] This specific approach teaches people to focus on the present and nonjudgmentally accept thoughts and feelings rather than avoiding them.[229] By staying in the present moment, Jack should become aware of his triggers and habits, which will boost the likelihood he will engage in poor health behaviors (e.g., overeating) and avoid positive health behaviors.[230,231] (e.g., exercise). This approach has been shown to dramatically improve people's ability to manage stress and engage, rather than avoid, potentially positive experiences (e.g., social experiences).[228] Thus, the skills Jack learns from this approach should help Jack to accept the anxiety he feels when deciding to attend social events as a widower and attend anyway—ultimately strengthening his social connections.[232]

Future Directions and Conclusion

The behaviors, social connections, and emotions that characterize people's lives shape their quality of life and physical health. Given the importance of lifestyle factors for preventing and treating chronic health conditions, lifestyle medicine holds considerable potential in shaping the future of healthcare. For the field to thrive in the era of evidence-based medicine, educating practitioners on the importance of taking *lifestyle medicine vital signs* and knowing how each indicator impacts disease processes will be critical. In addition to teaching and using evidence-based practices, practitioners must understand how the lifestyle pillars connect and influence each other and recognize the unique ways these connections manifest in each patient. With this background, tailored evidence-based treatment plans can be prescribed that address each patient's unique combination of lifestyle challenges. It will be necessary for the future of the field to educate other fields and the general public about what evidence-based practices mean and how they differ from an ever-increasing number of non-research-based practices sold to the public. A seemingly endless number of books and courses have espoused non-evidence-based practices without any basis in science. For the public to be able to differentiate these materials from evidence-based practices, we must work to educate the public and other practitioners. This will require a multidisciplinary approach. Finally, we should not forget the importance of lifestyle practitioners adopting healthy lifestyle practices themselves given the high rates of stress and burnout associated with the helping professions. In closing, although lifestyle medicine as a field is relatively new, it has made considerable progress. Indeed, in its short history, it has created and revised guidelines and training and been the subject of numerous books and articles. Challenges are ahead for the discipline but the future is bright.

References

1. Smith DS. Differential mortality in the United States before 1900. *J Interdiscip Hist.* 1983;*13*:735–759.
2. Armstrong GL, Conn LA, Pinner RW. Trends in infectious disease mortality in the United States during the 20th century. *JAMA.* 1999;*281*:61–66. https://doi.org/10.1001/jama.281.1.61
3. Atella V, Piano Mortari A, Kopinska J, et al. Trends in age-related disease burden and health-care utilization. *Aging Cell.* 2019;*18*:e12861. https://doi.org/10.1111/acel.12861
4. Kusnanto H, Agustian D, Hilmanto D. Biopsychosocial model of illnesses in primary care: a hermeneutic literature review. *J Family Med Prim Care.* 2018;*7*:497–500. https://doi.org/10.4103/jfmpc.jfmpc_145_17
5. Johnson NB, Hayes LD, Brown K, Hoo EC, Ethier KA, Centers for Disease Control and Prevention (CDC). CDC National Health Report: leading causes of morbidity and mortality and associated behavioral risk and protective factors—United States, 2005–2013. *MMWR Suppl.* 2014;*63*:3–27.
6. McCarthy M. A brief history of the World Health Organization. *Lancet.* 2002;*360*:1111–1112. https://doi.org/10.1016/S0140-6736(02)11244-X
7. Cueto M, Brown T, Fee E. *The World Health Organization: A History.* Cambridge University Press; 2019.
8. Adler RH. Engel's biopsychosocial model is still relevant today. *J Psychosom Res.* 2009;*67*:607–611. https://doi.org/10.1016/j.jpsychores.2009.08.008
9. Adams KM, Kohlmeier M, Zeisel SH. Nutrition education in US medical schools: latest update of a national survey. *Acad Med.* 2010;*85*:1537–1542. https://doi.org/10.1097/ACM.0b013e3181eab71b
10. Mogre V, Stevens FCJ, Aryee PA, Amalba A, Scherpbier AJJA. Why nutrition education is inadequate in the medical curriculum: a qualitative study of students' perspectives on barriers and strategies. *BMC Med Educ.* 2018;*18*:26. https://doi.org/10.1186/s12909-018-1130-5
11. Crowley J, Ball L, Hiddink GJ. Nutrition in medical education: a systematic review. *Lancet Planet Health.* 2019;*3*:e379–e389. https://doi.org/10.1016/S2542-5196(19)30171-8
12. Rippe JM. *Lifestyle Medicine.* 3rd ed. Taylor & Francis; 2019. Accessed January 25, 2023. https://www.taylorfrancis.com/books/edit/10.1201/9781315201108/lifestyle-medicine-third-edition-james-rippe
13. Rippe JM, ed. *Lifestyle Medicine.* CRC Press; 1999.
14. Pere D. Building physician competency in lifestyle medicine: a model for health improvement. *Am J Prev Med.* 2017;*52*:260–261. https://doi.org/10.1016/j.amepre.2016.11.001
15. Benigas S. American College of Lifestyle Medicine: vision, tenacity, transformation. *Am J Lifestyle Med.* 2019;*14*:57–60. https://doi.org/10.1177/1559827619881094
16. American College of Lifestyle Medicine. *6 Pillars of Lifestyle Medicine.* American College of Lifestyle Medicine; n.d. Accessed January 18, 2023. https://lifestylemedicine.org/
17. Woolf SH, Schoomaker H. Life expectancy and mortality rates in the United States, 1959–2017. *JAMA.* 2019;*322*:1996–2016. https://doi.org/10.1001/jama.2019.16932
18. Vargas AJ, Schully SD, Villani J, Ganoza Caballero L, Murray DM. Assessment of prevention research measuring leading risk factors and causes of mortality and disability supported by the US National Institutes of Health. *JAMA Netw Open.* 2019;*2*:e1914718. https://doi.org/10.1001/jamanetworkopen.2019.14718

19. Picard M, McManus MJ, Gray JD, et al. Mitochondrial functions modulate neuroendocrine, metabolic, inflammatory, and transcriptional responses to acute psychological stress. *Proc Natl Acad Sci U S A*. 2015;*112*:E6614–E6623. https://doi.org/10.1073/pnas.1515733112

20. Kotas ME, Medzhitov R. Homeostasis, inflammation, and disease susceptibility. *Cell*. 2015;*160*:816–827.

21. Saha S, Shalova IN, Biswas SK. Metabolic regulation of macrophage phenotype and function. *Immunol Rev*. 2017;*280*:102–111. https://doi.org/10.1111/imr.12603

22. Miller AH, Raison CL. The role of inflammation in depression: from evolutionary imperative to modern treatment target. *Nat Rev Immunol*. 2016;*16*:22–34. https://doi.org/10.1038/nri.2015.5

23. Meisinger C, Koenig W, Baumert J, Döring A. Uric acid levels are associated with all-cause and cardiovascular disease mortality independent of systemic inflammation in men from the general population. *Arterioscler Thromb Vasc Biol*. 2008;*28*:1186–1192. https://doi.org/10.1161/ATVBAHA.107.160184

24. Bonora M, Wieckowski MR, Sinclair DA, Kroemer G, Pinton P, Galluzzi L. Targeting mitochondria for cardiovascular disorders: therapeutic potential and obstacles. *Nat Rev Cardiol*. 2019;*16*:33–55. https://doi.org/10.1038/s41569-018-0074-0

25. Chaudhary KR, El-Sikhry H, Seubert JM. Mitochondria and the aging heart. *J Geriatr Cardiol*. 2011;*8*:159–167. https://doi.org/10.3724/SP.J.1263.2011.00159

26. Cordeiro M, Scaglia F, Da Silva SL, et al. The brain-heart connection in mitochondrial respiratory chain diseases. *Neuroradiol J*. 2009;*22*:558–563. https://doi.org/10.1177/197140090902200508

27. World Health Organization. Obesity and overweight. n.d. Accessed January 18, 2023. https://www.who.int/news-room/fact-sheets/detail/obesity-and-overweight

28. Bray GA, Kim KK, Wilding JPH, World Obesity Federation. Obesity: a chronic relapsing progressive disease process. A position statement of the World Obesity Federation. *Obes Rev*. 2017;*18*:715–723. https://doi.org/10.1111/obr.12551

29. Centers for Disease Control and Prevention. Defining adult overweight and obesity. 2022. Accessed January 18, 2023. https://www.cdc.gov/obesity/basics/adult-defining.html

30. Fontaine KR, Redden DT, Wang C, Westfall AO, Allison DB. Years of life lost due to obesity. *JAMA*. 2003;*289*:187–193. https://doi.org/10.1001/jama.289.2.187

31. Dobbins M, Decorby K, Choi BCK. The association between obesity and cancer risk: a meta-analysis of observational studies from 1985 to 2011. *ISRN Prev Med*. 2013;*2013*:680536. https://doi.org/10.5402/2013/680536

32. Institute for Health Metrics and Evaluation, University of Washington. Global Burden of Disease Study 2015 (GBD 2015) obesity and overweight prevalence 1980–2015. *GHDx*. n.d. Accessed January 18, 2023. https://ghdx.healthdata.org/record/ihme-data/gbd-2015-obesity-and-overweight-prevalence-1980-2015

33. Lemmer IL, Willemsen N, Hilal N, Bartelt A. A guide to understanding endoplasmic reticulum stress in metabolic disorders. *Mol Metab*. 2021;*47*:101169. https://doi.org/10.1016/j.molmet.2021.101169

34. Leventhal H. Fear appeals and persuasion: the differentiation of a motivational construct. *Am J Public Health*. 1971;*61*:1208–1224.

35. van 't Riet J, Ruiter RAC. Defensive reactions to health-promoting information: an overview and implications for future research. *Health Psychol Rev*. 2013;*7*:S104–S136. https://doi.org/10.1080/17437199.2011.606782

36. Edgar T, Volkman JE. Using communication theory for health promotion: practical guidance on message design and strategy. *Health Promot Pract.* 2012;*13*:587–590. https://doi.org/10.1177/1524839912450879

37. O'Connor DB, Thayer JF, Vedhara K. Stress and health: a review of psychobiological processes. *Annu Rev Psychol.* 2021;*72*:663–688. https://doi.org/10.1146/annurev-psych-062520-122331

38. Schulz R, Beach SR. Caregiving as a risk factor for mortality: the caregiver health effects study. *JAMA.* 1999;*282*:2215–2219. https://doi.org/10.1001/jama.282.23.2215

39. Öhlin B, Nilsson PM, Nilsson J-Å, Berglund G. Chronic psychosocial stress predicts long-term cardiovascular morbidity and mortality in middle-aged men. *Eur Heart J.* 2004;*25*:867–873. https://doi.org/10.1016/j.ehj.2004.03.003

40. Caserta MS, Lund DA. Toward the development of an inventory of daily widowed life (IDWL): guided by the dual process model of coping with bereavement. *Death Stud.* 2007;*31*:505–535. https://doi.org/10.1080/07481180701356761

41. Hahn EA, Cichy KE, Small BJ, Almeida DM. Daily emotional and physical reactivity to stressors among widowed and married older adults. *J Gerontol B Psychol Sci Soc Sci.* 2014;*69B*:19–28. https://doi.org/10.1093/geronb/gbt035

42. Lund D, Caserta M, Utz R, de Vries B. Experiences and early coping of bereaved spouses/partners in an intervention based on the dual process model (DPM). *Omega (Westport).* 2010;*61*:291–313.

43. Baban KA. Lifestyle medicine and stress management. *J Family Pract.* 2022;*71*:S24–S29. https://doi.org/10.12788/jfp.0285

44. Cohen S, Janicki-Deverts D, Doyle WJ, et al. Chronic stress, glucocorticoid receptor resistance, inflammation, and disease risk. *Proc Natl Acad Sci U S A.* 2012;*109*:5995–5999. https://doi.org/10.1073/pnas.1118355109

45. Cohen S, Tyrrell DAJ, Smith AP. Psychological stress and susceptibility to the common cold. *N Engl J Med.* 1991;*325*:606–612. https://doi.org/10.1056/NEJM199108293250903

46. Fagundes CP, Glaser R, Hwang B, Malarkey WB, Kiecolt-Glaser JK. Depressive symptoms enhance stress-induced inflammatory responses. *Brain Behav Immun.* 2012;*26*:S35. https://doi.org/10.1016/j.bbi.2012.07.151

47. Jaremka LM, Fagundes CP, Peng J, et al. Loneliness promotes inflammation during acute stress. *Psychol Sci.* 2013;*24*:1089–1097. https://doi.org/10.1177/0956797612464059

48. Cacioppo JT, Burleson MH, Poehlmann KM, et al. Autonomic and neuroendocrine responses to mild psychological stressors: effects of chronic stress on older women. *Ann Behav Med.* 2000;*22*:140–148. https://doi.org/10.1007/BF02895778

49. Glaser R, Robles TF, Sheridan J, Malarkey WB, Kiecolt-Glaser JK. Mild depressive symptoms are associated with amplified and prolonged inflammatory responses after influenza virus vaccination in older adults. *Arch Gen Psychiatry.* 2003;*60*:1009–1104. https://doi.org/10.1001/archpsyc.60.10.1009

50. Fagundes CP, Glaser R, Povoski S, et al. Social support and socioeconomic status interact to predict Epstein-Barr virus latency in women awaiting diagnosis or newly diagnosed with breast cancer. *Health Psychol.* 2012;*31*:11–19. https://doi.org/10.1037/a0025599

51. Fagundes CP, Murdock KW, LeRoy A, Baameur F, Thayer JF, Heijnen C. Spousal bereavement is associated with more pronounced ex vivo cytokine production and lower heart rate variability: mechanisms underlying cardiovascular risk? *Psychoneuroendocrinology.* 2018;*93*:65–71. https://doi.org/10.1016/j.psyneuen.2018.04.010

52. Bower JE, Irwin MR. Mind–body therapies and control of inflammatory biology: a descriptive review. *Brain Behav Immun.* 2016;*51*:1–11. https://doi.org/10.1016/j.bbi.2015.06.012

53. Dossett ML, Fricchione GL, Benson H. A new era for mind–body medicine. *N Engl J Med.* 2020;*382*:1390–1391. https://doi.org/10.1056/NEJMp1917461

54. Furukawa TA, Suganuma A, Ostinelli EG, et al. Dismantling, optimising, and personalising internet cognitive behavioural therapy for depression: a systematic review and component network meta-analysis using individual participant data. *Lancet Psychiatry.* 2021;*8*:500–511. https://doi.org/10.1016/S2215-0366(21)00077-8

55. Lynch D, Laws KR, McKenna PJ. Cognitive behavioural therapy for major psychiatric disorder: does it really work? A meta-analytical review of well-controlled trials. *Psychol Med.* 2010;*40*:9–24. https://doi.org/10.1017/S003329170900590X

56. Cooney G, Dwan K, Mead G. Exercise for depression. *JAMA.* 2014;*311*:2432–2433. https://doi.org/10.1001/jama.2014.4930

57. Anderson E, Durstine JL. Physical activity, exercise, and chronic diseases: a brief review. *Sports Med Health Sci.* 2019;*1*:3–10. https://doi.org/10.1016/j.smhs.2019.08.006

58. Stults-Kolehmainen MA, Sinha R. The effects of stress on physical activity and exercise. *Sports Med.* 2014;*44*:81–121. https://doi.org/10.1007/s40279-013-0090-5

59. Mata J, Thompson RJ, Jaeggi SM, Buschkuehl M, Jonides J, Gotlib IH. Walk on the bright side: physical activity and affect in major depressive disorder. *J Abnorm Psychol.* 2012;*121*:297–308. https://doi.org/10.1037/a0023533.

60. Meyer JD, Koltyn KF, Stegner AJ, Kim J-S, Cook DB. Influence of exercise intensity for improving depressed mood in depression: a dose-response study. *Behav Ther.* 2016;*47*:527–537. https://doi.org/10.1016/j.beth.2016.04.003

61. Troiano RP, Berrigan D, Dodd KW, Mâsse LC, Tilert T, Mcdowell M. Physical activity in the United States measured by accelerometer. *Med Sci Sports Exerc.* 2008;*40*:181–188. https://doi.org/10.1249/mss.0b013e31815a51b3

62. Booth F, Roberts C, Thyfault J, Ruegsegger G, Toedebusch R. Role of inactivity in chronic diseases: evolutionary insight and pathophysiological mechanisms. *Physiol Rev.* 2017;*97*:1351–1402. https://doi.org/10.1152/physrev.00019.2016

63. Carlson SA, Fulton JE, Pratt M, Yang Z, Adams EK. Inadequate physical activity and health care expenditures in the United States. *Prog Cardiovasc Dis.* 2015;*57*:315–323. https://doi.org/10.1016/j.pcad.2014.08.002

64. Kraus WE, Powell KE, Haskell WL, et al. Physical activity, all-cause and cardiovascular mortality, and cardiovascular disease. *Med Sci Sports Exerc.* 2019;*51*:1270–1281. https://doi.org/10.1249/MSS.0000000000001939

65. Islami F, Goding Sauer A, Miller KD, et al. Proportion and number of cancer cases and deaths attributable to potentially modifiable risk factors in the United States. *CA Cancer J Clin.* 2018;*68*:31–54. https://doi.org/10.3322/caac.21440

66. Mortimer JA, Stern Y. Physical exercise and activity may be important in reducing dementia risk at any age. *Neurology.* 2019;*92*:362–363. https://doi.org/10.1212/WNL.0000000000006935.

67. Sandercock GRH, Bromley PD, Brodie DA. Effects of exercise on heart rate variability: inferences from meta-analysis. *Med Sci Sports Exerc.* 2005;*37*:433–439. https://doi.org/10.1249/01.mss.0000155388.39002.9d

68. Segerstrom SC, Nes LS. Heart rate variability reflects self-regulatory strength, effort, and fatigue. *Psychol Sci.* 2007;*18*:275–281. https://doi.org/10.1111/j.1467-9280.2007.01888.x

69. Thayer JF, Lane RD. A model of neurovisceral integration in emotion regulation and dysregulation. *J Affect Disord.* 2000;*61*:201–216. https://doi.org/10.1016/S0165-0327(00)00338-4

70. Appelhans BM, Luecken LJ. Heart rate variability as an index of regulated emotional responding. *Rev Gen Psychol.* 2006;*10*:229–240. https://doi.org/10.1037/1089-2680.10.3.229

71. Mccraty R, Shaffer F. Heart rate variability: new perspectives on physiological mechanisms, assessment of self-regulatory capacity, and health risk. *Global Adv Health Med.* 2015;*4*:46–61. https://doi.org/10.7453/gahmj.2014.073

72. Thayer JF, Sternberg EM. Neural aspects of immunomodulation: focus on the vagus nerve. *Brain Behav Immun.* 2010;*24*:1223–1228. https://doi.org/10.1016/j.bbi.2010.07.247

73. Thayer JF, Fischer JE. Heart rate variability, overnight urinary norepinephrine and C-reactive protein: evidence for the cholinergic anti-inflammatory pathway in healthy human adults. *J Intern Med.* 2009;*265*:439–447. https://doi.org/10.1111/j.1365-2796.2008.02023.x

74. Schroeder EB, Liao D, Chambless LE, Prineas RJ, Evans GW, Heiss G. Hypertension, blood pressure, and heart rate variability: the Atherosclerosis Risk in Communities (ARIC) study. *Hypertension.* 2003;*42*:1106–1111. https://doi.org/10.1161/01.HYP.0000100444.71069.73

75. Mäkikallio TH, Huikuri HV, Mäkikallio A, et al. Prediction of sudden cardiac death by fractal analysis of heart rate variability in elderly subjects. *J Am Coll Cardiol.* 2001;*37*:1395–1402. https://doi.org/10.1016/S0735-1097(01)01171-8

76. Singh JP, Larson MG, O'Donnell CJ, et al. Association of hyperglycemia with reduced heart rate variability (the Framingham Heart Study). *Am J Cardiol.* 2000;*86*:309–312. https://doi.org/10.1016/S0002-9149(00)00920-6

77. Tsuji H, Venditti FJ, Manders ES, et al. Reduced heart rate variability and mortality risk in an elderly cohort. The Framingham Heart Study. *Circulation.* 1994;*90*:878–883. https://doi.org/10.1161/01.CIR.90.2.878

78. Schultze-Florey CR, Martínez-Maza O, Magpantay L, et al. When grief makes you sick: Bereavement induced systemic inflammation is a question of genotype. *Brain Behav Immun.* 2012;*26*:1066–1071. https://doi.org/10.1016/j.bbi.2012.06.009

79. Cohen M, Granger S, Fuller-Thomson E. The association between bereavement and biomarkers of inflammation. *Behav Med.* 2015;*41*:49–59. https://doi.org/10.1080/08964289.2013.866539

80. Cankaya B, Chapman BP, Talbot NL, Moynihan J, Duberstein PR. History of sudden unexpected loss is associated with elevated interleukin-6 and decreased insulin-like growth factor-1 in women in an urban primary care setting. *Psychosom Med.* 2009;*71*:914–919. https://doi.org/10.1097/PSY.0b013e3181be7aa8

81. Zulfiqar U, Jurivich DA, Gao W, Singer DH. Relation of high heart rate variability to healthy longevity. *Am J Cardiol.* 2010;*105*:1181–1185. https://doi.org/10.1016/j.amjcard.2009.12.022

82. Almeida-Santos MA, Barreto-Filho JA, Oliveira JLM, Reis FP, da Cunha Oliveira CC, Sousa ACS. Aging, heart rate variability and patterns of autonomic regulation of the heart. *Arch Geronto Geriatr.* 2016;*63*:1–8. https://doi.org/10.1016/j.archger.2015.11.011

83. Antelmi I, De Paula RS, Shinzato AR, Peres CA, Mansur AJ, Grupi CJ. Influence of age, gender, body mass index, and functional capacity on heart rate variability in a cohort of subjects without heart disease. *Am J Cardiol.* 2004;*93*:381–385. https://doi.org/10.1016/j.amjcard.2003.09.065

84. Fagundes CP, Murray DM, Hwang BS, et al. Sympathetic and parasympathetic activity in cancer-related fatigue: more evidence for a physiological substrate in cancer survivors. *Psychoneuroendocrinology.* 2011;*36*:1137–1147. https://doi.org/10.1016/j.psyneuen.2011.02.005

85. Kim DH, Lipsitz LA, Ferrucci L, et al. Association between reduced heart rate variability and cognitive impairment in older disabled women in the community: women's health and aging study I. *J Am Geriatr Soc.* 2006;*54*:1751–1757. https://doi.org/10.1111/j.1532-5415.2006.00940.x

86. Thayer JF, Sternberg E. Beyond heart rate variability: vagal regulation of allostatic systems. *Ann N Y Acad Sci.* 2006;*1088*:361–372. https://doi.org/10.1196/annals.1366.014

87. Reardon M, Malik M. Changes in heart rate variability with age. *Pacing Clin Electrophysiol.* 1996;*19*:1863–1866. https://doi.org/10.1111/j.1540-8159.1996.tb03241.x

88. Williams DP, Koenig J, Carnevali L, et al. Heart rate variability and inflammation: a meta-analysis of human studies. *Brain Behav Immun.* 2019;*80*:219–226. https://doi.org/10.1016/j.bbi.2019.03.009

89. Cooper TM, McKinley PS, Seeman TE, Choo T-H, Lee S, Sloan RP. Heart rate variability predicts levels of inflammatory markers: evidence for the vagal anti-inflammatory pathway. *Brain Behav Immun.* 2015;*49*:94–100. https://doi.org/10.1016/j.bbi.2014.12.017

90. Huston JM, Tracey KJ. The pulse of inflammation: heart rate variability, the cholinergic anti-inflammatory pathway and implications for therapy. *J Intern Med.* 2011;*269*:45–53. https://doi.org/10.1111/j.1365-2796.2010.02321.x

91. Lavie CJ, Ozemek C, Carbone S, Katzmarzyk PT, Blair SN. Sedentary behavior, exercise, and cardiovascular health. *Circ Res.* 2019;*124*:799–815. https://doi.org/10.1161/CIRCRESAHA.118.312669

92. Marzetti E, Calvani R, Tosato M, et al. Sarcopenia: an overview. *Aging Clin Exp Res.* 2017;*29*:11–17. https://doi.org/10.1007/s40520-016-0704-5

93. Executive summary of the clinical guidelines on the identification, evaluation, and treatment of overweight and obesity in adults. *Arch Intern Med.* 1998;*158*:1855–1867. https://doi.org/10.1001/archinte.158.17.1855

94. Bowden Davies KA, Sprung VS, Norman JA, et al. Short-term decreased physical activity with increased sedentary behaviour causes metabolic derangements and altered body composition: effects in individuals with and without a first-degree relative with type 2 diabetes. *Diabetologia.* 2018;*61*:1282–1294. https://doi.org/10.1007/s00125-018-4603-5

95. Dixon NC, Hurst TL, Talbot DCS, Tyrrell RM, Thompson D. Effect of short-term reduced physical activity on cardiovascular risk factors in active lean and overweight middle-aged men. *Metabolism.* 2013;*62*:361–368. https://doi.org/10.1016/j.metabol.2012.08.006

96. Bowden Davies KA, Sprung VS, Norman JA, et al. Physical activity and sedentary time: association with metabolic health and liver fat. *Med Sci Sports Exerc.* 2019;*51*:1169–1177. https://doi.org/10.1249/MSS.0000000000001901

97. US Department of Health and Human Services. Physical activity guidelines for Americans. 2nd ed. https://Health.Gov/Paguidelines/Second-Edition/Pdf/Physical_Activity_Guidelines_2nd_edition.Pdf. n.d. Accessed August 30, 2022.

98. Chekroud SR, Gueorguieva R, Zheutlin AB, Paulus M, Krumholz HM, Krystal JH, et al. Association between physical exercise and mental health in 1·2 million individuals in the USA between 2011 and 2015: a cross-sectional study. *Lancet Psychiatry* 2018;*5*:739–46. https://doi.org/10.1016/S2215-0366(18)30227-X.

99. Schuch FB, Vancampfort D, Firth J, et al. Physical activity and incident depression: a meta-analysis of prospective cohort studies. *Am J Psychiatry.* 2018;*175*:631–648. https://doi.org/10.1176/appi.ajp.2018.17111194

100. McDowell CP, Dishman RK, Gordon BR, Herring MP. Physical activity and anxiety: a systematic review and meta-analysis of prospective cohort studies. *Am J Prev Med.* 2019;*57*:545–556. https://doi.org/10.1016/j.amepre.2019.05.012

101. Masferrer L, Garre-Olmo J, Caparrós B. Is complicated grief a risk factor for substance use? A comparison of substance-users and normative grievers. *Addict Res Theory.* 2017;*25*:361–367. https://doi.org/10.1080/16066359.2017.1285912

102. Parisi A, Sharma A, Howard MO, Blank Wilson A. The relationship between substance misuse and complicated grief: a systematic review. *J Subst Abuse Treat.* 2019;*103*:43–57. https://doi.org/10.1016/j.jsat.2019.05.012

103. Angres DH, Bettinardi-Angres K. The disease of addiction: origins, treatment, and recovery. *Dis Mon.* 2008;*54*:696–721. https://doi.org/10.1016/j.disamonth.2008.07.002

104. Bagnardi V, Rota M, Botteri E, et al. Alcohol consumption and site-specific cancer risk: a comprehensive dose–response meta-analysis. *Br J Cancer.* 2015;*112*:580–593. https://doi.org/10.1038/bjc.2014.579

105. National Institute on Drug Abuse. Addiction and health. n.d. Accessed January 18, 2023. https://nida.nih.gov/publications/drugs-brains-behavior-science-addiction/addiction-health

106. Bahorik AL, Satre DD, Kline-Simon AH, Weisner CM, Campbell CI. Alcohol, cannabis, and opioid use disorders, and disease burden in an integrated health care system. *J Addict Med.* 2017;*11*:3–9. https://doi.org/10.1097/ADM.0000000000000260

107. Friedman H, Pross S, Klein TW. Addictive drugs and their relationship with infectious diseases. *FEMS Immunol Med Microbiol.* 2006;*47*:330–342. https://doi.org/10.1111/j.1574-695X.2006.00097.x

108. National Institute on Drug Abuse. Drug use and viral infections (HIV, hepatitis) drug facts. 2020. Accessed January 18, 2023. https://nida.nih.gov/research-topics/hiv

109. Friedman H, Newton C, Klein TW. Microbial infections, immunomodulation, and drugs of abuse. *Clin Microbiol Rev.* 2003;*16*:209–219. https://doi.org/10.1128/CMR.16.2.209-219.2003.

110. Centers for Disease Control and Prevention. CDC grand rounds: prescription drug overdoses—a US epidemic. 2012. Accessed January 18, 2023. https://www.cdc.gov/mmwr/preview/mmwrhtml/mm6101a3.htm

111. Hedegaard H, Miniño AM, Spencer MR, Warner M. *Drug Overdose Deaths in the United States, 1999–2020.* National Center for Health Statistics; 2021. NCHS data brief no. 428. https://doi.org/10.15620/cdc:112340

112. Urbanoski KA, Kelly JF. Understanding genetic risk for substance use and addiction: a guide for non-geneticists. *Clin Psychol Rev.* 2012;*32*:60–70. https://doi.org/10.1016/j.cpr.2011.11.002

113. Hatoum AS, Johnson EC, Colbert SMC, et al. The addiction risk factor: a unitary genetic vulnerability characterizes substance use disorders and their associations with common correlates. *Neuropsychopharmacology.* 2022;*47*:1739–1745. https://doi.org/10.1038/s41386-021-01209-w

114. Agrawal A, Lynskey MT. The genetic epidemiology of cannabis use, abuse and dependence. *Addiction.* 2006;*101*:801–812. https://doi.org/10.1111/j.1360-0443.2006.01399.x

115. Agrawal A, Lynskey MT. Are there genetic influences on addiction: evidence from family, adoption and twin studies. *Addiction.* 2008;*103*:1069–1081. https://doi.org/10.1111/j.1360-0443.2008.02213.x

116. Tsuang MT, Bar JL, Harley RM, Lyons MJ. The Harvard Twin Study of Substance Abuse: what we have learned. *Harv Rev Psychiatry.* 2001;9:267–279.

117. Lin S-Y, Fried EI, Eaton NR. The association of life stress with substance use symptoms: a network analysis and replication. *J Abnorm Psychol.* 2020;*129*:204–214. https://doi.org/10.1037/abn0000485

118. Boden JM, Fergusson DM. Alcohol and depression. *Addiction.* 2011;*106*:906–914. https://doi.org/10.1111/j.1360-0443.2010.03351.x

119. Enoch M-A. The role of early life stress as a predictor for alcohol and drug dependence. *Psychopharmacology (Berl).* 2011;*214*:17–31. https://doi.org/10.1007/s00213-010-1916-6

120. Oshri A, Sutton TE, Clay-Warner J, Miller JD. Child maltreatment types and risk behaviors: associations with attachment style and emotion regulation dimensions. *Pers Individ Dif.* 2015;*73*:127–133. https://doi.org/10.1016/j.paid.2014.09.015

121. Fletcher K, Nutton J, Brend D. Attachment, a matter of substance: the potential of attachment theory in the treatment of addictions. *Clin Soc Work J.* 2015;*43*:109–117. https://doi.org/10.1007/s10615-014-0502-5

122. Wyrzykowska E, Głogowska K, Mickiewicz K. Attachment relationships among alcohol dependent persons. *Alcohol Drug Addict.* 2014;*27*:145–161. https://doi.org/10.1016/S0867-4361(14)70010-0

123. Ralevski E, Petrakis I, Altemus M. Heart rate variability in alcohol use: a review. *Pharmacol Biochem Behav.* 2019;*176*:83–92. https://doi.org/10.1016/j.pbb.2018.12.003

124. Jang K-I, Shim M, Lee SM, et al. Increased beta power in the bereaved families of the Sewol ferry disaster: a paradoxical compensatory phenomenon? A two-channel electroencephalography study. *Psychiatry Clin Neurosci.* 2017;*71*:759–768. https://doi.org/10.1111/pcn.12546

125. Hardison HG, Neimeyer RA, Lichstein KL. Insomnia and complicated grief symptoms in bereaved college students. *Behav Sleep Med.* 2005;*3*:99–111. https://doi.org/10.1207/s15402010bsm0302_4

126. Eidelman P, Gershon A, McGlinchey E, Harvey AG. Sleep and psychopathology. In: Charles M. Morin and Colin A. Espie, eds. *The Oxford Handbook of Sleep and Sleep Disorders.* Oxford University Press; 2012:172–189.

127. Azza Y, Wilhelm I, Kleim B. Sleep early after trauma: a target for prevention and early intervention for posttraumatic stress disorder? *Eur Psychol.* 2020;*25*:239–251. https://doi.org/10.1027/1016-9040/a000401

128. Kronholm E, Laatikainen T, Peltonen M, Sippola R, Partonen T. Self-reported sleep duration, all-cause mortality, cardiovascular mortality and morbidity in Finland. *Sleep Med.* 2011;*12*:215–221. https://doi.org/10.1016/j.sleep.2010.07.021

129. Young T, Finn L, Peppard PE, et al. Sleep disordered breathing and mortality: eighteen-year follow-up of the Wisconsin Sleep Cohort. *Sleep.* 2008;*31*:1071–1078. https://doi.org/10.5665/sleep/31.8.1071

130. Korkalainen H, Töyräs J, Nikkonen S, Leppänen T. Mortality-risk-based apnea–hypopnea index thresholds for diagnostics of obstructive sleep apnea. *J Sleep Res.* 2019;*28*:e12855. https://doi.org/10.1111/jsr.12855

131. Redline S, Berger NA, eds. *Impact of Sleep and Sleep Disturbances on Obesity and Cancer.* Springer; 2014.

132. Cash RE, Crowe RP, Goldberg SA, et al. Association between sleep characteristics, ideal cardiovascular health, and systemic inflammation, NHANES 2017–2018. *J Sleep Res.* 2022;*31*:e13497. https://doi.org/10.1111/jsr.13497

133. Chaput J-P, McHill AW, Cox RC, et al. The role of insufficient sleep and circadian misalignment in obesity. *Nat Rev Endocrinol.* 2023;*19*:82–97. https://doi.org/10.1038/s41574-022-00747-7

134. Buxton OM, Cain SW, O'Connor SP, et al. Adverse metabolic consequences in humans of prolonged sleep restriction combined with circadian disruption. *Sci Transl Med.* 2012;*4*:129–143. https://doi.org/10.1126/scitranslmed.3003200

135. Morris CJ, Aeschbach D, Scheer FAJL. Circadian system, sleep and endocrinology. *Mol Cell Endocrinol.* 2012;*349*:91–104. https://doi.org/10.1016/j.mce.2011.09.003

136. Sequeira VCC, Bandeira PM, Azevedo JCM. Heart rate variability in adults with obstructive sleep apnea: a systematic review. *Sleep Sci.* 2019;*12*:214–221. https://doi.org/10.5935/1984-0063.20190082

137. Irwin MR. Sleep and inflammation: partners in sickness and in health. *Nat Rev Immunol.* 2019;*19*:702–715. https://doi.org/10.1038/s41577-019-0190-z

138. Travis RC, Balkwill A, Fensom GK, et al. Night shift work and breast cancer incidence: three prospective studies and meta-analysis of published studies. *J Natl Cancer Inst.* 2016;*108*:djw169. https://doi.org/10.1093/jnci/djw169

139. Truong T, Liquet B, Menegaux F, et al. Breast cancer risk, nightwork, and circadian clock gene polymorphisms. *Endocr Relat Cancer.* 2014;*21*:629–638. https://doi.org/10.1530/ERC-14-0121

140. Deng T, Lyon CJ, Bergin S, Caligiuri MA, Hsueh WA. Obesity, inflammation, and cancer. *Annu Rev Pathol.* 2016;*11*:421–449. https://doi.org/10.1146/annurev-pathol-012615-044359

141. Dimitrov S, Lange T, Tieken S, Fehm HL, Born J. Sleep associated regulation of T helper 1/T helper 2 cytokine balance in humans. *Brain Behav Immun.* 2004;*18*:341–348. https://doi.org/10.1016/j.bbi.2003.08.004

142. Fagundes CP, Murdock KW, Chirinos DA, Green PA. Biobehavioral pathways to cancer incidence, progression, and quality of life. *Curr Dir Psychol Sci.* 2017;*26*:548–553. https://doi.org/10.1177/0963721417720958

143. Chaput J-P, Dutil C, Sampasa-Kanyinga H. Sleeping hours: what is the ideal number and how does age impact this? *Nat Sci Sleep.* 2018;*10*:421–430. https://doi.org/10.2147/NSS.S163071

144. Bauman AE, Sallis JF, Dzewaltowski DA, Owen N. Toward a better understanding of the influences on physical activity: the role of determinants, correlates, causal variables, mediators, moderators, and confounders. *Am J Prev Med.* 2002;*23*:5–14. https://doi.org/10.1016/S0749-3797(02)00469-5

145. Anderson PL, Price M, Edwards SM, et al. Virtual reality exposure therapy for social anxiety disorder: a randomized controlled trial. *J Consult Clin Psychol.* 2013;*81*:751–760. https://doi.org/10.1037/a0033559

146. Levinson CA, Rodebaugh TL, Menatti AR, Weeks JW. Development and validation of the Social Exercise and Anxiety Measure (SEAM): assessing fears, avoidance, and importance of social exercise. *J Psychopathol Behav Assess.* 2013;*35*:244–253. https://doi.org/10.1007/s10862-012-9326-1

147. Luo Y, Hawkley LC, Waite LJ, Cacioppo JT. Loneliness, health, and mortality in old age: a national longitudinal study. *Soc Sci Med.* 2012;*74*:907–914. https://doi.org/10.1016/j.socscimed.2011.11.028

148. Hawkley LC, Cacioppo JT. Loneliness matters: a theoretical and empirical review of consequences and mechanisms. *Ann Behav Med.* 2010;*40*:218–227. https://doi.org/10.1007/s12160-010-9210-8

149. Yang YC, McClintock MK, Kozloski M, Li T. Social isolation and adult mortality: the role of chronic inflammation and sex differences. *J Health Soc Behav.* 2013;*54*:183–203. https://doi.org/10.1177/0022146513485244

150. Cacioppo JT, Cacioppo S, Capitanio JP, Cole SW. The neuroendocrinology of social isolation. *Annu Rev Psychol.* 2015;*66*:733–67.

151. Killam K. To combat loneliness, promote social health. *Scientific American.* January 23, 2018. Accessed January 25, 2023. https://www.scientificamerican.com/article/to-combat-loneliness-promote-social-health1/

152. Feller SC, Castillo EG, Greenberg JM, et al. Emotional well-being and public health: proposal for a model national initiative. *Public Health Rep.* 2018;*133*:136–141. https://doi.org/10.1177/0033354918754540

153. O'Sullivan R, Leavey G, Lawlor B. We need a public health approach to loneliness. *BMJ.* 2022;*376*:o280. https://doi.org/10.1136/bmj.o280

154. US Surgeon General. Our epidemic of loneliness and isolation. 2023. https://www.hhs.gov/sites/default/files/surgeon-general-social-connection-advisory.pdf

155. Cacioppo JT, Hawkley LC, Ernst JM, et al. Loneliness within a nomological net: an evolutionary perspective. *J Res Pers.* 2006;*40*:1054–1085. https://doi.org/10.1016/j.jrp.2005.11.007

156. Wilson C, Moulton B. *Loneliness Among Older Adults: A National Survey of Adults 45+.* AARP; 2010.

157. Cacioppo JT, Cacioppo S. Social relationships and health: the toxic effects of perceived social isolation. *Soc Personal Psychol Compass.* 2014;*8*:58–72. https://doi.org/10.1111/spc3.12087

158. Cacioppo S, Capitanio JP, Cacioppo JT. Toward a neurology of loneliness. *Psychol Bull.* 2014;*140*:1464–1504. https://doi.org/10.1037/a0037618

159. Holt-Lunstad J, Perissinotto C. Social isolation and loneliness as medical issues. *N Engl J Med.* 2023;*388*(3):193–195.

160. Kayaoğlu K, Okanlı A, Budak FK, Aslanoğlu E. The correlation between loneliness and substance use proclivity in child and adolescent substance users. *J Subst Use.* 2022;*27*:70–73. https://doi.org/10.1080/14659891.2021.1894495

161. Mannes ZL, Burrell LE, Bryant VE, Dunne EM, Hearn LE, Whitehead NE. Loneliness and substance use: the influence of gender among HIV+ Black/African American adults 50+. *AIDS Care.* 2016;*28*:598–602. https://doi.org/10.1080/09540121.2015.1120269

162. Holt-Lunstad J, Smith TB, Layton JB. Social relationships and mortality risk: a meta-analytic review. *PLoS Med.* 2010;*7*:e1000316. https://doi.org/10.1371/journal.pmed.1000316

163. Holt-Lunstad R, Smith TB, Baker M, Harris T, Stephenson D. Loneliness and social isolation as risk factors for mortality: a meta-analytic review. *Persp Psychol Sci.* 2015;*10*:227–237. Accessed January 29, 2023. https://journals.sagepub.com/doi/abs/10.1177/1745691614568352?journalCode=ppsa

164. Wilson SJ, Woody A, Padin AC, Lin J, Malarkey WB, Kiecolt-Glaser JK. Loneliness and telomere length: immune and parasympathetic function in associations with accelerated aging. *Ann Behav Med.* 2019;*53*:541–550. https://doi.org/10.1093/abm/kay064

165. Liu H, Zhang Z, Zhang Y. A national longitudinal study of marital quality and cognitive decline among older men and women. *Soc Sci Med.* 2021;*282*:114151. https://doi.org/10.1016/j.socscimed.2021.114151

166. Robles TF. Marital quality and health: implications for marriage in the 21st century. *Curr Dir Psychol Sci.* 2014;*23*:427–432. https://doi.org/10.1177/0963721414549043

167. Robles TF, Kiecolt-Glaser JK. The physiology of marriage: pathways to health. *Physiol Behav.* 2003;*79*:409–416. https://doi.org/10.1016/S0031-9384(03)00160-4

168. Robles TF. Marital quality and health: a meta-analytic review. *Psychol Bull.* 2014;*140*:140. https://doi.org/10.1037/a0031859

169. Kiecolt-Glaser JK. Stress, personal relationships, and immune function: health implications. *Brain Behav Immun.* 1999;*13*:61–72. https://doi.org/10.1006/brbi.1999.0552

170. Kiecolt-Glaser JK, Loving TJ, Stowell JR, et al. Hostile marital interactions, proinflammatory cytokine production, and wound healing. *Arch Gen Psychiatry.* 2005;*62*:1377–1384. https://doi.org/10.1001/archpsyc.62.12.1377

171. Graham JE, Glaser R, Loving TJ, Malarkey WB, Stowell JR, Kiecolt-Glaser JK. Cognitive word use during marital conflict and increases in proinflammatory cytokines. *Health Psychol.* 2009;*28*:621–630. https://doi.org/10.1037/a0015208

172. Troisi JD, Gabriel S. Chicken soup really is good for the soul: "comfort food" fulfills the need to belong. *Psychol Sci.* 2011;*22*:747–753. https://doi.org/10.1177/0956797611407931

173. Kiecolt-Glaser JK, Jaremka L, Andridge R, et al. Marital discord, past depression, and metabolic responses to high-fat meals: interpersonal pathways to obesity. *Psychoneuroendocrinology.* 2015;*52*:239–250. https://doi.org/10.1016/j.psyneuen.2014.11.018

174. Appelhans BM, Whited MC, Schneider KL, et al. Depression severity, diet quality, and physical activity in women with obesity and depression. *J Acad Nutr Diet.* 2012;*112*:693–698. https://doi.org/10.1016/j.jand.2012.02.006

175. Williams L. Turning down the nachos (aka managing grief and comfort eating). What's Your Grief? 2014. Accessed December 9, 2020. https://whatsyourgrief.com/managing-grief-and-comfort-eating/).

176. Cericola L. Our most comforting recipes in times of sorrow. *Southern Living.* 2017. Accessed December 9, 2020. https://www.southernliving.com/home-cooked-meals-comfort-food-grief-sorrow

177. Lyons L. Grief, depression & comfort eating: a common combination. Eating Disorder Hope. 2018. Accessed June 17, 2024. https://www.eatingdisorderhope.com/blog/grief-depression-comfort-eating

178. O'Brien S. A guide to the world's most comforting foods of grief. Atlas Obscura. 2020. Accessed December 9, 2020. http://www.atlasobscura.com/articles/funeral-foods-around-the-world

179. Van Der Meer E. This is how different cultures grieve with food. *HuffPost.* 2019. Accessed December 9, 2020. https://www.huffpost.com/entry/grieving-with-food_l_5c646722e4b0084c78e25df8

180. Kolb L. A widow's food guide to grief. *Washington Post.* March 27, 2018.

181. Oudenhove LV, McKie S, Lassman D, et al. Fatty acid–induced gut-brain signaling attenuates neural and behavioral effects of sad emotion in humans. *J Clin Investig.* 2011;*121*:3094–3099. https://doi.org/10.1172/JCI46380

182. Esmaillzadeh A, Kimiagar M, Mehrabi Y, Azadbakht L, Hu FB, Willett WC. Dietary patterns, insulin resistance, and prevalence of the metabolic syndrome in women. *Am J Clin Nutr.* 2007;*85*:910–918. https://doi.org/10.1093/ajcn/85.3.910

183. Lairon D, Lopez-Miranda J, Williams C. Methodology for studying postprandial lipid metabolism. *Eur J Clin Nutr.* 2007;*61*:1145–1161. https://doi.org/10.1038/sj.ejcn.1602749

184. Ting HJ, Stice JP, Schaff UY, et al. Triglyceride-rich lipoproteins prime aortic endothelium for an enhanced inflammatory response to tumor necrosis factor-α. *Circ Res.* 2007;*100*:381–390. https://doi.org/10.1161/01.RES.0000258023.76515.a3.

185. Baragetti A, Zampoleri V, Grigore L, et al. Triglycerides rich lipoproteins elicit cellular and endothelial inflammation. *Atherosclerosis.* 2019;*287*:e61. https://doi.org/10.1016/j.atherosclerosis.2019.06.173

186. Rodríguez-Carrio J, Alperi-López M, López P, et al. High triglycerides and low high-density lipoprotein cholesterol lipid profile in rheumatoid arthritis: a potential link among inflammation, oxidative status, and dysfunctional high-density lipoprotein. *J Clin Lipidol.* 2017;*11*:1043–1054.e2. https://doi.org/10.1016/j.jacl.2017.05.009

187. Mora S, Rifai N, Buring JE, Ridker PM. Fasting compared with nonfasting lipids and apolipoproteins for predicting incident cardiovascular events. *Circulation.* 2008;*118*:993–1001. https://doi.org/10.1161/CIRCULATIONAHA.108.777334

188. Stalenhoef AF, de Graaf J. Association of fasting and nonfasting serum triglycerides with cardiovascular disease and the role of remnant-like lipoproteins and small dense LDL. *Curr Opin Lipidol.* 2008;*19*:355–361. https://doi.org/10.1097/MOL.0b013e328304b63c

189. Freiberg JJ. Nonfasting triglycerides and risk of ischemic stroke in the general population. *JAMA.* 2008;*300*:2142. https://doi.org/10.1001/jama.2008.621

190. Patsch JR, Miesenböck G, Hopferwieser T, et al. Relation of triglyceride metabolism and coronary artery disease. Studies in the postprandial state. *Arterioscler Thromb.* 1992;*12*:1336–1345. https://doi.org/10.1161/01.ATV.12.11.1336

191. Iwagami M, Qizilbash N, Gregson J, et al. Blood cholesterol and risk of dementia in more than 1.8 million people over two decades: a retrospective cohort study. *Lancet Healthy Longev.* 2021;*2*:e498–e506. https://doi.org/10.1016/S2666-7568(21)00150-1

192. Dimache AM, Şalaru DL, Sascău R, Stătescu C. The role of high triglycerides level in predicting cognitive impairment: a review of current evidence. *Nutrients.* 2021;*13*:2118. https://doi.org/10.3390/nu13062118

193. Parthasarathy V, Frazier DT, Bettcher BM, et al. Triglycerides are negatively correlated with cognitive function in nondemented aging adults. *Neuropsychology.* 2017;*31*:682–688. https://doi.org/10.1037/neu0000335

194. Anstey KJ, Ashby-Mitchell K, Peters R. Updating the evidence on the association between serum cholesterol and risk of late-life dementia: review and meta-analysis. *J Alzheimers Dis.* 2017;*56*:215–228. https://doi.org/10.3233/JAD-160826

195. Feinkohl I, Janke J, Hadzidiakos D, et al. Associations of the metabolic syndrome and its components with cognitive impairment in older adults. *BMC Geriatr.* 2019;*19*:77. https://doi.org/10.1186/s12877-019-1073-7

196. He Q, Li Q, Zhao J, et al. Relationship between plasma lipids and mild cognitive impairment in the elderly Chinese: a case-control study. *Lipids Health Dis.* 2016;*15*:146. https://doi.org/10.1186/s12944-016-0320-6

197. Ouwens DM, Boer C, Fodor M, et al. Cardiac dysfunction induced by high-fat diet is associated with altered myocardial insulin signalling in rats. *Diabetologia.* 2005;*48*:1229–1237. http://dx.doi.org.ezproxy.rice.edu/10.1007/s00125-005-1755-x

198. Chiu GS, Maj MA, Rizvi S, et al. Pifithrin-μ prevents cisplatin-induced chemobrain by preserving neuronal mitochondrial function. *Cancer Res.* 2017;*77*:742–752. https://doi.org/10.1158/0008-5472.CAN-16-1817

199. Alberca RW, Oliveira LDM, Branco ACCC, Pereira NZ, Sato MN.Obesity as a risk factor for COVID-19: an overview. *Crit Rev Food Sci Nutr.* 2021;*61*(13):2262–2276.

200. US Department of Agriculture and US National Institutes of Health. *Dietary Guidelines for Americans, 2020–2025.* 9th ed. 2020. Accessed January 18, 2023. https://www.dietaryguidelines.gov/resources/2020-2025-dietary-guidelines-online-materials

201. Kiecolt-Glaser JK, Habash DL, Fagundes CP, et al. Daily stressors, past depression, and metabolic responses to high-fat meals: a novel path to obesity. *Biol Psychiatry.* 2015;*77*:653–660. https://doi.org/10.1016/j.biopsych.2014.05.018

202. Stoney CM, West S. Lipids, personality, and stress: mechanisms and modulators. In: Hillbrand M, Spitz RT, eds. *Lipids, Health, and Behavior.* American Psychological Association; 1997:47–66.

203. Le Fur C, Romon M, Lebel P, et al. Influence of mental stress and circadian cycle on postprandial lipemia. *Am J Clin Nutr.* 1999;*70*:213–220. https://doi.org/10.1093/ajcn.70.2.213

204. Stoney CM, West SG, Hughes JW, et al. Acute psychological stress reduces plasma triglyceride clearance. *Psychophysiology.* 2002;*39*:80–85.

205. Erridge C, Attina T, Spickett CM, Webb DJ. A high-fat meal induces low-grade endotoxemia: evidence of a novel mechanism of postprandial inflammation. *Am J Clin Nutr.* 2007;*86*:1286–1292. https://doi.org/10.1093/ajcn/86.5.1286

206. López-Moreno J, García-Carpintero S, Jimenez-Lucena R, et al. Effect of dietary lipids on endotoxemia influences postprandial inflammatory response. 2017;*65*:7756–7763. https://doi.org/10.1021/acs.jafc.7b01909

207. Blonstein AC, Yank V, Stafford RS, Wilson SR, Rosas LG, Ma J. Translating an evidence-based lifestyle intervention program into primary care: lessons learned. *Health Promot Pract.* 2013;*14*:491–497. https://doi.org/10.1177/1524839913481604

208. Onken LS, Carroll KM, Shoham V, Cuthbert BN, Riddle M. Reenvisioning clinical science: unifying the discipline to improve the public health. *Clin Psychol Sci.* 2014;*2*:22–34. https://doi.org/10.1177/2167702613497932

209. Golden SD, McLeroy KR, Green LW, Earp JAL, Lieberman LD. Upending the social ecological model to guide health promotion efforts toward policy and environmental change. *Health Educ Behav.* 2015;*42*:8S–14S. https://doi.org/10.1177/1090198115575098

210. Terry PE. A rose is a rose is a rose: reviewing definitions for and reimbursement for health promotion, lifestyle medicine, behavioral medicine, preventive medicine and population health. *Am J Health Promot.* 2022;*36*:1077–1082. https://doi.org/10.1177/08901171221106666

211. Bedimo-Rung AL, Mowen AJ, Cohen DA. The significance of parks to physical activity and public health: a conceptual model. *Am J Prev Med.* 2005;*28*:159–168. https://doi.org/10.1016/j.amepre.2004.10.024

212. Victor RG, Lynch K, Li N, et al. A cluster-randomized trial of blood-pressure reduction in black barbershops. *N Engl J Med.* 2018;*378*:1291–1301. https://doi.org/10.1056/NEJMoa1717250

213. Ferdinand KC, Graham RM. Uncontrolled hypertension in Black men. *Circulation.* 2019;*139*:20–23. https://doi.org/10.1161/CIRCULATIONAHA.118.038240

214. Saunders E. Hypertension in minorities: Blacks. *Am J Hypertens.* 1995;*8*:115S–119S. https://doi.org/10.1016/0895-7061(95)00309-6

215. Perry CK, Rosenfeld AG, Bennett JA, Potempa K. Heart-to-heart: promoting walking in rural women through motivational interviewing and group support. *J Cardiovasc Nurs.* 2007;*22*:304–312. https://doi.org/10.1097/01.JCN.0000278953.67630.e3

216. Lianov L, Rosenfeld R. The case for physician training and certification in lifestyle medicine. *Am J Lifestyle Med.* 2022;17(2):326–330. doi:10.1177/15598276221138087. PMID: 36896033; PMCID: PMC9989487.

217. Jani AA, Trask J, Ali A. Integrative medicine in preventive medicine education: competency and curriculum development for preventive medicine and other specialty residency programs. *Am J Prev Med.* 2015;*49*:S222–S229. https://doi.org/10.1016/j.amepre.2015.08.019

218. Lianov LS, Adamson K, Kelly JH, Matthews S, Palma M, Rea BL. Lifestyle medicine core competencies: 2022 update. *Am J Lifestyle Med.* 2022;*16*:734–739. https://doi.org/10.1177/15598276221121580

219. Lorencatto F, West R, Christopherson C, Michie S. Assessing fidelity of delivery of smoking cessation behavioural support in practice. *Implement Sci.* 2013;*8*:40. https://doi.org/10.1186/1748-5908-8-40.

220. Brownson RC, Baker EA, Deshpande AD, Gillespie KN. *Evidence-Based Public Health.* 3rd ed, Oxford University Press; 2017.

221. Friedman LM, Furberg CD, DeMets DL, Reboussin DM, Granger CB. *Fundamentals of Clinical Trials.* Springer International Publishing; 2015.

222. O'Bryan EM, Kraemer KM, McLeish AC. Using transdiagnostic mechanistic targets to advance prevention science. *Clin Psychol Sci Pract.* 2021;*28*:338–340. https://doi.org/10.1037/cps0000044

223. Sauer-Zavala S, Gutner CA, Farchione TJ, Boettcher HT, Bullis JR, Barlow DH. Current definitions of "transdiagnostic" in treatment development: a search for consensus. *Behav Ther.* 2017;*48*:128–138. https://doi.org/10.1016/j.beth.2016.09.004

224. Mansell W, Harvey A, Watkins E, Shafran R. Conceptual foundations of the transdiagnostic approach to CBT. *J Cogn Psychother.* 2009;*23*:6–19. https://doi.org/10.1891/0889-8391.23.1.6

225. Brierley M-EE, Thompson EM, Albertella L, Fontenelle LF. Lifestyle interventions in the treatment of obsessive-compulsive and related disorders: a systematic review. *Psychosom Med.* 2021;*83*:817–833. https://doi.org/10.1097/PSY.0000000000000988

226. McHugh RK, Murray HW, Barlow DH. Balancing fidelity and adaptation in the dissemination of empirically-supported treatments: the promise of transdiagnostic interventions. *Behav Res Ther.* 2009;*47*:946–953. https://doi.org/10.1016/j.brat.2009.07.005

227. Hayes SC, Luoma JB, Bond FW, Masuda A, Lillis J. Acceptance and commitment therapy: model, processes and outcomes. *Behav Res Ther.* 2006;*44*:1–25. https://doi.org/10.1016/j.brat.2005.06.006

228. Graham CD, Gouick J, Krahé C, Gillanders D. A systematic review of the use of acceptance and commitment therapy (ACT) in chronic disease and long-term conditions. *Clin Psychol Rev.* 2016;*46*:46–58. https://doi.org/10.1016/j.cpr.2016.04.009

229. Thompson EM, Destree L, Albertella L, Fontenelle LF. Internet-based acceptance and commitment therapy: a transdiagnostic systematic review and meta-analysis for mental health outcomes. *Behav Ther.* 2021;*52*:492–507. https://doi.org/10.1016/j.beth.2020.07.002

230. Stice E, Rohde P, Shaw H, Gau JM. Randomized trial of a dissonance-based group treatment for eating disorders versus a supportive mindfulness group treatment. *J Consult Clin Psychol.* 2019;*87*:79–90. https://doi.org/10.1037/ccp0000365

231. Brake CA, Sauer-Zavala S, Boswell JF, Gallagher MW, Farchione TJ, Barlow DH. Mindfulness-based exposure strategies as a transdiagnostic mechanism of change: an exploratory alternating treatment design. *Behav Ther.* 2016;*47*:225–238. https://doi.org/10.1016/j.beth.2015.10.008

232. Manlick CF, Cochran SV, Koon J. Acceptance and commitment therapy for eating disorders: rationale and literature review. *J Contemp Psychother.* 2013;*43*:115–122. https://doi.org/10.1007/s10879-012-9223-7

15
Professionalism and Conscientious Objection in Medicine

Mark Wicclair

Key Points

- When physicians conscientiously object to a medical service, their objections are based on their *moral convictions*.
- Accommodating physicians who conscientiously object to a medical service enables them to practice medicine without compromising their moral integrity.
- Whether conscientious objection is compatible with physicians' professional obligations is context dependent.

Introduction

This chapter examines conscientious objection from the perspective of medical professionals who have, or believe they have, a conscientious objection to a medical service; contemplate requesting an accommodation; and want to know whether conscientious objection is consistent with their professional obligations. The focus is on physicians and the medical profession. It provides answers to several important questions about conscientious objection in medicine. The following questions are addressed: (1) What does it mean for physicians to conscientiously object to a medical service? (2) What should members of the medical profession consider when deciding whether to conscientiously object and request an accommodation? (3) Should members of the medical profession be willing to inform and refer? (4) Should physicians be willing to explain their objections? (5) To whom, when, and how should members of the medical profession communicate their conscientious objections?

What Does It Mean to Conscientiously Object?

When members of the medical profession conscientiously object to a medical service, their objections are based on their *moral convictions*. Physicians' moral convictions can, but need not, be based on religious beliefs. Like people generally, members of the medical profession might not have any religious beliefs, but they can nevertheless have moral convictions that are the basis of conscientious objections. For example, their moral convictions might be influenced by the works of philosophers such as Aristotle, Mill, or Kant. Or their moral convictions can be based on commonly accepted moral principles that can be justified without appealing to religious beliefs. In some cases, conscientious objections can be based on a combination of religious and nonreligious moral beliefs. Notably, just as the Supreme Court held that to qualify for conscientious objector status, individuals' objections to military service need not be based on religious beliefs; so, too, physicians' conscientious objections to medical services need not be based on religious beliefs.[1]

Members of the medical profession can object to providing a medical service for a variety of other reasons. Objections that are not conscientious objections include the following:

1. Objections to providing a medical service because it is not clinically indicated.
   For example, a pediatrician refuses to provide a growth hormone when parents request it for their son who is well within the normal height range for his age. The parents want to increase their son's chances of becoming a basketball star. The pediatrician's reason for refusing the parents' request is a belief that providing growth hormone for a child within the normal height range is contrary to accepted clinical norms and standard of care.
2. Objections to providing a medical service to avoid a substantial risk of harm to the physician.
   Although refusing to provide or assist in providing abortions commonly is based on moral objections, there are other reasons. For example, in view of the violence that has been directed against abortion providers in the United States, practitioners who are not morally opposed to abortion might nevertheless refuse to terminate pregnancies out of a concern for their safety.
3. Objections to providing a medical service for financial reasons.
   For example, if physicians refuse to treat Medicaid patients due to low reimbursement rates, their refusals are not conscientious objections.
4. Objections to providing a medical service because it is illegal.
   For example, although Dr. Marta Goldstone believes that in certain circumstances it can be clinically appropriate and in the best interests of adolescents to provide gender-affirming care, she refuses to offer it because she practices in a state that prohibits it.[a]
5. Objections to providing a medical service because it is contrary to the profession's code of ethics.
   For example, if physicians who have no moral objection to active euthanasia refuse to provide it to patients who request it because it is contrary to the American Medical Association (AMA) Code of Medical Ethics, the refusal is not a conscientious objection.

[a] The pediatric endocrinologist might consider engaging in a different type of conscientious objection: providing legally prohibited medical services because physicians believe they have an ethical obligation to do so. This type of conscientious objection has been designated "conscientious commitment"[2,3] or "conscientious provision." Whereas conscientious commitment/provision involves "positive appeals to conscience," conscientious refusals involve "negative appeals to conscience."[4] This chapter will consider only conscientious *refusals*.

6. An objection to providing a medical service because it is beyond the scope of the practitioner's clinical competence.
   For example, if a general practitioner refuses to provide palliative services to patients in intractable pain because they lack the necessary training and expertise, the refusal is not a conscientious objection.

What Should Members of the Medical Profession Consider?

When deciding whether to conscientiously object, physicians should consider: (1) whether their objection is to a *medical service*; (2) whether the objection is "futility based"; (3) whether they believe that it is *morally wrong* to provide the medical service; (4) the importance to them of adhering to their moral beliefs; (5) whether refusing to provide the medical service is compatible with their professional obligations; and (6) how the refusal will impact other health professionals.

Does the Physician Object to a Medical Service?

Before deciding to conscientiously object, members of the medical profession should make sure that they are objecting to a *medical service* rather than to providing the service to a certain class of patients. It is one thing for physicians to object to providing a specific medical service (e.g., abortion, emergency contraception [EC], donation after circulatory determination of death [DCDD], or palliative sedation to unconsciousness) and quite another thing to object to providing a medical service to African American or Muslim patients and yet be willing to provide the same medical service to white or Christian patients. Professional codes of major health professions prohibit discrimination; it is a settled view—one based on defensible and widely shared conceptions of justice, equality, dignity, and respect–that racial, ethnic, religious, and gender-based prejudice or bias are ethically wrong. Objections based on such discriminatory beliefs are unprofessional and inappropriate—regardless of whether they are conscience based.

Is the Objection "Futility Based"?

Physicians sometimes object to providing a medical service on the grounds that it is "futile" or "potentially inappropriate." This claim implies a belief that providing the medical service would be unprofessional because it would violate clinical norms and therefore should not be offered by *any* healthcare professional.

Guidelines for responding to requests for treatment that is thought to be futile or potentially inappropriate endorsed by the American Thoracic Society (ATS) and several other professional organizations recommend a fair process approach when there is intractable disagreement.[5,b] Accordingly, rather than conscientiously objecting and requesting a personal exemption for themselves, physicians who believe that a medical

[b] This policy statement recommends "potentially inappropriate" rather than "futile."

service is futile or potentially inappropriate should initiate a fair process review. If that review upholds the physician's belief, then no physician is obligated to provide the medical service. On the other hand, if the review determines that it is not futile or potentially inappropriate and the physician continues to believe that providing it is morally wrong, they can conscientiously object and request a personal exemption. In such cases, physicians can reasonably expect to be accommodated only if other physicians are willing and able to provide the medical service.

Does the Physician Believe That It Is Morally Wrong?

The crucial question of whether the physician believes that a medical service is morally wrong is one that members of the medical profession should consider before concluding that they have a conscientious objection for which they will request an accommodation. Although physicians may initially think that they have a moral objection, on reflection they might realize that their objection is based on other reasons, such as those identified above. In addition, it is important to distinguish between feelings of unease or discomfort and moral objections. For example, it is understandable that withdrawing life support from infants and young children can be emotionally charged and a source of unease and discomfort. However, insofar as physicians do not believe that withdrawing life support in such situations is *morally wrong*, they do not have grounds for *conscientious objections*. They might seek some modification of their responsibilities to spare them from unease, discomfort, or moral distress. However, candor, professional integrity, and fairness to colleagues who might have similar feelings but do not request any modifications in their responsibilities—they might believe it would be unprofessional to do so unless they have genuine moral objections—require not intentionally or unintentionally misrepresenting other types of objections as conscientious objections. Notably, healthcare institutions typically have separate policies and procedures for managing conscientious objection and moral distress.

How Important Is It to the Physician?

Since refusing to provide medical services can negatively affect patients, colleagues, department heads, and institutions, physicians should consider the importance to them of adhering to their moral beliefs. Specifically, they should consider whether providing the medical service will undermine their *moral integrity*. If it will, physicians have a strong moral reason for conscientiously objecting, and accommodation gives them moral space in which to practice medicine without compromising their moral integrity.

Physicians' moral integrity is at stake only if the relevant ethical beliefs are among their most important core moral beliefs. One can violate peripheral ethical beliefs without undermining one's moral integrity. It is only when one violates one's most important, self-defining ethical beliefs that one fails to maintain one's moral integrity. For medical professionals, their conception of professional integrity can be among their self-defining ethical beliefs. Lynne McFall draws a useful distinction between defeasible and identity-conferring commitments.[6] The former can be "sacrificed without remorse" and without undermining one's integrity. By contrast, the latter "reflect what we take to be the most important and so determine, to a large extent, our identities."(p13) One's moral integrity is compromised only if one acts contrary to one's identity-conferring commitments. Case 15.1 and Case 15.2 illustrate this distinction:

> Case 15.1: An 89-year-old nursing home resident with advanced Alzheimer's is admitted to a hospital intensive care unit (ICU) after presenting at the emergency department (ED) with pneumonia and kidney failure. The patient's family members insist on providing life support. Dr. Edith Knowles, an intensivist, believes that providing life support would be wasteful and an unjust allocation of scarce resources. Although providing life support would be unjust in the eyes of Dr. Knowles, it would comprise an injustice of a type that she routinely tolerates rather than a perceived grave injustice, such as genocide and discrimination based on race or sexual orientation.

> Case 15.2: Dr. Samuel Freeman is an intensivist who is morally opposed to providing palliative sedation to unconsciousness. He believes that administering palliative sedation to unconsciousness is morally equivalent to unjustified killing. The belief that unjustified killing is wrong is among Dr. Freeman's most deeply held moral convictions. He also has a deep moral commitment to professional integrity, and he believes that providing palliative sedation to unconsciousness would undermine his professional integrity. Dr. Freeman would feel morally obligated to refuse to offer palliative sedation to unconsciousness even if he would thereby risk disciplinary action or dismissal. As he explains it: "Offering palliative sedation to unconsciousness is something I simply cannot do. I couldn't live with myself if I were to offer it." Offering palliative sedation to unconsciousness is contrary to Dr. Freeman's identity-conferring commitments and incompatible with maintaining his moral integrity.

Insofar as Dr. Freeman's moral integrity is at stake and Dr. Knowles's moral integrity is not, the former has a stronger reason for a conscience-based refusal. Understanding that her moral integrity is not at stake should prompt Dr. Knowles to consider means other than conscientious objection to address her moral concerns and potential moral distress. Since other members of the healthcare team may share Dr. Knowles's view about offering life support to the patient in Case 15.1, an option for her would be to seek institutional remedies, such as measures to alleviate moral distress and support staff who experience it.[7]

Is Refusing to Provide the Medical Service Compatible With Professional Obligations?

An essential factor to consider when physicians contemplate conscientious objection is their professional obligations. It is a generally recognized principle that physicians have an obligation to put patients' interests or well-being above their own self-interest—an obligation characteristic of fiduciary relationships. I refer to this as the patients' interests first principle (PIFP). What are the implications of the PIFP for conscientious objection?

Some bioethicists maintain that conscientious objection is incompatible with the PIFP.[8–11] However, this claimed incompatibility relies on an implausible understanding of the PIFP. That principle clearly prohibits physicians from considering their financial interests when making recommendations to patients. But beyond that, what are the scope and implications of the PIFP? Is there no significant ethical difference between a physician's financial interests and their interest in maintaining moral integrity? Are there no limits to the sacrifices of their own well-being that physicians are obligated to make for the sake of their patients' health or well-being? Surely, there must be limits or physicians would not be able to take vacations, refuse to make house calls, limit their practice hours, refuse to expose themselves to excessive financial losses or risks of harm, and so forth.

A more plausible interpretation of the PIFP is that physicians have an obligation to consider the impact of conscientious objection on their patients and avoid causing them excessive burdens or harm. The AMA Code of Medical Ethics offers a more plausible interpretation of the PIFP in relation to conscientious objection. The code endorses the PIFP: "Physicians' ethical responsibility [is] to place patients' welfare above the physician's own self-interest" (1.1.1).[12] However, it also explicitly denies that conscientious objection is incompatible with the obligations of physicians. It states that, with three specified limitations: "Physicians may be able to act (or refrain from acting) in accordance with the dictates of their conscience *without violating their professional obligations*" (1.1.7; emphasis added). The three specified limitations are: "Physicians are expected to provide care in emergencies, honor patients' informed decisions to refuse life-sustaining treatment, and respect basic civil liberties and not discriminate against individuals in deciding whether to enter into a professional relationship with a new patient" (1.1.7). The code includes the following additional guideline:

> Several factors impinge on the decision to act according to conscience. Physicians have stronger obligations to patients with whom they have a patient-physician relationship, especially one of long standing; when there is imminent risk of foreseeable harm to the patient or delay in access to treatment would significantly adversely affect the patient's physical or emotional well-being; and when the patient is not reasonably able to access needed treatment from another qualified physician. (1.1.7)

There may well be other plausible specifications of physicians' professional obligations in relation to conscientious objection.[c] However, it is indisputable that physicians contemplating conscientious objection have an obligation to consider the potential impact on patients and avoid causing them excessive burdens or harm.

Unfortunately, there is no algorithm for determining whether conscientious refusals will cause excessive harms or burdens. This is in part because their impact is context dependent. Among other factors, it depends on whether other physicians are willing and able to provide the service in a timely manner, the burdens patients experience when they attempt to find alternative providers, and the burdens patients experience when their care is transferred to another physician. For example, if an ED physician in a large metropolitan medical center has a conscientious objection to offering rape victims EC, patients may not be affected if triage personnel can direct patients to ED physicians who do offer EC. On the other hand, if the only ED physician in a rural community hospital conscientiously objects to offering EC, rape victims might have to travel at least 50 miles to receive it—arguably an excessive burden. Worse yet, if the patient is unable to get

[c] Elsewhere, I provide an in-depth analysis of professional obligations in relation to conscientious objection in healthcare.[13,14]

transportation to another ED, she might become pregnant—which she would consider a significant harm. Generally, finding another physician can be especially difficult for patients in rural areas with limited access to physicians and healthcare institutions. Preferred provider networks also can pose a significant obstacle to patients seeking alternative providers. Thus, compared to patients who are not subject to preferred provider network constraints, finding alternative providers can be substantially more burdensome for patients who are subject to those constraints. Moreover, even if patients can receive requested medical services from other providers, changing physicians can be emotionally stressful for patients, especially when they are more vulnerable due to illness or injury and a sense of relative powerlessness.

Whether burdens and harms are perceived as excessive by patients is in part subjective insofar as it can depend on an individual's distinctive response. Whereas some patients might perceive a delay of five hours or a transfer to another physician as an excessive burden, others might not. Unfortunately, there is no defensible general objective standard of excessiveness that objectors can use to assess whether expected burdens and harms are excessive. This is in part because whether burdens or harms are excessive can require weighing expected burdens and harms with expected benefits. To be sure, there can be clear cases of excessiveness and non-excessiveness. For example, it is an excessive burden if, due to an intensivist's conscientious objection, a terminally ill patient who refuses medically provided nutrition and hydration (MPNH) needs to be transported to another hospital to have their wishes followed; and it would be a risk of excessive harm if there is a high risk that a patient will not survive transport to another facility. Unfortunately, however, there is no bright line that separates excessiveness and non-excessiveness. In the gray area, objectors can minimize the risk that they will fail to meet their professional obligation to put patients' interests first by assuming that burdens will be excessive.

A fair deliberative process is an accepted decision-making procedure for situations when there is conflict or there are no bright lines. In institutional settings, interdisciplinary ethics committees that include one or more community members might offer an opportunity to subject accommodation decisions to a fair deliberative process. Thus, in institutional settings, ethics committee reviews of objectors' requests for accommodation might minimize the risk that objectors will fail to meet their professional obligations. Over time, committee decisions might provide case-based guidelines for future situations that can reduce the need for additional committee reviews.

In addition to the PIFP, another widely recognized professional obligation is to respect patient autonomy. Just as it is mistaken to maintain that conscientious objection is incompatible with the PIFP, it is no less mistaken to hold that conscientious objection is incompatible with respect for patient autonomy. That principle, first and foremost, requires physicians to receive patients' informed consent before initiating treatment. It does not entitle patients to demand and receive any medical service that they might want. Nevertheless, *obstructing* or *thwarting* patients' access to medical services to which physicians conscientiously object *is* incompatible with respect for autonomy. It is obstruction, for example, if an obstetrician/gynecologist who conscientiously objects to abortion fails to tell a pregnant patient of a suspected genetic fetal anomaly so that she will not request tests to determine whether to terminate the pregnancy. Generally, insofar as conscientious objectors are only attempting to maintain *their* moral integrity and are not attempting to thwart patients from acting in ways that violate the objectors' moral beliefs, they do not violate the principle of respect for autonomy.

How Will a Conscientious Objection Affect Other Health Professionals?

Just as conscientious refusals can affect patients, they can affect other health professionals. Refusing to provide a medical service or information about it can impose burdens on other health professionals, especially within healthcare organizations.

Depending on the specific circumstances, conscience-based refusals can impose substantial burdens on the health professionals who are called on to provide the services that an objector refuses to provide. For example, in hospitals that offer DCDD and palliative sedation to unconsciousness, conscience-based refusals to participate in either practice can require other clinicians to substitute for objectors. Other intensivists may be required to be on call more frequently, and their workloads may increase significantly. Such changes can be a substantial hardship. The burdensomeness can vary with the personal situation of the other intensivists. For example, it might be more of a burden to a physician who has other substantial responsibilities (e.g., family, research, teaching, and/or community service) than to a physician with substantially fewer other responsibilities.

Depending on the specific circumstances, conscience-based refusals in healthcare organizations can also impose substantial burdens on department heads, medical directors, and institutions. For example, to accommodate an intensivist with a conscience-based objection to offering palliative sedation to unconsciousness, an accepted procedure within a hospital, the department head might have to make significant modifications to the work assignments and on-call schedules of other ICU physicians. In smaller community hospitals, accommodation might even require hiring another intensivist, which can be burdensome to the institution. Moreover, as the frequency of conscientious objections increases, the burdens to nonobjecting physicians and the burdensomeness of making the necessary staffing and schedule changes can also increase.

Such burdens are a factor that physicians contemplating conscientious objection should consider. They should not expect to be exempt from providing a medical service if it would unfairly burden other health professionals and/or unreasonably burden their department head or institution. Although physicians should consider the impact of conscience-based refusals on others, typically department heads, medical directors, administrators, and/or ethics committees have the authority to decide when burdens are unfair or excessive and whether to grant or reject objectors' requests for accommodation. Optimally, objectors who are denied accommodation should have access to an appeals process.[d]

Should Physicians Be Willing to Inform and Refer?

Physicians have a professional responsibility to ensure that patients are not denied information about the range of clinically appropriate options because of a conscience-based objection to one or more of those options. Thus, even if objecting physicians believe that informing patients will make them complicit in a moral wrong, the professional obligation to put patients' interests first requires informing patients if it is necessary to ensure that they are aware of all clinically appropriate options. On the other hand, if

[d] Elsewhere, I discuss institutional mechanisms for managing conscientious objection.[15]

patients reasonably can be expected to receive information about the range of clinically appropriate options in a timely manner from other providers, objecting physicians do not have an obligation to provide it.

Consider the case of Dr. Shaheen Majumdar, who has a conscience-based objection to offering palliative sedation to unconsciousness. She cannot reasonably assume that patients who satisfy the clinical criteria and their surrogates know that palliative sedation to unconsciousness is an option. Does Dr. Majumdar have an obligation to inform patients who satisfy the clinical criteria, or their surrogates? She would not have that obligation if other members of the healthcare team accept responsibility for (1) reviewing the charts of her patients to identify those who meet the clinical criteria for offering palliative sedation to unconsciousness; (2) offering the procedure to patients who satisfy the clinical criteria or their surrogates; and (3) providing the procedure if it is requested by patients or their surrogates. On the other hand, if other members of the healthcare team are unwilling to either individually or collectively accept these responsibilities, Dr. Majumdar should inform.

Physicians have a professional responsibility to ensure that patients are not denied timely access to safe and effective medical services because of their conscience-based refusals. Thus, even if objecting physicians believe that referral will make them complicit in a moral wrong, the professional obligation to put patients' interests first requires referral if it is needed to ensure that patients will receive, in a timely manner, medical services that are safe and effective. On the other hand, if referral is not required, objecting physicians are not obligated to refer.

Consider the case of Dr. Oswald Trepke, an obstetrician/gynecologist in private practice, who has a conscience-based objection to abortion. When a patient requests an abortion, he informs her that he does not perform abortions or prescribe abortifacients. Agitated, the patient asks him to refer her to a physician who will help her terminate her pregnancy. When Dr. Trepke refuses, the patient becomes even more agitated and says that she will look on YouTube for information about self-termination. If Dr. Trepke is reasonably confident that the patient will attempt to self-abort and endanger her health, to meet his professional obligation to put the interests of patients first, he should be willing to refer her to a provider who can terminate the pregnancy safely and effectively.

Should Physicians Be Willing to Explain Their Objections?

When physicians request accommodations, the persons (e.g., department heads, medical directors, or supervisors) or entities (e.g., ethics committees) authorized to assess such requests might ask for an explanation. Requests for an explanation can serve a valuable function by giving objecting physicians an opportunity to reflect on their reasons and determine whether they object for moral or other reasons, and if they object for moral reasons, whether core or only peripheral moral conviction are at stake.

However, some writers require in addition that objectors explain their reasons and justify their moral objections. For example, Robert Card[16–19] proposes a "reasonableness" standard and maintains objectors should be accommodated "only if the practitioner makes the objection and its reasoned basis public, and the justification offered for the exemption is subjected to assessment."[18,p82] According to Card, "grounding reasons" must be (1) reasonable; (2) subject to evaluation in terms of their justifiability; and (3) based on reasonable conceptions of the good.

It is undoubtedly desirable for *anyone*, including physician conscientious objectors, to have basic critical thinking skills that enable them to reflect on their core moral convictions, critically assess them, and provide a justification. However, as desirable as it may be, it is doubtful that this ability is an appropriate criterion for accommodation. Physicians can have sincere and deeply held self-defining core moral convictions and yet lack the critical thinking skills that would enable them to provide a satisfactory justification of their grounding reasons, or they might opt to shield core convictions, especially if they are faith based, from public scrutiny. Requiring them to reveal their most intimate thoughts and beliefs might be an unjustified invasion of their privacy. In any event, it is unclear why an inability (or unwillingness) to provide a satisfactory public justification should disqualify physician conscientious objectors from being considered for accommodation.

In addition, it can be problematic to require physicians to provide a justification that will satisfy others (e.g., department heads, medical directors, or members of ethics committees). Insofar as other persons might not share an objector's moral and/or religious beliefs, this requirement risks introducing unwarranted arbitrariness and subjectivity and failing to respect the moral integrity of objectors.

Thus, although physicians should be willing to explain their objections, it is unreasonable to expect them to be willing and able to provide a justification of their conscience-based refusals that will satisfy others.

To Whom, When, and How Should Physicians Communicate Their Conscientious Objections?

A helpful rule of thumb for medical professionals is to provide advance notification of their conscientious objections whenever feasible and appropriate. This means that physicians should examine their core moral beliefs and consider whether there are any medical services within the scope of their clinical competencies and responsibilities that are incompatible with those beliefs. In other words, the time to recognize that one is conscientiously opposed to providing a specific medical service is not the first time one is asked to provide it.

For patients, advance notification can eliminate or significantly reduce burdens imposed on them by physicians' conscientious objections. For physicians in solo or group practices, whenever feasible and appropriate, patients should be informed prior to or at the initial visit. For example, if an obstetrician/gynecologist in a practice group is conscientiously opposed to abortion, prospective patients who call for a first appointment can be informed that a member of the practice does not perform abortions. That will give prospective patients who want an obstetrician/gynecologist who is willing to terminate pregnancies a chance to select a member of the practice group who is willing to terminate pregnancies or to find another practice group. It will also reduce the risk that once in the practice, patients will need to change their obstetrician/gynecologist if they want to terminate a pregnancy.

When advance notification is neither feasible nor appropriate prior to or during the initial visit, giving established patients "early warning" can give them more time and maximize their opportunity to find physicians who match their treatment preferences. It can also prevent the additional stress of needing to find and change physicians when one currently needs a medical service due to illness or injury. For example, internists conscientiously opposed to forgoing MPNH can give their patients "early warning" when reviewing their advance directives and end-of-life wishes. This may not eliminate the need for patients to change physicians, but at least patients will have an opportunity to take steps to ensure their end-of-life wishes will be respected while they retain the ability to do so. The timing of advance notifications can be important. For example, the time for physicians to give patients advance notification of their conscientious objection to forgoing MPNH is not when they first notify patients that they have stage 4 pancreatic cancer. Intended or not, that would only amplify patients' shock, anxiety, fear, and distress.

In healthcare organizations, advance notification can minimize disruptions in care and maximize the feasibility of implementing measures that will permit granting exemptions to physicians with conscientious objections. For example, if an intensivist knows that they are conscientiously opposed to DCDD, they should immediately inform the department head and not wait until being called on to participate in the procedure.

Advance notification is feasible when there is a specific medical service that a physician cannot in good conscience provide. But what about situations in which physicians do not have a blanket objection to a specific medical service? Instead, they only object to providing it in certain circumstances. Consider Dr. Emit Carnap, a neonatal ICU (NICU) physician, who has a conscience-based objection to continuing aggressive life support for Baby F, a preterm infant with an extremely poor prognosis. Dr. Carnap is not ethically opposed in principle to providing aggressive treatment to preterm neonates. After all, that is routine in the NICU. Rather, Dr. Carnap only is opposed to providing such care in cases like Baby F. Continued aggressive NICU care for Baby F is not clearly contrary to accepted clinical standards or NICU practice. It may be contrary to Dr. Carnap's conception of "good medicine," but it does not violate established professional norms and is not clearly outside the boundaries of "appropriate medical care." Dr. Carnap might be able to anticipate cases such as Baby F, articulate his standards, and communicate them to the department head and his colleagues. Doing so can help to minimize disruptions of care and maximize the likelihood that Dr. Carnap can be accommodated and exempted from caring for preterm infants like Baby F.

When informing patients that they are unable to provide a medical service, physicians should be mindful of their obligation as medical professionals to be respectful of patients. It is unprofessional to insult, embarrass, intimidate, or badger patients. As medical professionals, physicians also should refrain from expressing moral disapproval of patients or subjecting them to moral lectures. The primary aim of conscientious objection is to enable physicians to practice medicine without compromising their moral integrity, not to impose their moral beliefs on patients. Imposing their moral beliefs on patients is unprofessional.

To minimize the risk of disrespecting patients and expressing moral disapproval of them, physicians can avoid telling patients that they are unwilling to provide a medical service because they believe it is immoral. Instead, physicians can simply state that they are unable to offer it. If patients ask for a reason, and physicians opt to explain that they cannot in good conscience provide the service, physicians should clearly communicate that it is *their* conscience, and they understand that patients may not accept the physician's moral beliefs.

Conclusion

When physicians conscientiously object to providing a medical service, their objection is based on their *moral convictions*. Physicians' moral convictions can be secular in nature, based on their religious beliefs, or a combination of both.

When deciding whether to conscientiously object to providing a medical service, physicians should consider (1) whether their objection is to a *medical service* or to providing the service to a specified class of patients; (2) whether the objection is "futility based"; (3) whether they believe that it is *morally wrong* to provide the medical service; (4) the importance to them of adhering to their moral beliefs; (5) whether refusing to provide the medical service is compatible with their professional obligations; and (6) how the refusal will impact other health professionals.

Physicians have a professional responsibility to ensure that patients are not denied information about the range of clinically appropriate options because of their conscience-based objection to one or more of those options. Thus, objecting physicians should be willing to inform if it is necessary to ensure that patients are aware of all clinically appropriate options. On the other hand, if patients can reasonably be expected to receive information about the range of clinically appropriate options in a timely manner from other providers, objecting physicians do not have an obligation to provide it.

When physicians request accommodations, the persons (e.g., department heads, medical directors, or supervisors) or entities (e.g., ethics committees) authorized to assess such requests might ask for an explanation. Requests for an explanation can serve a valuable function by giving objecting physicians an opportunity to reflect on their reasons and determine whether they object for moral or other reasons, and if they object for moral reasons, whether core or only peripheral moral conviction are at stake. Thus, physicians should be willing to explain their objections. However, it is unreasonable to expect objecting physicians to be able and willing to provide a justification of their conscience-based refusals that can satisfy others.

Whenever feasible and appropriate, objecting physicians should provide advance notification of their conscientious objections. Advance notification can protect patients, minimize the impact on the healthcare team, and increase the likelihood of accommodation.

When informing patients that they are unable to provide a medical service, objecting physicians should be mindful of their obligation as medical professionals to be respectful of patients. It is unprofessional to insult, embarrass, intimidate, or badger patients. As medical professionals, physicians also should refrain from expressing moral disapproval of patients or subjecting them to moral lectures.

References

1. United States v. Seeger, 380 US 163 (1965); Welsh v. United Sates, 398 US 333 (1970).
2. Dickens BM, Cook RJ. Conscientious commitment to women's health. *Int J Gynecol Obstet.* 2011;113:163–166.
3. Harris LH. Recognizing conscience in abortion provision. *N Engl J Med.* 2012;367:981–983.
4. Wicclair MR. 2009. Negative and positive claims of conscience. *Camb Q Healthc Ethics* 18 (1):14–22.

5. Bosslet GT, Pope TM, Rubenfeld GD, et al. An official ATS/AACN/ACCP/ESICM/SCCM policy statement: responding to requests for potentially inappropriate treatments in intensive care units. *Am J Respir Crit Care Med.* 2015;191(11):1318–1330.
6. McFall L. Integrity. *Ethics.* 1987;98(1):5–20.
7. Lewis-Newby M, Wicclair M, Pope T, et al. An official American Thoracic Society policy statement: managing conscientious objections in intensive care medicine. *Am J Respir Crit Care Med.* 2015;191(2):219–227.
8. Stahl RY, Emanuel EJ. Physicians, not conscripts—conscientious objection in health care. *N Engl J Med.* 2017;376(14):1380–1385.
9. Savulescu J. Conscientious objection in medicine. *B M J.* 2006;332:294–297.
10. Savulescu J, Schuklenk U. Doctors have no right to refuse medical assistance in dying, abortion, or contraception. *Bioethics.* 2017;31(3):162–170.
11. Schuklenk U, Smalling R. Why medical professionals have no moral claim to conscientious objection accommodation in liberal democracies. *J Med Ethics.* 2017;43:234–240.
12. American Medical Association Council on Ethical and Judicial Affairs. *Code of Medical Ethics.* American Medical Association; 2017.
13. Wicclair MR. Is conscientious objection incompatible with a physician's professional obligations? *Theor Med Bioeth.* 2008;29(3):171–185.
14. Wicclair MR. *Conscientious Objection in Health Care: An Ethical Analysis.* Cambridge University Press; 2011.
15. Wicclair M. Managing conscientious objection in health care institutions. *HEC Forum.* 2014;26(3):267–283.
16. Card RF. Conscientious objection and emergency contraception. *Am J Bioeth.* 2007;7(6):8–14.
17. Card RF. Reasonability and conscientious objection in medicine: a reply to Marsh and an elaboration of the reason-giving requirement. *Bioethics.* 2014;28(6):320–326.
18. Card RF. The inevitability of assessing reasons in debates about conscientious objection in medicine. *Camb Q Healthc Ethics.* 2017;26:82–96.
19. Card RF. Reasons, reasonability and establishing conscientious objector status in medicine. *J Med Ethics.* 2017;43:222–225.

16

Spirituality and Professionalism

Gia Merlo

Key Points

- There is a distinction between religious and spiritual care. The development of spiritual care is a clinical skill that healthcare professionals should apply during clinical interactions.
- Spiritual and religious self-awareness and self-care by healthcare professionals are essential in the provision of patient care, particularly toward better understanding patients' needs, establishing patient rapport, and productive communication.
- There are several barriers to the development of effective spiritual care by healthcare professionals, including the lack of skills and knowledge training, time constraints in having spiritual care conversations with patients, and the lack of resources by healthcare instructions to help facilitate effective spiritual care.

Importance of Spirituality

The increasing diversity of cultural, social, religious, and spiritual backgrounds of patients calls for physicians to acquire greater skills and flexibility in order to meet the needs of each individual patient. In conjunction with the globalizing world, an ongoing coronavirus (COVID-19) pandemic began in the year 2020. Medical professionals and patients suffered moral injury due to the unprecedented deaths and loss of hope associated with the COVID-19 pandemic, leading to a heightened awareness and pursuit for religious and spiritual care.[1,2]

The high demands of spiritual care often pose difficulties for physicians during clinical interaction due to their perceived lack of competence and confidence in appropriately and effectively addressing the topic to improve the satisfaction and health outcomes of patients. It has been observed that the majority of physicians' barriers to discussing their patients' religions and spiritualities revolve on a lack of training and skill in these areas. Moreover, physicians often report concerns related to breaking therapeutic relationships by misaddressing a patient's religion and spirituality, which further hinders them integrating spiritual care into their daily practice.[3–5]

The purpose of this chapter is to address the role of physicians' spirituality in healthcare settings, as well as ways to address spiritual care for patients who undergo spiritual distress and psychosocial suffering.

History of Religion in Medicine

Religion, spirituality, and medicine have been bidirectionally intertwined throughout history, with religious beliefs often shaping medical practice and vice versa. The earliest known medical practices and healthcare systems were often closely associated with religious and spiritual ideologies. Many cultures adopted belief systems based on the concept that illness and health outcomes were the results of supernatural forces and could only be cured through spiritual interventions. Of note, the establishment of many hospitals and medical institutions were on the basis of religious orders. Moreover, various religious figures, including monks and nuns, were trained in providing medical care. The Enlightenment period largely marked the emergence of scientific medicine as a separate field from religion, which resulted in the decline of religious influence on medical practices. However, healthcare continues to be influenced by religious traditions and spiritual practices and beliefs. Religiosity and spirituality play an important role in today's healthcare climate. It has been noted that many patients seek spiritual support as a component of their medical care and treatment plan. Many healthcare organizations and hospitals recognize the importance of addressing patients' religious and spiritual needs and have worked to implement strategies that facilitate spiritual care. Additionally, some academic institutions and medical training facilities have made efforts to educate future clinicians on the intersection of religion, spirituality, and medicine, as well as how religion and spirituality can impact patients' quality of life, life satisfaction, and healthcare outcomes.

Primary care providers aim to provide comprehensive care that addresses not only physical health, but also mental, emotional, social, and spiritual well-being. Religious and spiritual beliefs and practices are critical components of holistic healthcare that can affect how patients cope with life challenges and poor health, make healthcare decisions, and find meaning, satisfaction, and purpose in life. Patient-centered care is a major focus of primary care medicine that involves recognizing, respecting, and addressing unique perspectives, preferences, values, and needs of patients. Spirituality and religiosity may play a significant role in shaping a patient's identity and outlook on life. Therefore, healthcare providers have a professional responsibility to collaborate and communicate with patients to identify their spiritual and religious beliefs and practices in order to appropriately incorporate them into their treatment plan and daily life in a health-promoting manner.

Spiritual Care

A clear distinction exists between religious and spiritual care, which is similar to the distinction between religion and spirituality. Religion "describes specific behavior patterns and practices that align with a traditional system of faith and worship,"[5] which indicates the confined nature of religious care to the already existing system of a religious framework.[5,6] Spirituality refers to the individual's connection between their life experiences to greater meaning, purpose, and transcendence.[7] Kuhn describes spiritual care as a derivative of spirituality, or "the caring for, i.e. enabling, preserving and protecting of a patient or health-care professional's personal identity in an existential crisis."[8,(p58)] Spiritual care is commonly used in the setting of palliative care, end-of-life circumstances, and other critical health diagnoses, such as cancer, to help patients spiritually reorient themselves and maintain a sense of fulfillment and purpose in the midst of challenging and potentially distressing times.

One can distinguish a patient who needs medical care versus spiritual care by understanding the difference between pain and suffering. Patients who display explicit abnormality in vital signs often immediately receive medical support to attenuate their symptoms. It is not uncommon for patients in spiritual distress to present with normal vital signs but still experience continued emotional and psychosocial suffering. The same level of support that is provided to patients regarding medical care may not be provided with regard to spiritual care, which may reduce their quality of life or adversely affect health outcomes. Physicians may facilitate the healing and recovery of their patients through emotional support and spiritual care in conjunction with conventional medical treatment. Spiritual care may be particularly essential in alleviating patient suffering in palliative and end-of-life care settings.[4,9]

For a clinical example, a patient, who recently lost his loved one from COVID-19, may walk into the emergency department claiming of chest pain and shortness of breath, while his physical examination results are normal. In this example, dismissing the patient due to lack of abnormality in examination results may indicate a physician's failure to practice spiritual care and, further, a failure to address their spiritual distress and moral injury from COVID-19. As explained by Büssing, an appropriate solution for this patient would be showing a compassionate presence.[9]

While the physician from the above example helped the patient by referring him to a therapist, the moral of the story goes far beyond a referral to another therapist or to a professional who can address mental and spiritual distress for patients. Spiritual care may involve the entire healthcare team in order to address and manage patients' spiritual distress and concerns and does not rely on a designated spiritual care provider. Spiritual care is a skill that any medical health professional should be able to apply during clinical interactions.[8]

Why Spiritual Care Is Necessary

Spiritual care is an ethical approach to addressing a fundamental aspect of human existence, which is the search for meaning, purpose, and connectedness.[10] Those who endure illness, injury, or death are often confronted with questions of meaning, value, and relationship. The provision of spiritual care may be considered a necessary component of healthcare that involves providing support and guidance to individuals in exploring their spiritual practices, beliefs, and values, as well as finding ways to integrate them into their daily lives. It is pertinent to note that healthcare professionals can adopt a respectful approach to addressing and honoring spiritual concerns and requests without compromising patient-provider relationships or interfering with the benefits of interventions provided by scientific medicine.[11]

Spiritual care is often an important component of palliative and end-of-life care. Healthcare providers who incorporate spiritual care into healthcare practice can help patients and what those patients care for and about by using strategies to foster comfort, meaning, and peace in the setting of illness, hardships, and death. Spiritual care is a patient-centered approach to holistic healthcare that recognizes and addresses the interconnectedness of the mind, body, and spirit in whole-person health. Moreover, spiritual care may promote healing and well-being in the face of life's challenges.

Professional Physician and Patient Interaction

A physician's professional role in spiritual care may be divided into intraprofessional care and ethics among physicians and interprofessional care between a physician and a patient.

Transdisciplinary/intraprofessional collaboration within the healthcare team, as well as a strong provider-patient relationship, is essential to the provision of spiritual care to allow for care focused on the needs of the patient.

Spiritual care can be delivered intraprofessionally through collaboration between healthcare professionals within the same discipline. The concept of intraprofessional spiritual care is based on the principle that healthcare professionals with different levels of experience and expertise in providing spiritual care can collaborate with others within the same discipline to improve quality and effectiveness of patient care. Intraprofessional spiritual care can leverage the shared knowledge and skills of healthcare professionals within the same discipline.

Interprofessional Care

Interprofessional execution of spiritual care involves transdisciplinary collaboration among healthcare professionals to provide comprehensive spiritual and medical care to patients. Providing interprofessional spiritual care can improve patient outcomes and quality of life by managing spiritual needs in a holistic and coordinated way.[12] An interprofessional approach to spiritual care considers the fact that spiritual care is a shared responsibility that is dependent on the contributions, expertise, and compassion of multiple healthcare professionals.[12] Healthcare professionals from different disciplines, such as social work and nursing, can collaborate to evaluate patients' spiritual and religious practices, beliefs, values, and interventional needs. An essential component of interprofessional spiritual care is shared goal setting, which is a transdisciplinary communication strategy that enables all professionals on a patient's healthcare team to work toward a common goal that has been tailored to the patient's individual preferences and needs.[9]

Physician's Skills to Practice Spiritual Care

As part of the educational requirement for physicians in training, some of the skill sets that are important to address are physicians' strong sense of their own religion and spirituality, spiritual self-care, and spiritual and cultural competence.[5,8]

Physician's Spiritual and Religious Self-Awareness

Spiritual and religious self-awareness is crucial for healthcare professionals to understand patients' needs, establish rapport with patients, and communicate productively with patients, which constitutes effective spiritual care. It has been noted that healthcare professionals should be aware of their own biases, beliefs, and limitations surrounding spirituality and religiosity in order to identify and appropriately manage personal ideology that may interfere with the provision of effective care.[8] Healthcare professionals who are self-aware are better equipped to provide compassionate and patient-centered care. Understanding the importance of respect and nonjudgment can foster a safe and open environment for patients to express themselves freely and deepen the patient-provider partnership.[13] Self-aware healthcare professionals can also communicate more effectively with patients about their spiritual and religious viewpoints.[14] It is possible to facilitate meaningful and respectful dialogue with patients by using appropriate language, context, and terminology that is sensitive to patients' beliefs and values.

Physician's Spiritual Self-Care

Healthcare professionals who engage in spiritual self-care may be better equipped to provide effective spiritual care to their patients.[8] Engaging in spiritual self-care can help clinicians enhance self-awareness of their own spiritual and religious beliefs, values, and needs. Increased self-awareness can improve providers' ability to respect, understand, and empathize with the spiritual needs of their patients. The practice of spiritual self-care may also facilitate improved communication with patients surrounding spirituality and religiosity. Spiritual self-care may allow healthcare professionals to translate their own experiences into better patient-provider connections and more meaningful conversations about religious and spiritual topics with patients. Additionally, this practice may buffer occupational emotional and psychological demands and burnout among healthcare professionals. Providers who experience burnout are often less likely to show empathy and provide effective spiritual care to patients. Therefore, spiritual self-care may facilitate the provision of quality healthcare by promoting the management of providers' spiritual needs.

Physician's Spiritual and Cultural Competence

The concept of cultural competence refers to the ability to understand and respect a wide range of practices, beliefs, and values of various cultures and religions, which can be achieved by self-awareness. Cultural competence facilitates the capacity of healthcare professionals to work effectively with patients from diverse backgrounds and provide patient-centered care that is adapted according to individual needs of patients.[15] Healthcare professionals who are culturally competent can provide more holistic care that addresses the physical, emotional, and spiritual needs of patients. Moreover, clinical cultural competence interventions may help to attenuate demographic/racioethnic disparities in healthcare and thereby improve healthcare on a population-level scale.[16]

Barriers to Providing Effective Spiritual Care

A variety of barriers may hinder the provision of effective spiritual care. Healthcare professionals often receive little to no training in spiritual care.[9] The lack of skills and knowledge that clinicians need to provide effective spiritual care can lead to feelings of incompetence or a lack of confidence around addressing spiritual concerns. Another commonly described barrier to spiritual care is time constraints.[17] Healthcare professionals are often bound by extreme time limitations, which may lead to a lack of attention to patients' spiritual needs. Additionally, healthcare facilities may not have the resources, training, or staff to provide effective spiritual care.[17–20] Lack of access to and availability of spiritual care providers or chaplains may hinder efforts to adequately support patients in their religious and spiritual journeys.[5] Personal spiritual beliefs, biases, and/or assumptions may prevent healthcare professionals from appropriately addressing the spiritual needs of their patients. Systemic lack of integration of spiritual care in overall treatment plans for patients may further impede the provision of attention to spirituality, religiosity, and effective spiritual care in comparison to other aspects of care.[5] It is crucial for healthcare professionals to recognize and address obstacles that may interfere with their ability to provide effective spiritual care to their patients.

Conclusion and Future Implications

Spiritual care and engagement may serve as a key strategy to improve patient health outcomes and quality of life, as well as enhance healthcare professionals' capacity to reduce their risk of burnout and provide effective, holistic, patient-centered care.[21] Incorporating these skill sets into systems of medical education for future medical students and physicians, principles like patient-centered care, and willingness to explore physicians' and patients' spiritual domain may help improve future spiritual care. Some examples of intervention may involve adopting a biopsychosocial-spiritual model in medical culture, or HoPES3 (a holistic care program for elderly patients to integrate spiritual needs, social activity, and self-care into disease management in primary care), which further engage patients with their religious and spirituality needs through a physician's "healing presence," which is unconditional support given to patients outside the designated spiritual care time.[19] Others may also include educational materials that provide workshops, physician collaboration and discussion around spiritual care, and training for patients to be comfortable addressing these topics and interacting with patients with spiritual care.

References

1. Ferrell BR, Handzo G, Picchi T, Puchalski C, Rosa WE. The urgency of spiritual care: COVID-19 and the critical need for whole-person palliation. *J Pain Symptom Manage.* 2020;60(3):e7–e11.
2. Rushton CH, Thomas TA, Antonsdottir IM, et al. Moral injury and moral resilience in health care workers during COVID-19 pandemic. *J Palliat Med.* 2022;25(5):712–719.
3. Anandarajah G, Roseman J, Mennillo L. G, Kelley B. Spirituality in primary palliative care and beyond: a 20-year longitudinal qualitative study of interacting factors impacting physicians' spiritual care provision over time. *J Pain Symptom Manage.* 2021;62(6):1216–1228.
4. Chahrour WH, Hvidt NC, Hvidt EA, Viftrup DT. Learning to care for the spirit of dying patients: the impact of spiritual care training in a hospice-setting. *BMC Palliat Care.* 2021;20(1):1–12.
5. Dillard V, Moss J, Padgett N, Tan X, Kennedy AB. Attitudes, beliefs and behaviors of religiosity, spirituality, and cultural competence in the medical profession: a cross-sectional survey study. *PLoS One.* 2021;16(6):e0252750.

6. Seybold KS, Hill PC. The role of religion and spirituality in mental and physical health. *Curr Dir Psychol Sci.* 2001;10(1):21–24.
7. Nolan S, Saltmarsh P, Leget C. Spiritual care in palliative care: working towards an EAPC Task Force. *Eur J Prev Cardiol.* 2011;18(2):86–89.
8. Kuhn E. Why me?–the concept of physicians' spiritual self-care: a contribution to professional and organisational ethics. In: *Ethical Challenges for Healthcare Practices at the End of Life: Interdisciplinary Perspectives*). Springer International Publishing; 2022:55–72.
9. Büssing A, ed. *Spiritual Needs in Research and Practice: The Spiritual Needs Questionnaire as a Global Resource for Health and Social Care.* Springer Nature; 2021.
10. Sulmasy DP. Ethical principles for spiritual care. In: Cobb MR, Puchalski CM, Rumbold B, eds. *Oxford Textbook of Spirituality in Healthcare.* Oxford University Press; 2012:465–472.
11. Astrow AB, Puchalski CM, Sulmasy DP. Religion, spirituality, and health care: social, ethical, and practical considerations. *Am J Med.* 2001;110(4):283–287.
12. Taylor EJ. Spiritual care: practical implications. In: Merlo, Gia and Berra, Kathy, eds. *Lifestyle Nursing.* CRC Press; 2022:417–427.
13. Dell'Aversana G, Bruno A. Different and similar at the same time. Cultural competence through the leans of healthcare providers. *Front Psychol.* 2017;8:1426.
14. Taylor EJ. Healing communication: a precision instrument for spiritual care. *Semin Oncol Nurs.* 2021;37(5):151213.
15. Mächler R, Straßner C, Sturm N, et al. GPs personal spirituality, their attitude and spiritual competence: a cross-sectional study in German general practices. *J Relig Health.* 2023;62(4):2436–2451. Published online 2022 Apr 27. doi:10.1007/s10943-022-01536-2.
16. Betancourt JR, Green AR, Carrillo JE, Owusu Ananeh-Firempong II. Defining cultural competence: a practical framework for addressing racial/ethnic disparities in health and health care. *Public Health Rep.* 2003;118(4):293–302. doi:10.1016/S0033-3549(04)50253-4.
17. Hathaway DB, de Oliveira e Oliveira FH, Mirhom M, Moreira-Almeida A, Fung WLA, Peteet JR. Teaching spiritual and religious competencies to psychiatry residents: a scoping and systematic review. *Acad Med.* 2022;97(2):300–310.
18. Jones KF, Paal P, Symons X, Best MC. The content, teaching methods and effectiveness of spiritual care training for healthcare professionals: a mixed-methods systematic review. *J Pain Symptom Manage.* 2021;62(3):e261–e278.
19. Kunsmann-Leutiger E, Straßner C, Schalhorn F, et al. Training general practitioners and medical assistants within the framework of HoPES3, a holistic care program for elderly patients to integrate spiritual needs, social activity, and self-care into disease management in primary care. *J Multidiscip Healthc.* 2021;14:1853–1861.
20. Rykkje L, Søvik MB, Ross L, McSherry W, Cone P, Giske T. Educational interventions and strategies for spiritual care in nursing and healthcare students and staff: a scoping review. *J Clin Nurs.* 2022;31(11–12):1440–1464.
21. White MS, Addison CC, Jenkins BW. Beliefs and practices regarding spirituality as a healthcare strategy. *Open J Prev Med.* 2022;12(3):59–72.

17
Managing Spiritual Issues in Catholic-Affiliated Health Systems

Elliott Louis Bedford and Jason T. Eberl

Key Points

- Spiritual care is an essential aspect of the holistic care provided in Catholic health systems.
- Medicine is fundamentally a healing profession comprising a moral community of professionals.
- Holistic end-of-life care includes appropriate forms of palliative and hospice care in which dying patients are accompanied by caregivers in their final days.
- Formation helps professionals working in Catholic health systems to understand and appreciate the spiritual nature and context of the system's healing ministry.
- Catholic health systems place a special emphasis on utilizing highly trained spiritual care professionals to provide care to patients, families, and clinical staff.

Introduction

In this chapter, we highlight some distinctive ways in which religiously affiliated health systems, specifically those of the Roman Catholic tradition, support and manage issues of spirituality in the provision of care, especially as they intersect issues of professionalism. Catholic healthcare institutions comprise a significant portion of the US healthcare system.[a,1] For such institutions, spirituality plays an explicit and distinguishing role in the mission, vision, and values of healthcare delivery. As one Catholic healthcare system defines their mission: "Our Catholic health ministry is dedicated to spiritually centered, holistic care which sustains and improves the health of individuals and communities."[2]

In the final two sections of this chapter, we highlight two different dimensions of this professional commitment to the spiritual dimension of healthcare. To begin, though, we draw attention to the philosophy of medicine that animates the identity and mission of Catholic healthcare, particularly as it is articulated and represented by the *Ethical and Religious Directives for Catholic Health Care Services* (*Directives*), the normative guide

[a] Approximately one in seven patients every day is cared for in a Catholic hospital.

for delivering mission-aligned care promulgated by the US Conference of Catholic Bishops.[3] These *Directives* serve as a professional formation guide, helping articulate the responsibilities of what it means to be a healthcare professional within a Catholic healthcare institution. We conclude by focusing on the specific practice of spiritual care, provided by professional chaplains, as a practical manifestation of the care of the whole person characteristic of the Catholic healthcare mission.

Catholic Healthcare's Philosophy of Medicine

Catholic healthcare is characterized by a distinctive philosophy of medicine and the medical profession, rooted in the ancient Hippocratic tradition, which has been modernized by scholars such as Edmund Pellegrino.[4] In this section, we elucidate this philosophy and how it informs the *Directives* that guide the professional practice of medicine within Catholic healthcare, focusing on end-of-life care.

Hippocratic Medicine Reconstructed

The birth of medicine as a *profession* is typically attributed to the formation of the Hippocratic school in ancient Greece, which distinguished itself from the Apollonian and Asclepian schools that allowed practitioners to utilize their skills either to heal or to wound or even kill for putatively humane reasons—a more modern example of the Apollonian model at work was Dr. Guillotine's invention of a "humane" method of execution.[5] The fundamental debate regarding what practices are congruent with the essential nature of medicine as a profession—even whether medicine has an "essential nature" or merely comprises a set of skills in which practitioners are trained—continues to this day. A primary example is whether physicians ought to offer euthanasia or medically aided death to terminally—or perhaps also chronically—ill patients. While many argue that physicians ought to use their skills and the pharmaceuticals at their disposal to aid or directly end a patient's life on their autonomous request,[6] others have contended that the practice of medicine does not entail simply acceding to patients' autonomous wishes or to aim at the promotion of one's overall well-being:

> The great temptation of modern medicine, not always resisted, is to move beyond the promotion and preservation of health into the boundless realm of general human happiness and well-being. The root problem of illness and mortality is both medical and philosophical or religious. "Why must I die?" can be asked as a technical, biological question or as a question about the meaning of life. When medicine tries to respond to the latter, which it is always under pressure to do, it moves beyond its proper role. . . . Medicine should try to relieve human suffering, but only that suffering which is brought on by illness and dying as biological phenomena, not that suffering which comes from anguish or despair at the human condition.[7]

This view of medicine as essentially a *healing* profession has been developed by Pellegrino and others into a comprehensive *philosophy of medicine*. Against those who contend that medical practitioners are merely service providers[8] or that medicine cannot be defined by any content-full moral ethos,[9] Pellegrino, inspired by the Hippocratic model, contends that medicine has an intrinsic teleological orientation toward restoring the healthy functioning of patient's bodies and minds in line with a view of what is *good* for the patient that includes, but is not limited to, the patient's own understanding of what is good for them.[b,2,10] With David Thomasma, Pellegrino has argued that medicine, as a profession, constitutes a "moral community" due to, among other factors, the *fiduciary* nature of the physician/patient relationship, the *nonproprietary* nature of medical knowledge, and the *self-effacing covenant* into which physicians enter on professing their oath.[c,11,12]

Catholic View of Health and Healing

The view just summarized of medicine's essential nature as a profession has been articulated and defended within a secular context; however, it is congruent with a Christian—and specifically Catholic—model of medicine's teleological orientation, internal morality, and specific virtues that physicians ought to cultivate.[13–15]

Foundationally, the Catholic Church grounds its healing ministry in the scriptural examples of Jesus's miraculous healings:

> Health in the biblical perspective means wholeness—not only physical, but also spiritual and psychological wholeness; not only individual, but also social and institutional wholeness. Jesus was the Divine Healer who came to restore this health. He healed people's physical and psychological ills; he healed them in the depth of their being. Through his life and ministry he proclaimed the kingdom of God on earth and reached out to touch and heal our wounded humanity. He came to the world to make us fully human, to help us to realize our human dignity as creatures made in the image of God. He came to bring us the fullness of life. . . . Members of the church follow the example of Jesus, therefore, when they carry out the work of healing—not only by providing care for the physically ill, but also by working to restore health and wholeness in all facets of the human person and the human community.[16(p4)]

It is important to note that the Catholic vision of healthcare ministry, which sometimes involves adhering to specific inviolable moral norms—such as respect for the intrinsic dignity of every human person from conception to natural death—does not entail a simplistic division between "reason" and "faith" or between "religion" and "science." In fact, the Church affirms the contributions that science and technological developments have made and continue to make in supporting its healing ministry:

> Through science the human race comes to understand God's wonderful work; and through technology it must conserve, protect, and perfect nature in harmony with God's purposes. Health care professionals pursue a special vocation to share in carrying forth God's life-giving and healing work.
>
> The dialogue between medical science and Christian faith has for its primary purpose the common good of all human persons. It presupposes that science and faith do not contradict each other. Both are grounded in respect for truth and freedom. As new

[b] For a congruent argument concerning the essential nature of medicine, see Reference 10.
[c] For further discussion of the "covenantal" nature of medicine, see Reference 12.

> knowledge and new technologies expand, each person must form a correct conscience based on the moral norms for proper health care.[3(General Intro p7)]

The Catholic healthcare ministry focuses on the healing of patients *holistically*, but not by reducing human well-being narrowly to the satisfaction of subjective desires, some of which may detract from the authentic flourishing of human persons. Let us now see how this vision of healthcare ministry is actualized in the context of end-of-life care.

Application—End-of-Life Care

The Catholic vision of healthcare shares the view espoused by Daniel Callahan and others (including the American Medical Association)[17] that intentionally ending the life of a terminally or chronically ill patient (euthanasia) or providing them with the means to end their own life (medically aided death) does not cohere with respect for the intrinsic dignity of human persons—for whom the fundamental good, necessary to pursue all other goods, is life—or with the essential nature of healthcare ministry as restoring a patient to their full humanity.[18]

Instead, Catholic healthcare has invested in the provision of quality *palliative* and *hospice care*, involving the holistic dimensions of physical (pain management), psychological (ameliorating depression), and spiritual (confronting existential distress) healing. In 2019, the Center to Advance Palliative Care (CAPC) published a report that illustrated "91% of Catholic hospitals offer palliative care, compared to 72 percent of hospitals overall."[19] In the words of Diane Meier, director of CAPC: "The Catholic hospitals have been way ahead of the rest of the hospitals since we started measuring and remain there."[19]

The aim of palliative and hospice care is not to restore health or functionality, but rather to *accompany* patients as they approach the end of their natural lives and prepare themselves for the life to come. Pope Francis has spoken repeatedly of the need for both professional and familial caregivers to accompany chronically ill and dying patients, particularly the elderly, as a form of "intergenerational solidarity":

> The objective of palliative care is to alleviate suffering in the final stages of illness and at the same time to ensure the patient appropriate human accompaniment. It is important support especially for the elderly, who, because of their age, receive increasingly less attention from curative medicine and are often abandoned. Abandonment is the most serious "illness" of the elderly and also the greatest injustice they can be submitted to: those who have helped us grow must not be abandoned when they are in need of our help, our love, and our tenderness.[20(p550)]

Pope Francis emphasizes a "culture of encounter," in opposition to the "culture of waste," in which we compassionately confront our own fragility and mortality by caring for those for whom the inherent limits of human life in this world have become manifest. Emphasizing the essential importance of *interpersonal encounter*, he echoes his predecessor Pope John Paul II:

> Here we are faced with one of the more alarming symptoms of the "culture of death" . . . marked by an attitude of excessive preoccupation with efficiency and which

> sees the growing number of elderly and disabled people as intolerable and too burdensome. These people are very often isolated by their families and by society, which are organized almost exclusively on the basis of criteria of productive efficiency, according to which a hopelessly impaired life no longer has any value.
>
> The request which arises from the human heart in the supreme confrontation with suffering and death, especially when faced with the temptation to give up in utter desperation, is above all a request for companionship, sympathy and support in the time of trial. It is a plea for help to keep on hoping when all human hopes fail.[d,21,22]

In this context, Pope Francis also offers a specific challenge to physicians and other healthcare professionals to live out their authentic vocation as healers:

> The doctor's identity and commitment depends not only on scientific knowledge and technical competence, but principally on the attitude of compassion and mercy towards those who suffer in body and spirit. Compassion does not mean pity, it means "suffering with." ... True compassion does not marginalize anyone, nor does it humiliate and exclude—much less considers the disappearance of a person as a good thing. You are well aware of the meaning of the triumph of selfishness, of this "throwaway culture" that rejects and dismisses those who do not comply with certain canons of health, beauty and utility.... Frailty, pain and infirmity are a difficult trial for everyone, including medical staff. They call for patience, for "suffering-with." Therefore, we must not give in to the functionalist temptation to apply rapid and drastic solutions, moved by false compassion or by mere criteria of efficiency or cost-effectiveness. The dignity of human life is at stake. The dignity of the medical vocation is at stake.[23]

Having elucidated congruent secular and Catholic perspectives on the essential nature of the medical profession and what it entails regarding the specific vocation of healthcare professionals, using end-of-life care as an example, let us now examine how the *institutional mission* of Catholic healthcare systems supports the *formation* of the professionals they employ to live out this vocation.

Institutional Mission and Formation

For the Catholic Church, there has been a historical commitment to provide an institutional ministry to the sick.[24] Thus, while individuals like St. Teresa of Calcutta responded personally to the Christian call to care for the sick and the poor, orders of religious men and women have a deep history of starting institutions such as hospitals, hospices, orphanages, and other social services organizations that are officially recognized and designated as corporate members of the institutional Church.[25] Given such officially recognized status as entities of the Church, these institutions, by their nature, fall under the same canonical and moral norms that govern the wider institutional Church.

Once this fundamental organizational connectivity is recognized, it becomes clear why the Church has always and will continue to affirm that Catholic healthcare—that is, care officially delivered on behalf of the Catholic Church—has an explicitly (albeit not exclusively) spiritual purpose. That is, since the Church has a spiritual mission, so does

[d] For further discussion, see Reference 22.

its health ministry. The "General Introduction" of the *Directives* makes the spiritual element of Catholic healthcare explicit:

> Jesus' healing mission went further than caring only for physical affliction. He touched people at the deepest level of their existence; he sought their physical, mental, and spiritual healing (Jn. 6:35, 11:25–27). He "came so that they might have life and have it more abundantly." (Jn. 10:10)[3(General Introduction, p6)]

Since Catholic healthcare claims it is the institutional continuation of Jesus's own healing ministry, the institutions that care for the sick and the poor in his name likewise view care for the spirit as intrinsic to their mission and practice.

The specific way that spirituality fits into the purpose, goals, and delivery of healthcare is likewise well established for Catholic healthcare. This is because of the theological anthropology—the vision of the human person—that animates and guides these institutions that care on behalf of the Church. As the *Catechism of the Catholic Church* states: "Every institution is inspired, at least implicitly, by a vision of man and his destiny, from which it derives the point of reference for its judgment, its hierarchy of values, its line of conduct."[26] At its most fundamental level, this means recognizing that human persons are composite beings, a unity of a material body and a spiritual (i.e., immaterial and rational) soul.[27] Such a vision is profoundly different from a reductive anthropology that understands human beings to be nothing more than graduate animals; purely material beings that happen to be more highly evolved than some of our fellow mammals. It also differs from a neo-Gnostic view of human beings as pure minds essentially distinct from our bodies, a view promoted by some "transhumanists," who envision the future possibility of uploading one's mind into a cybernetic mainframe.[28]

Inspired by this anthropological vision, Catholic healthcare provides a distinct context and purpose for care, in which the immaterial, spiritual dimension is an essential element for the person in need of care as well as the provider. This context highlights one of the ways in which the Catholic identity and mission of an organization shapes the way professionals recognize and address spiritual dimensions of care, referred to, within Catholic healthcare, as "formation."

Professionalism-in-Context

When healthcare professionals agree to provide care on behalf of a Catholic organization, they agree to discharge their professional responsibilities within a well-defined normative context. The *Directives* clearly outline the interrelationship:

> When the health care professional and the patient use institutional Catholic health care, they also accept its public commitment to the Church's understanding of and witness to the dignity of the human person. The Church's moral teaching on health care nurtures a truly interpersonal professional-patient relationship. This professional-patient relationship is never separated, then, from the Catholic identity of the health care institution.[3(p13)]

Thus, the Catholic institution serves as a party to the relationship between the professional and patient in a way that supports and promotes that relationship. The professional is never merely part of a relationship that is reducible to a mere economic exchange between employee and employer. As an agent who acts on behalf of the organization, the professional is a representative of the organization's identity.

Since the medical professional agrees to act on behalf of the Catholic institution and, in part, represents said institution, the *Directives* affirm the responsibility of the professional to act in accordance with institutional norms and values—in other terms, its "institutional conscience"[29]:

> Employees of a Catholic health care institution must respect and uphold the religious mission of the institution and adhere to these *Directives*. They should maintain professional standards and promote the institution's commitment to human dignity and the common good.[3(n9)]

In short, those who act on behalf of the institution should embody and represent the institution well. This fact highlights a few points worth noting.

First, adhering to the philosophy of medicine outlined above, the *Directives* view the demands and responsibilities of healthcare professionals as fundamentally congruent and complementary with the Catholic mission of the organization. This is noteworthy because this belief that the goals of medicine and the demands of medical professionalism are not incompatible with the mission of Catholic healthcare is not universally shared. For instance, consider organizations, such as the American College of Obstetricians and Gynecologists (ACOG), which hold that pregnancy terminations and contraceptive practices are intrinsically part of medicine and that medical professionalism requires offering them to patients.[30] Or consider arguments put forward by Julian Savulescu and others, who argue that conscientious refusals to provide such services are incompatible with the demands of medical professionalism.[31,32]

Second, it is precisely insofar as they "maintain professional standards" that healthcare professionals fulfill the mission of the Catholic organization to operate according to the highest standards of quality and excellence. Third, and finally, the *Directives* implicitly acknowledge and accept the responsibility that Catholic institutions must continually educate, train, and form medical professionals on how to provide care authentically within the context and on behalf of the Catholic mission. That is, the organization must help the professional understand how to be a professional "in this place" or "at a Catholic institution."

To meet this need for helping and enabling healthcare professionals to understand and discharge their responsibilities competently as a *professional-in-context*, Catholic healthcare ministries have developed a branch service referred to as "formation." The Catholic Health Association, the organization that collectively represents the majority of Catholic health systems in the United States, offers the following definition of ministry formation:

> Ministry formation creates experiences that invite those who serve in Catholic health care to discover connections between personal meaning and organizational purpose. These connections inspire and enable participants to articulate, integrate, and implement the distinctive elements of Catholic health ministry so that it flourishes now and into the future.[33]

Formation, as historically defined, is part of the process by which a postulant or initiate into a religious order is prepared and shaped into being part of the community and living out the charism of the order. Thus, formation also helps the postulant discern whether life with this particular order or community is appropriate; likewise, it helps the community discern if the postulant is a good fit for the community. The formation process cuts both ways to ensure best alignment between the parties.

As applied to a professional in a Catholic healthcare ministry, formation helps the participant understand and appreciate the spiritual nature and context of the ministry. Formation activities may include group programs that involve education, spiritual exercises, communal events, journaling and self-reflection, spiritual guidance, retreats, and spiritual reading. Participation in such formation does not require that the professional be Catholic or even Christian. In fact, many professionals that serve in Catholic hospitals are not themselves Catholic but, in their own spirituality, are able to find alignment with the spiritual values and goals of the organization. In other contexts, the formation process helps professionals clarify where there are points of incongruity. While this may lead to a parting of ways, such clarity about the spiritual culture of the organization helps clarify proactively why, for instance, such separation might be best for both parties since neither would be happy in the arrangement.

To help a clinician be the best professional-in-context, the *Directives* serve as a normative guide. The *Directives* articulate principles to help professionals make decisions in alignment with the values and norms of the organization. Thus, the more formed the professional is to acknowledge, understand, and appreciate the *Directives*—even in cases in which they do not personally agree with what a particular directive requires—the more capable they are to serve as a professional in the Catholic healthcare context. In some cases, this may mean avoiding the performance of specific interventions, such as direct pregnancy termination, sterilization, or medically aided death.[3(nn45,53,60)] However, taken as a whole, the *Directives* are predominantly positive obligations for professionals to accomplish, such as to ensure informed consent, be trained to look for signs of abuse, maximize patient comfort, promote research, exhibit particular care for victims of sexual assault, and so on.[3(nn4,26,35,36,61)]

As professionals come to learn and grow in their appreciation of the *Directives* and the culture and Catholic identity they represent, *ethics consultation* is a specific service that is available to help them interpret and apply the *Directives* in concrete situations. For example, one directive states:

> Catholic health care providers should be ready to offer compassionate physical, psychological, moral, and spiritual care to those persons who have suffered from the trauma of abortion.[3(n46)]

Note how this directive outlines the positive obligation of the Catholic healthcare professional to attend to the whole person who presents to them for care, including spiritual care. Thus, while pregnancy termination procedures are not performed at Catholic facilities under the *Directives*, those same *Directives* recognize that patients might receive those interventions elsewhere and that professionals formed to practice in Catholic healthcare nevertheless maintain a special, positive obligation to care for such patients should they desire care. In this way, Catholic healthcare systems form professionals to provide care on their behalf by forming and empowering the clinicians to act as professionals-in-context as representatives of the organization.

Spiritual Care as Whole-Person Care

Catholic healthcare systems place a special emphasis on utilizing highly trained spiritual care professionals (also called pastoral care professionals or chaplains) to provide care to patients, families, and clinical staff. Professional chaplains hold graduate-level academic degrees (generally in theology [MA, PhD, or ThD], divinity [MDiv], or ministry [DMin]), 1,600 hours of clinical pastoral education, and board certification through written and oral exams demonstrating specific competencies, plus 50 hours of continuing education each year. These highly trained professionals help patients and healthcare professionals navigate the spiritual dimensions of illness—especially vulnerability, frustration, and existential dread—that accompany experiences of profound suffering and dying.

In this final section of the chapter, we highlight two of these essential pastoral care services in which pastoral care professionals seek to address spiritual issues of concern for patients and families within the context of the *Directives*: The first is sacramental ministry, while the second is the specialized profession of spiritual care.

Sacramental Ministry

In the "Introduction to Part Two: The Pastoral and Spiritual Responsibility of Catholic Health Care," the *Directives* articulate the importance of spiritual care:

> Since a Catholic health care institution is a community of healing and compassion, the care offered is not limited to the treatment of a disease or bodily ailment but embraces the physical, psychological, social, and spiritual dimensions of the human person. The medical expertise offered through Catholic health care is combined with other forms of care to promote health and relieve human suffering. For this reason, Catholic health care extends to the spiritual nature of the person. Directed to spiritual needs that are often appreciated more deeply during times of illness, pastoral care is an integral part of Catholic health care.[3(Introduction to Part Two, p10)]

Thus, for Catholic health care, the delivery of services includes an irreducible commitment to care for the spiritual needs of patients, families, and staff, which manifests in very specific and targeted ways. For example, when a patient is approaching death and a family makes a request for sacramental services, the role of the chaplain is most often to facilitate the request to the appropriate resource. In the case of Catholic sacramental services, which include Anointing of the Sick, Reconciliation, and Eucharist, the first two can be administered only by an ordained priest. Eucharist can be, and often is during times of less intense care, brought to the patient through an extraordinary (i.e., unordained lay) minister. Participation in these sacraments is for not only the patient's spiritual benefit, but also all those involved in their care:

> For Catholic patients or residents, provision for the sacraments is an especially important part of Catholic health care ministry. Every effort should be made to have priests assigned to hospitals and health care institutions to celebrate the Eucharist and provide the sacraments to patients and staff.[3(n12)]

Within Catholic health systems, sacramental care is an essential service that is offered by specialized professionals to a targeted population. However, sacramental care is not exhaustive of the role. Indeed, the provision of spiritual care as part of a holistic approach to health and healing for all patients, families, and clinicians forms the basis of the general responsibility of professional chaplains in Catholic health systems.

Spiritual Care

According to the Pastoral Care Advisory Committee of the Catholic Health Association, fifteen essential services that a spiritual care department provides are given in Table 17.1 and divided into three subcategories.

As descriptions of these essential services illustrate, the spiritual care of patients, families, and clinicians involves a wide variety of activities. These services illustrate how pastoral care professionals are rightly considered as valuable contributors to the interdisciplinary medical team.

The broad scope of spiritual care services and necessary rigorous professional training is also recognized within the *Directives*. For instance, while they give special attention to sacramental ministry, the *Directives* are clear that spiritual care is not limited to Catholic patients or sacramental ministry:

Table 17.1 Spiritual Care Departments: Fifteen Essential Services[34]

	Triage patient/family pastoral support in critical care areas
Emergency and Crisis Care	Provide care and facilitate family interactions for level 1 and 2 trauma and code blue/cardiac/respiratory arrest activations during scheduled hours
	Facilitate initial grief and bereavement support at time of death
	Provide support to parents experiencing perinatal loss
	Collaborate with an interdisciplinary team to respond to referrals for high-risk spiritual distress
	Facilitate provisions of sacraments for Catholic patients on request
	Facilitate end-of-life rituals
Referrals and Sacramental Needs	Facilitate anticipatory grieving for palliative care patients
	Respond to referral requests from surgical and other patients
	Provide spiritual assessments, interventions, and documentation for palliative care patients
	Provide spiritual assessments, interventions, and documentation for other patients on referral
	Facilitate multidisciplinary team education for accurate spiritual screening
	Provide resilience support for staff following critical incidents
Education and Staff Support	Identify ethics concerns and make appropriate response/referrals
	Facilitate education for coworkers on how to provide basic spiritual support appropriate to their role

> A Catholic health care organization should provide pastoral care to minister to the religious and spiritual needs of all those it serves. Pastoral care personnel—clergy, religious, and lay alike—should have appropriate professional preparation, including an understanding of these Directives.[3(n10)]

While spiritual care professionals are certainly recognized for their professional training and competency, it is also important that they recognize their own professional limitations, especially in an effort to maximally support patients in their own faith traditions. For instance, concern for spiritual dimensions of care is not limited to only those professionals employed by the health system. In fact, the *Directives* place great emphasis on pastoral care professionals engaging and supporting community religious leaders' involvement in patient care.

> Pastoral care personnel should work in close collaboration with local parishes and community clergy. Appropriate pastoral services and/or referrals should be available to all in keeping with their religious beliefs or affiliation.[3(n11)]

Indeed, the *Directives* outline this collaborative nature between the internal resources of the health system and the community-based religious communities, showing that each has a mutually supportive role to play.

> Pastoral care encompasses the full range of spiritual services, including a listening presence; help in dealing with powerlessness, pain, and alienation; and assistance in recognizing and responding to God's will with greater joy and peace. It should be acknowledged, of course, that technological advances in medicine have reduced the length of hospital stays dramatically. It follows, therefore, that the pastoral care of patients, especially administration of the sacraments, will be provided more often than not at the parish level, both before and after one's hospitalization.[3(Introduction to Part Two, p10)]

By understanding the limits and boundaries of their own role and professional training, as well as their responsibility to help assist patients and others receive support from religious leaders within their respective faith tradition, these professionals serve an important role in facilitating a collaborative approach to the holistic health and healing journey of individuals.

Conclusion

Our aim in this chapter has been to articulate how the largest set of religiously affiliated health systems in the United States embodies in their institutional mission and values a distinctive philosophy of medicine, in which medicine is envisioned as essentially a holistic healing profession. This vision of medicine informs a set of *Directives* that guide the formation and practice of healthcare professionals charged with exercising the Catholic Church's healing ministry in a way that contributes to the authentic flourishing of patients, especially those diagnosed with a terminal illness and experiencing the physical, psychological, and existential dread that comes with confronting one's mortality. While all healthcare professionals working within Catholic healthcare institutions should maintain awareness of and sensitivity to their patient's spiritual needs, spiritual care professionals are specifically trained to attend to the sacramental (in the case of Catholic patients) and broader spiritual concerns of patients, especially those approaching the end of their earthly life, as well as those of their families and professional caregivers.

References

1. Catholic Health Association. US Catholic Health Care 2023. Accessed 2/28/2023. https://www.chausa.org/docs/default-source/default-document-library/the-strategic-profile.pdf
2. Ascension. Mission, Vision and Values. 2024. https://about.ascension.org/our-mission
3. US Conference of Catholic Bishops. *Ethical and Religious Directives for Catholic Health Care Services*, 6th ed. USCCB; 2018. https://www.usccb.org/resources/ethical-religious-directives-catholic-health-service-sixth-edition-2016-06_3.pdf
4. Pellegrino ED. *The Philosophy of Medicine Reborn: A Pellegrino Reader*. ed. Engelhardt HT Jr, Jotterand F. University of Notre Dame Press; 2008.
5. Cavanaugh TA. *Hippocrates' Oath and Asclepius' Snake: The Birth of the Medical Profession.* Oxford University Press; 2018.
6. Quill TE. A physician's position on physician-assisted suicide. *Bull N Y Acad Med.* 1997;74(1):114–118.
7. Callahan D. When self-determination runs amok. *Hastings Cent Rep*. 1992;22(2):55.
8. Schuklenk U. Conscientious objection in medicine: private ideological convictions must not supercede public service obligations. *Bioethics*. 2015;29(5):ii–iii.
9. Engelhardt HT Jr. *The Foundations of Bioethics*. 2nd ed. Oxford University Press; 1996.
10. Curlin F, Tollefsen C. *The Way of Medicine: Ethics and the Healing Profession* University of Notre Dame Press; 2021.
11. Pellegrino ED, and Thomasma DC., *The Virtues in Medical Practice*. Oxford University Press; 1993: ch. 3, pp. 31–50.
12. May WF. *The Physician's Covenant: Images of the Healer in Medical Ethics*. 2nd ed. John Knox Press; 2000.
13. Pellegrino ED, Thomasma DC. *The Christian Virtues in Medical Practice*. Georgetown University Press; 1996.
14. Engelhardt HT Jr. *The Foundations of Christian Bioethics*. Swets and Zeitlinger; 2000.
15. Ashley BM, deBlois J, O'Rourke KD. *Health Care Ethics: A Catholic Theological Analysis*. 5th ed. Georgetown University Press; 2006.
16. United States Catholic Conference. Health and Health Care: A Pastoral Letter of the American Catholic Bishops. November 19, 1981. https://www.usccb.org/issues-and-action/human-life-and-dignity/health-care/upload/health-and-health-care-pastoral-letter-pdf-09-01-43.pdf
17. American Medical Association. Code of medical ethics, Opinions E-5.7 and E-5.8. https://www.ama-assn.org/delivering-care/ethics/code-medical-ethics-caring-patients-end-life
18. Congregation for the Doctrine of the Faith. Declaration on euthanasia. May 5, 1980. https://www.vatican.va/roman_curia/congregations/cfaith/documents/rc_con_cfaith_doc_19800505_euthanasia_en.html

19. Eisenhauer L. Catholic hospitals out front in palliative care services. *Catholic Health World.* November 1, 2019. https://www.chausa.org/publications/catholic-health-world/archives/issues/november-1-2019/catholic-hospitals-out-front-in-palliative-care-services
20. Francis. Address to the Pontifical Academy for Life. *Natl Cathol Bioeth Q.* 2015;15(3):549–551.
21. John Paul II. Evangelium vitae. March 25, 1995, n. 64. https://www.vatican.va/content/john-paul-ii/en/encyclicals/documents/hf_jp-ii_enc_25031995_evangelium-vitae.html
22. Eberl JT. I am my brother's keeper: communitarian obligations to the dying person. *Christ Bioeth.* 2018;24(1):38–58.
23. Francis. Address to the medical orders of Spain and Latin America. June 9, 2016. https://press.vatican.va/content/salastampa/en/bollettino/pubblico/2016/06/09/160609a.html
24. Crislip AT. *From Monastery to Hospital: Christian Monasticism and the Transformation of Health Care in Late Antiquity.* University of Michigan Press; 2005.
25. Farren S. *A Call to Care: The Women Who Built Catholic Healthcare in America.* Catholic Health Association; 1996.
26. *Catechism of the Catholic Church.* n. 2244. 2003. https://www.vatican.va/archive/ENG0015/_INDEX.HTM
27. Eberl JT. *The Nature of Human Persons: Metaphysics and Bioethics.* University of Notre Dame Press; 2020.
28. Eberl JT. Enhancing the *Imago Dei*: can a Christian be a transhumanist? *Christ Bioeth.* 2022;28(1):76–93.
29. Bedford EL. The reality of institutional conscience. *Natl Cathol Bioeth Q.* 2016;16(2):255–272.
30. ACOG. Abortion Policy. https://www.acog.org/clinical-information/policy-and-position-statements/statements-of-policy/2022/abortion-policy
31. Savulescu J. Conscientious objection in medicine. *BMJ.* 2006;332: 294–297.
32. Savulescu J, Schuklenk U. Doctors have no right to refuse medical assistance in dying, abortion or contraception. *Bioethics.* 2017;31(3):162–170.
33. Catholic Health Association of the United States. Definition and description. n.d. https://www.chausa.org/ministry-formation/definition-and-description
34. Catholic Health Association of the United States. Acute care settings. 2019. https://www.chausa.org/pastoralcare/private---pastoral-care-standard-work-and-staffing

18
The Professionalism and Ethics of Medical Mission Work

Rachael Essig and Peter Angelos

Key Points

- Global medicine is a rapidly developing subspecialty of many medical divisions in which young trainees are eager to participate; therefore, an outline of professional conduct is imperative.
- Professional principles are sometimes shifted in times and locations of limited resources.
- Navigating novel professional issues while learning a new culture and processing available resources can be extremely daunting, but baseline principles, discussions with local providers, and "the rapid ethical decision-making model" can assist greatly in unburdening decisions.[1]

Medical Professionalism and Global Medicine

Professionalism in medicine is based on the ethical principles upheld by those collectively in the occupation. Medical professionalism is a vast topic, including morality, communication, responsibility, patient autonomy, and competence.[2,3] These principles are well known by those in medicine but can be tricky when applied to ever-varying clinical circumstances. Often clinicians are required to completely resolve the most complex of situations while lacking formal training. In the increasingly connected world and rise of global medicine, new occurrences are now even more complicated in an unfamiliar culture and unknown language. Those medical professionals entering the international setting to practice must be equipped with the knowledge of how to traverse these potentially perplexing professional quandaries.

Global medicine is a fast-growing area of medical practice with medical trainees stating increased interest in participation in international venues.[4–6] While international destinations provide excellent opportunities to gain diverse medical knowledge and nurture cultural sensitivity, there are many challenges that arise with minimal education on navigating them.[4,7] Highlighted challenges of medical professionalism novel to the international setting are communication with language and cultural barriers; patient autonomy, including the consent process; standard of care; questions of sustainability of care; and resource scarcity add significant complexity to an already unique situation.

These issues not only can negatively impact the patient but also can increase feelings of moral injury by the provider. Throughout this chapter we draw on examples to help highlight professional challenges. This provides a framework to assess and evaluate multiple possible scenarios in order to reach an ethically defensible position. Given our background as surgeons, many cases will be surgical in nature; however, the underlying principles will be applicable across various specialties.

Ethical Challenges of Medical Professionalism

Professionalism in surgery was not historically at the perceived forefront of surgeons' minds. Prior to the invention of safe, efficacious anesthesia around 1846, surgery was all about speed in attempt to mitigate the pain.[8] Another hurdle in surgical care was infection prevention. In the late 1860s, the first reports of antiseptic treatments emerged to less fanfare than the previous discovery of anesthetic medications.[8] Surgery went from a small portion of the medical community to a force of innovation, including establishing the predecessor committee to the Joint Commission for the Accreditation of Hospitals to focus on providing effective interventions.[8] It was necessary for the advances in patient care to occur to then have the profession look inward to assess what characteristics are necessary to be a surgeon.

For surgeons or proceduralists, patient autonomy is a cornerstone of professionalism. Without the patient's permission through the consent process to make an incision, what surgeons do in the operating room is not different from an assault on the streets. This aspect of surgical care in the international setting is complicated by communication and cultural barriers. Morals are a portion of professionalism, and ethics is the framework of morality in action.[9] Ethical principles in surgery are the same as other aspects of medicine (autonomy, beneficence, nonmaleficence, and justice) and are important for the ability to decipher a difficult situation.[10]

Autonomy refers to the principle of "respect for persons."[11] In practice this is demonstrated by tailoring therapies based on not only benefit but also incorporation of the patient's values, which can be difficult to ascertain with a potential language or cultural barrier.[11] Beneficence is the standard of doing what will improve the patient's medical condition.[11] The concept of nonmaleficence denotes not bringing further injury or illness to the patient.[11] The last principle, justice, can be applied to the healthcare system overall.[11] For the health system this can mean different things, including providing care in a consistent, evidence-based approach while also recognizing that sicker patients are treated first.[12] These principles are direct constructs of what the American society values and may have to be closely scrutinized in an international setting where medical volunteerism is common.[6]

It is important to investigate and understand the culture and belief systems that construct the society for which you will be providing medical care. "Ethical imperialism" is the concept of applying your own cultural beliefs on a local civilization.[5] This does a great disservice to the local population if the foreign medical providers feel as if they have the suitable solution and act on this without complete knowledge.[5] Norms are the established guidelines for professionalism, legality, and ethics in a society.[13] The norms of Western society are familiar as that is the society in which many of us live. When visiting a new community or society, it is important to understand these norms so that ethical issues can be reasoned with correct logic.[5,13,14]

There is almost always a concern for limitations to care due to scarcity of resources as this is usually the reason for the needed medical assistance; however, those limitations that the aid team might not even consider are that of their own feelings to need to care for the largest number of people.[13] Extending to provide these legions of persons follow-up places confines on care.[13] Having additional persons present, even if there to provide aid, can place further stress on an already taxed set of resources. To not add to the limitations, it is imperative to ask the local medical providers what supplies they need and actually procure those items.[6] Moreover, bringing personal protection equipment for the aid team is essential to not detract from the local stock.[6]

Weighing these above values in an unfamiliar location can feel overwhelming. A tool that can be used to assist with the unknown professional or ethical issue in the unaccustomed society is the rapid ethical decision-making model."[1] This tool is used to prevent "ethically incorrect" resolutions to an issue.[1] The first question to ask oneself is if this situation occurred before, and can one draw on those examples to help make a decision?[1] If this is a novel situation, then the next step is to attempt to buy time until the answer is required.[1] Often these situations do not lend themselves to delaying the answer. In the case of needing a more immediate answer, the provider must then assess with the "impartiality test." [1] "The impartiality test" asks the provider to determine if they would accept the choice if in the patient's position.[1] It is important to again note that the aid provider must try to separate their established ethical principles as they likely do not apply to a different culture.[14] There can be many variances in other cultures, which creates a decision-making paradigm that is hard to replicate. This can include a shifting of what we perceive as autonomy and having a family member or community leader decide outcomes.[15] Additional challenging aspects are language barriers.[1,15]

The next portion of the model is the "universalizability test," which asks the aid provider to assess their level of comfort with the intended action if it was to be performed by all clinicians in similar situations.[1] In this section of the model, an uncomfortable topic is raised, namely, luck. Clinicians spend lifetimes trying to provide appropriate and just care to patients and try not to believe luck plays a role in treatment. For those providing aid in a less-resourced area, luck often comes into play. It is auspicious that providers are present who are able to deliver what is seen as specialty care for the region; however, simply their presence does not mean reduced resources should be stressed, consequently compromising an entire community's care.[1] This step highlights the frequently encountered limited resources, but this must be heavily weighed as a decision that would divert precious resources to an ineffective treatment for the region. Limited resources change the medical goals, but this varies with the circumstance.[1] Even in the Western world, it is considered ethical not to offer those interventions deemed to not realistically benefit the patient; however, those situations are usually due to overwhelming medical conditions and not lack of resources.[16]

The last piece of the model is the "interpersonal justifiability test." [1] With this test the provider must consider if the proposed endeavor can be defended in a public format in both the aid location and at home.[1] Often the last two tests can bring to the forefront the moral injury of the aid provider conjecturing a patient could be saved if only in their home location.[5] It is hard for a clinician to fathom withholding interventions based on lack of resources, but it is an important part of distributive justice when supplies are limited.[15]

Informed Consent: The Intersection of Autonomy, Communication, Cultural Differences, and the Standard of Care

A young female arrives at the hospital complaining of abdominal pain and lack of regular menses for the past seven weeks followed by significant vaginal bleeding today. She is having signs of peritonitis on abdominal examination, with distention and rebound tenderness. As luck would have it, you are at the hospital as a provider. The patient's urine dipstick pregnancy test is positive. You are concerned for an ectopic pregnancy and wish to treat the patient with a surgical procedure. Those that complete procedures in their clinical roles in Western medicine understand the importance of obtaining accurate informed consent. Both ethics and legality are important. There is abundant literature about the concept of informed consent and the many layers that this entails. The key concepts are providing education on the benefits and risks of the procedure while detailing other options.[11] While providing care in a low- to middle-income country (LMIC) as a general surgeon, a patient arrives at the hospital and is diagnosed with an ectopic pregnancy. Ectopic pregnancies, instead of being intrauterine, reside most commonly within the fallopian tubes and have a great risk of rupture, leading to intra-abdominal hemorrhage and the most common cause of first trimester maternal deaths.[17] The treatment of this condition is an emergency operation to remove the extrauterine pregnancy and the fallopian tube if residing in that location.[17]

The professionalism of the physicians requires that informed consent be obtained from the patient. What are the minimum standards for the consent process? The aid surgeon wants the patient to be well informed of their clinical condition, including the pathophysiology, lasting issues, and treatment. If that treatment involves a procedure the patient should be cognizant of the basic overview, benefits, risks, and long-term concerns. Concerning potential complications, having knowledge of the local resources available is important. When there is time and ability to educate the patient on all aspects of the above topics, the surgeon feels more at ease with proceeding. The legal issues that plague Western society are not as prominent in LMIC. However, documentation of consent and the subsequent procedure is extremely important for follow-up care.

Luckily the patient is awake, alert, and able to communicate. While able to communicate, they speak a different language from the surgeon. If there are not any dedicated medical translators, the barrier to appropriate translation can be treacherous. Do you accept a family member or a member of the healthcare team you know is not suitable as a translator? Would this meet the minimum standards for the consenting process? These questions are hard to answer, especially when managing a time-sensitive medical problem. A dedicated translator is found for you to educate the patient on their condition and proposed treatment. They defer their consent to both the head of their family and community leader as is tradition.[15] What are the next steps if these individuals are not present or readily available? It is tempting to be medically paternalistic, but professionalism requires cultural sensitivity and respect for the patient's wishes as long as the provider feels that the patient is adequately educated on the medical consequences.

Given that this is a condition that traditionally a general surgeon would not attend to in a location with varied specialty providers, what is the professional responsibility to inform the patient of the surgeon's usual scope of practice? Are you the correct provider to complete this procedure? There are varying thoughts on this topic. Some believe that given the emergent nature of the condition and lack of another more specialized caregiver in this location, it is reasonable to proceed if the provider feels comfortable, while others consider it unethical to operate in a capacity that is not the provider's norm.[15] Education for international surgical rotations is highly recommended to include the forty-four essential pathologies for providers in other specialties to help mitigate stress and guilt physicians may experience when in this type of position.[6,15] How does this case change if a surgical resident is completing a procedure within their own specialty? Often there is expanded autonomy on the trainee's part while providing care in LMIC. Is it ethical for a trainee to independently perform an entire procedure that they could only do under supervision at their home institution? The Accreditation Council for Graduate Medical Education (ACGME) approved trainees partaking in international rotations in 2011 if the trainee is in the senior portion of their general surgery residency.[6] This change was designed to provide bidirectional education. Remember that while education is important, educating the local providers about therapies that are unavailable in that region is an ineffective endeavor.[5]

Fortunately, the patient survives the ectopic pregnancy and recovers well from their operation. Lack of follow-up is common in LMIC and can contribute to poor sustainability of volunteer medical care.[15] The portion of the informed consent about long-term issues should be reiterated after the patient recovers. In addition to providing patient education, the local providers should also be educated on the potential complications and the resources required to manage them as they will be providing the follow-up care. This case highlights the challenges to the professionalism of physicians arising from the informed consent process, the aid providers scope of practice boundaries, increased autonomy of trainees, and the limitations on follow-up care. It is imperative that at the forefront of the aid provider's thoughts is to be flexible and respectful regarding cultural differences throughout this process. Doing so involves close work with the local providers and community leaders to be able to have a sustainable system and provide maintainable solutions to problems.[5]

Disaster States: The Intersection of Autonomy, Standard of Care, Resource Scarcity, and Care Sustainability

Disaster situations are a common reason for medical aid to be provided to another location. You travel to a tsunami-ravaged area; it is important to recognize that the values in this situation have shifted. A much greater number of patients will require medical attention, making scarce resources even harder to find in an already resource poor region. During this high-stakes time, ethical principles shift toward a more utilitarian-based approach.[5] This promises to maximize the benefit to the local population as a whole.[5,18] As the utilitarian approach suggests, the individual does not play as large a role. Triaging is an important tool when the medical system is being overwhelmed.

At some point, if care is in such high demand, there will have to be rationing of treatments.[12] It can feel as though one is shirking one's professional responsibilities to triage patients knowing that in other circumstances patients with similar injuries could have been saved.[12]

In disaster situations, the four standard ethical principles our profession bases care around change from autonomy, beneficence, nonmaleficence, and justice to fidelity, veracity, autonomy, justice, and beneficence (Table 18.1). [12] Fidelity describes the trust relationship between the provider and the patients with the knowledge less acutely ill patients will be deferred treatment until those with life-threatening conditions are stabilized.[12] Throughout the triage process, it can be difficult to know how much to disclose to a critically ill patient. The principle of veracity is the expectation a provider will divulge the truth to the patient; however, this does not require providers to explicitly tell each person that their death is imminent but a responsibility to the group as a whole.[12] As previously stated, this situation can exacerbate symptoms of moral injury a clinician may be sensing. While respect for autonomy remains important, the relative importance varies with the circumstance.[12] It has been noted that during extraordinary settings, many people may express their autonomy in an unusual way—namely with the request for those more injured to be treated before them.[12] This is a selflessness and acquiescent nature that often allows triage to occur with equitable composure. A person should not demand care that infringes on the utilitarian mindset of a disaster triage situation. Moreover, while in this position, the person's autonomy can be respected without acting in the best interest of the individual.[12] Justice in this case is a distributive justice of resources in relation to the injury.[12,15] Returning to our tsunami scenario, decisions such as not resuscitating a child that has been impaled in the chest with a tree branch while simultaneously applying a tourniquet to a bleeding extremity in the midst of fifty other severely wounded persons is overwhelming to even imagine, let alone live through.[19] These split-second decisions have an immense impact on a population. The professionalism of the physician may require these quick decisions be made by only one person. Such decision-making may fall victim to bias or even indecision, but it is the unfortunate nature of such challenging situations.[12,19]

For the greater good of the community, there must be a plan for how to transition care once the medical aid team leaves. Models can be thought of prior to even being in the situation so that there are several possibilities. Practically, once the aid team arrives there should be an assessment of the barriers to transition of care and a plan initiated.[5] Being proactive prevents the concept of "medical adventurism," where there is only doing and

Table 18.1 Changes to Ethical Principles Based on Location, Resources, and Situations

Standard Ethical Principles	Disaster States Ethical Principles
Autonomy	Fidelity
Beneficence	Veracity
Non-maleficence	Autonomy
Justice	Justice
	Beneficence

no education, which discourages local clinician confidence.[5] Furthermore, the professionalism of physicians demands an assessment of benefit to the local population rather than feeding the love of adventure by some caregivers. While most think of this as an issue that would only plague LMIC, this is a situation that could easily happen anywhere where a natural disaster, war, or terrorist attack could take place. Due to the potentially universal nature of this risk, it is imperative that all healthcare providers have the basic foundation for the professionalism and ethics associated with medical triage in disaster settings.

Long-Term Follow-Up: The Concern for Sustainability of Care

A middle-aged man arrives at the local hospital complaining of nausea, vomiting, and abdominal pain. On examination, his heart rate is elevated, and his abdomen is rigid and distended, with rebound tenderness, and is tympanitic on percussion. The local hospital is able to obtain a plain film chest radiograph that demonstrates pneumoperitoneum. This patient is whisked to the operating room, where one large and several small gastric ulcers are found. Given the multiple ulcers, the patient undergoes a gastric resection. Thankfully the patient recovers over the next few weeks and is able to be sent home. This procedure, while a standard one that all general surgical providers should be able to complete, is fraught with potential complications both during the immediate recovery and afterward.[20] Your time as an aid physician ends after the patient is discharged. What are the plans that should be completed to ensure the best follow-up care for the patient?

It is known that there are around 2.1 million deaths during the postoperative period in LMIC, which leads to a significant amount of lost productivity each year.[15] These are staggering figures. Providers should keep these in mind when performing procedures to match the operative techniques to the resources of the area.[15] This patient needs to not only follow up for basic postoperative milestones but also be educated on the signs and symptoms they may encounter and the need for lifelong acid suppression medication (not needed if a vagotomy is performed). Due to this lack of personal presence for the patient's health, there must be a program of follow-up care. While it is tempting to mimic the practice setting or treatment strategies that one might have in their home location, this often will not be beneficial to the local population.[5] There is a common theme of early involvement and education of the local practitioners. This is key to establishing any long-term sustainability in a region. The local community and providers know what the region needs and what aspects will be able to be supported by the resources available. The general principles of follow-up of any procedure or treatment should be education regarding prevention of future complications, recognition of those complications, and knowing when and how to elevate to a higher tier hospital if needed. If not educated, even extremely low-risk medications can have unintended complications, such as children eating numerous multivitamins and suffering vitamin toxicity.[21] Additionally, education on therapies that are not able to be offered due to resource limitations are not beneficial to the local care providers or community.[5] This includes things that are apparent, such as advanced trauma life support to more of what we believe to be essential diagnostic tests like reading an electrocardiogram to monitor Qtc-prolonging medications when an electrocardiographic machine is not available at the local hospital.

The Injured Individual: Intersection of Autonomy, Standard of Care, and Resource Scarcity

Previously, there was discussion of a disaster situation. This case pertains to a single trauma patient at an international aid site. An older gentleman farmer arrives at the local hospital with his right lower extremity missing from the midshin distally after an accident with his plow. The neighbors wound cloth around the leg, but the bandage is saturated with blood. He is tachycardic and pale, and his blood pressure is difficult to auscultate. Fluid boluses are given and a tourniquet is applied to the right lower extremity. At this point the patient unfortunately loses consciousness. A non-rebreather is placed on the patient to supply oxygen, but he continues to worsen, with bradycardia and eventual loss of pulses. He is pronounced dead minutes later. This situation feels different from the disaster scenario. Here, we have only one patient. Physicians may have thoughts that if only this scene had been played out in the home hospital of the aid provider, then the patient might have lived.[5] In the provider's head is the thought that we could have intubated, transfused blood products, taken the patient to the operating room immediately to control bleeding, or completed cardiopulmonary resuscitation (CPR). But in a region with extremely limited resources at a local hospital, you quickly realize to what end would you be doing these action items and with what equipment? The nearest ventilator might be 100 miles away. There might be only one blood product available. Is this the person to use that precious resource with the knowledge that the patient's injury is likely too great for him to survive in this location? If one wanted to complete an operation, it would be hard without surgical tools and an operative theater. One can argue that an amputation may be one of the easier action items to complete with little resources, but again, to what end when the other issues are unable to be corrected. Last, if you cannot intervene with any of the aforementioned issues, then completing CPR is not upholding the principle of nonmaleficence.

In this situation, utilitarianism is in play, but not the triage ethics of the previous case. Since the local hospital lacks the capacity to provide the care this patient needs, professionalism necessitates that there must be a different "standard of care" to medical treatments.[5] This again can feel morally wrong. As the provider in an unusual setting, you cannot hold yourself to the ideal standard of care philosophy of one's home hospital. It is important to always provide care that aligns with professional standards; however, it must be within the confines of institutional practice standards, which vary based on location, resources, and situation.

Conclusions

As mentioned in the disaster scenario section, most think of these professionalism concerns while in an LMIC; however, this is not the only place where they are important to consider. There can be situations of resource scarcity within a self-professed affluent nation, whether it is due to geographic isolation, an unfortunate natural disaster, or a worldwide pandemic. This makes critical thinking of ethical issues during limited resources not simply a concern for those that cross overseas, but a potential concern in a healthcare system near you.

It is important to have an understanding of the basic ethical principles. While these do not always pertain in settings of scarce resources, each concept is helpful to apply in many such situations. The rapid ethical decision-making model is a helpful tool that can be used when novel ethical choices must be rapidly made.[1] It is not enough to provide aid, but the team must also have a suitable plan for education of the local healthcare team. This is the first step to having a sustainable system in that region. The plan, like shared decision-making with patients, requires input from both the aid and local team to succeed.

More and more healthcare professionals are participating in global medicine. This chapter enhances the understanding of professionalism of physicians in international situations by providing a framework for decision-making. Following this framework through unknown situations will uphold the core ethical principles while maintaining the professionalism needed in adapting to a culture or society in order to provide complete care to those individuals.

References

1. Iserson K. The rapid ethical decisionmaking model: what critical medical interventions to use in resource-poor environments. *Camb Q Healthc Ethics.* 2011;20:1–7. doi:10.1017/S0963180110000678
2. Lotfi A. Aspiring doctors and professionalism in medicine. *US News.* February 16, 2021. Accessed November 17, 2022. https://www.usnews.com/education/blogs/medical-school-admissions-doctor/articles/professionalism-in-medicine-what-every-aspiring-physician-should-know
3. Goddard A, Patel M. The changing face of medical professionalism and the impact of COVID-19. *Lancet.* 2021;397:950–952. doi.org/10.1016/S0140-6736(21)00436-0
4. DeCamp M, Rodriguez J, Hecht S, Barry M, Sugarman J. An ethics curriculum for short-term global health trainees. *Global Health.* 2013;9(5). doi:10.1186/1744-8603-9-5
5. Iserson K, Biros M, Hollman C. Challenges in international medicine: ethical dilemmas, unanticipated consequences, and accepting limitations. *Acad Emerg Med.* 2012;19(6):683–692. doi:10.1111/j.1553-2712.2012.01376.x
6. Sherif Y, Choudhury T, Makasa E, Rosengart T, Davis R, Kaseje N. ethics of educating American global surgeons: an approach to conscientious training on the individual, departmental, and institutional levels." *J Am Coll Surg.* 2022;234(2):239–246. doi:10.1097/XCS.0000000000000026
7. Alcauskas M. From medical school to mission: the ethics of international medical volunteerism. *AMA J Ethics.* 2006;8(12):797–800. doi:10.1001/virtualmentor.2006.8.12.fred1-0612
8. Gawande A. Two hundred years of surgery. *N Engl J Med.* 2012;266:1716–1723. doi:10.1056/NEJMra1202392
9. Velji A, Bryant J. Global health ethics. In: *Understanding Global Health.* 2nd ed. McGraw Hill Medical; 2014: Chap 21, pp. 463–486 .
10. Hellsten S. Global bioethics: utopia or reality? *Dev World Bioeth.* 2008;8(2):70–81. doi:10.1111/j.1471-8847.2006.00162.x
11. Jonsen A, Siegler M, Winslade W. *Clinical Ethics: A Practical Approach to Ethical Decisions in Clinical Medicine.* 8th ed. McGraw-Hill Education; 2015.
12. Repine T, Lisagor P, Cohen D. The dynamics and ethics of triage: rationing care in hard times. *Mil Med.* 2005;170(6):505–509. doi:10.7205/milmed.170.6.505

13. Wall A. *Ethics for International Medicine: A Practical Guide for Aid Workers in Developing Countries.* Dartmouth College Press; 2012.

14. Ijsselmuiden C, Faden R. Research and informed consent in Africa—another look. *N Engl J Med.* 1992;326(12):830–833. doi:10.1056/NEJM199203193261212

15. Agochukwu-Mmonu N, Chung K. Ethics in global surgery." *Hand Clin.* 2019;35(4):421–427. doi:10.1016/j.hcl.2019.07.013

16. Nonbeneficial ("futile") emergency medical interventions. *Ann Emerg Med.* 2017;70(1):117–118. doi:10.1016/j.annemergmed.2017.03.056

17. Goyaux N, Leke R, Keita N, Thonneau P. Ectopic pregnancy in African developing countries. *Acta Obstet Gynecol Scand.* 2003;82(4):305–312. doi:10.1034/j.1600-0412.2003.00175.x

18. Baker R, Strosberg M. Triage and equality: an historical reassessment of utilitarian analyses of triage. *Kennedy Inst Ethics J.* 1992;2(2):103–123. doi:10.1353/ken.0.0035

19. Moskop J, Iserson K. Triage in medicine, part II: underlying values and principles. *Ann Emerg Med.* 2007;49(3):282–287. doi:10.1016/j.annemergmed.2006.07.012

20. McCord C, Ozgediz D, Beard J, Debas H. General surgical emergencies [Essay]. In: Haile T. Debas, Peter Donkor, Atul Gawande, et al., eds. *Disease Control Priorities: Essential Surgery.* 3rd ed. World Bank; 2015:61–76.

21. Decamp M. Scrutinizing global short-term medical outreach. *Hastings Cent Report.* 2007;37(6):21–23. doi:10.1353/hcr.2007.0096

19
Special Considerations for Military and Veterans

Ronald Place and Steven G. Sugden

Key Points

- Military medicine is categorically different from the provision of medicine in civilian populations.
- Principles of military medical professionalism and medical ethics support the integration of lessons from military medicine and civilian-based medical care.
- Despite differences in the provision of care in military medicine, the training of military effectively mirrors the medical training they would receive outside of their military duty.

> The U.S. Military's purpose is to protect our Nation and win our wars. We do this through military operations to defend the homeland, build security globally, and project power and win decisively. Our military supports diplomatic, informational, and economic activities that promote our enduring national interests.[1]

Introduction

For centuries, communities have relied on armed forces to defend their homeland, build security within their regions, or project power toward their neighbors. Since its initial revolution, the United States has relied on its military to provide these services. Historically, however, the United States did not have a standing military until the twentieth century. Following this, social scientists like Samuel Huntington and Morris Janowitz started defining the characteristics of professionalism within military service.[2] These characteristics are summarized in the following concepts: "expertise, jurisdiction, and legitimacy."[2] The purpose of this review is to show how these principles create the uniqueness of the medical military profession and how this profession has influenced healthcare.

Military Medicine Expertise

Military medicine is a complex, diverse, mobile, and highly unpredictable specialty of medicine that has a unique role in maintaining and preserving the health of *Soldiers* (this term is used generically here to include Soldiers, Sailors, Marines, Airmen, and Airwomen. The expertise of military medicine incorporates the mastery of all medical specialties.[2,3] Additionally, these services can be provided in traditional brick-and-mortar hospitals that are affiliated with military bases or in mobile, austere environments. The ability to provide this level of diverse care is considered a force multiplier, as it improves the overall health of the Soldier and helps the military achieve its mission. The final aspect of expertise is using the mastery of knowledge to benefit those around them.[2] By operating in this unique environment, the U.S. military has developed expertise in trauma care, infectious disease, and public health and has used its expertise to shape healthcare.

Advancement in Trauma Care

Due to the nature of armed conflicts, traumatic injury has been a significant cause of Soldier mortality on the battlefield. In addition to the operation art that the Napoleonic wars brought, Dominique Jean Larrey, surgeon in chief of French armies, introduced criteria for triage and the "flying ambulance" as a means to quickly evacuate wounded Soldiers to a centralized location to receive more definitive treatment.[4] Despite the adoption of triage and the eventual use of helicopters, the U.S. military still noted a 91% prehospital mortality rate during the Korean War and 88% prehospital mortality rate during the Vietnam War.[5] The majority of these deaths were due to hemorrhaging from extremity wounds.[6]

Within the U.S. military community, a pragmatic, continuous approach can be adopted in lieu of waiting for a randomized clinical trial to determine standards of care.[7] For example, during the Mogadishu conflict, U.S. Special Forces medics faced a dilemma about how to attend to their fellow Soldiers, who were hemorrhaging from extremity wounds and could not be evacuated for more than 15 hours. They reintroduced tourniquet use as an effective and safe means to stop bleeding. Their "lessons learned" became critical in developing tactical combat casualty care (TCCC), which is now the foundation of trauma care within the U.S. military combat doctrine as well as first responders within the United States.[8] This process reduced the prehospital mortality rate to less than 10% among U.S. Soldiers, and it has improved trauma care within the United States.[9]

Advancement in Infectious Disease

Next, the U.S. military has developed expertise in the identification of infectious diseases and parasites and the development of vaccines and prophylaxis treatments as a means to protect its soldiers. The Spanish-American War of 1898 was a relatively brief conflict that was mostly fought in Cuba. Although there were 260 U.S. fatalities from combat-related injuries, records indicate that nearly 1,600 U.S. Soldiers died from typhoid and yellow fever. MAJ Walter Reed led the commission that studied these diseases. He found how typhoid, typically a waterborne illness, had spread due to human-to-human and fly contact.[10] Later, MAJ Reed determined how yellow fever had been spread by the *Aedes aegypti* mosquitoes.[11] Improved sanitation[9] and vector eradication measures were implemented to protect Soldiers.[11] In 1909, MAJ Fredrick Russell developed the first typhoid vaccine.[11]

Although World War I (WWI) broke out in 1914, the United States did not officially enter the war until 1917. As U.S. Soldiers were drafted and prepared for war, many encountered a more deadly agent, the Spanish flu, than the actual combat. Of the 115,660 reported casualties among U.S. military, more than half were due to the Spanish flu.[12] Additionally, between 20% and 40% of all U.S. military were impacted by the Spanish flu.[12] Military medical officers treated soldiers, conducted epidemiological surveys, and tried implementing social distancing and sanitation standards. It was not until the 1930s that the influenza pathology could be identified. Even though the U.S. military has not suffered from infectious disease and parasites, it has made significant contributions to knowledge of trench fever, pneumococcus, hepatitis A and B, rubella, Japanese encephalitis, leishmaniasis, schistosomes, malaria, anthrax, Ebola, and COVID-19 (see References 11, 13, and 14).

Advancements in Public Health

Ensuring the health of an army's soldiers has been a critical aspect of military strategy. The U.S. military uses the term force health protection (FHP) to encompass aspects of public health within the context of all potential global health challenges. The importance of public health, particularly sanitation, has been traced back to Romans, who laid out camps and maintained latrines downstream from their soldiers.[4] Yet, within the U.S. military, FHP was first initiated within the Continental Army, under General George Washington. During a smallpox epidemic, Washington ensured that his Soldiers were inoculated for smallpox and effectively started the first immunization campaign within the U.S. military.[11] Following the discovery of the typhoid vaccine in 1909, all U.S. military were required to receive the vaccine prior to deploying to WWI.[11] As new vaccines are developed, the U.S. military continues to address the importance of vaccination as a vital component of FHP [15] This campaign has continued through COVID-19. Not only has the U.S. military advocated for the administration of the COVID-19 vaccination among soldiers, but has also helped distribute and administer COVID-19 vaccinations throughout the United States.[16]

During the winter of 1777–1778, the Continental Army struggled to survive its winter encampment at Valley Forge, Pennsylvania. Benjamin Rush, the newly appointed surgeon general of the Continental Army, found the sanitation conditions "deplorable," and he exhorted General Washington to make improvements to the encampment sanitation, which included: improving the soldiers' dress, diet, cleanliness, encampment (sanitation), and exercise.[17] Rush's initial demands continue to be at the center of the U.S. military FHP.

Since the humble beginning of the Continental Army, the U.S. military has incorporated the importance of sanitation within its doctrine.[18] Through every campaign since then, the U.S. military has attempted to incorporate sanitation as part of its encampment setup (see References 19–21). Similarly, following WWI, the U.S. military has developed a standard of physical fitness. Each branch has developed its own unique requirements based on the service's needs.[22] Finally, dietary needs have long been a logistic challenge for the U.S. military throughout every campaign. Due to the diversity of deployable environments and the potential scarcity of adequate caloric intake, the U.S. military has relied heavily on highly processed foods. This may account for the high rates of Soldiers with prediabetes[23] and the doubled rate of type 2 diabetes among U.S. veterans compared to the normal population.[24] To address both fitness and dietary needs, the U.S. military has developed the Total Force Fitness program,[25] in conjunction with the U.S. Air Force's Lifestyle and Performance Medicine Initiative to further address these needs.

Military Medicine Jurisdiction

As noted, military medicine has developed its expertise in the domain where it is practiced, which is the professional definition of jurisdiction.[2] The actual entity by which the U.S. military provides care is the Military Health System (MHS), operated by the Department of Defense (DOD). The DOD has a legal obligation to provide healthcare to a diverse population of almost 10 million Americans, ranging from infants to the elderly. While the central purpose of the MHS is to ensure the medical readiness of the U.S. military personnel, they also provide care for the family members of active-duty Soldiers and retired military Soldiers and family members. The MHS operates worldwide—with brick-and-mortar military hospitals and clinics throughout the United States and its territories and in a number of overseas countries, including the United Kingdom, Belgium, Germany, Spain, Italy, Turkey, Greece, Japan, South Korea, Cuba, and other operating locations in support of U.S. Soldiers throughout the world.

Military Medicine Legitimacy

Finally, to claim that military medicine is a legitimate profession and adheres to a professionalism code, it needs to be shown that the U.S. military provides a unique education and adherence to ethical codes.

Education and Development of Military Medical Professionals

From the onset of the Continental Army, the U.S. military relied heavily on medical professionals, but it was not until 1818, when the US Congress made the Medical Department a permanent component of the military, that it did not have to be stood down after each campaign. Later, in 1847, medical professionals were given rank, and finally, in 1909, the "Medical Corp" became a permanent branch. During WWI, it was estimated that up to 30% of the U.S. total medical providers were serving within the military.[12] Though the overall percentage of U.S. healthcare providers who serve in the US military is lower than in WWI, there are currently over 10,000 active-duty providers,[26] and this is significantly higher when U.S. Reservist and National Guard providers are taken into consideration.

Today, medical professionals enter military service from a variety of backgrounds and education routes. For the purposes of this chapter, the principal focus is on physician accession and professional development, but the pathways for other medical professionals—pharmacists, psychologists, nurses, administrators, and others—follow a similar pathway.

Though a small number of medical professionals begin their undergraduate education within the military academies—the U.S. Military Academy (West Point), the U.S. Naval Academy (Annapolis), or the U.S. Air Force Academy (Colorado Springs)—the majority of military medical professionals receive their undergraduate medical education from either state or private schools. Some will have participated in university-supported Reserve Officer Training Corps (ROTC), but many others will pursue military service without ROTC experience and access military service through direct commissioning programs and Officer Candidate School (OCS) or Officer Training School (OTS).

For prospective medical school students emerging from undergraduate programs, however, there are two principal pipelines for those interested in military service. The first avenue is through the Uniformed Services University of the Health Sciences (USU), located in Bethesda, Maryland. Self-described by DOD leaders as "the nation's federal health professions academy," similar to the U.S. military academies at West Point, Annapolis, and Colorado Springs. Just like the academies, medical students are not charged tuition, and they repay their tuition through time in service. Furthermore, medical students are commissioned as officers and given the rank of Second Lieutenant (Army or Air Force) or Ensign for their four-year schooling—the most junior officer rank possible. The differentiating element of the USU curricula, as opposed to civilian educational institutions, is the added focus on military medical leadership and medical operations in deployed locations. USU graduates approximately 175 medical students each year, and USU graduates comprise approximately 25% of all physicians on active duty.[27]

The second avenue—and representing the largest pool for military physician accessions—is through medical school education financed through the Health Professions Scholarship Program (HPSP). Through this route, medical school tuition is paid by the sponsoring military department—the Army, Navy, or Air Force. Tuition and a stipend for incidental expenses (books, equipment, supplies) are paid. Students may obtain two-, three-, or four-year scholarships and incur a service obligation that is commensurate with the length of the scholarship. However, HPSP scholarship students are commissioned as U.S. Reserve component officers and do not receive a salary while in medical school. Specialized annual military training is required for HPSP students, and they are paid for their time in this training.

On graduation from medical school, students are competitively selected for residency programs. These residencies may be completed at any number of military medical centers and hospitals around the world or—depending on the specialty—completed at civilian institutions in the United States. On residency completion, most newly credentialed physicians will begin practicing in military medical facilities or within Reserve or National Guard units.

Regardless of the entry point, military medical professionals are expected to complete the same level of professional military education as their nonmedical counterparts. Here, they are taught further military leadership and how their role enhances the overall military function. They are also expected to maintain their medical board certifications. For those military medical professionals who are not active-duty members, they participate in monthly weekend training and annual yearly training and stand ready to respond to future deployments.

Military Medical Ethics

Military physicians adhere to the fundamental tenets of medical ethics. There are numerous circumstances, however, in which military medical professionals may be placed that may create challenges unknown to civilian practitioners. To address these concerns, the DOD issued the DOD Instruction 6025.27, "Medical Ethics in the Military Health System." Within this document, the DOD outlined ten principles, which expanded the American Medical Association's eight principles. Key differences center on the unique missions and the unique role of US national security.[28]

The executive summary from the Defense Health Board captures those areas where different ethical considerations may emerge and later outlines steps to address them:

> Military health care professionals serve in a variety of settings, more diverse than is typically found in the civilian environment. . . . Military health care professionals are also expected to care for detainees, enemy combatants, nonstate actors, local nationals, and coalition forces. In addition, U.S. military personnel are often deployed to assist in humanitarian missions, such as natural disasters, or to provide care to local citizens in combat zones. . . . Conflicting roles and expectations of how one fills multiple responsibilities and obligations can place the health care professional in a difficult and ambiguous situation. Potential ethical conflicts between professional standards and other values, commitments, or interests can become even more acute when health care professionals work in military environments. . . . For the military health care professional, it can be more pronounced in the combat or detainee setting. As a health care provider, the professional is obligated to preserve life, attend the sick and wounded, and minimize suffering, even on behalf of the enemy. On the other hand, the health care professional, as a Service member, is obligated to support the mission, maintain military readiness, and support military operations. Tensions can arise if the demands of the mission or line command are at odds or in tension with the duties to attend to the health of those needing care. . . . This type of decision-making structure can be challenging to health care professionals who are facing ambiguous or uncharted territory that requires them to rely on their judgment, discretion, and in accordance with nonmilitary professional standards.[29]

Conclusion—Challenges and Opportunities Ahead

This chapter is intended to introduce the military medical profession and to familiarize the reader with information on the DOD legacy, services, and programs to care for those in uniform today and those who have served in the past.

In 2016, the National Academies of Sciences highlighted this demand with their seminal report: *A National Trauma Care System: Integrating Military and Civilian Trauma Systems to Achieve Zero Preventable Deaths After Injury.*[30] This report pointed out that both systems can benefit from greater sharing of best practices and clinical processes. The advances made in wartime need to be shared more rapidly with civilian counterparts. Conversely, in peacetime, military medical professional's exposure to trauma cases naturally goes down—and learning shifts to civilian experiences.

Technology advances, to include significant leaps forward in clinical simulation, provide a platform for improved performance across American medicine. Nonetheless, there are opportunities for deeper partnerships in graduate medical education, resource sharing in select communities, and opportunities for civilian medical professionals to practice in medical institutions. These partnerships can only be achieved through better understanding of the unique populations served by federal healthcare providers; by familiarity with the individuals who serve in federal health systems; and by ongoing communication and legal frameworks that permit greater sharing of resources, talent, and learnings. This chapter is a first step on this path. Readers are encouraged to reach out nationally or locally to investigate how partnerships can be strengthened and grown in the years ahead.

References

1. The national military strategy of the United States of America. 2015. Accessed 25 February 2023. https://www.jcs.mil/Portals/36/Documents/Publications/2015_National_Military_Strategy.pdf
2. Burk J. Expertise, jurisdiction, and legitimacy of the military profession. In: Snider DM, Matthews LJ, eds. *The Future of the Army Profession*. 2nd ed. McGraw Hill Custom Publishing; 2005:19–38.
3. Raeeszadeh M, Goodarzi H, Moghaddam JA, Machian MSB, Gooshki HS, Khoshi A. The role of military medicine and the significance of training military medicine. *J Family Med Prim Care*. 2022;11(8):4184–4189. doi:10.4103/jfmpc.jfmpc_80_22.
4. Van Way C 3rd. War and trauma: a history of military medicine. *Mo Med*. 2016;113(4):260–263.
5. Rasmussen TE, Baer DG, Cap AP, Lein BC. Ahead of the curve: sustained innovation for future combat casualty care. *J Trauma Acute Care Surg*. 2015;79(4 suppl 2):S61–S64. doi:10.1097/TA.0000000000000795
6. Bellamy RF. The causes of death in conventional land warfare: implications for combat casualty care research. *Mil Med*. 1984;149(2):55–62.
7. Elster EA, Butler FK, Rasmussen TE. Implications of combat casualty care for mass casualty events. *JAMA*. 2013;310(5):475–476. doi:10.1001/jama.2013.167481
8. Butler FK Jr, Hagmann JH, Richards DT. Tactical management of urban warfare casualties in special operations. *Mil Med*. 2000;165(4 suppl):1–48.
9. Bailey JA, Morrison JJ, Rasmussen TE. Military trauma system in Afghanistan: lessons for civil systems? *Curr Opin Crit Care*. 2013;19(6):569–577. doi:10.1097/MCC.0000000000000037
10. Gotschlich EC. Bullets and bacilli. The Spanish-American War and military medicine. *J Clin Invest*. 2005;115(1):3. doi:10.1172/JCI24100
11. Artenstein AW, Opal JM, Opal SM, Tramont EC, Peter G, Russell PK. History of US military contributions to the study of vaccines against infectious diseases. *Mil Med*. 2005;170(4 suppl):3–11. doi:10.7205/milmed.170.4s.3
12. Byerly CR. The US military and the influenza pandemic of 1918–1919. *Public Health Rep*. 2010;125(Suppl 3):82–91.
13. Crum NF, Aronson NE, Lederman ER, Rusnak JM, Cross JH. History of US military contributions to the study of parasitic diseases. *Mil Med*. 2005;170(4 suppl):17–29. doi:10.7205/milmed.170.4s.17
14. Biselli R, Nisini R, Lista F, et al. A historical review of military medical strategies for fighting infectious diseases: from battlefields to global health. *Biomedicines*. 2022;10(8):2050. doi:10.3390/biomedicines10082050
15. Grabenstein JD, Pittman PR, Greenwood JT, Engler RJ. Immunization to protect the US Armed Forces: heritage, current practice, and prospects. *Epidemiol Rev*. 2006;28:3–26. doi:10.1093/epirev/mxj003

16. Gibson-Fall F. Military responses to COVID-19, emerging trends in global civil-military engagements. *Rev Int Stud.* 2021;47(2):1–16. doi:10.1017/S0260210521000048
17. Carlson ET. Benjamin Rush on revolutionary war hygiene. *Bull N Y Acad Med.* 1979;55(7):614–635.
18. Joint Health Service. Joint Publication 4.02. *Joint Chiefs of Staff,* 17 Dec 2017. Accessed 25 Feb 2023.
19. Blaisdell FW. Medical advances during the Civil War. *Arch Surg.* 1988;123(9):1045–1050. doi:10.1001/archsurg.1988.01400330021001
20. Lewis, JJ. Sanitary Commission (USSC). ThoughtCo. August 26, 2020. thoughtco.com/sanitary-commission-ussc-3528670
21. Czerw RJ. Perspective. Force health protection. *US Army Med Dep J.* 2009;April–June:1–5.
22. Knapik JJ, East WB. History of United States Army physical fitness and physical readiness training. *US Army Med Dep J.* 2014;April–June:5–19.
23. Clutter CA, Beckman DJ, Wardian JL, Rittel AG, True MW. Are we missing an opportunity? Prediabetes in the US military. *Mil Med.* 2022;July 4:usac197. doi:10.1093/milmed/usac197
24. Davis PJ, Liu M, Sherman S, et al. HbA1c, lipid profiles and risk of incident type 2 diabetes in United States Veterans. *PLoS One.* 2018;13(9):e0203484. doi:10.1371/journal.pone.0203484
25. United States Army. *Field Manual 7.22.* 2020. Accessed 25 February 2023.
26. Cole R, Rudinsky S, Conley SP, et al. The impact of medical school on military physicians' readiness for their first deployment. *Mil Med.* 2022;187(7–8):e995–e1006. doi:10.1093/milmed/usac049
27. Uniformed Services University. Home page. https://www.usuhs.edu. Accessed 25 February 2023.
28. Thomas R, Lough F, Girton J, Casciotti JA. A code of ethics for military medicine. *Mil Med.* 2020;185(5–6):e527–e531. doi:10.1093/milmed/usaa007
29. Defense Health Board Report, Ethical Guidelines and Practices for US Military Medical Professionals. March 3, 2015. Accessed 25 February 2023.
30. Committee on Military Trauma Care's Learning Health System and Its Translation to the Civilian Sector; Board on Health Sciences Policy; Board on the Health of Select Populations; Health and Medicine Division; National Academies of Sciences, Engineering, and Medicine. *A National Trauma Care System: Integrating Military and Civilian Trauma Systems to Achieve Zero Preventable Deaths After Injury.* Berwick D, Downey A, Cornett E, eds. National Academies Press; 2016 Sep 12.

20
Cultivating Professionalism Through Difficult Conversations

Nathan Carlin

Key Points

- Samuel Shem's *The House of God* was—and remains—controversial.
- Once contextualized and understood, *The House of God* is useful in encouraging the professional identity formation of medical interns and residents because it gives voice to their suffering.

Introduction

While few would doubt the importance of teaching professionalism to interns and residents, there is perhaps less consensus on the best way to teach it. In general, the didactic lecture has fallen out of favor in medical education,[1] with a growing preference for more active and experiential learning, such as team-based learning or problem-based learning modules in undergraduate medical education.[2] Also, within the literature on professionalism, there has been a movement toward the term *professional identity formation* to focus on the inner lives of trainees, beyond discussions of behavior and compliance.[3,4] Medical humanities,[5] and specifically the subfields of literature and medicine and narrative medicine,[6] have made the case for the use of memoir, fiction, poetry, and other genres; arts; and media for the teaching of ethics and professionalism on the grounds that these can offer a thicker or richer account of human experience than other approaches (e.g., clinical case presentations).[7]

In this chapter, I use literature to engage in professional identity formation. Specifically, I focus on Samuel Shem's *The House of God*.[8] I do so for three reasons. First, the book is so controversial that it is inevitable that it will generate discussion. Second, the book raises a striking number of professionalism issues, many of which remain relevant since its publication in 1978. And third, in a unique way the novel gives voice to the suffering of interns. By reading the novel and reflecting on the issues it raises in their own lives, the book can be used to host difficult conversations with interns and residents about their own experiences and identities in a way that is unlikely to occur with other pedagogical methods.

A Word About Difficult Conversations in Medical Education

Generally, in medical education—both undergraduate and graduate—the idea of difficult conversations refers to communication skills with patients and their families, or what used to be called bedside manner. The topic that gets the most attention in this regard is how to deliver bad news to patients.[9] The literature is weighted toward end-of-life conversations,[10] and it is specialty specific.[11,12] Other important topics that have received attention include discussions about error disclosure[11] and, more recently, conversations about implicit bias.[13]

What *The House of God* offers is that it can enable a different kind of difficult conversation within medical education, one that cuts to its very heart. If the literature on difficult conversations within medical education tends to focus on improving how clinicians interact with patients, *The House of God* invites—no, *requires*—us to look at the soul of the profession and ask: What if we are doing it all wrong? This is indeed a very difficult conversation to have when our jobs, identities, and lives are on the line.

The House of God

Samuel Shem is the pen name of Stephen Bergman (b. 1944). Trained as a psychiatrist, though he no longer identifies as such, preferring instead the more general title of "doctor," Shem gained international acclaim for *The House of God*, which fictionalized his intern year at Beth Israel Hospital, affiliated with Harvard Medical School.

In "The Satiric Image: Healers in *The House of God*,"[14] Kathryn Montgomery Hunter situates the novel within a broad historical and literary context, observing that what makes Shem's *The House of God* unique is that it is the first novel to criticize via humor the medical profession *from the inside*. She writes: "*The House of God* attacks the profession itself and its sacred center: the process by which ordinary young men and women become expert practitioners."[14(p137)] She suggests that the force of the novel is its timeliness, for "many of our moral questions are currently expressed in the medical arena." [14(p145)] While "medicine cannot answer these questions," she writes, "it [also] cannot ignore them." [14(p145)]

The novel is set in the 1970s at a teaching hospital (the House of God) in Boston, Massachusetts, following the training of Roy Basch, who graduated from Best Medical School. As noted, Shem himself graduated from Harvard Medical School and completed his intern year at Beth Israel Hospital. Thus, the House of God stands for Beth Israel Hospital and Best Medical School stands for Harvard Medical School. Shem has indicated in interviews that much of what he writes is based on modified real events, what he calls "imagined autobiography" or "a half step off real."[a,15]

Roy begins his internship with a feeling of apprehension, fearing that medical school did not really prepare him for residency. The first resident that he encounters is named the Fat Man, who, at first, seems cynical, eccentric, and unethical. However, during the course of the year the Fat Man is revealed to be correct on just about every matter. He turns out to be deeply compassionate as well. As such, the Fat Man is a kind of moral guide for Roy. The Fat Man offers a number of Laws of the House of God to Roy and the other interns, and, during the course of the year, Roy adds to the Laws as well.[b] These Laws are examined below.

[a] Personal conversation, October 29, 2020.
[b] See, for example, Law 10 (Shem, *The House of God*, 123).

During his intern year, Roy becomes disillusioned with the way that medicine works. He learns about turfing (the practice of finding a way to get a patient out of your service as quickly as possible) and bouncing (the practice of sending patients back to the service from which they were turfed). He is disappointed to discover that so much of medicine seems to be about billing. When the basic model is fee for service, there is a built-in incentive to do procedures, but, as the Fat Man taught the interns, less is often more in medicine, for interventions can cause more harm than good.

So, the Fat Man taught the interns to do as little as possible and to lie in charting (which is fraud) to disguise the fact that they were doing nothing. When the interns did this, the patients did, in fact, do better. While his patients loved him, the Fat Man was an outsider, and neither the hospital administrators nor the other rule-following residents liked him much.

The novel progresses by detailing the grueling nature of internship, both its physical and emotional demands. In the 1970s (prior to duty hour restrictions for residents), it was not uncommon for residents to work over 100 hours in a week. But, after the death of Libby Zion in 1984, who died at the age of 18 because of, as alleged by her father, neglect from overworked residents, limits on the number of hours that residents can work were put in place.[16] Usually, residents are not permitted to work more than 80 hours a week, though there is some flexibility in surgical specialties. *The House of God* also likely played a role in the creation of duty hour restrictions as well, as it gave voice to these struggles prior to Zion's death.

Why did *The House of God* gain so much popularity? Why does it continue to sell well? I think the reason is this: Shem gave voice to the brutal conditions of medical training, and, while there has been reform, internship is still physically and emotionally difficult. As Roy puts it: "This internship—this whole training—it destroys people," and, as Berry responds: "Yes. It's a disease. The kind of stress you are under, unless you can find some safety, some caring, you've got only a few choices: kill yourself, go crazy, kill someone else."[8(p311)] I asked a department chair at a medical school about this recently, and he said: "Things are better than they used to be, but there is no way around it—internship is hard."[c]

The theme of burnout is a major one in Shem's book, and, due to a lack of institutional support, a fellow intern does die by suicide in *The House of God*. In an interview, Shem once noted that writing "kept me from suicide."[16]Because physicians are still today at great risk of suicide—more so than the general population[17]—Shem remains timely.

Toward the end of the book, Berry suggests to Roy that he should become a psychiatrist, feeling that psychiatry would seem to suit him and make him happy, offering him a chance at curing people in a different way. Roy is persuaded by this idea, and so, too, are several other interns. The novel can be read as a kind of rebuke of internal medicine in general and of internship in particular. Roy is hopeful to find something better in psychiatry.

Shem's Use of Satire

In "*The House of God*: Another Look," Delese Wear [18] offers an insightful discussion on the anger directed at Shem over the years, suggesting that this has been the result of a

[c] I have chosen to leave this quotation unattributed.

basic lack of understanding of satire in Shem's writings. If Montgomery Hunter situated *The House of God* as satire, Wear explores the fact that this nevertheless has not been appreciated. In part, this could be because, as she points out, Shem resisted the label of satire on the grounds that satire "implies a departure from reality," whereas Shem insists that what he has written is true, though sometimes exaggerated for the sake of humor. Still, Wear writes: "Without aiming to write satire, Shem achieves its intent," for "its goal is social correction." She continues:

> Shem takes very ordinary, recognizable characters—the intern, the attending, the nurse, the patient—and depicts them in ways no one dared to do before.... He uses one tool of satire—humor—to portray how, in the hospital, those in power act inhumanely toward those without power—attendings act inhumanely toward trainees, doctors at all levels act inhumanely toward patients. It is this wit, this often macabre humor, that keeps the novel from falling into a direct expression of bitterness and anger. Further, good satire is the *engine* of anger rather than its direct expression, but it may produce anger in its readers.[18(p499)]

Because Shem is writing fiction, he is able to use satire in a way that other forms of teaching—such as a didactic lecture—cannot. Also, the topics that he is writing about are very painful for interns, so his use of humor enables one to talk about these matters in a way that may feel safer for trainees than if they were to offer cases from their own clinical practice outside of the context of discussing this novel.

It is also important to realize that Shem is not at all cynical. This is widely misunderstood. In an interview Shem noted:

> Some have said that *The House of God* is cynical. And yet in rereading, it has a constant message that I was dimly conscious of in writing: being with the patient. In the words of the hero of the novel, the Fat Man, "I make them feel that they're still part of life, part of some grand nutty scheme, instead of alone with their diseases. With me, they still feel part of the human race." And as the narrator Roy Basch realized, "What these patients wanted was what anyone wanted: the hand in their hand, the sense that their doctor could care."[19]

Relatedly, in another interview, this one on Shem's *Man's 4th Best Hospital*, the issue of cynicism and idealism was noted to be a key feature of his current writing:

Interviewer: Speaking of the Fat Man and his idealism, one of the lines he says caught my attention. He says to a resident, "I'm so idealistic, to you I sound cynical." I felt that's how the book started—a little cynical—but by the end I realized that, yeah, this book *is* idealistic. That one line seemed to capture everything.

Shem: As a writer, you don't plan to write a line like that. It came out of God, out of the Divinity, you know, not me.[20]

Of note, Shem sees himself as an optimist, and he pointed out to me that all of his novels have an arc where the main character plunges into despair, but, by the end, they are saved in some way, which, he added, is rooted in his spirituality.[21]

Using the Laws of *The House of God* to Teach Professionalism

The House of God is a fairly long novel. One way to get a handle on it for use in teaching is by focusing on the Laws. I offer some discussion of these Laws, noting in a table some of professionalism issues that they raise. The Laws are as follows:

1. Gomers don't die.
2. Gomers go to ground.
3. At a cardiac arrest, the first procedure is to take your own pulse.
4. The patient is the one with the disease.
5. Placement comes first.
6. There is no body cavity that cannot be reached with a #14 needle and a good strong arm.
7. Age + BUN = Lasix dose.
8. They can always hurt you more.
9. The only good admission is a dead admission.
10. If you don't take a temperature, you can't find a fever.
11. Show me a BMS who only triples my work and I will kiss his feet.
12. If the radiology resident and the BMS both see a lesion on the chest X ray, there can be no lesion there.
13. The delivery of medical care is to do as much nothing as possible.[8(p361)]

For anyone outside of medicine—and also for persons unfamiliar with this novel—the reader is left with certain impressions when encountering these Laws for the first time. One is that these Laws are filled with many inside references or jokes. What is a gomer? What is a #14 needle? What does the equation about the Lasix dose mean? Another is that the list, at times, is obviously cynical ("the only good admission is a dead admission"). While both of these impressions are true, the Laws also are filled with good advice and, on deeper reflection, idealism.

Let's begin with the first Law: "Gomers don't die." GOMER stands for the feeling a resident has when a chronically ill older person enters the emergency department: "Get out of my emergency room!"[8(p28)] In an interview, Shem noted that he did not coin the term *gomer*. This is something that he heard being used during his clinical training. But he added that he *did* coin the French feminine form of the term: *Gomere*.[8(364),15] In any case, the term, of course, is ageist, mean, and uncompassionate. One would be deeply offended if one's parent or grandparent were referred to as a gomer by a health professional. And this is why Shem's use of satire is so controversial. Readers wonder: Is he being ageist by writing this way or is he criticizing ageism? Is Shem acting like a mirror, reflecting back to medicine the ageism that he witnessed, or is he partaking in it?

As intimated above, the same question of Shem holds for other categories of identity: race, gender, class, able-bodied-ness, fatness, and more. Clearly, the medical culture of the 1970s was ageist, racist, sexist, classist, ableist, and biased against fat persons. Shem has faced a great deal of criticism over these issues of identity politics and humor.[20] Indeed, some years ago Shem publicly addressed these criticisms at a conference on *The House of God* when some of the discussion of the book focused on its sexism.[22] While, to his credit, Shem admitted that *The House of God* is sexist, he does not regret what he wrote because he feels that it was important to describe the sexism of the times.

In a recent interview, Mara Gordon picked up on this criticism. Here is an excerpt:

Gordon: One of the major criticisms of *The House of God* is that it's sexist. It seems like your hero, Dr. Basch, has gotten a little more enlightened by the time of *Man's 4th Best Hospital.* Does this reflect a change you've also experienced personally?

Shem: I was roundly criticized for the way women were seen in *The House of God.* I remember the first rotation I had as a medical student at Harvard [Medical School] was at Beth Israel, doing surgery. It got to be late at night, and I was trailing the surgeon around, and he went into the on-call room. There was a bunk bed there, and he started getting ready to go to bed. And I said, "Well, I'll take the top bunk." And he said, "You can't sleep here." So I left, and in walked a nurse. I was shocked. Things have changed, and I am very, very glad. I don't know if it seems conscious—I was very pleased to have total gender equity in the Fat Man Clinic [where the characters in *Man's 4th Best Hospital* work] by the end of the book.[23]

The issue of gomers is different from other categories of identity, for, as Shem points out via the Fat Man, gomers are created by modern medicine because of the ambiguous advancements of medical technology: we can (and are) living longer, but our quality of life gains have not kept pace with our increases in life expectancy.[24] Thus, the very existence of gomers raises basic questions in the philosophy of medicine: What should our goals of medical care and scientific research be? How long should we extend life, life span, and life expectancy? To what extent does quality of life matter? So, while the term is ageist and should not be used, the philosophical critique implied by the term is legitimate.

The second Law is "Gomers go to ground." By this, the Fat Man means that these chronically ill older persons will find a way to fall out of their hospital beds no matter how many precautions are taken. The Fat Man, apparently, is trying to alleviate the distress that the interns will feel when they see this happen. In point of fact, this is a very serious problem.[25] The clinical term today is "falls risk." Thus, by satirically writing about something that he, no doubt, witnessed, Shem was throwing light on a problem in medicine that, apparently, no one seemed to care about then, at least not enough to do anything much about it.

Laws 3 and 4 are meant as helpful advice to interns. Law 3 ("At a cardiac arrest, the first procedure is to take your own pulse"), while humorous, is simply an injunction to calm down and focus when an emergency strikes. Likewise, Law 4 ("The patient is the one with the disease") is meant to counter medical student syndrome,[26] an experience in which a trainee becomes convinced that they have the disease that they are studying or treating.

Law 5 is a critique again: "Placement comes first." This refers to the practice of turfing. It is puzzling to Roy because, he wonders, how can one place a patient *before* diagnosing them? While appearing to be cynical, it is an acknowledgment that residents are overworked and are bound by institutional constraints. Likewise, Law 9 ("The only good admission is a dead admission") is deeply cynical, but, at the same time, it is an honest expression of the physical and emotional exhaustion that residents feel. It is a cry from the soul. Relatedly, Law 10—"If you don't take a temperature, you can't find a fever"—is a humorous act of resistance, but one that is more lighthearted than Law 9.

Laws 6, 7, 11, and 12 are inside jokes. They also are affirmations of practical wisdom in medicine. That is, there are many things to know that are useful in residency that have not been taught in medical school, even though they do not seem to make sense and do not have an evidence base. Laws 11 and 12 speak to the frustrations (from the point of view of residents) of working with medical students. Medical students need a lot of time to learn, and residents have no time to give. To be sure, if these laws were written from the perspective of medical students, they would make fun of residents.

Law 8, "They can always hurt you more," is a kind of moral warning, a counter to the idea that there is only so much suffering one can be asked to endure in life. There are aphorisms in life that people live by or assume (e.g., "Whatever doesn't kill you makes you stronger") that are obviously false on even just a moment of serious reflection.[27] Here, Shem is giving voice to the relentlessness of residency.

Law 13 is the most important: "The delivery of medical care is to do as much nothing as possible." Originally, Shem had written the law as follows: "The delivery of medical care is to do nothing."[d] But he felt that this was too cynical and also not quite right. Sometimes, things have to be done, and medicine really does save lives. However, the spirit of Shem's Law is a critique that modern doctors often intervene too much, causing more harm than good.[28] In bioethics, the principle of nonmaleficence is meant to guard against overintervention. Also, Shem, via the Fat Man, is affirming the body's innate capacity to heal itself when it is left to do so.

Practical Application

Because medical education has, as noted, been moving toward more active learning models, I suggest that a good way to use *The House of God* for interns and residents is to have them read the novel and discuss it in small groups. These groups should be encouraged to pick themes or passages from *The House of God* that are important to them, but, for the sake of ease, I have organized in table form some possible issues for discussion.

Influenced by theological education,[29] professional identity formation in medical education pays attention to the inner lives of trainees. These discussion questions, therefore, are meant to engage interns and residents emotionally so that this exercise is a meaningful experience for them. This means that some of the questions may not seem directly related to professionalism, but this is intentional, for the key objective is to encourage reflection on identity.

Taken together, the Laws of *The House of God* are a fierce defense of interns who live and work in a brutal system. The Laws are a plea for mercy to hospital administrators for things to change. This novel legitimizes their pain so that it can be talked about rather than merely suffered and subsequently inflicted on someone else.

Teaching Tips for Program Directors in Graduate Medical Education

1. The book should be read after the interns have had significant clinical experience (at least six months in hospital settings).
2. Provide some protected time for interns or residents to read the book.
3. Dedicate a three-hour block for discussion.

[d] Shem disclosed this in an online class seminar on November 16, 2020.

4. Ask an intern or resident to lead the discussion. The conversation should be among equals (no attendings, program directors, senior residents, etc.).
5. Use the Table 20.1 for the basis of discussion.
6. The facilitator should steer the conversation toward these two strategies for the future:
   a. Are there things we can do to help each other?
   b. Are there key issues that we want leadership to know about, things that should change?
7. Watch Samuel Shem, "How to Stay Human in Residency," on YouTube.

Table 20.1 Issues for Discussion in Residency Education

Law	Professional Identity Formation Question
Gomers don't die.	Where do you see ageism in the hospital? To what extent do we overtreat? What do you think about the use of nicknames for patients?
Gomers go to ground.	How often do you see patients fall? Has this problem been solved since 1978?
At a cardiac arrest, the first procedure is to take your own pulse.	When have you found yourself anxious or otherwise emotional in a clinical encounter? How have your emotional reactions changed over time?
The patient is the one with the disease.	What is your experience with medical student syndrome? To what extent do you find yourself thinking of patients as "other," as though disease is not something that can or will happen to you, because you are a healer?
Placement comes first.	Is this still true today? Do you find that services "turf" and "bounce"? Assuming money and time are no issue, how would you design the admissions process?
There is no body cavity that cannot be reached with a #14 needle and a good strong arm.	When is humor a mature defense mechanism, used for coping? When is it malicious? How do we know when humor is helpful or harmful?
Age + BUN = Lasix dose.	What are the truisms in residency that you were not taught in medical school? Do these truisms have an evidence base?
They can always hurt you more.	What are the mantras that you hold onto (e.g., "Everything happens for a reason")? To what extent have your own personal mantras been challenged by your clinical experience?
The only good admission is a dead admission.	Have you ever felt this way? What are the worst feelings you have ever felt toward a patient? Why do you think you felt this way? Do you think you have changed as a person because of your medical training?
If you don't take a temperature, you can't find a fever.	In what ways do you find yourself cutting corners?
Show me a BMS who only triples my work and I will kiss his feet.	How has your perspective changed as you have progressed in your training? What did you think as a medical student that now, as a resident, you disavow?
If the radiology resident and the BMS both see a lesion on the chest X ray, there can be no lesion there.	What are some things that you have witnessed that seem to have no medical or rational explanation?
The delivery of medical care is to do as much nothing as possible.	Is this Law true? Why or why not?

References

1. Hurtubise L, Hall E, Sheridan L, Han H. The flipped classroom in medical education: engaging students to build competency. *J Med Educ Curric Dev.* 2015;2:JMECD–S23895.
2. Burgess A, Bleasel J, Haq I, et al. Team-based learning (TBL) in the medical curriculum: better than PBL?" *BMC Med Educ.* 2017;17(1):1–11.
3. Holden M, Buck E, Luk J, et al. Professional identity formation: creating a longitudinal framework through TIME (Transformation in Medical Education). *Acad Med.* 90, no. 6 (2015): 761–767.
4. Wald H, Anthony D, Hutchinson TA, Liben S, Smilovitch M, Donato AA. Professional identity formation in medical education for humanistic, resilient physicians: pedagogic strategies for bridging theory to practice. *Acad Med.* 2015;90(6):753–760.
5. Cole T, Carlin N, Carson R. *Medical Humanities: An Introduction.* Cambridge University Press; 2015.
6. Charon R. *Narrative Medicine: Honoring the Stories of Illness.* Oxford University Press; 2006.
7. Elliott C. *A Philosophical Disease: Bioethics, Culture, and Identity.* Routledge; 2014.
8. Shem S. *The House of God.* Berkley; 2010.
9. Colletti L, Gruppen L, Barclay M, Stern D. Teaching students to break bad news. *Am J Surg.* 2001;182(1): 20–23.
10. Marcus J, Mott FE. Difficult conversations: from diagnosis to death. *Ochsner J.* 2014;14(4):712–717.
11. Brown S, Callahan MJ, Browning DM, et al. Radiology trainees' comfort with difficult conversations and attitudes about error disclosure: effect of a communication skills workshop. *J Am Coll Radiol.* 2014;11(8):781–787.
12. Jeffrey Chipman J, Gregory J. Beilman GJ, Constance C. Schmitz CC, and Susan C. Seatter SC., "Development and pilot testing of an OSCE for difficult conversations in surgical intensive care,". *Journal of Surgical Education.* 2007;64, no. (2 ()2007): 79–87.
13. Sherman M, Ricco J, Nelson S, Nezhad S, Prasad. Implicit bias training in a residency program: aiming for enduring effects. *Fam Med.* 2019;51(8): 677–681.
14. Hunter KM. The satiric image: healers in *The House of God. Lit Med.* 1983;2(1):135–147.
15. Claire Brash C,. "An interview with Samuel Shem, author of *The House of God,. London Journal of Primary* Care, 2017; 9(4): 46–48.
16. Lerner B. A life-changing case for doctors in training. *New York Times,* March 3, 2009. https://www.nytimes.com/2009/03/03/health/03zion.html. Accessed June 3, 2024.
17. Gerada C. Doctors and suicide. *Br J Gen Pract.* 2018;68(669):168–169.
18. Wear D. *The House of God*: another look. Acad Med. 2002; 77(6):495–501.
19. Shem S. Samuel Shem, 34 years after *The House of God. Atlantic,* November 28, 2012. https://www.theatlantic.com/health/archive/2012/11/samuel-shem-34-years-after-the-house-of-god/265675/.
20. Murphy J. *House of God* author discusses new sequel in exclusive interview. *MDLinx,* December 13, 2019. https://www.mdlinx.com/article/-house-of-god-author-discusses-new-sequel-in-exclusive-interview/6btdHvC7wrZp5UlstqV3HA.
21. Personal interview, March 10, 2021.
22. Kohn M, Donley C, eds. *Return to* The House of God: *Medical Resident Education, 1978–2008.* Kent State University Press; 2008.

23. Gordon M. Novelist doctor skewers corporate medicine in *Man's 4th Best Hospital*. NPR, November 13, 2019. https://www.npr.org/sections/health-shots/2019/11/13/777688384/novelist-doctor-skewers-corporate-medicine-in-mans-4th-best-hospital.

24. Emanuel E. Why I hope to die at 75." *Atlantic*, October 2014. https://www.theatlantic.com/magazine/archive/2014/10/why-i-hope-to-die-at-75/379329/.

25. Oliver D, Daly F, Martin FC, McMurdo MET. Risk factors and risk assessment tools for falls in hospital in-patients: a systematic review. *Age Ageing*. 2004;33(2):122–130.

26. Waterman L, Weinman J. Medical student syndrome: fact or fiction? A cross-sectional study. *JRSM Open*. 2014;5(2):2042533313512480.

27. Hitchens C. *Mortality*. Twelve; 2012:59–75.

28. Lagu T. "Less is more" and *The House of God*: Was the Fat Man Right Again? *JAMA Intern Med*. 2015;175(3):459–460.

29. Carlin N, Cole T, Strobel H. Guidance from the humanities for professional formation. In: Puchalski C, Rumbold B, eds. *Oxford Textbook of Spirituality in Healthcare*. Oxford University Press; 2012:443–450.

21

Professionalism in Engagement and Patient/Family Communication

Ryan Pferdehirt and Brian S. Carter

Key Points

- Professionalism requires the physician be self-aware.
- Professionalism requires a recognition of a power differential between the physician and patient and work to mitigate its constraining effects on effective engagement.
- The principle of autonomy (respect of persons) and virtues of veracity, empathy, and humility help to equip the physician with requisite skills to esteem and engage patients toward shared decision-making.

Introduction

Healthcare professionals (HCPs) of all disciplines undergo rigorous training to acquire the requisite life-saving skills and care competencies for their practice as healers. Physicians undergo years of both basic and laboratory education followed by more experiential clinical and specialty training. Beyond discipline-specific education and training, it is incumbent on all physicians and other HCPs to be able to communicate effectively. At the same time, professionalism is demonstrated when the physician displays confidence and competence with other HCPs, patients, and families. The character in the physician's presentation to, and behaviors with, the patient is telling.

In this chapter, we discuss matters of professional communication, demeanor, AND virtue characteristics of and a disposition toward service to the patient's needs. The professional acknowledges and must accommodate a certain distance between themselves as well-educated and highly trained specialists that hold an element of power in being the gatekeeper of healthcare. Halpern refers to this as "detached concern" and provides a structure for how one might move toward a posture of empathy.[1] The latter is more helpful in accomplishing real communication with the vulnerable, ill, or dying patient and the patient's family.[2]

We discuss professionalism in the context of both adult and pediatric patient interactions.

Engaging With Family

An important aspect of clinical professionalism displayed in patient care is the ability for clinicians to engage with patients and families both effectively and compassionately. It is often not enough for the clinician to have outstanding clinical knowledge, but the clinician must also be able to communicate that knowledge effectively with patients and families. Failing to do so can create challenges and complicate the delivery of patient care. Poor communication may result in a perception of uncaring that may be a barrier to the development of trust. Trust is fundamental for an effective clinical relationship.

Code of Ethics and Moral Authority

Historically, the Hippocratic oath has guided the practice of Western medicine and shaped physician ethics and actions. Often attributed to the oath is the phrase, "first do no harm," but this is in error. The Latin translation of the original Greek to "first do no harm" does not come from the Hippocratic oath but from other writings of the Hippocratic Corpus (those writings attributed to Hippocrates) and from the Hippocratic treatise on epidemics. There it is said: "In illnesses one should keep two things in mind, to be useful rather than cause no harm."[3] Yet most educated citizens would state that their expectations are that physicians, indeed, cause no harm. What the Hippocratic writings, and oath, provide for is an appeal to a higher moral source than oneself in the pursuit of doing good for the patient. The oath and its influence on the practice of Western medicine dates back more than 2,000 years. Similar oaths exist in the Indian Sanskrit writings that address ayurveda (Indian traditional medicine), the Chinese tradition, the oath of Maimonides (Jewish tradition), and more recently the oath of an Islamic physician that reflects a composite of thought and writings of physicians in the Islamic world.[4]

There are several benefits of the practice of oaths and codes in medicine with two prominent ones being their inclination toward establishing a base level of trust between the physician and the patient and minimizing the individual physician as the sole source of moral authority.

When a patient enters a physician-patient relationship with the knowledge of the moral obligations of that physician, the patient will have a higher sense of trust toward that physician acting in their best interest and that the physician is not morally compromised. This type of trust engenders meaningful dialogical engagement that grows with successive interactions and the physician demonstrating they are worthy of the patient's trust. But with the nature and practice of much of modern Western medicine, this is often not possible. This can be due to the necessary urgency seen in emergency medicine, or the prominent specialization of medical practice within an outpatient or inpatient clinical setting. Ensuring that all physicians take a shared oath facilitates the public's expectation of and inclination toward an initial level of trust. In turn, the trust that the public hold in physicians needs to be respected and strengthened through actions void of abuse or carelessness that would see to the dissolution of trust. Medical codes also help to establish the method of *argumentum ad verecundiam*, or an argument from authority. This is when an argument is "accepted out of deference for the prestige, stature, or presumed expertise of a person, institution, or office holder."[5(p93)] But for argument from authority to be valid, the qualifications of the authority must be established. This is a reason arguments from authority have a bad reputation "because of its frequent misuse and because it was used in the wrong context . . . or without proper qualification."[5(pp93–94)]

While codes in medicine can be beneficial, they can present several challenges. Codes establish a moral authority and impart a reputation for moral authority. This authority can become difficult to overcome, especially when trying to empower the patient and respect the patient's right to self-determination.

And moral codes are only as good as the person who adheres to the code, as Pellegrino states: "Any moral code must be translated into a moral act by a human person, and that moral act will reflect the moral values and sensitivities of that agent."[5(p103)] They can give a sense of infallibility that can devalue and dismiss a patient's concerns that are not in line with the opinion of the physician. Physicians need to recognize this potential sense of moral superiority that can be created toward patients and move beyond it in order that they have meaningful engagement with patients. Patient engagement requires mutual respect, consideration, and agreement that may not be attainable if a physician inserts an air of moral authority that is falsely attributed to moral codes.

Power Dynamics

Due in part to the high degree of specialization in modern medicine, there is a large social divide between patient and physician.[6] There are several reasons for this divide, some being the differences in medical education, social expectations, and authority.[7] This social divide contributes to the power dynamic seen across members of the profession of medicine and the patients they serve, but not in a uniform manner. For several reasons, not all medical practices exist across wide social and power divides. For example, in a 2016 study on the nature of power dynamics between patient and physician, Nimmon and Stenfors-Hayes found: "Although trained within the same institutional and organizational culture of medicine, physicians' varying interpretations of power relations in this study suggest that there is a crucial intersection of agency, context, time, training, and practice which are linked to perceptions of social space and/or the social position an individual possesses."[7(p6)] And while there are many factors that contribute to this divide, the result is the creation of an uneven power dynamic between physician and patient. While it might be foreseeable, or even natural, that a power dynamic between the physician and patient would exist, unrecognized or unchecked by the physician it can expectantly yield a negative effect on the physician-patient relationship, patient engagement, and trust.

Indeed, this power divide can often go unnoticed. In a 2016 study of the impact on the handling of power in the physician-patient relationship, most physicians were unaware this power discrepancy existed. Many physicians were "surprised by the interview questions that inquired into their perceptions of power relations in the context of teaching their patients. Many physicians asking us to restate the question or repeating back to us the word power for clarification: 'what . . . sorry . . . power?' "[7(p4)] That there is often such a vast difference in the level of education between physicians and their patients most certainly contributes to at least a perceived power differential. Physicians have on average ten to twelve years of postsecondary school education, while "some patients have such limited knowledge bases that communication about alien or novel situations is exceedingly difficult, especially if physicians introduce new concepts and cognitive constructs."[8]

This education gap is an obstacle that needs to be accounted for and cannot be ignored. While patients cannot be expected to fully comprehend all their medical decisions, they should always be allowed to retain their sense of individualism and identity and expect that physicians acknowledge this—giving voice to the ethical principle of respect of persons, or the autonomy of the patient. This becomes complicated in several different scenarios, such as when a patient makes poor choices (as judged by their physician's recommendations) or a decision that may have potentially harmful consequences. In these scenarios, it is understandable that a physician would want to act in a way that prioritizes the principle of beneficence and act in a paternalist manner. In such challenging scenarios, some HCPs prioritize respect for autonomy by not interfering beyond education and persuasion, while other professionals attempt to protect the patient against these potentially harmful consequences and act in a more beneficent manner.[8(p132)] But professionalism requires more than a simple hierarchical application of principles and not merely "focus on how to specify or balance these principles, which principle to follow under which conditions, and how to intervene in the decisions and affairs of such patient when intervention is warranted."[8(p132)] While the physician does need to balance their intent to do good (beneficence) and the need to always respect their patient's autonomy, left alone these principles may remain in great ethical tension. The professionalism sought by patients is such that they be seen, heard, understood, and respected.[9] Hence, the resolution of this contest of principles requires an incorporation of the patient's narrative—who they are, what is most meaningful to them in both a values clarification and a desired quality of life, and how they might express their own goals of care. In such situations, professionalism leads the physician to employ empathic inquiry in order to better understand the patient and make decisions with and for them.[10,11] At other times, such as when there is a long-standing physician-patient relationship in which mutual trust has developed, the path forward may be so clear as to make choices that are aligned with patient values readily identifiable, and the physician acts most professionally when employing a shared decision-making (SDM) model that respects the patient's goals and values while providing necessary and appropriate clinical counsel and guidance toward a mutually identified process forward. Identifiable portrayals of professionalism in such cases include discussing with the patient how desirable SDM is, what options exist for managing the patient's condition, exploring the patient's own preferences, and thinking through choices, then making a well-discussed decision together.[12]

The SDM model respects patient autonomy and mitigates unguarded paternalism, even when such paternalism is vested in the patient's welfare as best understood by all the available evidence. For indeed, as noted by Hoffman and colleagues: "Without shared decision-making, EBM can turn into evidence tyranny."[13] With the SDM approach, because the physician either knows (by virtue of long-standing relationship) or inquires of the patient in order to know (empathic inquiry) how the physician can best choose both with and for the patient's benefit in a trustworthy manner.

Engagement

In view of the many factors that can potentially create harmful power dynamics that result in a divide between the physician and the patient, it is important to find meaningful ways to engage with patients so that the physician can more properly practice the healing arts. Such engagement is foundational to quality patient care and is a requirement to build trust. Excellent communication is important as it facilitates engagement—either nurturing it or foreclosing opportunities when there is insensitivity in word choice, poor listening skills, and reflection and clarification. Excellence in communication is increasingly recognized by professional societies as well as medical schools, including communication via telehealth technologies.[14,15] As stated by the American Thoracic Society and the Society for Critical Care Medicine, "multiple professional societies . . . define communication with families as a key component of high-quality critical care. Effective physician-patient communication improves measurable outcomes including decreased ICU length of stay and may reduce distress amongst patients' families."[16] Being able to effectively communicate delicate and difficult information requires a different skill set than the standard medical knowledge, but it is a requisite skill of the professionalism demanded by the public that enhances both the abilities and understanding of the physician. In a word, it makes the physician kind.

Humility

Many distinct factors within the education and training of physicians, as well as the healthcare system itself, can contribute to challenges for physicians in their efforts to develop a beneficial relationship with the patient. Patient encounters and engagement may be brief, constrained by time and competing commitments, fraught, or fractured. One way to minimize such challenges is through incorporation and focus on physician humility. It is important to have both the physician and the patient/family acting on equal terms—with mutual respect. Such mutuality is required to accomplish SDM, which can be defined as "an approach where clinicians and patients make decisions together using the best available evidence. Patients are encouraged to think about the available screening, treatment, or management options and the benefits and harms of each so that they can communicate their preferences and help select the best course of action for them."[17] This is supported by the principles of respect for autonomy and patient engagement. But it is only achievable when patients feel empowered and capable of expressing their opinion and medical preference. If the patient feels, either consciously or unconsciously, that a divisive power dynamic exists between themselves and the physician, it is possible that there would be only a tentative sense of mutual respect, an unease in truly establishing trust, and a reticence to honestly express their goals and values. Hubris on the part of the physician will impede patient engagement and entering into the SDM process. As Elwyn et al. state: "Achieving shared decision making depends on building a good relationship in the clinical encounter so that information is shared, and patients are supported to deliberate and express their preferences and views during the decision-making process."[18] Without the virtue of humility, described by Coulehan to be "the medical virtue most difficult to understand and practice,"[19] professionalism may be unattainable by physicians.

To employ humility, Coulehan characterizes the virtue as having four important components. First, the physician must be able to practice with unpretentious openness. The physician must make an honest appraisal of personal knowledge, skills, and abilities, as well as cultural inclinations and spiritual or philosophic beliefs—self-awareness.[20] Second, the physician who portrays professionalism via the virtue of humility does so by avoiding any semblance of arrogance. Third, humility requires honesty—of both an intellectual nature (knowing one's limits) and responsibility and accountability. Such is seen in the physician owning personal mistakes and medical errors and working toward both error prevention and the mitigation of any associated harm. Last, humility requires the physician to avoid self-interest, to practice self-effacement, and to act in service to the patient (and society) in an altruistic manner. Coulehan captures the long shadow cast by the highly esteemed physician and ethicist Edmund Pellegrino and philosophers David Thomasma and Al Jonsen, who characterized this facet of humility in the tension between self-interest and the patient's best interest. He appeals to Aristotle's Golden Mean as a measure of morally appropriate balance of interests. And as he notes: "The good doctor embodies compassion, respect, and fidelity precisely because she is sufficiently reflective and motivated to down-regulate her personal interests (e.g., convenience, peer approval, pleasure, financial gain, power, or prestige) when it is in her patients' best interests to do so."[19(p212)]

Humility is reflected in the physician's need to remain conscious of the power dynamics that can impact patient engagement, the provision of care, and even how effective patient education can be. Respect of persons must entail respect for their education and understanding, recognizing that there may be cultural, linguistic, or numeracy constraints. These would require the physician to jettison jargon, incorporate interpreter services, or use visual aids to communicate numerical information more clearly than might be accomplished with citing statistics, frequencies, or rates. Certainly, the physician must not assume that the patient has the same knowledge, comprehension, or facility with words or numbers as they might hold themselves. It is both an act of humility and respect for the physician to ask the patient how they like to hear about facts and figures and how detail oriented they might be and communicate accordingly.

In a 2022 study on the perceived value of humility in clinical practice, Wadhwa and Mahant (2022) found that physicians identified humility to be an important driver for excellence in clinical practice. They further identified several themes and concepts for humility that were interconnected and interdependent.[21] These include inward or intellectual perspectives, which include one's ability and limits, self-confidence, and intellectual openness and adaptability. And outward or social perspectives, including appreciation for the larger system, openness to others, and valuing the patient's experience.[21] It is important to acknowledge that embracing humility and working to be "at the patient's level" is not an act of lowering a physician's sense of ability or dropping their self-confidence, but rather the pursuit of attaining a "fine balance" and the self-confidence to be able to acknowledge one's limitations while having confidence in one's ability.[21(p5)]

Veracity

In addition to humility, another fundamental component of a beneficial physician-patient relationship is the principle of veracity. This can be understood as the accurate, timely, objective, and comprehensive transmission of information that goes toward the fostering of the patient's understanding.[8(p303)] While often closely related to the principle of autonomy as a means for patients to make an informed decision, there are some subtleties that make veracity its own principle.

It is important for patients to be informed regarding their medical condition so that they can make decisions that are as informed as possible. Before patients can give informed consent to any medical intervention, they should know "the *nature* of the intervention, the expected *benefits*, the *risks*, and the likely *consequences*."[22] Without this information, patients are not able to make optimal decisions and therefore not able to truly exercise their liberty rights that respect their autonomy. But for patients to know the nature, benefits, risks, and consequences of an intervention, they are often completely reliant on that information being discussed with them by the physician. This illustrates the importance of ensuring that the physician is acting with veracity. The placebo effect is an example of a situation that some might argue is acceptable for veracity and truth-telling to be ignored. They might argue that if patients benefit, then full truth and disclosure is not required. This is prioritizing the principle of beneficence in a most domineering manner over autonomy. Countering this, Singh and Ernst believe that even "white lies" in medicine can have long-term negative effects: "These opponents would feel that white lies are acceptable if they improve the health of patients. We would counter that routine peddling of placebos would lead to a widespread culture of deception in medicine, which would in turn result in a series of corrosive consequences for the medical profession."[23] Patients need to trust that the information being discussed with a physician is the truth, and any action that may compromise that trust should be avoided due to the long-term damage to patient-physician relationships going forward.

Trust

Several things contribute to successful patient engagement. These include excellent communication skills, minimizing differentials in power dynamics, acting with humility, and prioritizing veracity. But all these rest on the importance of truthfulness within the relationship. Without a base of truth between patient and physician, the relationship cannot be one of trust, and it will not be successful. The patient needs to trust that the physician is providing truthful information and acting in the patient's best interest, while the physician needs to trust that the patient is informed and sharing all relevant information truthfully. As stated in the American Medical Association's Code of Medical Ethics:

> The health and well-being of patients depends on a collaborative effort between patient and physician in a mutually respectful alliance. Patients contribute to this alliance when they fulfill responsibilities they have, to seek care and to be candid with their physicians. Physicians can best contribute to a mutually respectful alliance with patients by serving as their patients' advocates and by respecting patients' rights.[24]

The physician who acts with humility and attempts to mitigate or balance power differentials is endeavoring to establish and uphold trust.

Adults

While they both share the importance of proper patient engagement, including elimination of power dynamics, value of humility, and establishing trust, there are many factors that differentiate actions between physicians and adult patients with whom they seek engagement and those in which pediatric patient (or parent) engagement is sought. The biggest difference comes in terms of capacity.

The nature of sickness and hospitalization can create barriers to mutually beneficial patient engagement. Patients often have a feeling of powerlessness,[25,26] which can impact their ability to engage with their provider. As their narrative has been interrupted by illness, feelings of unfairness often accompany being sick. As patients accommodate feelings of being powerless, lacking control, and being rendered dependent on others due to their disease or condition, the existential concerns of the meaning of illness and the inevitability of death put these matters foremost in the minds of many patients. These feelings of powerlessness may also be heightened when patients do not feel heard. While actions can be done to minimize these matters, it is not possible to have them eliminated entirely. Hence, physicians might find patients acting in ways that are against the patient's best interests or even against the patient's own stated goals of care. This can come in the form of being nonadherent to treatment plans, to the patient changing their mind on decisions, and variations in the level of participation in their own treatment. It can also come through the patient's attitude toward the individual physician or the medical team, with the patient acting in what is often described as a "difficult" manner.[27,28] What should be understood is this can simply be a person attempting to assert some semblance of control or ownership over their own life and circumstances. This is a fundamentally important aspect of human dignity and needs to be recognized.

In the state of Washington, through its program of Death with Dignity, or medical aid in dying (MAID), one of the most frequently stated reasons for engaging in physician-assisted death has been the patient's sense of loss of their own autonomy. In 2020, 89.6% of so involved patients cited that as a reason. This was equal to another common reason: "Less able to engage in activities making life enjoyable" at 90.6% but greater than "Loss of control of bodily functions" at 48.8 %.[29] It is intrinsically part of human nature to pursue what is self-determined as being able to engage meaningfully with one's environment and to retain some level of control over oneself and that environment. Physicians need to be able to understand the patient's feeling of powerlessness and loss of autonomy and utilize techniques and conversation to break down the barriers that this imposes and fully engage with the patient.

A lack of control or sense of not being heard is also experienced by patient surrogate decision-makers, particularly around medical staff communication with them.[30] This can be frustrating and create feelings of animosity and powerlessness as: "Surrogate decision makers are often displeased with the frequency of communication, the limited availability of attending physicians, and report feeling excluded from discussion."[31]

One method of minimizing these feelings of powerlessness and establishing trust and respect for a patient is to give them "little wins" in terms of their care. This means creating situations with minimum risk and allowing the patient to express their preferences and immediately acceding to those preferences. This can be as easy as when entering a patient room, the physician states she wants to have a conversation and asks if this is a suitable time. If the patient would prefer having it at a later time, the physician should work to accommodate that, giving the patient a sense of control. In giving the patient this control and freedom to exercise it, the physician models humility, and this can help to establish trust and minimize the patient's feelings of powerlessness. By giving patients little wins, they can regain a sense of ownership and control. They and their family members or surrogate decision-makers may see that they are being heard and respected. This facilitates trust and mutual respect between the patient and physician and provides greater likelihood of SDM and a positive impact in the patient's care. When the patient feels able to communicate on an equal basis with the physician, the patient is more likely to express personal medical preferences. This proves beneficial when conversations turn toward more complicated and medically pressing topics, such as end-of-life decisions. By allowing the patient to have some control, and certainly respect, they are more likely to engage in meaningful conversations and express themselves knowing that the physician will listen to and respect the decision they make. Sharing power (control) and demonstrating mutual respect also adds value when the physician expresses concern over a chosen course of treatment or in situations such as the continuation or cessation of life-sustaining treatments or other aggressive measures. Odero and colleagues have recently elaborated on this phenomenon in a model that they call the "patient-as-partner approach."[32] They note that certain prerequisites exist in order to attain and implement patient partnership in healthcare: embracing the values held by patients and by physicians and cultivating these parties' mutual competencies around relevant knowledge and skills, interactional skills and behaviors, attitudes, and cognitive capacities. In sharing power as partners, the physician demonstrates humility and respect, while the patient is empowered by the respect shown and allowance to contribute toward a truly shared decisional process. This is patient-centered care.

Ensuring that medicine is patient centered "affords far greater priority to the personal relationship between doctor and patient, based on psychotherapeutic developments around the concept of the `therapeutic alliance'" but also but require core attitudes of "empathy, congruence, and unconditional positive regard are both necessary and sufficient for effecting therapeutic change in clients ."[33(p1090)] Additional aspects related to these core attitudes, seen to be important aspects of the professional/patient relationship, include "(a) the patient's perception of the relevance and potency of interventions offered, (b) agreement over the goals of treatment, and (c) cognitive and affective components, such as the personal bond between doctor and patient and perception of the doctor as caring, sensitive and sympathetic."[33(p1090),34]

Pediatrics

While some adult patients may lose capacity and the ability to express their medical preferences, in pediatric medicine and surgery, the patient often does not have the ability to make medical decisions. This makes for sometimes challenging interactions. Children are, by their nature, dynamic and growing physically and cognitively throughout the pediatric age spectrum. They may be said to start with a tabula rasa, a blank slate,[35] when it comes to decisional capacity, but in time they come to understand facts, situations, choices, and the ramifications of their choices. This is accomplished at varying rates and ages and impacted by circumstances of illness, chronic conditions, and adult facilitation of maturation or impediments to it.[36,37] Hence, while all children should be spoken to, addressed with respect, and allowed to know and understand their health to the best of their ability, for sociocultural, historical, legal, and moral reasons the child's parent or legal guardian is the foremost encountered decision-maker.

For the adolescent and young adult (AYA), it remains important to understand the differences in their direct involvement in medical decisions and that of adults who truly decide for themselves. Barring cognitive impairments or a state impacting an adult's decisional capacity, the adult patient is the de facto medical decision-maker and the one that the physician needs to engage. If the patient lacks capacity, then the patient's surrogate decision-maker becomes involved and becomes the one making medical decisions. AYA patients can be said to have an evolving autonomy and capacity to understand and engage in medical decision-making. The distinct need to address parental engagement in pediatric and AYA decision-making renders all medical decision-making a process requiring a surrogate. The guiding principle in decision-making for children and AYA is that of seeking the child's best interest, and certainly to mitigate or avoid harm. Such efforts may result in some conflicting ideas about just what, precisely, might constitute the "best" interest of the child. Stakeholders such as parents, the child, and the medical team may all have an opinion, but reasonableness should prevail.[38]

Valuable professionalism takes an approach to patient engagement that focuses on the family unit and understands that the decisions made and actions taken can reverberate through the relationship between all of those involved. Such an awareness is important for all physicians to incorporate into their professional encounters with children, AYA, and parents as the professional environment of the pediatric clinic or hospital is so different from that of adults and requires it. In many instances, pediatric clinicians of several disciplines, including physicians, may choose to adopt an approach in clinical decision-making that is more focused on the valued relationship(s) within a family.[39] In such instances, expectations of professionalism require that the physician will add to a personal repertoire of conduct engaging the child and showing interest and respect while simultaneously engaging the adult parent in a manner like the described in the patient-as-partner approach. The major difference in this pediatric encounter is that the parental partnership is one that works toward the best interests of the child/AYA rather than the adult's interests per se. Such engagement requires humility on the part of the medical professional, respect (for the child and the parent), veracity, and empathy. Parental determinants in the decision-making process are at once contingent on family values, the child/AYA's health needs and interests, and the physician's ability to communicate effectively and represent reasonable choices.

The pediatric clinician that centers professionalism toward honoring and sustaining valued relationships across and between family members, the child, schoolmates, sports team members, civic clubs and organizations, and religious and faith communities does so by employing principles and virtues that facilitate trust. The pediatrician serves the family by attending to the child's health and serves the broader community and society by attending to social justice, public health, and safety. While motivated by the pursuit of being the "good physician," as noted by Cohen, it may well be humanism, a way of being, "provides the passion that animates professionalism."[40] This is most evident in the clinical encounter of the pediatrician with the patient and the patient's parent. In few places in medicine can the physician display professionalism by acting funny and engaging the patient—with respect—in play. But such is the expectation of the pediatrician's manner of being. Even the process of narrative enquiry seems most natural in relating to a child and parent's story of immigrating to their new home.

It is often said that pediatricians never grow up—or grow old—as they continue to engage in youthful interaction and discourse. Indeed, a pediatrician that is arrogant or self-aggrandizing will likely not be in practice long. Regis and colleagues noted in their study of parental expectations of professionalism in pediatricians that the most frequently family-identified characteristics were evidence of care and concern, good communication skills, appropriate knowledge and skill, and reliable honesty and a good attitude.[41]

Conclusion

Medical professionals often meet families during some of their most challenging times, including during the decline and loss of a loved one, a new diagnosis, or health struggles of a child. During moments like these, patients are not only looking for facts and information, but also seeking the humanistic aspects of the practice of medicine. It is not enough to deliver information to a patient or family; the ability to provide information with compassion, empathy, and humility is a defining characteristic of professionalism in medicine.

Inherent in the physician/patient relationship is an imbalance of power. This power imbalance comes from the differences in education, knowledge, and experience, and it can negatively impact communication between physicians and patients. While it may be impossible to eliminate this imbalance entirely, the physician who employs humility and veracity and looks to the power of virtues and principles to inform and shape decision-making through respectful engagement with the patient will find his or her professionalism well received. Medical professionalism moves beyond the mere set of knowledge and skills retained by the physician; it is the "habitual and judicious use of communication, knowledge, technical skills, clinical reasoning, emotions, values, and reflection in daily practice for the benefit of the individual and community being served."[42]

Beneficial and meaningful engagement with patients and families is a cornerstone of professional behavior, and the key to this level of engagement is primarily through trust—a trust that can only come from physicians acting with veracity and humility. Since the time of Hippocrates, the practice of medicine is understood through the perspective of virtue ethics. This means that the character of the physician is as important as the physician's knowledge and abilities. The character of a physician is easily revealed by how that physician engages with patients. All physicians need to understand that they are a part of a great tradition created for the benefit of all people, a tradition that understands the importance of each and every individual physician embodying the virtues of medicine and conducting himself/herself with the highest level of professionalism.

References

1. Halpern J. *From Detached Concern to Empathy: Humanizing Medical Practice.* Oxford University Press; 2001.
2. Halpern J. What is clinical empathy? *J Gen Intern Med.* 2003;18(8):670–674. http://doi.org/10.1046/j.1525-1497.2003.21017.x
3. Retsa S. *BMJ* 2019 in response to Abbasi K, "First Do No Harm: The Impossible Oath?" *BMJ.* 2019;366:l4734 https://doi.org/10.1136/bmj.l4734
4. Gupta SK. Hippocrates and the Hippocratic oath. *J Pract Cardiovasc Sci.*2015;1(1):81.
5. Pellegrino ED. Codes, virtue, and professionalism. *Meth Med Ethics.* 2010;91–108.
6. Verlinde E, De Laender N, De Maesschalck S, Deveugele M, Willems S. The social gradient in doctor-patient communication. *Int J Equity Health.* 2012;11:12. https://doi.org/10.1186/1475-9276-11-12
7. Nimmon L, Stenfors-Hayes T. The "handling" of power in the physician-patient encounter: perceptions from experienced physicians. *BMC Med Educ.* 2016; 16:114. https://doi.org/10.1186/s12909-016-0634-0

8. Beauchamp TL, Childress JF. *Principles of Biomedical Ethics.* Oxford University Press; 2001:132.
9. Sari MI, Prabandari YS, Claramita M. Physicians' professionalism at primary care facilities from patients' perspective: the importance of doctors' communication skills. *J Family Med Prim Care.* 2016;5(1):56–60. https://doi.org/10.4103/2249-4863.184624
10. Halpern J. What is clinical empathy? *J Gen Intern Med.* 2003;18(8):670–674. http://doi.org/10.1046/j.1525-1497.2003.21017.x
11. Jeffrey D. Empathy, sympathy, and compassion in healthcare: is there a problem? Is there a difference? Does it matter? *J Royal Soc Med.* 2016;109(12):446–452. https://doi.org/10.1177/0141076816680120
12. Baghus A, Giroldi E, Muris J, et al. Identifying entrustable professional activities for shared decision making in postgraduate medical education: a national Delphi study. *Acad Med.* 2021;96(1):126–133. https://doi.org/10.1097/ACM.0000000000003618
13. Hoffman TC, Montori VM, Del Mar C. The connection between evidence-based medicine and shared decision making. *JAMA.* 2014; 312(13):1295. https://doi.org/10.1001/jama.2014.10186
14. Kelly S, Smyth E, Murphy P, et al. A scoping review: virtual patients for communication skills in medical undergraduates. *BMC Med Educ.* 2022;22:429. https://doi.org/10.1186/s12909-022-03474-9
15. Noronha C, Lo MC, Nikiforova T. et al. Telehealth competencies in medical education: new frontiers in faculty development and learner assessments. *J Gen Intern Med.* 2022;37:3168–3173. https://doi.org/10.1007/s11606-022-07564-8
16. McFarlin J, Tulsky JA, Back AL, Arnold RM. A talking map for family meetings in the intensive care unit. *J Clin Outcomes Manage.* 2017;24(1):15.
17. Elwyn G, Laitner S, Coulter A, Walker E, Watson P, Thomson R. Implementing shared decision making in the NHS. *BMJ.* 2010;341:971. https://doi.org/10.1136/bmj.c5146
18. Elwyn G, Frosch D, Thomson R, Joseph-William N, Lloyd A, Kinnersley P. Shared decision making: a model for clinical practice. *J Gen Intern Med.* 2012;27(10):1361. https://doi.org/10.1007/s11606-012-2077-6
19. Coulehan J. "A gentle and humane temper": humility in medicine. *Perspect Biol Med.* 2011;54(2):206. https://doi.org/10.1353/pbm.2011.0017
20. Reichel W. Physician, know thyself. *J Am Board Fam Pract.* 1999;12(3):258–259.
21. Wadhwa A, Mahant S. Humility in medical practice: a qualitative study of peer-nominated excellent clinicians. *BMC Med Educ.* 2022;22(1):1–9.
22. Lo B. *Resolving Ethical Dilemmas: A Guide for Clinicians.* Lippincott Williams & Wilkins; 2009:20.
23. Singh S, Ernst E. *Trick, or Treatment: The Undeniable Facts About Alternative Medicine.* WW Norton & Company; 2008:246.
24. American Medical Association. Opinion 1.1.3 Patient rights. *Code of Medical Ethics.* https://www.ama-assn.org/delivering-care/patient-rights. Accessed June 3, 2024.
25. Sheridan NF, Kenealy TW, Kidd JD, et al. Patients' engagement in primary care: powerlessness and compounding jeopardy. A qualitative study. *Health Expect.* 2015;18(1):32–43. https://doi.org/10.1111/hex.12006
26. Batho D. Experiences of powerlessness and the limits of control in healthcare. *Intern J Philos Theol.* 2022:83(5):405–415. https://doi.org/10.1080/21692327.2022.2137565

27. Aronson L. "Good" patients and "difficult" patients—rethinking our definitions. *N Engl J Med.* 2013;369:796–797. https://doi.org/10.1056/NEJMp1303057

28. Launer J. Dealing with difficult patients—by dealing with difficult doctors. *Postgrad Med J.* 2022;98:649–650. https://doi.org/10.1136/postgradmedj-2022-141976

29. Washington State Department of Health. 2020 Death With Dignity Act Report. October 21, 2021. https://doh.wa.gov/sites/default/files/2022-02/422-109-DeathWithDignityAct2020.pdf?uid=6283d0d11ed2f) Accessed June 3, 2024

30. Su Y, Yuki M, Hirayama K. The experiences and perspectives of family surrogate decision-makers: a systematic review of qualitative studies. *Pat Educ Counsel.* 2020;103(6):1070–1081. https://doi.org/10.1016/j.pec.2019.12.011

31. McFarlin J, Tulsky JA, Back AL, Arnold RM. A talking map for family meetings in the intensive care unit. *J Clin Outcomes Manage.* 2017;24(1):15.

32. Odero A, Pongy M, Chauvel L, et al. Core values that influence the patient-healthcare professional power dynamic: steering interaction towards partnership. *Int J Environ Res Public Health.* 2020;17(22):8458. https://doi.org/10.3390/ijerph17228458

33. Mead N, Bower P. Patient-centredness: a conceptual framework and review of the empirical literature. *Soc Sci Med.* 2000;51(7):1090.

34. Roth, A., Fonagy, P., Parry, G., Target, M., et al. (1996). *What works for whom? A critical review of psychotherapy research.* Guilford Press..

35. Duschinsky R. "Tabula rasa" and human nature. *Philosophy.* 2012;87(342):509–529.

36. Grootens-Wiegers P, Hein IM, van den Broek JM, de Vries MC. Medical decision-making in children and adolescents: developmental and neuroscientific aspects. *BMC Pediatr.* 2017;17(1):120. https://doi.org/10.1186/s12887-017-0869-x

37. Sawyer K, Rosenberg AR. How should adolescent health decision-making authority be shared? *AMA J Ethics.* 2020;22(5):E372–E379. https://doi.org/10.1001/amajethics.2020.372

38. Hester DM, Salter EK. Reasonableness as a relational principle: an integrated framework for pediatric decision-making. *J Pediatr.* 2022;251:30–35. https://doi.org/10.1016/j.jpeds.2022.06.002

39. Pettersen T. The ethics of care: normative structures and empirical implications. *Health Care Anal.* 2011;19(1):51–64. https://doi.org/10.1007/s10728-010-0163-7

40. Cohen JJ. Viewpoint: linking professionalism to humanism: what it means, why it matters. *Acad Med.* 2007;82(11):1029. https://doi.org/10.1097/01.ACM.0000285307.17430.74

41. Regis T, Steiner MJ, Ford CA, Byerley JS. Professionalism expectations seen through the eyes of resident physicians and patient families. *Pediatrics.* 2011;127(2):317–324.https://doi.org/10.1542/peds.2010-2472

42. Epstein RM, Hundert EM. Defining and assessing professional competence. *JAMA.* 2002;287(2:226).

22

Medical Leadership, Professionalism, and Vulnerable Populations

S. Monty Ghosh

Key Points

- Individuals who experience homelessness are a diverse group where there is an intersection of health and social determinants of health that impacts overall wellness.
- Adverse childhood experiences often contribute to poor health outcomes, and a trauma-informed lens is important in dealing with vulnerable populations.
- Care must be taken when working with vulnerable populations, and clinicians are encouraged to incorporate strategies to understand behavioral complexities and concerns where possible.

Introduction

When working with vulnerable populations, it is important to understand that people experiencing homelessness, while referring to someone who does not have a home, includes a diverse population of individuals experiencing different forms of housing insecurity that is nonubiquitous in nature. It can refer to a diversity of individuals who are without accommodation, living in unstable housing or shelters, sleeping outside in encampments, living in their cars, or occupying public spaces not meant for habitation. It can also include insecure accommodation, such as individuals who are couch surfing, living with family, or living in homes unfit or unsanitary for habitation.[1] These populations often have multiple comorbid conditions involving complex mental health/psychiatric concerns, substance use, and medical concerns that compound their vulnerability.[2] In addition, they may have significant physical or cognitive disabilities complicated by ableism or experience marginalization due to their race, gender, economic status, or sexuality. Add in the possible intersectional confines of the sex trade or justice concerns, and the complexity of this population only heightens.

As such, when providing healthcare-associated leadership and professionalism within the vulnerable populations sector, it is incredibly important to approach all activities with a holistic lens. One must look beyond a client's health needs to understand the complexities of the population. This includes examining wellness through a trans-sectoral lens within the realms of social and criminal justice, social services, and politics.

There are several factors that cause individuals to enter homelessness.[3] As health professionals, understanding what these factors are can help mitigate them and ensure we avoid precipitating homelessness in those most vulnerable. Factors causing homelessness include structural aspects such as lack of income, affordable housing, and discrimination preventing access to essential resources. They include systems failures, especially during life or health transitions such as people leaving child welfare, coming out of corrections or hospital, or new immigrants, refugees, and other migrants transitioning to a new country. They equally include significant individual events such as house fires, job loss, domestic violence, or significant injury or illness.[4]

Health and homelessness are intricately intertwined. Indeed, health problems can lead to homelessness, such as personal injury leading to job loss and income insecurity, perpetuating into losing one's property and wealth. Homelessness can worsen health problems, with individuals facing food insecurity leading to malnutrition or hygiene and sanitation concerns leading to infection as well as other associated health outcomes. The status of homelessness can lead to discrimination and other barriers to accessing timely healthcare and other support, such as a lack of transportation to health and social services, further worsening health outcomes.[5]

Despite increased barriers, healthcare utilization is also high in this population, with frequent emergency visits, admissions, and hospital recidivism. Additionally, two studies demonstrated that the length of stay in hospital for someone experiencing homelessness compared to a housed individual range between 2.3 and 4.1.[6,7] Likewise, mortality rates among those who are unsheltered and sleeping rough are 9.8 times higher than that of the general population and 3 times higher than individuals who are homeless yet access shelters.[8] Discrimination and implicit bias in the healthcare system toward vulnerable populations often lead to situations where client needs are ignored, and the risk of misdiagnosis, underdiagnosis, or inappropriate treatment of both mental and physical health is high.[9]

Social Determinants of Health and an Integrated Approach to Care

As mentioned, individuals experiencing homelessness, mental health, and substance use concerns often intersect with multiple different systems outside of health. As medical clinicians we often focus on the health aspects of patients, but a key piece to the overall wellness of these individuals includes the upstream social determinants of health, including access to housing and income support. Social determinants of health, as defined by the World Health Organization (WHO), are "the conditions in which people are born, grow, live, work and age."[10] These conditions are further influenced by the distribution of resources available in particular areas and communities, which create societal stratification and inequities .[11] It is these inequities that lead to various health outcomes in particular populations, which self-perpetuate. For instance, poor health, whether physical or mental, resulting from health inequity and marginalization, may lead to the inability of an individual to access educational and income opportunities. This limited access in turn may lead to further inequity and marginalization. While approaching these clients, a staunch focus on addressing these social determinants is key to improving their overall health outcomes.

Indeed, it is estimated that nearly half of all deaths in the United States are attributable to behavioral factors, which are in turn influenced by social determinants, including education, employment, and income.[12] As a population's social circumstance improves, so does their overall health, indicating the need to elevate the overall social wellness of vulnerable and marginalized populations.[13] Economically advantaged populations have better access to support networks, custom health resources, and safety amenities.

Understanding social determinants of health helps inform what barriers clients may be facing in regard to wellness. For instance, individuals experiencing extreme vulnerabilities often have competing priorities. The necessity to focus on basic survival requirements, such as attempting to find food, shelter, or seeking safety can impede working on improving their health, making appointments, or taking their medications. As such, "meeting clients where they are at" is a key principle to providing appropriate care, where healthcare professionals recognize these barriers and meet the clients either physically where they are located or meet them where they are at mentally or emotionally with their wellness.

To ensure overall health and wellness, a focus on basic needs is imperative. This includes ensuring individuals have adequate food security, housing, income support, and sense of personal safety. As studies have demonstrated that spending on social services may have a greater impact on population health than spending on healthcare itself, it should be a strong focus by health leaders.[14] It involves strong collaboration and coordination with the social service sectors, and potentially other sectors, in regard to patient care.

For example, to ensure management of complex diabetes, a focus on food security is essential to manage their blood glucose. This not only involves finding and providing food support but also ensuring the food has adequate nutritional value. Additionally, coupling support with access to housing and income support can help with affordable food storage and preparation.

The sheer number of resources vulnerable populations need to access can be daunting and time consuming. Navigating the complex system of multiple systems such as social services, health, and justice can be overwhelming. As such, it is critical to integrate multiple aspects of health and wellness to a single point of care. Where possible, providing integrated foot care, dental, medical, psychological, social services, and substance use management is key. Providing this integrated care within a low-barrier and collaborative model can streamline often disparate services.[15] The likelihood of individuals accessing care where multiple needs are managed and met is highest in "one-stop shop" facilities, reducing barriers such as transport, cost, and time.

Where one-stop shop options are not possible, other creative strategies can be employed. These include using navigation resources such as peer navigators or intensive case management to help individuals reach various community resources.[16] Bringing services physically to where clients are located, such as encampments, as opposed to having them come to services is another option. This forms the basis of the street medicine approach: providing easy access to care for the most vulnerable.[17]

Where multiple professionals are interacting with vulnerable clients, strong coordination between groups can help support client care and remove duplication of services. One strategy for coordination is creating communities of practice, whether informal or formal, that not only can discuss specific clients and their needs, but also create opportunities to share knowledge and care approaches between practitioners. It promotes patient-centric care and collaboration and provides a space to access evidence-based practices.

Last, advocacy, which is a key piece to the work of clinicians, cannot end with advocating only for health-related concerns. Advocacy must also address the social inequities that exist in our communities. Advocacy cannot end with health alone but must incorporate other intersectional inequity concerns.

Professional Development and Vulnerable Populations

There has been a paucity of professional education around the needs of those experiencing homelessness.[18] Exposure to vulnerable populations during professional training can be limited, and as such, it is strongly encouraged that professionals who plan to work with people experiencing housing insecurity seek opportunities to improve their understanding of vulnerable populations and social determinants of health. Education and exposure to homelessness, while important, should be done with consideration of the population at hand and an understanding that they are not simply a training opportunity. Professional development around this sector must include community experts and people with lived experience to provide front-line context to the complexities and hurdles this population faces.

One overlooked aspect of care for vulnerable populations includes one's own inherent biases and discrimination. Open discussion on inherent biases around this population should be explored by clinicians with a focus on how these biases may impact their own approaches to providing care for this group. Critical ongoing self-reflection is necessary. It can be done informally through independent journaling or discussion with colleagues or via a more formal process through professional evaluations within academic settings and requirements. It is an active process with an appreciation and willingness to learn from one's challenges and successes.[19] Interdisciplinary learning and professional development among various allied professions who intersect with this population may be helpful in gaining further insight of the complexities these clients face, while also providing greater understanding around the multidisciplinary aspects of patient care. This approach can help clinicians best understand how to leverage their collective strength to support the client's needs and how to coordinate care.[20]

Additionally, clinicians must be prepared to see complex disease processes at late stages rarely seen in modern medicine, as many individuals with these conditions rarely access appropriate care.[21] These late-stage presentations, while providing unique learning opportunities, must be approached through a lens of understanding the structural and societal barriers that prevented individuals from accessing care in the first place, as well as barriers that may persist to impede healthy outcomes for these individuals. Exploration of these barriers and finding ways to remove them is key.

Working with vulnerable populations can often impact the personal wellness of providers. Providers with limited exposure to conditions of homelessness and shelter/encampment life may be overwhelmed by the state of perceived hopelessness and degree of disparity their clients may face. Working with these populations provides unique challenges to professionals, including self-reflective feelings of guilt for their client, sadness, and defeat.[22] These emotions can be complex to navigate and often lead to feelings of jadedness and emotional burnout. These can complicate clinician and client relationships. Additionally, as the vulnerable population sector is often resource limited, requiring practitioners to do duties typically left to allied health professionals to do in other areas of healthcare.

When working with vulnerable populations and facing the magnitude of system-wide inequities, professionals may face moral distress or moral injury. Professionals will feel that they cannot provide high-quality care while working in low-resource environments. Moral injury is often defined as an insult that pierces a person's identity, sense of morality, and relationship to society.[23] Ensuring professionals have autonomy and support to make decisions in their client's best interests despite limitations in resources can be helpful in minimizing this sense of defeat when it comes to patient care. Focused self-care and wellness are crucial to avoid burnout. Thoughtful strategies to manage these emotions include awareness of personal vulnerabilities in dealing with these patients and the employment of effective coping strategies, including sleep, exercise, team building and regular team debriefing, and emotional support can help mitigate concerns. To augment self-care, team care is crucial. The collective wellness of the team can keep morale high. Understanding that within a difficult and often broken system, it is often unrealistic to expect an individual or even a team to change a biased system or structure, but through collective self-work and external advocacy, they can come to peace knowing that they are doing what they can, in the best and feasible way possible.

Health and Justice Intersectionality

Vulnerable populations invariably struggle with the justice system as a structural consequence of their very vulnerability. Often, they are unfairly targeted due to their racial or ethnic background, due to the criminalization of their substance use, or because of their need to commit minor crimes in order to survive due to a lack of shelter and income support.[24,25] The complexity of the justice system can weigh heavily on the mental health of many clients and add more bureaucracy to their lives while they attempt to navigate basic needs on top of health needs. Arrest cycles cause issues such as missed work, job loss, and future difficulties accessing housing and work due to criminal records. It can cause family separation and loss of child custody and induce trauma. It can also lead to feelings of shame, fear, and hopelessness, which can fuel self-medication through substance use. It can further isolate and institutionalize individuals.

Once incarcerated, individuals may have worsened health outcomes. For example, individuals in corrections have been found to have worse psychological and mental health outcomes, cardiac concerns, obesity, hypertension, and poor glucose control to matched nonincarcerated individuals.[26] Despite this, correctional facilities are often deemed "the hospitals of last resort." It is often the only constitutionally protected space where individuals have direct access to health and wellness supports.[27] Correctional facilities present a unique opportunity to provide care to a population that otherwise "slips through the cracks."[28] It provides an environment to stabilize substance use and health concerns for individuals.

Special attention must be paid to individuals when exiting corrections. Individuals leaving corrections and transitioning to community experience a 12.5 times higher risk of mortality due to factors such as loss of opioid tolerance and subsequent overdose, violence, and suicidality.[29] Ensuring interconnectedness between the justice system and community health services can help prevent these poor outcomes. Additionally, screening for justice concerns with clients can help circumvent interruptions to community-based medical care when individuals are incarcerated.

Trauma-Informed Professionalism and Leadership

Trauma-informed leadership and professionalism is a relatively new concept borne from the general approach of trauma-informed care. The basis of a trauma-informed approach consists of an understanding, awareness, and tolerance of psychological traumas that underlie numerous health and wellness issues.[30]

Much of trauma-informed care stems from recent advances in the understanding of adverse childhood experiences (ACEs), which are ten experiences in early childhood that predispose someone to future adverse harms, including a risk of increased mental health and substance use concerns, HIV, teenage pregnancy, and decreased access to educational and income opportunities. These key experiences include physical, emotional, and sexual abuse; physical or emotional neglect; and family-based dysfunction, including domestic violence, substance misuse, mental health concerns, separation and divorce, and a parent who was incarcerated. Recognizing these factors helps one understand that many of our societal concerns and problems as well as concerns we traditionally associate as individual behavioral or emotional dysregulation are actually born from ACEs. When leading, understanding that one's clients, colleagues, and people of lived experience are operating from a traumatized background helps one to appreciate one's own vulnerability and the ongoing impacts of trauma and helps one lead from a place of understanding and compassion. While ACEs can cause harm, resiliency factors can minimize their impact. They include providing and encouraging safe and nurturing relationships, supportive and nurturing parent relationships, parent overall health and wellness, supportive community and neighborhoods, and close parent-child relationships.[31]

Substance Abuse and Mental Health Service Administration (SAMSHA) provides a simplified take on trauma, as the three e's, or event, experience of the event, and its effect. The event is described as the actual threat or extreme threat of harm. The interpretation of this event is the experience of the event, which can differ from person to person even with the same event. These in turn manifest into the effect, or the ultimate manifestation of trauma. These can manifest immediately or have a slower insidious onset. The effect is influenced by various factors, including the individual's baseline wellness, number of traumatic experiences they've had, as well as support post-traumatic event.

SAMHSA's trauma informed approach can be pivoted to support leadership and professionalism in systems.[32] This includes the following:

1. ***Realizing*** the widespread impact of trauma and understanding potential paths for recovery and how it can impact group, families, organizations, and communities: Practically speaking, this means understanding trauma at an individual, community, and systems-based level. For example, understanding if someone's behavior at work may be related to domestic violence, that a group of substance users' reluctance to work with healthcare providers stems from previous negative interactions with the healthcare system, or why a whole Indigenous community may be cautious about working with the government due to generational colonial aggressions and their ongoing impacts. These types of realizations can help one understand the baseline apprehension, concern, or behavior of the stakeholder and determine a more appropriate approach to working together.
2. ***Recognizes*** the signs and symptoms of trauma in clients, families, staff, organizations, and others involved with the system:

These signs and symptoms are nonspecific and can vary based on the background of the individual or group, their gender, age, and setting.

3. ***Responds*** by fully integrating knowledge about trauma into policies, procedures, and practices:
   The impact of trauma can permeate all levels of an organization, from clients, to staff, to leaders. The effects of trauma can be both direct and indirect, and efforts should be made by leaders to help foster an understanding of the effects of trauma among all groups and stakeholders and ensure the lens of trauma is understood and applied where necessary to bring a more meaningful understanding, especially in conflict situations. A focus on healing from trauma and increasing resiliency against future trauma can help build cohesiveness and overall wellness.
4. ***Seeking*** to actively resist *retraumatization:*
   When working with vulnerable populations, there is an inadvertent risk of causing further trauma to already traumatized individuals. There is also a risk of compounding existing stress many staff and stakeholders have by baseline trauma by new situations and stressful situations worsening their baseline wellness. Conscious efforts are necessary to avoid retraumatizing individuals, organizations, and communities.

As resiliency factors can be used to help minimize the impact of ACE and other traumas, they can also be used to improve relationships and wellness within groups. They should be promoted as much as possible when working with vulnerable populations and the organizations that serve them. These factors form the basis of a trauma-informed approach to leadership and professionalism.

1. Safety: As safe and nurturing relationships are a key resiliency factor for minimizing the impact of ACE, they should continue to be applied to all traumas. Creating both safe spaces and psychological safety is paramount. This also includes understanding how various stakeholders perceive safety and ensuring those perceptions are understood and promoted. As professionals we should always promote a sense of safety with all interactions.
2. Trustworthiness and Transparency: All professional activities, including decisions and activities, should be conducted with transparency with a key goal of promoting and fostering trust.
3. Collaboration and Mutuality: Within all levels of stakeholders, partnerships, and organizations, professionals should promote equality and leveling of power differentials. Power and decision-making are shared among groups, and a leader understands that all stakeholders have a role to play in promoting wellness and establishing and utilizing a trauma-informed approach.
4. Cultural, Historical, and Gender Support: Professionals should respect and understand cultural, historical, and gender differences without bringing in biases or stereotypes. They should also promote these differences in policies, procedures, and protocols.

The last two approaches include peer support and empowerment, which are discussed below.

Peer-Focused Leadership and Empowerment

Peer-based leadership and empowerment are two approaches espoused within the framework of trauma-informed care. Peer support functions with the understanding that peers, defined as people with lived experience of trauma, are best at navigating and supporting their own needs and the needs of others who may have also experienced trauma or the consequences of trauma leading to shared lived experience of homelessness, mental health concerns, and substance use. Because peers have "walked the walk," they can "talk the talk" and are better equipped to support individuals who have experienced trauma or live with similar conditions. The utilization of peers increases trust within the population they are meaning to serve.

Professionalism in this context involves ensuring that people of lived experience and peers are involved in every process of activity that intersects with them. For instance, with research, we incorporate peer expertise at every stage: research concept development, methodology review, evaluation, and interpretation of results. With program implementation, this would mean engaging with peers around the planning process, fundraising, implementation of any service programming, and last, developing a joint evaluation and knowledge translation plan around the successes and limitations of the service. With knowledge translation in particular, there needs to be a focus on reporting the results back to the peers in a method that's understandable and appreciable by them.

Empowerment

Leadership and professionalism strongly involve empowering the voice of those most vulnerable. Due to the structural consequences of society, individuals who are most vulnerable are often left out of any sort of decision-making around their own needs, sometimes due to competing priorities and sometimes from the lack of engagement from care teams. As such, it is crucial that teams engage and empower individuals to take charge of their own wellness. This approach encompasses the trauma-informed lens by upholding the belief that individuals who experience trauma and achieve recovery are best able to support the healing of others. Shared decision-making is encouraged, as is providing nonjudgmental choice for the client. Similarly, encouraging self-advocacy while also providing the tools for self-advocacy is a key component to ensuring people of lived experience are successful in their overall wellness goals.

A Lens of Harm Reduction

Harm reduction is defined as an evidence-based, client-centered approach that seeks to reduce the health and social harms associated with addiction and substance use, without necessarily requiring people who use substances from abstaining or stopping.[33] Many of the principles of harm reduction overlap with trauma-informed approaches, with the paramount aspects of utilizing nonjudgmental and noncoercive strategies to minimize harm to individuals to ensure they live safer and healthier lives.

Harm reduction acknowledges that individuals experiencing extreme vulnerabilities may not be able to actively engage with their own wellness to a level society deems as acceptable. An example of this is the requirement for individuals to abstain from substance use, which is not a reality for many. As such, the goal of harm reduction is to improve the overall quality of life for an individual, whatever that means for an individual, including access to housing, income support, and food security, but also access to sterile supplies, naloxone kits, and safer consumption sites to avoid unintentional drug poisonings.[34]

Harm reduction as an approach can be difficult for healthcare professionals to comprehend due to the inherent need for many clinicians to solve/cure/treat disease states. With harm reduction, professionals must come to the understanding that while they cannot stop substance use, they can encourage overall wellness and support improvements in quality of life and ensure avoidance of worsening someone's clinical state. An example of this is the day-to-day utilization of seat belts, bike helmets, and life jackets. All these activities have inherent risk of morbidity and death, but these risks can be minimized without stopping individuals from engaging with these activities.

When providing harm reduction support, a focus on information sharing and education should provide individuals with the ability to make personal autonomous informed decisions on their health and their needs without placing judgment or conditions around their care. Clinicians should try to determine the individual goals of clients and respectfully provide support for clients to reach those goals, with a focus on supporting wellness and minimizing harms.

Practical Tips to Approaching Patients With Vulnerabilities

A clinical approach to those experiencing vulnerabilities such as homelessness is often more involved than those who are stably housed due to the various intersectional complexities clients face. Traditionally, this was seen as beyond the scope of most practitioners; however, addressing these key elements helps with the overall health of clients. Some key aspects to note and incorporate include the following[35]:

- Maintaining flexibility: Structured timed appointments are not a reality for many clients who may have to travel distances to see you or deal with competing priorities of survival. Having the ability to accommodate walk-in appointments or accepting clients who are early or late for their appointments is crucial for their engagement in their care.
- Ensure a broad evaluation of baseline cognition of clients, screen for mental health and substance use concerns, and examine their housing, income, food security, and safety concerns.
- Screen for justice concerns and ensure support is provided via referral to legal guidance.
- Ensure appointments are kept short and simple to a maximum of 30 minutes where possible.
- Limit physical exams to an as needed basis as they can retrigger traumatic experiences such as physical assault in the past.
- Medication insurance and flexibility: Medications are often not covered by health insurance and may be unaffordable for clients. Determining what a client can afford and ensuring the appropriate and reasonably effective medication meets the needs of the client is crucial. This may require gaining compassionate access to certain medications. Additionally, try to ensure medication adherence by not providing complex regimens but rather simplified regimens (i.e., antibiotics once a day instead of four times a day).

When dealing with problematic behaviors, concerns such as nonadherence to medications, or missed appointments, taking a step back and revaluating the situation can be beneficial. Using the "5 whys" technique can clarify the root cause of the concern and also provide ideas on how to manage it.[36] For example, if someone continues to miss appointments, ask the following:

1. Why did they miss their appointment? They were unable to reach their bus on time and had to walk to the clinic.
2. Why did they miss their bus? They had to work extra hours to afford child care so as to not have to bring their children to the clinic.
3. Why did they not just bring their children with them? Because the clinic has a strict no children policy.
4. Why does the clinic have a no children policy? Clinic policies dictated this not realizing it was a barrier to patient access and care.

While we did not need to ask a fifth "why," we were able to determine that it was the clinic's own inherent policy that prevented the patient from coming to the clinic and created stress and barriers for them.

The strategies above only outline possible ways to approach clients with vulnerabilities and navigate common issues and concerns that may arise during your professional interactions with them.

Conclusion

Within our clinical practices, we will inevitably encounter situations in which we intersect with individuals who are highly vulnerable, whether it is from homelessness, mental health concerns, or substance use. Health and homelessness are intricately intertwined, and a core understanding and reflection of our inherent biases and judgments can go a long way to help reduce stigma this population faces and further reduce health disparities. Placing ourselves in their shoes can further expand understanding of the unique barriers the population faces, further enhancing our clinical understanding.

While working with vulnerable populations, an understanding of social determinants of health, the impact of trauma, and a focus on wellness around harm reduction and quality of life are key approaches that need to be incorporated into care. These aspects can improve provider-client relationships and improve the overall wellness of this highly stigmatized and marginalized population. Professional development with trauma-informed principles must be underscored, as well as an understanding of the complex intersectionality seen between health, social services, justice, and the political system.

These key leadership strategies and principles for working with this population can also extend to professional relationships, strategic management, and overall organizational leadership. Indeed, incorporating trauma-informed care into every aspect of leadership can greatly increase collaboration, create greater connectivity among the team, and further overall strategic outcomes for this population. Last, empowering the population we serve can be one of the most powerful ways to enhance the health, autonomy, and self-resiliency with those who are highly vulnerable.

References

1. Gaetz S, Barr C, Friesen A, et al. *Canadian Definition of Homelessness.* Canadian Observatory on Homelessness Press; 2012.
2. Hwang SW. Homelessness and health. *CMAJ.* 2001;164(2):229–233.
3. Gaetz S, Donaldson J, Richter T, Gulliver T. *The State of Homelessness in Canada 2013.* Canadian Homelessness Research Network Press; 2013.
4. Nilsson SF, Nordentoft M, Hjorthøj C. Individual-level predictors for becoming homeless and exiting homelessness: a systematic review and meta-analysis. *J Urban Health.* 2019;96(5):741–750. doi:10.1007/s11524-019-00377-x
5. Darkwah V, Yamane H, Richter S, Caine V, Maina G, Chambers T, and Johnson L. A systematic review on the intersection of homelessness and healthcare in Canada. *J Nurs Care.* 2012;1:5. doi:10.4172/2167-1168.1000115
6. Hwang SW, Weaver J, Aubry T, Hoch JS. Hospital costs and length of stay among homeless patients admitted to medical, surgical, and psychiatric services. *Med Care.* 2011;49(4):350–354. doi:10.1097/MLR.0b013e318206c50d
7. Salit SA, Kuhn EM, Hartz AJ, Vu JM, Mosso AL. Hospitalization costs associated with homelessness in New York City. *N Engl J Med.* 1998;338(24):1734–1740. doi:10.1056/NEJM199806113382406
8. Roncarati JS, Baggett TP, O'Connell JJ, et al. Mortality among unsheltered homeless adults in Boston, Massachusetts, 2000–2009. *JAMA Intern Med.* 2018;178(9):1242–1248. doi:10.1001/jamainternmed.2018.2924
9. Bowen EA, Quenette L, Walton LQ. Disparities and the social determinants of mental health and addictions: opportunities for a multifaceted social work response. *Health Soc Work.* 2015;40(3):e59–e65. https://doi.org/10.1093/hsw/hlv034
10. Social determinants of health. World Health Organization. Accessed March 1, 2023. https://www.who.int/teams/social-determinants-of-health
11. Board on Environmental Change and Society; Committee on Population; Division of Behavioral and Social Sciences and Education; Board on Life Sciences; Division on Earth and Life Studies; National Research Council. *Can Earth's and Society's Systems Meet the Needs of 10 Billion People? Summary of a Workshop.* National Academies Press; August 7, 2014. Resource Distribution and Global Inequality. https://www.ncbi.nlm.nih.gov/books/NBK253872/
12. Mackenbach JP, Stronks K, Kunst AE. The contribution of medical care to inequalities in health: differences between socio-economic groups in decline of mortality from conditions amenable to medical intervention. *Soc Sci Med.* 1989;29:369–376.
13. Braveman PA, Cubbin C, Egerter S, Williams DR, Pamuk E. Socioeconomic disparities in health in the United States: what the patterns tell us. *Am J Public Health.* 2010;100(suppl 1):S186–S196.
14. Bradley EH, Canavan M, Rogan E, et al. Variation in health outcomes: the role of spending on social services, public health, and health care, 2000–09. *Health Aff (Millwood).* 2016;35(5):760–768. doi:10.1377/hlthaff.2015.0814
15. Sullivan MM, Lazowy EE, Roncarati JS, Koh HK, O'Connell James J. Training clinicians to care for patients where they are. *AMA J Ethics.* 2021;23(11):E852–E857. doi:10.1001/amajethics.2021.852
16. Corrigan PW, Kraus DJ, Pickett SA, et al. Using peer navigators to address the integrated health care needs of homeless African Americans with serious mental illness. *Psychiatr Serv.* 2017;68(3):264–270. doi:10.1176/appi.ps.201600134

17. Doohan NC, Mishori R. Street medicine: creating a "classroom without walls" for teaching population health. *Med Sci Educ.* 2019;30(1):513–521. doi:10.1007/s40670-019-00849-4

18. McNeil R, Guirguis-Younger M, Dilley LB, Turnbull J, Hwang SW. Learning to account for the social determinants of health affecting homeless persons. *Med Educ.* 2013;47(5):485–494.

19. Essentials of professionalism and ethics. Canadian Center of Substance Use and Addiction. https://www.ccsa.ca/sites/default/files/2019-04/CCSA-Professionalism-Ethics-Summary-2017-en.pdf

20. Buchanan D, Rohr L, Kehoe L, Glick SB, Jain S. Changing attitudes toward homeless people. *J Gen Intern Med.* 2004;19(5, pt 2):566–568.

21. Gardner J, Emory J. Changing students' perceptions of the homeless: a community service-learning experience. *Nurse Educ Pract.* 2018;29:133–136.

22. Sedhom R. Taking our oath seriously: compassion for patients. *AMA J Ethics.* 2016;18(1):69–72. doi:10.1001/journalofethics.2017.18.1.mnar1-1601

23. Talbot S Dean W. Physicians' aren't burning out, they're suffering from moral injury. *Stat News.* July 26, 2018. https://www.statnews.com/2018/07/26/physicians-not-burning-out-they-are-suffering-moral-injury/

24. Binswanger IA, Redmond N, Steiner JF, Hicks LS. Health disparities and the criminal justice system: an agenda for further research and action. *J Urban Health.* 2012;*89*(1):98–107. doi:10.1007/s11524-011-9614-1

25. Sugiharti L, Purwono R, Esquivias MA, Rohmawati H. The nexus between crime rates, poverty, and income inequality: a case study of Indonesia. *Economies.* 2023;*11*:62. https://doi.org/10.3390/economies11020062

26. Massoglia M. Incarceration as exposure: the prison, infectious disease, and other stress-related illnesses. *J Health Soc Behav.* 2008;49(1):56–71. doi:10.1177/002214650804900105

27. Cloud D, Dougherty M, May RL 2nd, Parsons J, Wormeli P, Rudman WJ. At the intersection of health and justice. *Perspect Health Inf Manag.* 2014;11(Winter):1c.

28. Draine J, Herman DB. Critical time intervention for reentry from prison for persons with mental illness. *Psychiatr Serv.* 2007;58:1577–1581.

29. Binswanger IA, Stern MF, Deyo RA, et al. Release from prison—a high risk of death for former inmates. *N Engl J Med.* 2007;356:157–165.

30. Tweedy D. Trauma informed leadership: an approach to healthcare. Accessed October 17, 2022. https://healthadministrationdegree.usc.edu/blog/trauma-informed-leadership/

31. Crouch E, Radcliff E, Strompolis M, Srivastav A. Safe, stable, and nurtured: protective factors against poor physical and mental health outcomes following exposure to adverse childhood experiences (ACEs). *J Child Adolesc Trauma.* 2019;12:165–173. doi:10.1007/s40653-018-0217-9

32. Substance Abuse and Mental Health Services Administration. *SAMHSA's Concept of Trauma and Guidance for a Trauma-Informed Approach.* Substance Abuse and Mental Health Services Administration; 2014. HHS publication no. (SMA) 14-4884. https://store.samhsa.gov/sites/default/files/d7/priv/sma14-4884.pdf

33. Thomas G. *Harm Reduction Policies and Programs Involved for Persons Involved in the Criminal Justice System.* Canadian Centre on Substance Use; 2005.

34. Pires R, Yeoman R, Allen T, et al. Engaging users, reducing harms. Collaborative research exploring the practices and results of harm reduction. United Way Report. 2007. http://ekonomos.com/wp-content/uploads/2014/03/Harm-Reduction-Report.pdf

35. Davies A, Wood L. Homeless health care: meeting the challenges of providing primary care. *Med J Aust.* September 3, 2018.

36. Card AJ. The problem with "5 whys." *BMJ Qual Saf.* 2017;26:671–677.

23
Well-Being
An Essential Element of Medical Professionalism

Joseph Carrese and Gia Merlo

Key Points

- There is an inextricable link between physician well-being and medical professionalism.
- Sub-optimal well-being is detrimental to patient care and ultimately leads to lapses in medical professionalism.
- Addressing concerns about well-being in clinical practice requires addressing well-being from a systems perspective and is insufficiently addressed when the focus is solely on individual physicians.

This chapter addresses the relationship between well-being and medical professionalism. While we use the language of well-being, we acknowledge several other, to some extent over lapping, terms are used to address this general concept, including wellness, mental health, and more recently brain health.[1,2] While each of these concepts includes somewhat distinct elements and considerations, typically their definitions are quite similar and include reference to each other. In some formulations, well-being is considered the overarching construct, while in other formulations well-being is subsumed within wellness, mental health, and brain health. We cannot address these three concepts and their respective relationships in depth in this chapter, but have included references to facilitate further exploration.

The relationship between well-being and medical professionalism is fraught. Historically, physicians' well-being has suffered, due to both the stressful nature and circumstances of their work and the relationship of that work to the rest of their lives.

The nature and circumstances of physicians' work involves repeated exposure to the suffering and trauma of others, which can lead to empathic strain and compassion fatigue.[3] This is compounded by other work-related factors, such as overall workload, burdensome administrative tasks and challenges associated with use of technology.[4] All of this can undermine well-being.

Regarding the relationship of physician's work to the rest of their lives, key tenets of professionalism include "responsiveness to patient needs that supersedes self-interest"[5(p20)] and the primacy of patient welfare.[6] Consistent with these principles, typically professionalism has been operationalized as subordination of self, family, and other important personal relationships to professional responsibilities. While this formulation is understandable and appropriate up to a point, taken to an extreme it can result in a level of self-sacrifice that undermines or even neglects well-being. In this way, well-being becomes a casualty of professionalism.

Self-sacrifice leading to neglect of well-being, the demanding nature of the work, as well as the burden associated with the circumstances of the work, together can be associated with dissatisfaction, cynicism, emotional exhaustion, depersonalization, loss of meaning, and ultimately burnout.[7,8,9] Other harmful outcomes may follow, including but not limited to impairment (e.g., substance use disorders), depression, divorce, and even suicide.[10,11,12] Beyond the harm to individual providers and their relationships, there may be other consequences: substandard patient care (affecting safety and quality) and lapses in professionalism.[13,14] For example, residents with low well-being reported having fewer or even inappropriate interactions with patients, increased conflict with colleagues, and feeling indifferent at work.[15] In addition, because physicians who suffer from burnout are suboptimal teachers and role models, learners may be harmed.[16(pxiv)]

If anything, the work of healthcare has become more complex, demanding, and stressful in recent years—and this was true before the coronavirus pandemic. During the pandemic "health care teams and public health workers experienced extraordinary fear, fatigue, isolation, and moral distress and injury."[17(p51)] Recent survey data indicate nearly 63% of physicians experience at least one manifestation of burnout.[18]

In contrast to the conventional approach to professionalism, where well-being may be sacrificed, an alternative conceptualization of professionalism, one that is arguably healthier and more sustainable, considers well-being as an essential element. The goal of this latter approach is to create and maintain balance in one's life and career, to serve with joy and meaning and guard against personal outcomes that may lead to lapses in professionalism and in turn suboptimal outcomes for patients and substandard educational experiences for learners.

Accordingly, well-being must be a major focus of medical education and training; a core component of professional identity formation; and an essential element of professionalism throughout one's career.

So, then, what is well-being? According to one conceptualization, focusing on work and career: "Professional well-being is a function of being satisfied with one's job, finding meaning in work, feeling engaged at work, having a high-quality working life, and finding professional fulfillment in work."[17(pxiv),19,20] Another definition, from the American Psychological Association, defines well-being as "a state of happiness and contentment, with low levels of distress, overall good physical and mental health and outlook, or good quality of life."[21]

In thinking about the project of addressing well-being, it is critical to appreciate that well-being is undermined by occupational stress secondary to high job demands and systems-level factors.[16(p1)] While only a small part of the problem is under the control of and modifiable by individuals,[22,23] solutions for burnout typically focus on the individual rather than the system. [17(p51)] As the 2022 National Academy of Medicine (NAM) report notes: "It does not matter if resilience is instilled in individual future health workers if they enter systems that diminish their abilities to thrive."[17(p61)]

Therefore, the goal of addressing well-being as an essential element of a robust and sustainable version of professionalism cannot be accomplished only by individual physicians motivated to protect themselves, the health of their patients, and the best interests of their learners. It must also be a priority of other stakeholders who drive much of the problem: healthcare organizations and actors in the larger, external environment.

We must "institutionalize well-being as a long-term value" in order to be successful in addressing the problem.[17(p6)]

The NAM presents a conceptual model of well-being that depicts a systems-level approach when considering this issue (Figure 23.1).

In order to address the systems-level dimensions of the problem, steps must be taken, among other things, to create positive work environments; reduce administrative burdens and workplace inefficiencies; modify technology so it helps rather than exacerbates the problem; and provide support to clinicians to facilitate attention to emotional health and well-being.[16(Box S-2,p9)] Many organizations have created Offices of Well-Being and named chief wellness officers to facilitate these changes, accomplished in part by creating needed resources and making them available to employees.[24]

Systems also must be modified in other fundamental ways to address well-being. For example, by aligning organizational structures, policies, and processes with mutually agreed on values that prioritize well-being; having leadership committed to this effort; and redesigning the work experience to enhance meaning and purpose, provide adequate resources, and facilitate a collaborative approach to patient care.[16(Box S-1,p7)]

Beyond the institutional level, several societal factors play a role. The NAM report presenting the systems model states the following: "The third level of the system model is the external environment, which includes political, market, professional, and societal factors. This level contains opportunities and constraints that influence decisions and actions at the health care organization level and the work done by clinicians at the frontline care delivery level."[16(Box S-1,p6)] Examples of actors in the external environment include the Center for Medicare and Medicaid Services; other government agencies/regulators; state governments; and state licensing boards.

Well-being/wellness at the individual level is multidimensional. According to one popular conceptualization, wellness includes six dimensions (Figure 23.2).

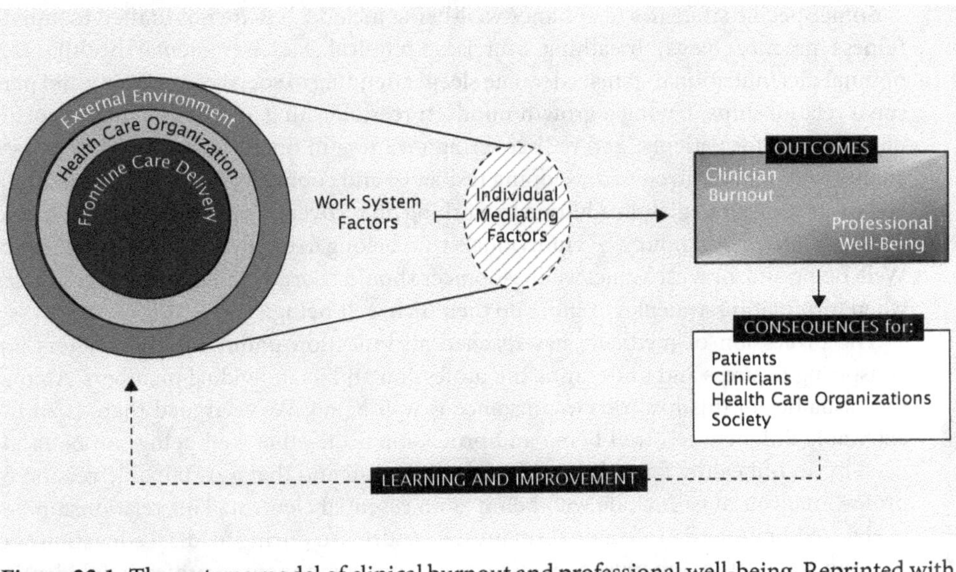

Figure 23.1 The systems model of clinical burnout and professional well-being. Reprinted with permission from the National Academies of Sciences, Engineering, and Medicine.

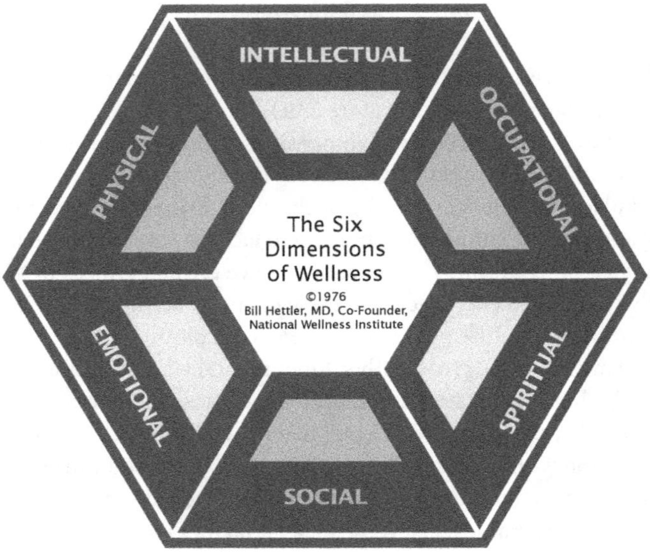

Figure 23.2 The six dimensions of wellness. Reprinted with permission from the National Wellness Institute, Inc., NationalWellness.org.

Individuals can and should be taught during their education/training to prioritize their well-being and engage in self-care strategies that attend to each of these multiple dimensions, perhaps prioritizing areas most important to them and that address their individual needs best. The objective of achieving well-being is an ongoing project that must be consistently attended to throughout one's career. Individuals should also appreciate that their personal efforts are only part of the solution, given, as has been already pointed out, the prominent role institutions, systems, and the broader external environment play in the status of physicians' well-being.

Some specific strategies to enhance well-being include, but are not limited to, mindfulness practice; yoga; breathing exercises; physical exercise; mental health care; optimal diet/nutritional status; adequate sleep; attending to social connectivity and personal relationships; having a growth mindset; reestablishing and optimizing opportunities to care for patients; and rediscovering meaning in one's work.[25,26,27,28,29,30] Also, attention should be given to developing resilience and coping by employing prevention and protection strategies, in addition to working on recovery from moral distress, moral suffering, and moral injury.[31,32] Individuals who belong to organizations with Offices of Well-Being and/or with a chief wellness officer should take advantage of these resources when formulating strategies to shore up their own well-being.

The profession of medicine has reached an inflection point: Multiple factors are conspiring to stress and undermine the profession and its individual members. Among the casualties of this historic circumstance is well-being. We've argued there is an inextricable link between well-being and professionalism—that well-being can be sacrificed by an unhealthy formulation of professionalism and that a sustainable version of professionalism must include well-being as an essential element. This relationship between well-being and professionalism must be addressed during medical education and training, and well-being must be included as a core component of professional identity formation and professionalism throughout one's career. We've also argued that focusing exclusively on individual physicians and what they can do for themselves will not adequately address the magnitude of this problem. Systems factors at multiple levels, involving multiple actors, must be simultaneously attended to in order for a robust state of well-being that supports a high level of professionalism to be achieved. To be successful, all of us must be committed to this project for the long haul.

References

1. Merlo G, Sugden S, Abascal L. Introduction to lifestyle psychiatry. In: Rippe JM, ed. *Lifestyle Medicine.* 4th ed. Taylor & Francis; 2024.
2. Chapman SB, Robertson IH, Zientz J, et al. The neuroscience of brain health. In: Rippe JM, ed. *Lifestyle Medicine.* 4th ed. Taylor & Francis, 2024.
3. Cocker F, Joss N. Compassion fatigue among healthcare, emergency and community service workers: a systematic review. *Int J Environ Res Public Health.* 2016;13(6):618.
4. National Academies of Sciences, Engineering, and Medicine. *Taking Action Against Clinician Burnout: A Systems Approach to Professional Well-Being.* National Academies Press; 2019: Preface, xiv. https://doi.org/10.17226/25521
5. ACGME Common Program Requirements (Residency). 2022. Accessed May 17, 2023. https://www.acgme.org/what-we-do/accreditation/common-program-requirements/
6. Project of the ABIM Foundation, ACP–ASIM Foundation, and European Federation of Internal Medicine. Medical professionalism in the new millennium: a physician charter. *Ann Intern Med.* 2002;136:243–246.
7. Spickard A Jr, Gabbe SG, Christensen JF. Mid-career burnout in generalist and specialist physicians. *JAMA.* 2002;288:1447–1450.
8. Dyrbye LN, West CP, Satele D, et al. Burnout among US medical students, residents, and early career physicians relative to the general population. *Acad Med.* 2014;89:443–451.
9. Sexton JB, Adair KC, Proulx J, et al. Emotional exhaustion among US health care workers before and during the COVID-19 pandemic, 2019–2021. *JAMA Netw Open.* 2022;5(9):e2232748. doi:10.1001/jamanetworkopen.2022.32748
10. Berge KH, Seppala MD, Schipper AM. Chemical dependency and the physician. *Mayo Clin Proc.* 2009;84(7):625–631. doi:10.1016/S0025-6196(11)60751-9
11. Ly DP, Seabury SA, Jena AB. Divorce among physicians and other healthcare professionals in the United States: analysis of census survey data. *BMJ.* 2015;350:h706.
12. Harvey SB, Epstein RM, Glozier N, et al. Mental illness and suicide among physicians. *Lancet.* 2021;398:920–930.
13. Dyrbye LN, Massie FS, Eacker A, et al. Relationship between burnout and professional conduct and attitudes among US medical students. *JAMA.* 2010;304:1173–1180.
14. McTaggart LS, Walker JP. The relationship between resident physician burnout and its' effects on patient care, professionalism, and academic achievement: a review of the literature. *Health Sci Rev.* 2022;4:100049. https://doi.org/10.1016/j.hsr.2022.100049
15. Ratanawongsa N, Wright SM, Carrese JA. Well-being in residency: effects on relationships with patients, interactions with colleagues, performance, and motivation. *Patient Educ Couns.* 2008;72(2):194–200.
16. National Academies of Sciences, Engineering, and Medicine. *Taking Action Against Clinician Burnout: A Systems Approach to Professional Well-Being.* 2019: Preface, xiv.

17. National Academy of Medicine. *National Plan for Health Workforce Well-Being.* National Academies Press; 2022:51. https://doi.org/10.17226/26744

18. Shanafelt TD, West CP, Dyrbye LN, et al. Changes in burnout and satisfaction with work-life integration in physicians during the first 2 years of the COVID-19 pandemic. *Mayo Clin Proc.* 2022;97(12):2248–2258.

19. Danna K, Griffin RW. 1999. Health and well-being in the workforce: a review and synthesis of the literature. *J Manage.* 1999;25(3):357–384. https://doi.org/10.1177/014920639902500305

20. Doble SE, Santha JC. Occupational well-being: rethinking occupational therapy outcomes. *Can J Occup Ther.* 2008;75(3):184–190. https://doi.org/10.1177/000841740807500310

21. American Psychological Association. *APA Dictionary of Psychology.* Well-being. Accessed May 25, 2023. https://dictionary.apa.org/well-being

22. Dyrbye L, Shanafelt T. A narrative review on burnout experienced by medical students and residents. *Med Educ.* 2016;50(1):132–149.

23. Williams ES, Konrad TR, Linzer M, et al. Physician, practice, and patient characteristics related to primary care physician physical and mental health: results from the Physician Worklife Study. *Health Serv Res.* 2002;37(1):121–143.

24. Pipas CF, Courand J, Neumann SA, et al. *The Rise of Wellness Initiatives in Health Care: Using National Survey Data to Support Effective Well-Being Champions and Wellness Programs.* AAMC; 2021.

25. Horn DJ, Johnston CB. Burnout and self care for palliative care practitioners. *Med Clin N Am.* 2020;104:561–572.

26. Ellin A. Doctors, facing burnout, turn to self-care. *New York Times.* January 26, 2021. Accessed 5/22/2023.

27. Beckman HB, Wendland M, Mooney C, et al. The impact of a program in mindful communication of primary care physicians. *Acad Med.* 2012;87:1–5.

28. Kopacz D, Houghton L. A new paradigm for growth. *Closler.* October 2022. https://closler.org/lifelong-learning-in-clinical-excellence/a-new-paradigm-for-growth. Accessed 5/23/2023.

29. Schwenk TL. Physician well-being and the regenerative power of caring. *JAMA.* 2018;319(15):1543–44. doi:10.1001/jama.2018.1539.

30. Morris A, Do D, Gottlieb-Smith R, et al. Impact of a fitness intervention on medical students. *South Med J.* 2012;105:12:630–634.

31. Rushton C, Swoboda S, Reimer T, et al. The Mindful Ethical Practice & Resilience Academy (MEPRA): sustainability of impact. *Am J Crit Care.* 2023;32(3):184–194. doi:10.4037/ajcc2023236

32. Rushton CR (ed.). *Moral Resilience: Transforming Moral Suffering in Healthcare.* Oxford University Press; 2018. https://doi.org/10.1093/med/9780190619268.001.0001

24
Professionalism Considerations in Social Media Use

John Spandorfer

Key Points

- The professional and personal use of social media by physicians is widespread.
- Despite the potential risks to medical professionalism that come with social media use (e.g., violations of patient privacy), there are notable benefits to the utilization of social media among the medical professions.
- Several medical professional societies offer guidance for the professional use of social media, including guidance regarding the content of publicly viewable social media posts.

Social Media—Types and Prevalence of Use

As of January 2022, 58% of the world's population has been found to use social media.[1] The prevalence of physicians and other healthcare providers that use social media, for both private and professional use, is also widespread. Types of social media they may use include social networking, video hosting, discussion forums, blogging or microblogging, and consumer review networks (Table 24.1).

In a 2021 study of European healthcare professionals, 18.5% of respondents used social media exclusively for professional purposes, 17.5% only for private purposes, and 64.0% for both.[2] The most widely used social media for professional use found in this study are LinkedIn (60.8%), Twitter (55.1%), Facebook (49.5%), YouTube (28.3%), Instagram (24.7%), personal blogs (3.1%), and TikTok (0.5%).

In a 2021 study of Australian healthcare providers, Facebook, YouTube, Twitter, and LinkedIn are the most popular social media applications.[3] In this study, Facebook was found to be the most frequently used platform 47% were regular users of it. YouTube was the second most popular platform among health professionals (45%). This is followed by 25% of respondents frequently using Twitter and 21% of respondents' access LinkedIn. Of respondents, 15% employ various other social media platforms for personal use. Concerning the professional use of social media, however, 25% use YouTube, 21% use LinkedIn, 19% use Facebook, 12% use Twitter, 7% use blog sites, and 11% use other platforms.

In a 2017 study of 366 Texas healthcare workers, 88% indicated that they used social media.[4] Not surprisingly, those under 40 were significantly more likely to use social media than those over 40.

Table 24.1 Types of Social Media and Their Examples

Types of Social Media	Examples
Social networking	Facebook, LinkedIn, Instagram, Doximity, SERMO
Video hosting	YouTube, TikTok, Vimeo
Discussion forums	Reddit
Blogging or microblogging	Twitter, Kevin MD
Consumer review networks	Yelp

Table 24.2 Benefits of Social Media in Medicine[3,5,6]

Ability of professional organizations to connect with members
Ability of professionals to rapidly communicate health information to peers and patients
Collective sourcing of advice on challenging medical cases
Contribute to public health research and service
Enhance professional development/learning
Networking
Social support

Benefits of Social Media

Appropriate use of social media in medicine has many potential advantages (Table 24.2). In the United Kingdom's General Medical Council's guidance on doctors and social media, the authors note many areas of benefits of using social media, including the rapid dissemination to peers of new developments, position statements, and upcoming meetings; collective sourcing of advice on challenging medical cases; and the ability of professional organizations to connect with its members.[5] In a survey of healthcare professionals, respondents listed the following as potential benefits: networking, health communication, social media as a form of social support, learning, and health promotion.[3] Finally, others have described the benefits of social media to improve communication with patients, enhance professional development, and contribute to public health research and service.[6]

Risks of Social Media

While there are many potential benefits to the appropriate use of social media, there are also many professionalism risks, such as violations of privacy and professional codes of conduct.

Privacy Violations on Social Media

A resident posted to his social media site a photograph that was of him being hugged by his patient and holding the patient's infant child. The photo, taken by a nurse and emailed to the resident, was of the mother and infant at the time of discharge, which followed a prolonged hospitalization that involved a premature birth and 2-month hospitalization of the newborn in the newborn intensive care unit. The resident had cared for the child over the past month. Below the photograph, he wrote: "So excited and proud to be involved in this family's care! Finally going home after being born at 28 weeks!"

A medical student, on an emergency medicine rotation, was on the trauma team that cared for six patients who were victims of a mass shooting. Three patients died of their injuries. Following the shift that evening, the student posted on her social media site a photo taken of the x-ray of the pelvis containing the bullet that pierced the pelvis of the patient who had survived. The name on the x-ray was redacted. In addition to posting the photo, the student wrote: "Sad story from the ED [emergency department] last night. Three patients died in a mass shooting; this patient survived. We need better gun safety laws!"

Although stories of the Health Insurance Portability and Accountability Act (HIPAA) violations on social media have been reported widely in the press,[7] the true incidence of these breaches are unknown. While considering whether a social media post is a violation of confidentiality, it is useful to consider whether the post violates a standard of legal conduct or more generally violates a standard of professional or ethical conduct. [8,9] In the United States, the HIPAA Privacy Rule stipulates the legal standard for using confidential information. The HIPAA statute notes: "There are no restrictions on the use or disclosure of de-identified health information. De-identified health information neither identifies nor provides a reasonable basis to identify an individual."[9] The Privacy Rule describes the process of de-identifying medical information:

There are two ways to de-identify information: (1) a formal determination by a qualified statistician; and (2) the removal of specified identifiers of an individual and of the individual's relatives, household members, and employers is required, and is adequate only if the covered entity (such as a physician or student) has no actual knowledge that the remaining information could be used to identify the individual.

In the first example above, although probably well meaning, the post was a HIPAA violation (assuming no permission from the mother was given) as it contained protected health information (see Table 24.3). It is understandable how this oversight may occur. While not considering the privacy violation, the resident was caught in the emotional success of caring for a complex patient and wanted to share this sentiment with his online followers.

In the example of the student's post about the trauma patient, whether this was a legal violation of the HIPAA statute is not as clear as the first example. There was no name on the x-ray, and there was more than one patient who survived the shooting. Nevertheless, the student has no ability to assess whether viewers of the post were able to identify who sustained a bullet injury to the pelvis. Between news accounts of the incident and other information that may become known either publicly or privately, it is conceivable a highly motivated individual who viewed the post could associate the x-ray with the specific shooting victim.

Compared to sharing the same story with a single confidant or presenting the story at an educational meeting, sharing the story on social media, with its ability to disseminate information to an unlimited number of viewers, leads to a greater risk of privacy violation. The student in the example above may believe that the post will be viewed by a limited number of individuals (his followers), and as stipulated in the HIPAA statute may

Table 24.3 18 HIPAA Identifiers

Name
Address (all geographic subdivisions smaller than state, including street address, city, county, and zip code)
All elements (except years) of dates related to an individual (including birthdate, admission date, discharge date, date of death, and exact age if over 89)
Telephone numbers
Fax numbers
Email address
Social Security number
Medical record number
Health plan beneficiary number
Account number
Certificate or license number
Vehicle identifiers and serial numbers, including license plate numbers
Device identifiers and serial numbers
Web URL
Internet Protocol (IP) address
Finger- or voiceprint
Photographic, not limited to images of the face
Other characteristics that could uniquely identify the individual

have "no actual knowledge that the remaining information could be used to identify the individual." However, on social media, users must realize that any risk for a privacy violation is magnified as the post can be easily forwarded to an unlimited number of viewers. Once forwarded, the post may also be taken out of context. Therefore, the individual who posts may not be violating a legal threshold such as HIPAA but may be violating a standard of professional or ethical conduct.

Other Inappropriate Posts

An anesthesiologist posts on a medical social media site: "It's unbelievable how many obese patients we have in our hospital! Always a challenge to intubate. Had one today that was close to exceeding the weight limit of our table. I have an idea—how about we stop any fatty over 300 pounds from having elective surgery!"

A resident physician posts a video on a social media site of an end-of-year house staff party in which he and many peers were drinking and making sexist comments about residents in another specialty of the same hospital. Along with the video, the resident wrote: "We worked our asses off this year; it was great to finally unwind with the best residents in the world."

Institutional and specialty professional codes of conduct stipulate that those in the medical profession should not engage in activity that erodes trust of patients or harms the reputation of colleagues. Recommendations from multiple specialty organizations give guidance on this topic. Specifically, guidelines from the American College of Surgeons describe:

> It is never appropriate to post derogatory comments about patients or colleagues. Surgeons should be careful not to post in anger or under the influence of any substance. Although it is acceptable to disagree with colleagues via social media, such posts should be respectful, collegial, and reflect positively on the profession. Statements about a colleague's abilities, experience, or outcomes intended in jest may be appropriate for the surgeon's lounge, yet entirely inappropriate for public consumption. A practice of "pausing before posting" is likely to prevent regretful posts in this vein.[10]

Any post that disparages patients erodes the trust that the post's readers would have in that physician. The Physician Charter, endorsed by professional organizations worldwide, describes that "professionalism is the basis of medicine's contract with society."[11] The charter further states that "essential to this contract is public trust in physicians which depends on the integrity of both individual physicians and the whole profession" and that "professionalism demands placing the interest of patients above those of the physician." The post about the obese patient places the needs of the physician ahead of the patient and shows a clear lack of integrity as well as empathy toward this group of patients.

Appropriate Posts on Social Media

If each of the examples above illustrates inappropriate social media posts, could the posts be revised to contain the same sentiments and without any concerns of professionalism violations?[8] Stevenson and Peck, as well as Chretien and Kind, propose a model, using the double-effect reasoning, when justifying social media posts. The authors recommend the following criteria[12,13]:

1. The social media post considered separately from its unintended harmful effect is in itself not wrong.
2. The writer intends only the good and does not intend harm as an end or as a mean.
3. The writer reflects upon his/her relevant duties, considering accepted norms and takes due care to eliminate or alleviate any foreseen harm through his/her act.

Though the physician posting about obese patients met none of these criteria, many respectfully written posts by health care providers may. Prior to writing on social media about a patient, permission from that patient should be sought. When patients are informed about the good intent of the post and assured they would not be identified (unless the patient chooses to be identified), they may consent to having their story made public.

As suggested by Chretien and Kind, the types of posts that consider the intent of the writer meet the criteria above and may be justified are shown in Table 24.4.

Table 24.4 Suggestions for Modifying the Content of Social Media Posts

Intent of Writer	Suggested Modification of Social Media Post Examples	Example Post
Stimulate understanding or empathy without intention to harm	The resident instead writes about the difficulties patients born premature have and how it is a privilege to be involved with their care.	A photo of the resident and a colleague in front of the hospital with the caption: "We are inspired by many of our patients who have been through so much. Thrilled to be involved in their care!"
Fulfill the role of teacher	The student instead writes at the conclusion of her emergency medicine rotation about the many injuries she has seen related to gun violence.	"After caring for gun violence victims in the ER during my rotation, I am even more committed to advocating for gun safety."
Reflection about the provider's struggles and professional and ethical duties	The physician instead writes about the challenges that morbidly obese patients have during perioperative care.	"With increasing numbers of morbidly obese patients in our hospitals, we need to have better training and equipment for their specific needs. It's frustrating when we don't."

Boundaries Violations in Social Media

A neurologist evaluated a patient for migraine headaches. By the second visit, the neurologist and patient realized they had children of similar ages who went to the same school. That evening, the neurologist received a friend request from the patient.

Following a first visit with a 45-year-old man, a family doctor was curious about the personal life of his patient and searched for information about the patient on various social media platforms. While viewing these sites over 10 minutes, the physician learned of the patient's family, recent vacations they had been on, as well as his views on various political issues.

Accepting the Friend Request

As a general rule, physicians should not engage in extramedical social interactions with patients, such as meeting them for meals or drinks, calling them for personal advice, or actively involving themselves in the social lives of patients.[14] Developing a relationship with a patient online, beyond the scope of the professional relationship, is such an extramedical social interaction. During their care, patients may develop an emotional attachment to their physician or other healthcare provider and may desire to continue to stay connected when away from the clinical setting. Following an accepted friend request, invitations from the patient to personal gatherings or other overtures to strengthen the relationship may continue. But such blurring of boundaries may create challenges in balancing the role of authority required in future professional interactions.[15] Will the physician give preferential treatment of the patient who she has a relationship with outside of the office? Would the extra effort needed to maintain the outside professional relationship strain the work-life balance of the physician? And would any rejection of social interaction with the patient affect the future therapeutic relationship? These challenging questions should give the physician pause before accepting the friend request.

Managing a friend request or other social media connections may be more challenging when there is already an established social relationship with the patient, which may occur more often in rural settings where members of the community have less choice in choosing their physician. An open dialogue with the patient about the potential pitfalls of a dual relationship, such as risks to patient confidentiality and preferential treatment, should be reviewed. If the physician senses that there may be substandard care or a risk for professional violations, the physician should consider referring that patient to a colleague.

Searching for Patient Information on Social Media

In early 2010, of practicing physicians, 16% acknowledged having visited a patient's online profile or that of a patient's family member.[16] With increased use of social media since 2010, the prevalence of this may now be higher.

In 2017, the American Psychiatric Association Ethics Committee noted that performing targeted internet searches on a patient is not, in and of itself, unethical.[17] However, the committee states this type of search should only be done in the interests of promoting patient care and well-being and not to satisfy the curiosity or other needs of the clinician. It is also important to consider how this could influence treatment decisions. And, in the name of transparency, the committee recommends the clinician should disclose to a patient that such a search took place.

The family physician in the vignette should first consider how such an online search may help the patient. If after doing so, the physician concludes the reason for the search is not for the patient's interest and rather only for the physician's curiosity, it would be prudent to avoid the internet search.

Recommendations From Medical Organizations

In addition to guidelines from the American College of Surgeons noted above, many organizations have published recommendations on how physicians should use social media.

In their Code of Medial Ethics, Opinion 2.3.2, the American Medical Association recommends physicians consider seven elements when maintaining a presence online[18]:

1. Physicians should be cognizant of standards of patient privacy and confidentiality that must be maintained in all environments, including online, and must refrain from posting identifiable patient information online.
2. When using social media for educational purposes or to exchange information professionally with other physicians, follow ethics guidance regarding confidentiality, privacy, and informed consent.

3. When using the internet for social networking, physicians should use privacy settings to safeguard personal information and content to the extent possible, but should realize that privacy settings are not absolute and that once on the internet, content is likely there permanently. Thus, physicians should routinely monitor their own internet presence to ensure that the personal and professional information on their own sites and, to the extent possible, content posted about them by others, is accurate and appropriate.
4. If they interact with patients on the internet, physicians must maintain appropriate boundaries of the patient-physician relationship in accordance with professional ethics guidance just as they would in any other context.
5. To maintain appropriate professional boundaries, physicians should consider separating personal and professional content online.
6. When physicians see content posted by colleagues that appears unprofessional they have a responsibility to bring that content to the attention of the individual, so that he or she can remove it and/or take other appropriate actions. If the behavior significantly violates professional norms and the individual does not take appropriate action to resolve the situation, the physician should report the matter to appropriate authorities.
7. Physicians must recognize that actions online and content posted may negatively affect their reputations among patients and colleagues, may have consequences for their medical careers (particularly for physicians in training and medical students) and can undermine public trust in the medical profession.

The Federation of State Medical Boards, the organization that is charged with sanctioning physicians who are found to use social media inappropriately, published their recommendations on appropriate use of social media and social networking in medical practice. Their recommendations included the following[19]:

1. Physicians should only have online interaction with patients when discussing the patient's medical treatment within the physician-patient relationship, and these interactions should never occur on personal social networking or social media websites.
2. Social networking websites may be useful for physicians to gather and share their experiences. While using such networks may be useful, it is the responsibility of the physician to ensure that professional networks for physicians are secure and that only verified and registered users have access to the information.
3. While physicians may post their experiences on nonclinical sites, they should never provide any information that could be used to identify patients.
4. Physicians should always act professionally and take caution not to post information that is ambiguous or that could be misconstrued or taken out of context.
5. Use separate personal and professional social networking sites.
6. Report any unprofessional behavior that is witnessed to supervisory and/or regulatory authorities.
7. Always adhere to the same principles of professionalism online as you would offline.
8. Refer as appropriate to an employer social media or social networking policy for direction on the proper use of social media and social networking in relation to their employment.

References

1. Chaffey D. Global social media statistics research summary 2023. Accessed December 15, 2023. https://www.smartinsights.com/social-media-marketing/social-media-strategy/new-global-social-media-research/
2. Guerra F, Linz D, Garcia R, et al. The use of social media for professional purposes by healthcare professionals: the #intEHRAct survey. *Europace.* 2022;24(4):691–696.
3. Khan MI, Saleh MA, Quazi A. Social media adoption by health professionals: a TAM-based study. *Informatics.* 2021; 8(1): 6.
4. Surani Z, Hirani R, Elias A, et al. Social media usage among health care providers. *BMC Res Notes.* 2017;10(1), 1–5.
5. General Medical Council. *Doctors' Use of Social Media.* General Medical Council; 2013.
6. George DR, Rovniak LS, Kraschnewski JL. Dangers and opportunities for social media in medicine. *Clin Obstet Gynecol.* 2013;56(3), 453–462.
7. Becker's Health IT & CIO Review. Going "social": monitoring and addressing HIPAA violations on social media. 2012, April 16. Accessed August 14, 2022. http://www.beckershospitalreview.com/healthcare-information-technology/goingqsocialq-monitoring-and-addressing-hipaa-violations-on-social-media.html
8. Spandorfer J. Confidentiality and social media. In: Cooper N, Frain A, Frain J, eds. *ABC of Clinical Professionalism.* John Wiley & Sons; 2018:29–34.
9. U.S. Department of Health & Human Services. Summary of the HIPAA Privacy Rule. 2003. Accessed June 6, 2024. https://www.hhs.gov/sites/default/files/ocr/privacy/hipaa/understanding/summary/privacysummary.pdf. P. 4.
10. Logghe HJ, Boeck MA, Gusani NJ, et al. Best practices for surgeons' social media use: statement of the Resident and Associate Society of the American College of Surgeons. *J Am Coll Surg.* 2018;226(3):317–327.
11. ABIM Foundation; ACP-ASIM Foundation; European Federation of Internal Medicine. Medical professionalism in the new millennium: a physician charter. *Ann Intern Med.* 2002;136(3):243–246.
12. Chretien KC, Kind T. Social media and clinical care. Ethical, professional, and social implications. *Circulation.* 2013;127:1413–1421.
13. Stevenson SE, Peck LA. "I am eating a sandwich now": intent and foresight in the Twitter age. *J Mass Media Ethics.* 2011;26(1):56–65.
14. Appel JM. Engagement without entanglement: a framework for non-sexual patient–physician boundaries. *J Med Ethics.* 2023;49(6):383–388.
15. Wiener L, Crum C, Grady C, Merchant M. To friend or not to friend: the use of social media in clinical oncology. *J Oncol Pract.* 2012;8(2):103–106.
16. Bosslet GT, Torke AM, Hickman SE, et al. The patient-doctor relationship and online social networks: results of a national survey. *J Gen Intern Med.* 2011;26:1168–1174.
17. Select opinions of the Ethics Committee on the Principle of Medical Ethics of particular relevance to trainees and early career psychiatrists. American Psychiatric Association. Accessed December 15, 2023. APA-Ethics-Committee-Opinions-Trainees-Early-Career-Psychiatrists.pdf
18. American Medical Association (AMA). Professionalism in the Use of Social Media, 2.3.3. In: *Code of Medical Ethics.* AMA; 2017:42–43.
19. Federation of State Medical Boards. Model policy guidelines for the appropriate use of social media and social networking in medical practice. *J Med Regul.* 2012;98(2):27–33.

25

How Physicians Demonstrate and Maintain Professionalism Through Communication

Nathan Houchens

> **Key Points**
>
> - Relationship-centered care is epitomized by mutual respect, trust, and confidence in the other.
> - Physicians contribute to meaningful connections with patients through their words, behaviors, actions, and attire. Effective communication is paramount when approaching and responding to challenging situations involving stereotype threat, bias, harassment, discrimination, and microaggressions.
> - Physicians can employ relationship-centered communication skills to proactively mitigate their own biases, repair relationship ruptures, and demonstrate support for themselves and other members of the healthcare team.

Foundations of Relationship-Centered Communication

Relationships between physician and patient are a cornerstone in effective healthcare delivery. As it has been for centuries, the ways in which these two individuals connect may lead to shared understanding and empathy, deep meaning making, and improved experiences and outcomes or it may lead to challenged information exchange, lack of trust, poorer outcomes, and disengagement.[1]

Prior conceptual frameworks of centeredness in healthcare have described "physician-centered" or "patient-centered" approaches to care.[2] The latter evolved as a way for physicians to implement the biopsychosocial "whole-health" model more tangibly and incorporate important nonbiological dimensions of health such as spirituality, psychology, and social networks.[3] More recently, an alternative framework known as "relationship-centered" care has emerged. This framework recognizes how relationships of all kinds can impact the healthcare experience and patient outcomes.[4–6] Rather than placing the focus exclusively on the physician or the patient, it is instead about the complex interplay between the two that is central to good health.

The relationship-centered care model is based on four key principles: (1) Personhood matters; (2) affect and emotion are important; (3) relationships do not occur in isolation; and (4) maintaining genuine relationships is necessary for health and recovery and is morally valuable.[7] Effective relationships are predicated on mutual respect, trust between the parties, confidence in abilities, and care and even love for the other. The description of love by Laura Hendricks reflects these characteristics: "[Love] is quiet, mutual confidence, sharing, and forgiving. It is loyalty through good and bad times. It settles for less than perfection and makes allowances for human weaknesses. . . . It is the day-in and day-out chronicles of irritations, problems, compromises, small disappointments, big victories, and working toward common goals."[8]

A multitude of benefits to patients have been shown to be associated with a relationship-centered approach to healthcare. It is worth noting that not all of these benefits are subjective; in fact, a number of empiric patient health outcomes have demonstrated improvement. Patients note enhanced comprehension and recall; trust; sense of self-efficacy; satisfaction with care; adherence with treatment plans; self-management of chronic conditions; symptom improvement or resolution (e.g., improvement in blood pressure readings, reductions of hemoglobin A_{1c} values for patients with diabetes mellitus); functional improvement; better health status and quality of life; fewer 30-day hospital readmissions; and less risk of death.[9–15]

Important benefits of relationship-centered care are not limited solely to patients but extend also to the physicians providing that care. Indeed, physicians note improved diagnostic accuracy, work efficiency, self-confidence, and job satisfaction and engagement.[16–19] Likewise, physicians also note reductions in burnout, costs of care, and malpractice claims.[16,20,21] These benefits are particularly noteworthy since approximately half of all physicians in the United States noted at least one symptom of professional burnout.[22] It is worth highlighting that these data were collected prior to the COVID-19 pandemic. Indeed, research in 2022 has determined that burnout increased, with 62.8% of physicians reporting at least one manifestation of burnout during the first two years of the pandemic.[23]

The complexity of all the various elements that inform and comprise the patient-physician relationship cannot be overstated. As with any relationship, the exchange between patient and physician is bidirectional, with contributions from both parties. It may be seen as an intricate dance in which both individuals exert influence and, it is hoped, align toward a common goal. The patient and physician enter into the relationship with their respective intersecting identities on display, a concept that may lead to trust, empathy, and connection or that may predispose to bias, stereotype threat, and microaggressions.

Along with both parties' identities, a multitude of other variables exert influence on this interplay. Among many others, these include the many domains of verbal and nonverbal communication between the parties, physician technical ability, patient's perceptions of level of agency and locus of control in healthcare, level of physician facilitation in shared medical decision-making, mental health factors of both parties, health literacy levels, and even external media representation of healthcare institutions and physicians.[24–26]

Finally, a critical element that impacts the patient-physician relationship is professionalism, an area with many distinct and overlapping facets. The American Board of Internal Medicine describes physicians' professionalism as "not only their personal commitment to the welfare of their patients but also collective efforts to improve the health care system for the welfare of society."[27] This chapter explores the ways in which physicians contribute to meaningful relationships, specifically how they demonstrate professionalism with patients through their communication. Particular emphases are placed on physicians' words (verbal) and actions (nonverbal communication techniques, including bodily positioning and the attire worn and most appreciated by patients). The chapter concludes by examining ways in which physicians may work to prevent their own biases and maintain professionalism when confronted with challenging situations and inappropriate behaviors from patients.

Principles of Relationship-Centered Communication

Many models have been described that enumerate key skills of effective relationship-centered communication.[28–31] Despite their sheer number, these models generally outline many of the same core principles and techniques that help to foster relationships with patients. The skills are, somewhat artificially, divided into categories in the following sections, starting with verbal and then nonverbal communication.

Verbal Communication

Connect With the Patient

The first set of skills encourages the physician to connect with the patient by recognizing emotional cues that may arise at any point in an encounter and responding in the moment with empathy and compassion. The physician may wish to clarify with the patient if the emotion is unclear, perhaps through naming the perceived emotion or exploring with the patient how they are feeling. They should work to avoid judgment and refrain from trying to "fix" or reassure, particularly when delivering serious news. The physician may wish to embrace pauses and welcome silence during moments of intensity or gravity. A variety of categories of verbal empathic statements and responses to emotion have been put forth, but a common system known as **NURSE** is illustrative: **N**ame the emotion, seek to **U**nderstand the lived experience, demonstrate **R**espect, show **S**upport, and **E**xplore the emotion.[32] NURSE statements, coupled with an awareness and appreciation of their own emotional responses and a desire to simply be present with the patient, allow the physician to create shared intimacies.

Especially powerful moments between parties have been defined as "sacred moments," brief but highly memorable periods of time in which the individuals involved experience qualities of transcendence, boundlessness, deep interconnectedness, and spiritual emotions.[33] They have been described as a deep sense of connection, as if time stood still, and imparting individuals with a sense of joy, peace, and empathy for the other person.[34] In fact, research in psychotherapy has demonstrated that these sacred moment experiences may have positive effects on individuals' well-being and stress levels.[35,36]

Create a Safe and Supportive Care Environment

Within a very brief amount of time, physicians can effectively create a care environment that is safe, supportive, and inviting. They may establish rapport by conveying value and respect through a variety of techniques. For instance, if they have the time and are in a position to do so, physicians may wish to review the medical chart in advance to familiarize themselves with the patient's history so that time may be spent in other ways than reviewing details. As much as feasible, the physician can attempt to minimize disruptions and interruptions in the conversation. The physician can show respect by knocking on the door to the hospital or examination room and inquiring if it is acceptable to enter. A warm welcome along with a smile, culturally appropriate salutation, and inquiry about the patient's preferred name will make the encounter inviting from the outset.

If the physician is accompanied by other individuals on the care team (e.g., registered nurse, social work, residents, or medical student learners), it is reasonable to make introductions and describe the roles of everyone in the room, including how the roles relate to the care of the patient and to each other. The physician should ensure that the physical environment is conducive to the comfort and privacy of the patient while removing any literal or metaphorical barriers to communication. For instance, if a computer will be utilized during the encounter, strategies could include introducing the computer and providing the rationale for and benefits of its use. The physician can do this while maintaining eye contact with the patient and including the patient in review of the images and diagnostic studies as much as possible. Physicians may wish to eschew the typical opening inquiring about the purpose of the visit or the chief concern and instead engage the patient in a humanistic comment or question. These types of nonmedical, social interactions do much to put patients at ease and promote rapid rapport.

Cultivate Stories

Physicians can use techniques to ensure conversations with their patients are dialogue rather than monologue and that patients' stories are heard. The physician may start by collaboratively setting the agenda for the visit or the day, which entails co-creating a list of agenda items by asking "What else?" repeatedly, prioritizing the agenda list if necessary, summarizing and repeating back to confirm accuracy, and obtaining patient agreement.

Once the agenda is established, the physician may begin with open-ended questions to invite the patient to tell their story, without interruption whenever possible. By exploring the patient experience domains (e.g., their cultural and religious/spiritual beliefs and background, concerns, values, prior and current experiences, companions, community) and using reflective listening to show they have heard what has been said, the physician demonstrates curiosity about the person (not just the patient) and builds rapport.

Coach for Success

As the encounter progresses to the counseling and planning portion in which diagnostic tests or treatment plans are discussed, physicians may coach their patients for success in achieving the best health possible. The very best plans will likely falter if the patient is not a partner in care, so it is incumbent on the physicians to ensure they are explaining concepts well and that the patient is engaged and understanding. Physicians may inquire about health literacy using validated questions and incorporate the patient's preferred learning style. Using clear and concise language devoid of medical jargon helps to keep the information accessible, and framing the information in the patient's context (particularly referencing the patient's original concerns) helps to keep it meaningful. Physicians may consider using pauses in conversation liberally, small portions of information at a time with a focus on the big picture, and cognitive aids (e.g., visual representations of disease processes) to help in the explanation of complex medical concepts.

Just as physicians collaboratively set the agenda with patients, so, too, should they collaboratively set the treatment plan. Unlike the paternalistic plans put forth from prior generations of physicians, shared decision-making between physician and patient is at the heart of effective treatment. Key steps include: (1) discussing the rationale, goals, and options with risks, benefits, and alternatives for each; (2) using motivational interviewing, if needed, to harness a patient's internal goals that will help propel and sustain lifestyle changes; (3) assessing the patient's motivation, preferences, concerns, and ability, and integrating them into a mutually agreeable plan; (4) and reviewing the expected course, potential adverse effects, and any resources/plans, such as written materials that may assist the patient. After summarizing key points and reviewing next steps together, physicians should assess patient understanding using techniques such as the "teach-back" method.[37] Assuming patients will have questions and to be as inviting as possible, it behooves the physician to pose inquiries like "What questions can I address?" rather than the dichotomous "Do you have any questions?" since the latter may lead to less meaningful patient engagement. The physician can signal further respect by committing to the partnership, affirming the patient's contributions during the encounter, and closing with appreciation and gratitude.

Nonverbal Communication

The practice of communication between physician and patient encompasses not just *what* is shared, the words and ideas that flow between the two parties, but also *how* communication occurs, the movements, actions, and subtleties that are often just as impactful. The physician's body positioning and posture, gestures, eye contact, and chosen attire, among many others, all play a role in how interactions unfold and whether and to what extent rapport is developed and maintained[38]—in essence, how the physician makes the patient feel. Indeed, nonverbal communication affects patient adherence to care, satisfaction, trust, and important clinical outcomes.[39,40] Each aspect of nonverbal communication has been studied in the medical literature, and a portion of this research is presented here to inform how physicians may demonstrate professionalism through their actions.

Hierarchies and power differentials are inherent in healthcare environments. For physicians and their patients, one way that power differential may be influenced is through the physician's bodily positioning and posture. Patients are often seated or lying supine, and physicians have the option of standing over the patient or positioning themselves at eye level with the patient. In one study, among hospitalized patients with cancer who viewed videos of physicians standing and sitting, 81% indicated a preference that favored the seated physician.[41] In another, hospitalized patients who had undergone elective spine surgery indicated more positive interactions and a greater understanding of their health condition when the physician sat compared to when the physician stood.[42] Likewise, these patients also perceived that the physician was physically present at the bedside for a longer period of time when they sat despite the fact that the actual time spent at the bedside was not different between physicians who sat and stood. The authors hypothesized that patients did not feel the physician was rushed when they sat and that being physically closer and perhaps making better eye contact increased the physician's expression of empathy. Finally, in another study designed to evaluate whether physicians were performing "etiquette-based medicine" in the hospital, observers recorded specific behaviors of hospitalists, one of which was sitting down while interacting with patients.[43] The authors demonstrated that hospitalists only sit at any point during the encounter approximately one in five times. Yet, this same study identified that sitting was associated with higher scores on a composite rating of physician quality as assessed through national patient perception surveys.

Nonverbal communication encompasses a plethora of different behaviors. Researchers have noted associations between patient satisfaction and nonverbal indicators of interest shown by physicians. These include more nuanced bodily posture such as forward-leaning torso, open arms, greater number of head nods and hand gestures, and less interpersonal distance between the parties.[44] Likewise, the amount of time, including actual time and time relative to the entire encounter, spent maintaining eye contact and gaze with the patient has been found to predict greater patient satisfaction.[45,46] As a corollary, less time spent reviewing the patient's chart with a computer in the room was also associated with greater satisfaction, presumably due to enhanced eye contact.[44] A noteworthy systematic review examining curricula for training around empathy and compassion identified 52 studies in which curricula demonstrated improvement in patient perception of physician empathy or compassion.[38] The authors suggested several key behaviors for these curricula to be effective, including detecting patients' nonverbal cues of emotion and nonverbal communication of caring, such as through eye contact.

Physician Attire

The clothing a physician wears is another form of nonverbal communication. Given its impacts on patient satisfaction, experience, and the patient-physician relationship, many studies have sought to better understand physician attire.[47] In particular, researchers have focused on patient perceptions and their most preferred forms of physician dress. These studies, conducted over many years, have varied greatly in terms of geographic locations, clinical contexts, healthcare settings, and patient populations. The following paragraphs represent a nonexhaustive attempt to summarize much of the existing knowledge gathered about the complex topic of physician attire.

It is challenging to directly compare the results obtained from the array of studies on physician attire because of the different measurement tools utilized and outcomes assessed. As such, the findings in the medical literature are diverse and often conflicting. For instance, a number of articles across continents have demonstrated strong patient preference for white coats,[48–55] often viewed as a traditional symbol or marker of the medical profession.[56] Yet, some studies indicated that patients do not have a significant preference for the white coat,[57,58] and still others showed higher levels of patient tension that results from the white coat.[59]After education about the potential risk of infectious microorganisms that could be transmitted from the white coat, some studies have shown a decrease in patient preference for this piece of attire,[51,60] while others showed no change.[61] In some articles, patients have demonstrated preference for specific forms of attire in specific circumstances (e.g., scrubs in gastroenterology suites[62] and emergency situations[63]). And finally, some studies have shown that older patients feel that physician attire is more important than those who are younger.[64,65]

Despite the diverse findings within the scholarly literature, a few themes have emerged that may help to guide physicians, policymakers, and healthcare systems in deciding what to suggest or require for physician dress. While not universal, multiple studies have demonstrated that patients indicate physician attire is important to them and influences their experience, their perceptions of physician empathy and quality of care received, and their satisfaction.[48,49,53,65–69] Patients often feel that chosen clothing affects their confidence and trust in the physician.[48,49,53,61] Certain attire, often a version of formal/professional dress with a white coat, causes patients to feel more comfortable, better able to communicate, and more willing to share personal, intimate pieces of information about themselves[48,49,70]—this rapport and these details are critical, as they may be a deciding factor in arriving at the correct diagnosis or deriving a mutually agreed treatment approach.

The literature has repeatedly demonstrated that considering the context of care is paramount when considering nonverbal communication like physician attire. Patient viewpoints depend on a host of different factors, including type of care and physician and even time of day. For instance, Switzerland is one of the only countries that touts a national healthcare uniform of white scrubs and white coat, a phenomenon that likely has led to expectations of and strong preferences for this form of dress.[71] In the United States, parents of children who are being assessed in one pediatric emergency department were more likely to prefer physicians wearing scrubs—yet this was only the case if the child was experiencing a surgical emergency.[72] In the same study, parents who visited the emergency department during the day preferred formal dress, while those who visited during the night preferred less formal attire.[72] Last, preferences have sometimes been demonstrated to deviate from cultural norms or established national dress. In one study, patients seeking care in family medicine clinics in Saudi Arabia were more likely to follow medical advice and return to the clinic in the future if the physician was dressed in Western clothing.[65] However, the same population was more willing to discuss personal issues (e.g., psychological and social problems) with a physician wearing Saudi national dress.[65]

In a more recent study, a group of researchers set out to better understand patient preferences for physician attire in different contexts of care and within different geographic regions and countries using a twenty-two-item standardized survey instrument.[73] This survey tool allowed direct comparisons and contrasts across diverse geographic regions, populations, physician types, and clinical contexts and alleviated some of the heterogeneity and limitations inherent in prior studies. In this multicenter, cross-sectional study, a convenience sample of over 9,000 adult patients in twenty hospitals or healthcare centers in four countries (Italy, Japan, Switzerland, and the United States) completed surveys. Participants were seeking care in academic hospitals, general medicine clinics, specialty clinics, and ophthalmology practices. Survey questions elicited preferences regarding photographs of medical providers wearing seven distinct forms of attire: casual, casual with white coat, scrubs, scrubs with white coat, formal, formal with white coat, and business suit. Professional photographs were taken with specific attention paid to constant facial expressions and consistent visual cues (e.g., lighting, background, posture).

Perhaps not surprisingly, the results were both consistent in some ways and divergent in others. The highest rated form of attire differed across countries, but all most strongly preferred a white coat with any attire. Indeed, among all respondents, approximately three out of four preferred some form of attire with a white coat. Patients in the United States more strongly preferred all types of formal attire compared with patients in Italy, Japan, and Switzerland. When considering emergency department physicians and surgeons specifically, there was greater preference for scrubs-based attire than other forms; conversely, for primary care and hospital-based physicians, patient preferences varied, both among and within countries. With some exceptions, patients tended to dislike attire extremes, such as casual or business suit. In terms of respondent age, patients 65 years and older rated casual attire, formal attire, formal attire with white coat, and business suit more highly than younger patients in Japan and the United States. In contrast, no differences in preferences were noted when comparing patients of different age groups.

Physician attire is one nonverbal form of communication that influences the patient experience. Research has demonstrated that a single type of attire is unlikely to reflect the desires and expectations of patients in varying geographies and contexts. Physicians can use the results of individual studies to decide what they should wear based on what form patients prefer most. This may help to cultivate the patient-physician relationship and in turn enhance satisfaction, trust, confidence, and important health outcomes.

Maintaining Professionalism in Challenging Situations

Understanding is a two-way street.

—Eleanor Roosevelt

Relationship-centered communication is not solely about the patient or solely the provider, but about the complex interplay between them. This is the two-way street of understanding in healthcare. Physicians and patients perceive each other through identities that are on display. As such, physicians may approach patients with bias and stereotype threat, and patients may approach physicians with the same. Challenging scenarios may arise when the two parties are communicating across differences.

Physicians may harbor problematic biases toward patients. These may take the form of conscious/explicit stereotypes or unconscious/implicit biases. Two systematic reviews of the literature from 2015 and 2017 were conducted with the goal of examining prevalence of implicit bias in healthcare professionals toward patients. Evidence for implicit bias was found in fourteen of fifteen articles reviewed[74] and thirty-five of forty-two articles reviewed, respectively.[75] The implicit bias scores noted in healthcare professionals were similar to those in the general population.[74] Regardless of the nature of the bias, there are also myriad deleterious effects for patients that stem from physician bias. In these same studies, implicit bias was significantly associated with patient-provider interactions, treatment decisions and adherence, and health outcomes.[74,75] In other words, the more implicit bias the physician held, the lower the quality of care delivered.

While they cannot control the belief systems, biases, and stereotypes of others, physicians may strive to employ communication skills to proactively mitigate their own stereotype threats and thus prevent misunderstandings and challenge. These skills are also useful to help repair any relationship ruptures that may occur, and in fact, they parallel the foundational relationship-centered communication skills, albeit through a slightly different lens. Physicians may start with a personal awareness of what preconceived notions and conceptual frameworks they bring when about to engage with a patient who may not share their same array of intersecting identities. Using language that acknowledges differences and validates the patient's lived experience and emotions is an important strategy to maintain rapport. During the conversation, patients may name particular barriers, such as unequal treatment because of race, ethnicity, gender, age, or any number of other sociodemographic or personal characteristics. In these moments, reflective listening and humble inquiry may assist the physician. For instance, reflecting a patient's own language accomplishes two goals: It demonstrates true listening, and it lowers the extent to which assumptions are imposed.

Rather than avoiding charged topics altogether, physicians may recognize and directly respond to cues of concern about bias. This approach works to normalize the topic and invite dialogue in a constructive way. Creating a welcoming environment with positive affect and warm verbal and nonverbal cues throughout the conversation may reduce any tensions and allow space for forthright conversation. It is especially important to have unrushed behaviors, such as slow pacing of speech and sitting with appropriate eye contact; all of these skills demonstrate that the physician cares and has time for the patient. Physicians may respond to concerns of stereotype threat and bias by normalizing the patient's anxiety and prior difficulties, recognizing and respecting their strengths, communicating confidence in their capacity to reach health goals, using language of partnership, and consistently ensuring shared decision-making. When a relationship rupture or negative event occurs, it is often wise to momentarily pause the physician's conversation, shift focus away from the agenda, and instead listen openly and respond with empathy. Acknowledging frustrations and concerns, clarifying wants and needs, and seeking ways for the physician to earn the patient's trust are all strategies that may help to repair the relationship and signal allyship.

At times, patients and their family members may be the sources of inappropriate behavior, such as bias, harassment, discrimination, and microaggressions. These behaviors may be targeted toward physicians, medical learners, healthcare employees, or other patients. Some brief definitions are warranted: Harassment refers to unwanted verbal or physical actions that are meant to be offensive, humiliating, or intimidating. Discrimination refers to unjust, unfair, or prejudicial actions based on personal characteristics such as race, color, national origin, religion, gender identity, sexual orientation, age, or disability or for the purpose of retaliation. Microaggressions are brief and commonplace verbal, behavioral, or environmental indignities, whether intentional or unintentional, that communicate hostile, derogatory, or negative slights or insults.

The prevalence, scope, and negative effects of these actions on healthcare providers cannot be overstated. Most medical trainees have experienced at least one form of harassment or discrimination during their training, and patients and their families are a commonly cited source.[76] In one study conducted at an academic medical center, nearly two in three female faculty and nearly half of male faculty reported sexual harassment from patients and their families.[77] Another study found that surgical residents who report exposure to discrimination, abuse, or harassment at least a few times per month were more likely to report symptoms of burnout and suicidal thoughts.[78] This same study also found that patients and their families were the most frequent sources of gender and racial discrimination.[78]

How might physicians respond to inappropriateness from patients or their family members? For many, addressing problematic behaviors in real time is a challenge because the sentiments are inherently uncomfortable, surprising, and perhaps disarming. The goal is not necessarily to change the patient's thought process or belief structure, but rather to curb inappropriate culture and demonstrate support for team members and the self. Luckily, a few studies have provided guidance.[79,80] Key steps that physicians can take, alone or with other members of the healthcare team, are found in Table 25.1. The first step is to prepare for the fact that inappropriate behaviors will occur before encountering them. This opens the lines of communication and establishes a culture of respect and support. The second step is to assess the situation for safety and stability and to address the behavior in real time. A menu of some possible response options to consider is found in Table 25.2. The address step may require multiple responses or departing the room if the behavior persists or escalates. The third step is to debrief with team members after any and all problematic encounters to ensure safety, evaluate how the plan was executed, and discuss ways to improve for future instances.

Table 25.1 Steps and Key Skills Physicians May Employ to Prepare for, Respond to, and Debrief After Inappropriate Behaviors

Step	Key Skill	Details
Prepare	Set the stage	Acknowledge that team members may experience inappropriate behaviors
		Create a culture of respect by opening lines of dialogue
	Invite input	Decide who will respond to inappropriate comments when they occur
		Identify verbal or nonverbal cues a team member will use if they want another to interject in real time
	Make the plan explicit	Use input from team members to individualize the team's approach
		Recognize own fallibility to keep the dialogue open if the plan does not unfold as prepared
		Allow team members space and permission to step in if the plan is not being followed
	Show commitment	Invite team members to commit to their roles
		Agree to debrief after all problematic encounters
Address	Assess safety	Consider both physical and emotional safety of all team members
		If unsafe, the team should immediately leave the room, report the behavior and/or contact security, and debrief
	Evaluate stability	If the patient is not clinically stable, it is up to the judgment of the physician as to whether to address the inappropriate behavior in real time
		Recognize that words and actions of any patients, stable or unstable, can create trauma; debrief after the event
	Address the behavior	Address in real time and avoid silence, minimizing, and jokes/banter
		Use the menu of response options, which includes be direct, redirect, clarify roles, challenge stereotype, describe, and probe
Debrief	Ensure team safety	Check in with team members to assess level of trauma; follow up with particularly traumatized individuals
		Consider connecting team members with institutional mental health resources
	Acknowledge the challenge	Verbalize the ways in which the encounter was problematic
		Invite team members to reflect and interpret areas in which the plan went well and areas in which it did not work as intended
	Discuss ways to improve	Invite team members to consider ways to improve
		Update the plan according to the feedback and recommit

Table 25.2 Menu of Response Options to Address Inappropriate Behaviors

Category	Example
Be direct	That is not okay to say.
	I am surprised you thought that was appropriate to say.
	Please avoid comments that are disrespectful.
	We do not tolerate that kind of speech here.
Redirect the conversation	Let's keep this professional.
	We are here to focus on your health.
Clarify roles	We are your team of doctors.
	We all completed the same training and expected to be treated with the same respect.
	[Name] is the medical student on our team.
Challenge stereotypes	That stereotype is not fair.
	I do not think you would have said that to a white/male/older physician.
Describe the situation	When you said that, it made me uncomfortable.
	You are putting forth some problematic ideas.
	Comments like that make us feel unsafe and do not allow us to care for you to the best of our ability.
Probe for more information	What did you mean by that?
	What was your goal with that comment?
	Tell me more about why you said that.

Everyone deserves to feel safe, welcome, and respected in their careers. If patients and families explicitly or implicitly undermine that respect, it is important for the physician to respond—indeed, it is a marker of medical professionalism to do so. Dedicated practice, reflection, and feedback may be useful in honing these skills so that physicians may effectively advocate for themselves and other members of the healthcare team.

References

1. Lelorain S, Brédart A, Dolbeault S, Sultan S. A systematic review of the associations between empathy measures and patient outcomes in cancer care. *Psychooncology*. 2012;21(12):1255–1264. doi:10.1002/pon.2115
2. Hughes JC, Bamford C, May C. Types of centredness in health care: themes and concepts. *Med Health Care Philos*. 2008;11(4):455–463. doi:10.1007/s11019-008-9131-5
3. Levenstein JH, McCracken EC, McWhinney IR, Stewart MA, Brown JB. The patient-centred clinical method. A model for the doctor-patient interaction in family medicine. *Fam Pract*. 1986;3(1):24–30. doi:10.1093/fampra/3.1.24
4. Boissy A, Windover AK, Bokar D, et al. Communication skills training for physicians improves patient satisfaction. *J Gen Intern Med*. 2016;31(7):755–761. doi:10.1007/s11606-016-3597-2
5. Rider EA. Advanced communication strategies for relationship-centered care. *Pediatr Ann*. 2011;40(9):447–453. doi:10.3928/00904481-20110815-08

6. Massey Z, Rising SS, Ickovics J. CenteringPregnancy group prenatal care: promoting relationship-centered care. *J Obstet Gynecol Neonatal Nurs.* 2006;35(2):286–294. doi:10.1111/j.1552-6909.2006.00040.x
7. Beach MC, Inui T; Relationship-Centered Care Research Network. Relationship-centered care. A constructive reframing. *J Gen Intern Med.* 2006;21(suppl 1):S3–S8. doi:10.1111/j.1525-1497.2006.00302.x
8. Hendricks L. Wedding reading by Laura Hendricks.https://www.thewedplanners.co.uk/blog-content/wedding-reading-laura-hendricks. Accessed June 11, 2024.
9. Barbosa CD, Balp MM, Kulich K, et al. A literature review to explore the link between treatment satisfaction and adherence, compliance, and persistence. *Patient Prefer Adherence.* 2012;6:39–48.
10. Boulding W, Glickman SW, Manary MP, et al. Relationship between patient satisfaction with inpatient care and hospital readmission within 30 days. *Am J Manag Care.* 2011;17:41–48.
11. Jha AK, Orav EJ, Zheng J, et al. Patients' perception of hospital care in the United States. *N Engl J Med.* 2008;359:1921–1931.
12. Manary MP, Boulding W, Staelin R, et al. The patient experience and health outcomes. *N Engl J Med.* 2013;368:201–203.
13. O'Malley AS, Forrest CB, Mandelblatt J. Adherence of low-income women to cancer screening recommendations. *J Gen Intern Med.* 2002;17:144–154.
14. Jin J, Sklar GE, Min Sen Oh V, et al. Factors affecting therapeutic compliance: a review from the patient's perspective. *Ther Clin Risk Manag.* 2008;4:269–286.
15. Zolnierek KB, Dimatteo MR. Physician communication and patient adherence to treatment: a meta-analysis. *Med Care.* 2009;47:826–834.
16. Marvel MK, Epstein RM, Flowers K, Beckman HB. Soliciting the patient's agenda: have we improved? *JAMA.* 1999;281(3):283–287. doi:10.1001/jama.281.3.283
17. Mauksch LB, Dugdale DC, Dodson S, Epstein R. Relationship, communication, and efficiency in the medical encounter: creating a clinical model from a literature review. *Arch Intern Med.* 2008;168(13):1387–1395. doi:10.1001/archinte.168.13.1387
18. Roter DL, Stewart M, Putnam SM, Lipkin M Jr, Stiles W, Inui TS. Communication patterns of primary care physicians. *JAMA.* 1997;277(4):350–356.
19. Weng HC, Hung CM, Liu YT, et al. Associations between emotional intelligence and doctor burnout, job satisfaction and patient satisfaction. *Med Educ.* 2011;45(8):835–842. doi:10.1111/j.1365-2923.2011.03985.x
20. Beckman H, Markakis K, Suchman A, Frankel R. Getting the most from a 20-minute visit. *Am J Gastroenterol.* 1994;89(5):662–664.
21. Levinson W, Roter DL, Mullooly JP, Dull VT, Frankel RM. Physician-patient communication. The relationship with malpractice claims among primary care physicians and surgeons. *JAMA.* 1997;277(7):553–559. doi:10.1001/jama.277.7.553
22. Shanafelt TD, Hasan O, Dyrbye LN, et al. Changes in burnout and satisfaction with work-life balance in physicians and the general US working population between 2011 and 2014. *Mayo Clin Proc.* 2015;90(12):1600–16513. doi:10.1016/j.mayocp.2015.08.023. Erratum in: *Mayo Clin Proc.* 2016;91(2):276.
23. Shanafelt TD, West CP, Dyrbye LN, et al. Changes in burnout and satisfaction with work-life integration in physicians during the first 2 years of the COVID-19 pandemic. *Mayo Clin Proc.* 2022;97(12):2248–2258. doi:10.1016/j.mayocp.2022.09.002

24. Hamelin ND, Nikolis A, Armano J, Harris PG, Brutus JP. Evaluation of factors influencing confidence and trust in the patient-physician relationship: a survey of patient in a hand clinic. *Chir Main.* 2012;31(2):83–90. doi:10.1016/j.main.2012.01.005

25. Liang CY, Wang KY, Hwang SJ, Lin KC, Pan HH. Factors affecting the physician-patient relationship of older veterans with inadequate health literacy: an observational study. *Br J Gen Pract.* 2013;63(610):e354–e360. doi:10.3399/bjgp13X667222

26. Qiao T, Fan Y, Geater AF, Chongsuvivatwong V, McNeil EB. Factors associated with the doctor-patient relationship: doctor and patient perspectives in hospital outpatient clinics of Inner Mongolia Autonomous Region, China. *Patient Prefer Adherence.* 2019;13:1125–1143. doi:10.2147/PPA.S189345

27. ABIM Foundation. Physician charter. https://abimfoundation.org/what-we-do/physician-charter. Accessed June 11, 2024.

28. Makoul G. The SEGUE Framework for teaching and assessing communication skills. *Patient Educ Couns.* 2001;45(1):23–34. doi:10.1016/s0738-3991(01)00136-7

29. Frankel RM, Stein T. Getting the most out of the clinical encounter: the four habits model. *J Med Pract Manage.* 2001;16(4):184–191.

30. Makoul G. Essential elements of communication in medical encounters: the Kalamazoo consensus statement. *Acad Med.* 2001;76(4):390–393. doi:10.1097/00001888-200104000-00021

31. ACOG Committee Opinion No. 587: effective patient-physician communication. *Obstet Gynecol.* 2014;123(2 Pt 1):389–393. doi:10.1097/01.AOG.0000443279.14017.12

32. Responding to emotion: respect. VitalTalk. 2019. https://www.vitaltalk.org/guides/responding-to-emotion- respecting/. Accessed June 11, 2024.

33. Lomax JW, Kripal JJ, Pargament KI. Perspectives on "sacred moments" in psychotherapy. *Am J Psychiatry.* 2011;168(1):12–18. doi:10.1176/appi.ajp.2010.10050739

34. Pargament KI, Lomax JW, McGee JS, Fang Q. Sacred moments in psychotherapy from the perspectives of mental health providers and clients: prevalence, predictors and consequences. *Spiritual Clin Pract.* 2014;1:248–262.

35. Goldstein ED. Sacred moments: implications on well-being and stress. *J Clin Psychol.* 2007;63:1001–1019.

36. Wachholtz AB, Pargament KI. Is spirituality a critical ingredient of meditation? Comparing the effects of spiritual meditation, secular meditation, and relaxation on spiritual, psychological, cardiac, and pain outcomes. *J Behav Med.* 2005;28:369–384.

37. Ha Dinh TT, Bonner A, Clark R, Ramsbotham J, Hines S. The effectiveness of the teach-back method on adherence and self-management in health education for people with chronic disease: a systematic review. *JBI Database System Rev Implement Rep.* 2016;14(1):210–247. doi:10.11124/jbisrir-2016-2296

38. Patel S, Pelletier-Bui A, Smith S, et al. Curricula for empathy and compassion training in medical education: a systematic review. *PLoS One.* 2019;14(8):e0221412. doi:10.1371/journal.pone.0221412

39. Roter DL, Frankel RM, Hall JA, Sluyter D. The expression of emotion through nonverbal behavior in medical visits. Mechanisms and outcomes. *J Gen Intern Med.* 2006;21(suppl 1):S28–S34. doi:10.1111/j.1525-1497.2006.00306.x

40. Mast MS. On the importance of nonverbal communication in the physician-patient interaction. *Patient Educ Couns.* 2007;67(3):315–318. doi:10.1016/j.pec.2007.03.005

41. Strasser F, Palmer JL, Willey J, et al. Impact of physician sitting versus standing during inpatient oncology consultations: patients' preference and perception of compassion and duration. A randomized controlled trial. *J Pain Symptom Manage.* 2005;29(5):489–497. doi:10.1016/j.jpainsymman.2004.08.011

42. Swayden KJ, Anderson KK, Connelly LM, Moran JS, McMahon JK, Arnold PM. Effect of sitting vs. standing on perception of provider time at bedside: a pilot study. *Patient Educ Couns.* 2012;86(2):166–171. doi:10.1016/j.pec.2011.05.024

43. Tackett S, Tad-y D, Rios R, Kisuule F, Wright S. Appraising the practice of etiquette-based medicine in the inpatient setting. *J Gen Intern Med.* 2013;28(7):908–913. doi:10.1007/s11606-012-2328-6

44. Hall JA, Harrigan JA, Rosenthal R. Nonverbal behavior in clinician-patient interaction. *Appl Prev Psychol.* 1995;4:21–37.

45. Larsen KM, Smith CK. Assessment of nonverbal communication in the patient-physician interview. *J Fam Pract.* 1981;12(3):481–488

46. Bensing J. Doctor-patient communication and the quality of care. *Soc Sci Med.* 1991;32(11):1301–1310. doi:10.1016/0277-9536(91)90047-g

47. Petrilli CM, Mack M, Petrilli JJ, Hickner A, Saint S, Chopra V. Understanding the role of physician attire on patient perceptions: a systematic review of the literature—Targeting Attire to Improve Likelihood of Rapport (TAILOR) investigators. *BMJ Open.* 2015;5(1):e006578. doi:10.1136/bmjopen-2014-006578

48. Rehman SU, Nietert PJ, Cope DW, et al. What to wear today? Effect of doctor's attire on the trust and confidence of patients. *Am J Med.* 2005;118(11):1279–1286. doi:10.1016/j.amjmed.2005.04.026

49. Jennings JD, Ciaravino SG, Ramsey FV, et al. Physicians' attire influences patients' perceptions in the urban outpatient orthopaedic surgery setting. *Clin Orthop Relat Res.* 2016;474(9):1908–1918. doi:10.1007/s11999-016-4855-7

50. Mun HW, Kim JH, Ahn JH, et al. Patient's preference on neurosurgeon's attire and appearance: a single center study in Korea cross-sectional study. *Biomed Res Int.* 2019;2019:3893049. doi:10.1155/2019/3893049

51. Zahrina AZ, Haymond P, Rosanna P, et al. Does the attire of a primary care physician affect patients' perceptions and their levels of trust in the doctor? *Malays Fam Physician.* 2018;13(3):3–11.

52. Major K, Hayase Y, Balderrama D, et al. Attitudes regarding surgeons' attire. *Am J Surg.* 2005;190(1):103–106. doi:10.1016/j.amjsurg.2005.04.003

53. Yamada Y, Takahashi O, Ohde S, et al. Patients' preferences for doctors' attire in Japan. *Intern Med.* 2010;49(15):1521–1526. doi:10.2169/internalmedicine.49.3572

54. Gallagher J, Waldron Lynch F, Stack J, et al. Dress and address: patient preferences regarding doctor's style of dress and patient interaction. *Ir Med J.* 2008;101(7):211–213.

55. McNaughton-Filion L, Chen JS, Norton PG. The physician's appearance. *Fam Med.* 1991 Mar-Apr;23(3):208–11. PMID: 2016013.

56. Karnieli-Miller O, Frankel RM, Inui TS. Cloak of compassion, or evidence of elitism? An empirical analysis of white coat ceremonies. *Med Educ.* 2013;47(1):97–108. doi:10.1111/j.1365-2923.2012.04324.x

57. Cha A, Hecht BR, Nelson K, et al. Resident physician attire: does it make a difference to our patients? *Am J Obstet Gynecol.* 2004;190(5):1484–1488. doi:10.1016/j.ajog.2004.02.022

58. Varnado-Sullivan P, Larzelere M, Solek K, et al. The impact of physician demographic characteristics on perceptions of their attire. *Fam Med.* 2019;51(9):737–741. doi:10.22454/FamMed.2019.650493

59. Ikusaka M, Kamegai M, Sunaga T, et al. Patients' attitude toward consultations by a physician without a white coat in Japan. *Intern Med.* 1999;38(7):533–536. doi:10.2169/internalmedicine.38.533

60. Hueston WJ, Carek SM. Patients' preference for physician attire: a survey of patients in family medicine training practices. *Fam Med.* 2011;43(9):643–647.

61. Landry M, Dornelles AC, Hayek G, et al. Patient preferences for doctor attire: the white coat's place in the medical profession. *Ochsner J.* 2013;13(3):334–342.

62. Clark M, Shuja A, Thomas A, et al. Patients' perceptions of gastroenterologists' attire in the clinic and endoscopy suite. *Ann Gastroenterol.* 2018;31(2):237–240. doi:10.20524/aog.2017.0223

63. Van De Car W, Starostanko A, Wendling A. Rural patient preference for physician attire. *PRiMER.* 2017;1:3. doi:10.22454/PRiMER.2017.1.3.

64. Kurihara H, Maeno T, Maeno T. Importance of physicians' attire: factors influencing the impression it makes on patients, a cross-sectional study. *Asia Pac Fam Med.* 2014;13(1):2. doi:10.1186/1447-056X-13-2.

65. Batais MA. Patients' attitudes toward the attire of male physicians: a single-center study in Saudi Arabia. *Ann Saudi Med.* 2014;34(5):383–389. doi:10.5144/0256-4947.2014.383

66. Petrilli CM, Saint S, Jennings JJ, et al. Understanding patient preference for physician attire: a cross-sectional observational study of 10 academic medical centres in the USA. *BMJ Open.* 2018;8(5):e021239. doi:10.1136/bmjopen-2017-021239

67. Chung H, Lee H, Chang DS, et al. Doctor's attire influences perceived empathy in the patient-doctor relationship. *Patient Educ Couns.* 2012;89(3):387–391. doi:10.1016/j.pec.2012.02.017

68. Al Amry KM, Al Farrah M, Ur Rahman S, Abdulmajeed I. Patient perceptions and preferences of physicians' attire in Saudi primary healthcare setting. *J Community Hosp Intern Med Perspect.* 2018;8(6):326–330. doi:10.1080/20009666.2018.1551026.

69. Aldrees T, Alsuhaibani R, Alqaryan S, et al. Physicians' attire. Parents preferences in a tertiary hospital. *Saudi Med J.* 2017;38(4):435–439. doi:10.15537/smj.2017.4.15853

70. Trowbridge RE, Pearson R. Impact of military physician rank and appearance on patient perceptions of clinical competency in a primary care setting. *Mil Med.* 2013;178(9):994–1001. doi:10.7205/MILMED-D-13-00197

71. Zollinger M, Houchens N, Chopra V, et al. Understanding patient preference for physician attire in ambulatory clinics: a cross-sectional observational study. *BMJ Open.* 2019;9(5):e026009. doi:10.1136/bmjopen-2018-026009

72. Gonzalez Del Rey JA, Paul RI. Preferences of parents for pediatric emergency physicians' attire. *Pediatr Emerg Care.* 1995;11(6):361–364. doi:10.1097/00006565-199512000-00007

73. Houchens N, Saint S, Petrilli C, et al. International patient preferences for physician attire: results from cross-sectional studies in four countries across three continents. *BMJ Open.* 2022;12(10):e061092. doi:10.1136/bmjopen-2022-061092

74. Hall WJ, Chapman MV, Lee KM, et al. Implicit racial/ethnic bias among health care professionals and its influence on health care outcomes: a systematic review. *Am J Public Health.* 2015;105(12):e60–e76. doi:10.2105/AJPH.2015.302903

75. FitzGerald C, Hurst S. Implicit bias in healthcare professionals: a systematic review. *BMC Med Ethics.* 2017;18(1):19. doi:10.1186/s12910-017-0179-8

76. Fnais N, Soobiah C, Chen MH, et al. Harassment and discrimination in medical training: a systematic review and meta-analysis. *Acad Med.* 2014;89(5):817–827. doi:10.1097/ACM.0000000000000200

77. Vargas EA, Brassel ST, Cortina LM, Settles IH, Johnson TRB, Jagsi R. #MedToo: a large-scale examination of the incidence and impact of sexual harassment of physicians and other faculty at an academic medical center. *J Womens Health (Larchmt).* 2020;29(1):13–20. doi:10.1089/jwh.2019.7766

78. Hu YY, Ellis RJ, Hewitt DB, et al. Discrimination, abuse, harassment, and burnout in surgical residency training. *N Engl J Med.* 2019;381(18):1741–1752. doi:10.1056/NEJMsa1903759

79. Viglianti EM, Oliverio AL, Meeks LM. Sexual harassment and abuse: when the patient is the perpetrator. *Lancet.* 2018;392(10145):368–370. doi:10.1016/S0140-6736(18)31502-2

80. Shankar M, Albert T, Yee N, Overland M. Approaches for residents to address problematic patient behavior: before, during, and after the clinical encounter. *J Grad Med Educ.* 2019;11(4):371–374. doi:10.4300/JGME-D-19-00075.1

26
Special Considerations for Clinical Research

Marie Nicolini and Christine Grady

Key Points

- While the activities of clinical care and clinical research are ultimately the same—improving health—the professional and ethical norms that guide clinical research are different from those in clinical care.
- Although the scientific approach is a necessary condition for establishing professionalism in clinical research, it is not sufficient. There are additional relevant conditions physician-researchers must adhere to for the sake of medical professionalism.
- Norms of professionalism in clinical research also require physicians be guided by relevant virtues and responsibilities, as well as adequate knowledge of the nature, ethics, and challenges of clinical research.
- Professionalism in clinical research also requires understanding and appreciating the organizational culture and structure of the health systems in which research is being conducted.

Medicine and Research Adhere to Distinct Standards, Norms and Methods

Clinical care is inextricably linked with clinical research. Some clinicians actively pursue research in their careers, and many if not all will need to evaluate the latest research findings in their field to deliver optimal clinical care and to decide with patients about appropriate referrals to clinical trials. This chapter describes what constitutes ethical clinical research and what it means for clinicians involved in research to act professionally. We focus on the clinician-scientist as the paradigm case for discussing ethical and professionalism standards, bearing in mind that these considerations apply to all clinicians[a] who, in one way or another, are involved in clinical research.

Clinical practice and research share a common goal of improving health. However, the ethical standards and norms that govern the two endeavors are very different. The landmark National Commission's Belmont Report recognized the distinction between research and practice by stating in its opening paragraph that "it is important to distinguish between biomedical and behavioral research, on the one hand, and the practice of accepted therapy on the other."[1(p3)] How are clinicians to reconcile wearing two

[a] We use the term *clinician* to include all health professionals.

hats—that of the clinician and that of the scientist—with the prevailing view that clinical research and clinical care are fundamentally different? And what does this mean for how we define professionalism standards for clinicians who engage in research?

In what follows, we first establish the relationship between professionalism and ethics. Second, we outline the ethical standards that govern clinical research, following the prevailing conceptual model of "the scientific approach" to clinical research. Third, we describe why the scientific approach to clinical research is necessary but not sufficient to ground the standards for professionalism in clinical research and outline additional relevant considerations. Finally, we conclude with two current examples that illustrate how clinician-scientists can ensure continued ethical and professionalism standards as they engage in and with clinical research.

The Relation Between Ethics and Professionalism

A helpful starting point is to clarify how the relationship between professionalism and ethics applies to clinicians involved in research. Professionalism standards are rooted in ethics standards: The standards for professional behavior build on the ethical foundations of a given moral enterprise.[2,3] In short, ethics precedes professionalism. To define what professionalism for clinicians involved in research means we need to first characterize the ethical standards that govern clinical research. The focus here will be on clinical research involving human subjects, as this is the type of research most relevant for the purpose of defining professionalism standards and the type that practicing clinicians are most likely to engage with. It will *not* focus on other types of research, such as basic and preclinical research involving nonsentient research materials and sentient nonhuman animals. Having established what the ethical norms for clinical research are, we then define what it means for a clinician-scientist to possess professional integrity characterized as a "coherent moral identity."[3(p1452)] That is, for a moral identity to be coherent, it needs to apply across the spectrum of clinical research, which includes studies of interventions that might be therapeutic as well as studies and interventions and procedures that are nontherapeutic. The therapeutic versus nontherapeutic research distinction has been found unhelpful in determining professionalism standards for a number of reasons, not least because it obfuscates the fact that all research is, essentially, nontherapeutic.[4]

Ethical and Professionalism Standards for Clinician-Scientists

The widely accepted view is that clinical research requires a set of ethical standards distinct from those that govern clinical practice.[5–8] This view, also referred to as "the scientific approach" to clinical research, grounds the relationship between the clinician-scientist and the patient-subject in science—rather than in a therapeutic orientation as between clinician and patient.[5(p34)] The scientific approach recognizes that, while both clinical practice and clinical research share a common ultimate goal of improving health, the purposes of the two endeavors are distinct: clinical practice aims at promoting individual patients' health and medical best interests, while Clinical research aims at generating socially valuable knowledge about health and disease.[5,6] What, then, are the ethical standards that govern clinical research? In thinking about the ethical standards for justifying and designing clinical research, the following requirements have been described—in order of importance: social or scientific value, scientific validity, fair subject or participant selection, and risk/benefit assessment.[9,10] Four other requirements are important for the ethical implementation of clinical research: collaborative partnership, informed consent, independent review, and respect for enrolled persons or communities.

Social and scientific value refer to the potential of clinical research to generate socially valuable knowledge useful for improving or better understanding health or well-being.[9,11] This requirement is fundamental to justify inviting people to participate in clinical research and in considering risks and benefits in clinical research.[12] "Without social value, research exposes people to risk for no good reason, and wastes resources."[10(p127)] While scientific and social value are often considered together, considerable discussion continues regarding how the concept of social value should be conceived, assessed, and enforced. Some have questioned whether it is a necessary and operationalizable requirement, arguing against the desirableness and usefulness of the social value requirement because it is difficult to predict, can be understood in different ways (i.e., according to a subjective or an objective account), and is not enforceable.[13] Others have argued against research with no social value and in favor of social value especially for net-risk research.[14] Despite these unsettled issues, the social value requirement continues to be considered of paramount importance for the ethics of clinical research.[15]

Scientific validity of research requires that the scientific principles and methods be reliable and valid. Scientific validity is necessary to enable the first requirement that the research carry social and scientific value, and that the study design and methods are rigorous, reliable, valid, and feasible and can realize the study objectives. One concept important to scientific validity is clinical equipoise, the requirement for a "null hypothesis" in randomized trials, such that there is *uncertainty* among the scientific community about the relative merits of the interventions being studied.[16] If a given intervention is known to be better than standard of care, there is no "null hypothesis" and hence no clinical equipoise. As we discuss below, the clinical equipoise requirement is another controversial concept—one that not everyone recognizes is necessary for ethical clinical research and that may exclude research that is not necessarily unethical.

Fair subject or participant selection refers to considerations and decisions regarding who should be included and excluded in the research to answer the socially or scientifically valuable question and to ensure a fair distribution of research-related benefits and burdens. Fair subject selection requires that the scientific goals be the basis for subject recruitment—rather than unrelated considerations, such as ease of access or privilege. Selection among those who could meet scientific goals is further informed by considerations of minimizing risk, enhancing benefit, and protecting vulnerable participants. Mackay and Saylor have distinguished four subprinciples to further characterize fair subject selection: fair inclusion, fair burden sharing, fair opportunity, and fair distribution of third-party risks.[17] Clarifying these distinct subprinciples is useful for study design and for the justification of inclusion and exclusion criteria, in a way that enables a fair distribution of burden and benefits to both research participants and the communities the research is intended to benefit.

A favorable risk-benefit ratio encompasses key ethical principles of nonmaleficence and beneficence. Risk-benefit evaluations help to ensure that research interventions and studies do not pose excessive risks of harm to participants for the benefit of others. Unlike in clinical practice, clinical research risks are not weighed solely against direct benefits to individual subjects. Rather, they are considered in light of any potential benefits to participants as well as the social and scientific value of the research, that is, the potential to generate knowledge that will improve health. A favorable risk-benefit ratio is fundamental to avoid exploitation in research. Rid and Wendler have described a framework for evaluating the risk-benefit ratio of a given study, consisting of ensuring the study's social value; identifying the research interventions and procedures in question; assessing and reducing risks to participants; evaluating and enhancing benefits to participants; evaluating whether the intervention poses net risks (i.e., risks that outweigh potential individual benefits); evaluating whether the net risks are justified by the potential benefits of other interventions in the study; and evaluating whether remaining net risks are justified by the study's social value.[18]

Collaborative partnership, independent review, informed consent, and respect for enrolled participants are the remaining requirements for ethical clinical research. Collaborative partnership recognizes that research is not done *to* people but *with* people. Collaborative partnership demands respect for the important contributions of many collaborators, such as participants, clinicians, research teams, funders, policymakers, and communities. Independent review of research is carried out by institutional review boards or research ethics committees and by independent data safety monitoring boards and is crucial for ensuring social accountability of research as a social and moral enterprise. Independent review ensures that a clinical study complies with the ethical requirements outlined in regulatory guidance, that the risk-benefit profile is favorable to the research participant and that it avoids undue harm to them. Institutional review boards historically emerged after the infamous and blatantly unethical research experiments and research scandals of the twentieth century, such as those perpetuated during World War II and the US studies of syphilis in Tuskegee. Today, independent institutional review, required by most codes of ethics and national regulations, functions as an additional safeguard against misuse of research subjects and ensures that research is enacted in an ethical manner, which is of utmost importance to preserve public trust in research.

Informed consent is of central importance for ethical research and consists of presenting relevant study information and relying on three key conditions: (1) understanding; (2) decision-making capacity; (3) and voluntariness. Informed consent is a foundational requirement, one that is morally transformative in that it permits acts that would otherwise be considered a moral violation.[19–21] For example, to perform an investigational procedure on someone without their consent is a clear violation of that person's bodily integrity and hence a moral wrong—providing consent transforms the act into one that is permissible. Exactly how much understanding is required for valid informed consent in the context of clinical research remains debated.[22–26] Finally, respect for research participants throughout the research is ensured by allowing subjects to withdraw from the study, protecting their privacy and confidentiality, adequately informing them of newly discovered risks and benefits as well as relevant study findings, and ensuring participants' welfare throughout the study.[9]

The ethical requirements described above have proven to be a useful framework for thinking through ethical clinical research. Recognizing clinical research and clinical practice as different allows us to make sense of why similar ethical principles apply in a fundamentally different way in the two endeavors. For example, in clinical practice, risks should not outweigh benefits to the patient, as per the proportionality requirement. The proportionality requirement applies to clinical research in a different way since the risks need to be outweighed by the social value of the study in addition to any benefits to the participant. Hence risk-benefit assessments in clinical practice differ from those in research, and an intervention that would not be justified in clinical research due, for example, to its high risk might be justified in clinical practice when the prospect of benefit outweighs the risks.

The scientific approach also helps clarify key concepts and address commonly described problems for clinical research. Concrete examples are the concept of therapeutic misconception and randomization to placebo. Therapeutic misconception, as defined in the original article that coined the term, is "to deny the possibility that there may be major disadvantages to participating in clinical research that stem from the nature of the research process itself."[27(p20)] It is important to bear in mind that therapeutic misconception is not limited to research participants and can also apply to clinician-scientists.[28–30] Clinician-scientists can endorse and promote therapeutic misconceptions in many ways, such as when they overstate—or are vague about—the prospect of medical benefit of trial participation or when they refer a patient to a trial assuming that patient benefit will be equal to or greater than what she would receive otherwise.[29,31] Various other types of misconceptions in research have been described, such as therapeutic misestimation and therapeutic optimism.[32] The prevailing view is that endorsing a scientific approach to clinical research, which recognizes an ethically relevant distinction between clinical research and practice, can help to identify and resolve tensions and responsibilities—although this remains a topic of debate.[33,34] Randomization to placebo is another example of a concept that can be ethically justified according to the scientific approach to clinical research, while the use of placebo typically would not be justifiable in clinical practice as it brings no direct benefit to the individual patient. Randomization to placebo can be justified in clinical research when using a placebo-controlled design would enable the generation of socially valuable knowledge that would not otherwise be obtainable—provided, among other methodological reasons, there is no proven effective treatment available and/or the risks of withholding an intervention do not pose excessive harm to the research subjects.[6,35] These and other key concepts that continue to be debated show that while the scientific approach is most suited to understanding the ethics of clinical research, it is not without remaining challenges. While the view that the ethics of clinical research is distinct from that of clinical practice has proven helpful in thinking about debated issues like therapeutic misconception and placebo-controlled trials, not everyone agrees that this approach settles the disputes, and some commentators believe that clinical equipoise is a necessary ethical requirement for all research.

Professionalism in Clinical Research

Ethical constraints on clinical research are useful for thinking in a principled and systematic manner about the justification for and the design and conduct of clinical research. Yet the role of the clinician-scientist remains ill-defined and debated.[36] What duties does a clinician-investigator have, beyond ensuring that research is scientifically valid, socially valuable, and fair? While the scientific approach to clinical research offers a necessary framework for ethical constraints, it is not sufficient to define the standards for professionalism. The reason is that attention to participants' well-being and clinical needs is necessary throughout the process of participation in research, requiring an expanded understanding of the clinician-scientists' duties toward the patient-subject. Given that clinical research requires clinical judgment, defining professional integrity in clinical research is crucial. Key transition points when clinician-scientists are expected to guide the patient-subject are, for example, when deciding whether to enroll or refer a patient for research, when transitioning a patient to research and later back to clinical care, when deciding whether to withdraw an individual participant, provide ancillary care, stop a trial due to serious adverse effects, or when determining post-trial responsibilities toward research participants.[37–39] What exactly, in this complex dual role, does it mean for a clinician-scientist to act professionally?

Miller has argued that "the roles of clinician and scientist must be integrated to manage conscientiously the ethical complexity, ambiguity, and tensions between the potentially competing loyalties of science and care of volunteer patients."[3(p1450)] He proposes a hybrid model that integrates the clinician and scientists' roles, drawing from the relationship between the scientist and research participant: Both parties need to be clear about the nature of clinical research and the scope of the exchange, while fostering a therapeutic alliance. In what follows, we first discuss the central issue of the clinician-scientist's dual role and the inherent tension between therapeutic and scientific obligations. Next, we discuss relevant moral considerations for the clinician-scientist when therapeutic and scientific obligations conflict and what virtues are important for clinical-scientists' professional integrity.

The Inherent Conflict of Interest

The clinician-scientist's dual role carries an inherent conflict of interest between attending to research interests and ensuring adequate protection of research participants, while also attending to their rights and welfare. While it might be straightforward to understand how clinician-scientists should address financial conflicts of interests (e.g., adequate disclosure, prioritizing research and patient welfare interests over sponsor interests), navigating the inherent conflict of interest that the dual role entails is more murky terrain.

The pervasiveness of the inherent tension is exemplified in the problem of therapeutic misconception, as described previously, as well as in the concept of clinical equipoise, and the question of who should obtain consent for research. For example, scientifically and methodologically justified and rigorous randomized controlled trials permit clinicians to do scientifically valid research while ensuring their therapeutic obligation toward research participants. As such, this can satisfy clinical equipoise as an ethical constraint on study design as well as a professional integrity issue. Yet some have argued that by requiring clinical equipoise one fundamentally endorses a misguided therapeutic approach to research, in a way that conflates clinical research and clinical care and therefore poses a problem for the professional integrity of the clinician-scientist.[6] A better way, according to this view, is to recognize that clinical equipoise is not a necessary normative requirement and to allow for adequately informed prospective participants to waive their right to standard medical care when consenting to ethically designed and justifiable research.[6] Another example concerns the question of when it is permissible for clinician-scientists to obtain consent from their own patients to enroll in a research trial. Some have argued that mere disclosure of the inherent conflict of interest is sufficient, while others have stated that informed consent should be obtained from an independent third party.[40–42] Because the inherent conflict of interest cannot be eliminated, the main question is how to manage the tension—a tension that, some have argued, can be adequately managed by requiring that the treating clinician be different from the scientist-investigator, except in some cases where the practical advantage of a dual role is important[42] or where research participation more closely approximates usual clinical care.[43] However, while discussions have revolved mainly around clinician-scientists who are also the treating clinician,[42–44] the question of clinician-scientists who are *not* the treating clinician yet face a conflict between scientific and therapeutic obligation remains underexplored.[45]

When Scientific and Therapeutic Obligations Conflict

Professional integrity means tending to the scientific and therapeutic obligations that arise in clinical research in a way that ensures the integrity of the research as well as the safety and welfare of research participants. The scientific obligations entail that a researcher adopt the course of action that is most conducive to scientific validity of the trial. The therapeutic (protective) obligations mean that there is a duty to protect research subjects from research-related undue harms. When scientific and therapeutic obligations conflict, professional integrity toward research participants requires that, as a default, participants' safety be guaranteed and undue research-related harms avoided: protective duty trumps scientific duty. Empirical research shows that nearly all clinician-scientists report facing this conflict of obligations and that their default in these situations is to revert to their protective duty—yet sometimes at the cost of negatively influencing the validity of their research.[46] In some protocol-specific cases, it might be permissible to prioritize scientific overprotective duty (e.g., a clinical trial studying asthma exacerbation) provided adequate informed consent has been obtained beforehand.[47] In the hard cases where both scientific and protective duties are equally compelling, Merritt has alternatively argued that the priority strategy can be to appeal to a third moral consideration, namely the research participant's interest in achieving their personal goals for participation.[47] This differs from the participants' welfare or medical interests in that it is about what the participant considers a research-related goal for themselves. For example, they might feel engaged or derive an altruistic feeling of worth or pride from contributing to research that will benefit others with a similar disease. Similarly, they might benefit from attending a well-resourced research institution and interact with experts on their disease. An appeal to the participant's interest in contributing to a project that is valuable to them can be an additional justification for an adult participant to be exposed to net risks for the benefit of others.[4] The value of patient engagement in research has been recognized and formalized through professional research organizations such as the Patient-Centered Outcomes Research Institute (PCORI).[48]

Defining the Virtuous Clinician-Scientist

Given that the ethics of clinical research differs from the ethics of clinical care, it is not a simple task to define what integrity in clinical research means in terms of professional identity and character.[3,37] The scientific approach enables applying appropriate and rigorous methods while minimizing risks to research participants and maximizing the social value of the research. But clinician-scientists face several important steps throughout any research study that require professional integrity, such as the responsibility to attend to the participants' clinical status and the requirement for honest data collection, analysis, and reporting. Clearly, then, adhering to the ethical restraints and focusing on protection alone is insufficient. Similar to professionalism in clinical practice, virtues play a role in defining professionalism standards in clinical research.[37] Henry Beecher famously stated, in his landmark 1966 article "Ethics and Clinical Research," that two components are the most important to guarantee ethical clinical research: first, adequate informed consent, and second, "the more reliable safeguard provided by the presence of an intelligent, informed conscientious, compassionate, responsible investigator."[49(p1354)] The role of virtues as part of the internal morality of medicine—such as benevolence, intellectual honesty, courage, compassion, prudence, and truthfulness—have received ample attention in the literature.[50–54] Given the view that the ethics of the relationship between clinician-scientist and patient-subject is grounded in *science*, which set of virtues should the clinician-scientist possess?

A set of six virtues has been proposed as crucial for clinician-scientists' delicate task of skillfully balancing therapeutic and research obligations while ensuring adequate protective duties toward research participants: integrity, trustworthiness, discernment, conscientiousness, compassion, and intellectual honesty.[37] Integrity refers to the duty of clinician-scientists to stand up for what they believe is right, for example, by refusing to enroll a patient who they think could be harmed by enrollment or by being transparent about financial conflict of interests and prioritizing scientific and participants' interests above financial interests of the study sponsors. Trustworthiness in the context of research means being dependable and accountable for the integrity of the study data, as well as for the clinical status of the research participant. Discernment refers to the use of good clinical judgment throughout the study, particularly when addressing conflicts between scientific and therapeutic obligations. Conscientiousness means being careful and vigilant, compassion refers to genuine care for participants, and intellectual honesty refers to honesty in the acquisition, analysis, and application of ideas and data and reporting of the findings. Taken together, these virtues safeguard the welfare and interests of people participating as human subjects in research.[37]

Challenges and Opportunities for Clinician-Scientists: Two Examples

Professionalism in clinicians is fostered across the tripartite mission of clinical care, clinical research, and medical education. In what follows, we use two examples to illustrate how ethical requirements for clinical research relate to and inform professionalism standards for clinician-scientists. A first example relates to navigating clinician-scientists' dual role in two cases: (1) when enrolling or referring their own patients for clinical research and (2) when engaging in embedded research or learning health systems. A second example focuses on professional education of clinician-scientists to promote structural competence, a concept that focuses on how clinicians can foster skills to recognize and address social and structural determinants of health.

The Clinician-Scientists' Dual Role in Practice

The ethics of enrolling and referring one's own patients for research continues to be debated and offers a good opportunity to reflect on professionalism standards for clinician-scientists. Arguments against enrolling one's own patients and obtaining their consent are the role conflict for the clinician-scientist, possible compromise of the voluntariness of participants' consent, and the promotion of therapeutic misconception.[43] Morain and colleagues have argued that revising the position against dual-role consent is desirable for three reasons: (1) increased interest in integrating research and care to advance evidence-based medicine and to support socially valuable research; (2) patients' preference to discuss research participants with their treating clinician, as per empirical evidence; and (3) mismatch between policy and practice, where policies typically do not explicitly state who should obtain consent (rather, they focus on what consent should include) and practice instead often relies on treating clinicians' judgment.[43] Therefore, they argue that it can be ethically permissible, and in fact desirable, for clinician-scientists to obtain consent if research participation approximates standard care. According to this view, obtaining dual consent is permissible in the case of randomized comparative effectiveness trials but might still be impermissible in the case of early placebo-controlled trials.

A similar question, albeit more straightforward ethically speaking, relates to clinicians' decision-making about referring a patient for a clinical trial. Empirical research has shown that reasons for primary care physicians not to refer their patients are more likely related to practical reasons (e.g., preferring to leave this to a specialist or being unaware of any available trials) and lack of knowledge, rather than ethical concerns related to patient participation.[55] A survey assessing the willingness of primary care physicians to refer their patients to a preventive vaccine trial shows that limited knowledge and education about clinical research in general is the main obstacle to patient referral.[56] These studies suggest that, contrary to concern about the ethics of dual-role consent, clinicians are less concerned about the ethics of referring a patient for research—provided that the research itself is done ethically. Rather, to be able to evaluate when to refer their own patients for participation in research, prospective clinicians need to receive adequate training about clinical research in their medical education.

The increasing use of learning health systems or embedded research—research incorporated in clinical care—poses distinct challenges and opportunities for clinician-scientists' dual role and for the distinction between practice and research more broadly.[57–59] Learning health systems offer a unique opportunity for continued quality improvement and comparative effectiveness research.[57] They also provide a potential response to the key challenge of justifying the risks to research participants for the benefit of others: Risks can be justified by regarding research risks as an essential component of learning health systems, designed to continuously evaluate clinical care.[4,57] Specific challenges arise regarding the ethical distinction between clinical research and clinical care, while conducting research that is, by its very design, embedded in clinical care. In learning health systems, waiving of individual informed consent sometimes can be justified for methodological reasons, providing there is an ethically robust oversight system.[60–62] Yet this poses novel unsettled questions, such as what it means to promote respect for patient-participants independently of informed consent or the assessment and disclosure of risks involved in comparing standard-of-care interventions.[61,63]

Fostering Clinician-Scientists' Structural Competence

Clinical care and research are embedded in larger societal processes, and clinicians need to be able to navigate these intersections in a way that avoids harming patients and their communities and promotes their welfare.[64] Whether clinicians have an additional duty to promote social justice has been a long-standing topic of debate.[65,66] Yet there has been a *prise de conscience* ("realization") over the last decade that clinicians have a duty to recognize the social and systemic inequities that affect their patient's health outcomes.[67,68] The previously prevailing concept of "cultural competency" as an essential part of medical education is being replaced by the emerging model of "structural competency."[69,70] This emerging model, increasingly used in clinical training programs across the United States, focuses on recognizing and addressing how structural inequities operate in clinical care.[68,71,72] The approach consists of training clinicians in five core competencies to develop the ability to (1) recognize the structures that shape clinical interactions; (2) use a language of structure; (3) rearticulate "cultural" formulations in structural terms; (4) observe and conceive of structural interventions; and (5) foster structural humility.[68]

A starting point for thinking about structural, particularly racial, inequities in medicine is to gain awareness of the complex categorization of race in clinical practice and research.[73,74] The structural competence model raises novel and underexplored questions about the ramifications for clinicians who engage in clinical research and for the research community more broadly. Importantly, the concept of structural competence offers new opportunities for clinician-scientists to ask socially valuable research questions that will counter systemic and structural inequities and contribute to a more just healthcare system. In determining research priorities and socially valuable research questions about a given disorder and its symptoms, structural competency enables the clinician-scientist to discern the symptoms from their upstream social and structural determinants of health. In addition, the structural competence model may guide fair participant selection and recruitment strategies, monitoring participant welfare, and planning for appropriate transition at the end of a clinical trial. Avenues for how to foster structural competency in clinician-scientists are emerging,[75] yielding novel opportunities for meaningful engagement toward structural change.

Conclusion

Clinical practice and clinical research share a common goal of improving health. Yet, the two endeavors are governed by different ethical standards and norms, and there are inherent tensions in the roles played by clinician-scientists. In this chapter, we reviewed the ethical norms that govern clinical research, emphasizing the scientific approach to clinical research, and recognized that additional considerations are critical to defining the ethical and professional obligations of clinician-scientists to patients and research participants. Professionalism norms in clinician-scientists should be guided by relevant virtues and responsibilities, as well as adequate knowledge about the nature, ethics, and challenges of clinical research. Finally, concepts such as learning health systems and structural competence pose novel questions for the ethics of clinical research and professionalism norms in clinician-scientists. They yield promising avenues for clinical practice and research's shared commitment to improving health.

Disclaimers

The views expressed here are those of the authors and do not necessarily reflect the policies of the National Institutes of Health, the Department of Health and Human Services, or the federal government. The authors report no financial conflict of interests.

References

1. National Commission for the Protection of Human Subjects of Biomedical and Behavioral Research. *The Belmont Report: Ethical Principles and Guidelines for the Protection of Human Subjects of Research.* 1978. https://www.hhs.gov/ohrp/regulations-and-policy/belmont-report/read-the-belmont-report/index.html
2. Dudzinski DM. Integrity in the relationship between medical ethics and professionalism. *Am J Bioeth.* 2004;4(2):26–27.
3. Miller FG. Professional integrity in clinical research. *JAMA.* 1998;280(16):1449–1454.
4. Wendler D. The ethics of clinical research. In: Zalta EN, ed. *The Stanford Encyclopedia of Philosophy.* Metaphysics Research Lab, Philosophy Department, Stanford University; 2021. https://plato.stanford.edu/entries/clinical-research/
5. Joffe S, Miller FG. Bench to bedside: mapping the moral terrain of clinical research. *Hastings Cent Rep.* 2008;38(2):30–42.
6. Miller FG. Revisiting the distinction and the connection between research and practice. *Perspect Biol Med.* 2020;63(2):277–292.
7. Beauchamp TL, Saghai Y. The historical foundations of the research-practice distinction in bioethics. *Theor Med Bioeth.* 2012;33(1):45–56.
8. Miller FG, Rosenstein DL. The therapeutic orientation to clinical trials. *N Engl J Med.* 2003;348(14):1383–1386.
9. Emanuel EJ, Wendler D, Grady C. What makes clinical research ethical? *JAMA.* 2000;283(20):2701–2711.
10. Emanuel EJ, Grady C, Crouch RA, Lie RK, Miller FG, Wendler DE. *The Oxford Textbook of Clinical Research Ethics.* Oxford University Press; 2008.
11. Rid A, Shah SK. Substantiating the social value requirement for research: an introduction. *Bioethics.* 2017;31(2):72–76.
12. Rid A. Judging the social value of health-related research: current debate and open questions. *Perspect Biol Med.* 2020;63(2):293–312.
13. Wertheimer A. The social value requirement reconsidered. *Bioethics.* 2015;29(5):301–308.
14. Wendler D, Rid A. In defense of a social value requirement for clinical research. *Bioethics.* 2017;31(2):77–86.
15. Habets MG, Van Delden JJ, Bredenoord AL. The social value of clinical research. *BMC Med Ethics.* 2014;15(1):66.
16. Freedman B. Equipoise and the ethics of clinical research. *N Engl J Med.* 1987;317(3):141–145.
17. Mackay D, Saylor KW. Four faces of fair subject selection. *Am J Bioeth.* 2020;20(2):5–19.
18. Rid A, Wendler D. A framework for risk-benefit evaluations in biomedical research. *Kennedy Inst Ethics J.* 2011;21(2):141–179.

19. Millum J, Bromwich D. Informed consent: what must be disclosed and what must be understood? *Am J Bioeth.* 2021;21(5):46–58.
20. Millum J, Bromwich D. Understanding, communication, and consent. *Ergo.* 2018;(5):45–68.
21. Beauchamp TL. Informed consent: its history, meaning, and present challenges. *Camb Q Healthc Ethics.* 2011;20(4):515–523.
22. Grady C. Enduring and emerging challenges of informed consent. *N Engl J Med.* 2015;372(22):2172.
23. Shepherd L, Macklin R. Erosion of informed consent in US research. *Bioethics.* 2019;33(1):4–12.
24. Sugarman J. Examining provisions related to consent in the revised common rule. *Am J Bioeth.* 2017;17(7):22–26.
25. Greenblum J, Hubbard R. The common rule's "reasonable person" standard for informed consent. *Bioethics.* 2019;33(2):274–277.
26. Dickert NW, Eyal N, Goldkind SF, et al. Reframing consent for clinical research: a function-based approach. *Am J Bioeth.* 2017;17(12):3–11.
27. Appelbaum PS, Roth LH, Lidz CW, Benson P, Winslade W. False hopes and best data: consent to research and the therapeutic misconception. *Hastings Cent Rep.* 1987;17(2):20.
28. Henderson GE, Churchill LR, Davis AM, et al. Clinical trials and medical care: defining the therapeutic misconception. *PLoS Med.* 2007;4(11):e324.
29. Dresser R. The ubiquity and utility of the therapeutic misconception. *Soc Philos Policy.* 2002;19(2): 271–294.
30. Miller FG, Brody H. A critique of clinical equipoise. Therapeutic misconception in the ethics of clinical trials. *Hastings Cent Rep.* 2003;33(3):19–28.
31. Henderson GE, Davis AM, King NMP, et al. Uncertain benefit: investigators' views and communications in early phase gene transfer trials. *Mol Ther.* 2004;10(2):225–231.
32. Horng S, Grady C. Misunderstanding in clinical research: distinguishing therapeutic misconception, therapeutic misestimation, and therapeutic optimism. *IRB.* 2003;25(1):11–16.
33. Appelbaum PS, Lidz CW. Twenty-five years of therapeutic misconception. *Hastings Cent Rep.* 2008;38(2):5–6; author reply: 7.
34. Appelbaum PS, Lidz CW, Grisso T. Therapeutic misconception in clinical research: frequency and risk factors. *IRB.* 2004;26(2):1–8.
35. Millum J, Grady C. The ethics of placebo-controlled trials: methodological justifications. *Contemp Clin Trials.* 2013;36(2):510–514.
36. Jansen LA. Doctor vs. scientist? *Hastings Cent Rep.* 2008;38(2):3.
37. Grady C, Fauci AS. The role of the virtuous investigator in protecting human research subjects. *Perspect Biol Med.* 2016;59(1):122–131.
38. Grady C. The challenge of assuring continued post-trial access to beneficial treatment. *Yale J Health Policy Law Ethics.* 2005;5(1):425–435.
39. Richardson HS, Belsky L. The ancillary-care responsibilities of medical researchers. An ethical framework for thinking about the clinical care that researchers owe their subjects. *Hastings Cent Rep.* 2004;34(1):25–33.
40. Sollitto S, Hoffman S, Mehlman MJ, Lederman RJ, Youngner SJ, Lederman MM. Intrinsic conflicts of interest in clinical research: a need for disclosure. *Kennedy Inst Ethics J.* 2003;13(2):83–91.

41. Levinsky NG. Nonfinancial conflicts of interest in research. *N Engl J Med.* 2002;347(10):759–761.

42. Brody H, Miller FG. The clinician-investigator: unavoidable but manageable tension. *Kennedy Inst Ethics J.* 2003;13(4):329–346.

43. Morain SR, Joffe S, Largent EA. When is it ethical for physician-investigators to seek consent from their own patients? *Am J Bioeth.* 2019;19(4):11–18.

44. Shah A, Porter K, Juul S, Wilfond BS. Precluding consent by clinicians who are both the attending and the investigator: an outdated shibboleth? *The Am J Bioeth.* 2015;15(4):80–82.

45. Nicolini ME, Wendler D. Inherent conflict of interest in clinical research: a call for effective guidance. *Am J Bioeth.* 2020;20(10):94–96.

46. Lidz CW, Appelbaum PS, Joffe S, Albert K, Rosenbaum J, Simon L. Competing commitments in clinical trials. *IRB.* 2009;31(5):1–6.

47. Merritt M. Moral conflict in clinical trials. *Ethics.* 2005;115(2):306–330.

48. PCORI. Patient-Centered Outcomes Research Institute. About PCORI. Accessed Nov 2022. https://www.pcori.org/about/about-pcori

49. Beecher HK. Ethics and clinical research. *N Engl J Med.* 1966;274(24): 1354–1360.

50. Pellegrino ED. The internal morality of clinical medicine: a paradigm for the ethics of the helping and healing professions. *J Med Philos.* 2001;26(6):559–579.

51. Symons X. Pellegrino, MacIntyre, and the internal morality of clinical medicine. *Theor Med Bioeth.* 2019;40(3):243–251.

52. Miller FG, Brody H. The internal morality of medicine: an evolutionary perspective. *J Med Philos.* 2001;26(6): 581–599.

53. Veatch RM. The impossibility of a morality internal to medicine. *J Med Philos.* 2001;26(6):621–642.

54. MacIntyre A. *After Virtue.* University of Notre Dame Press; 1981.

55. Crosson K, Eisner E, Brown C, Ter Maat J. Primary care physicians' attitudes, knowledge, and practices related to cancer clinical trials. *J Cancer Educ.* 2001;16(4):188–192.

56. Detoc M, Touche C, Charles R, Lucht F, Gagneux-Brunon A, Botelho-Nevers E. Primary physicians' attitudes toward their patients receiving a proposal to participate in a vaccine trial. *Hum Vaccin Immunother.* 2019;15(12):2969–2979.

57. Faden RR, Kass NE, Goodman SN, Pronovost P, Tunis S, Beauchamp TL. An ethics framework for a learning health care system: a departure from traditional research ethics and clinical ethics. *Hastings Cent Rep.* 2013;Spec No:S16–S27.

58. Kass NE, Faden RR, Goodman SN, Pronovost P, Tunis S, Beauchamp TL. The research-treatment distinction: a problematic approach for determining which activities should have ethical oversight. *Hastings Cent Rep.* 2013;Spec No:S4–S15.

59. Morain S, Largent E. Think pragmatically: investigators' obligations to patient-subjects when research is embedded in care. *Am J Bioeth.* 2022;23(8), 10–21.

60. Pletcher MJ, Lo B, Grady D. Informed consent in randomized quality improvement trials. *JAMA Intern Med.* 2014;174(5):668.

61. Morain SR, Kraft SA, Wilfond BS, et al. Toward meeting the obligation of respect for persons in pragmatic clinical trials. *Hastings Cent Rep.* 2022;52(3):9–17.

62. Faden RR, Beauchamp TL, Kass NE. Informed consent, comparative effectiveness, and learning health care. *N Engl J Med.* 2014;370(8):766–768.

63. Kim SYH, Kimmelman J. Practical steps to identifying the research risk of pragmatic trials. *Clin Trials.* 2022:19(2):211–216.

64. Burson RC, Familusi OO, Clapp JT. Imagining the "structural" in medical education and practice in the United States: a curricular investigation. *Soc Sci Med.* 2022;300:114453.

65. Wear D, Kuczewski MG. The professionalism movement: can we pause? *Am J Bioeth.* 2004;4(2):1–10.

66. Twohig PL, MacDonald C. Professionalism and the social role of medicine. *Am J Bioeth.* 2004;4(2):3–5.

67. Khazanchi R, Keeler H, Strong S, et al. Building structural competency through community engagement. *Clin Teach.* 2021;18(5):535–541.

68. Metzl JM, Hansen H. Structural competency: theorizing a new medical engagement with stigma and inequality. *Soc Sci Med.* 2014;103:126–133.

69. Hansen H, Braslow J, Rohrbaugh RM. From cultural to structural competency—training psychiatry residents to act on social determinants of health and institutional racism. *JAMA Psychiatry.* 2018;75(2):117-118.

70. Drevdahl DJ. Culture shifts: from cultural to structural theorizing in nursing. *Nurs Res.* 2018;67(2):146–160.

71. Neff J, Holmes SM, Knight KR, et al. Structural competency: curriculum for medical students, residents, and interprofessional teams on the structural factors that produce health disparities. *MedEdPORTAL* 2020;16:10888.

72. Hansen H, Metzl JM. New medicine for the US health care system: training physicians for structural interventions. *Acad Med.* 2017;92(3):279–281.

73. Shim RS. Dismantling structural racism in academic medicine: a skeptical optimism. *Acad Med.* 2020;95(12):1793–1795.

74. Gutin I. Essential(ist) medicine: promoting social explanations for racial variation in biomedical research. *Med Human.* 2019;45(3):224–234.

75. Udemgba C, Jefferson AA, Stern J, Khoury P. Toolkit for developing structural competency in health disparities in allergy and immunology training and research. *J Allergy Clin Immunol Pract.* 2022;10(4):936–949.

PART C: EPILOGUE

REHAB

Thomas S. Inui

As fans of the HBO series *The Wire* or readers of *Public Health Reports* know, Baltimore City has long had a major problem with heroin/cocaine/crack/smack—opioids in every form imaginable. Starting sometime in the late 1940s, by the 1960s the Centers for Disease Control and Prevention reported that there were so many addicts in the metropolitan population that Bawlmer, the city of my birth, had the highest per capita addiction rate of any American city. I might have guessed this was the situation from my experience in medical school and medical residency 1965–1974. Overdose presentations to Hopkins Hospital's Emergency Room (ER) were commonplace in the evenings and overnight. "Presentations" rather dignifies these events. A car would roar up the ER drive, a door open, and a body would be rolled out. We'd run out a gurney, pick up the person, and administer Narcan. After evaluation and observation, only a select few would be admitted to hospital—the dead to the morgue, those with aspiration and/or fever to the medical service. Drawing blood for any purpose was a bitch—they had long since blown all their veins, some even using their groins for access. In the ER and in the hospital, they were angry patients, sometimes because we kept them from wrestling with our medical stuff, and sometimes because they were in withdrawal, sweating like pigs and in pain.

And these addicts were dangerous. I still have the knife I took from a patient in the ER before he could create any havoc. One snowy night, as I tried to walk home from the hospital, two guys with small pupils and a gun took everything I had in my pockets. It was the second time I had been robbed just outside the hospital. It made me so mad I ran after them for a block or two after they melted into the dark neighborhood where the streetlights were all out, until my better self spoke ("What are you **doing**? They had a GUN!"), and I wrote off the loss as part of the cost of living close to the hospital. We all knew that Hopkins students and residents had been murdered in the neighborhood. Students lived in high-rise dormitories with controlled access. Residents lived behind high security fences in a unit called "The Compound," a term that somehow suggested that they might be considered prisoners of war. What war?

But these addicts were also helpless. Slaves to their habit. Doing anything they had to do to keep their stash going. In the ER or on the wards, it was clear that there was nothing I could do to help them escape the morass of addiction and its associated abuse of self and others. It seemed to me that the conditions we treated—the pneumonias, cellulitis, endocarditis, phlebitis—were the least of their troubles. The day we discharged them from the hospital was high risk for reappearances in the ER drive with an overdose. We had kept them long enough in the hospital that they had partially detoxified, and the usual bags on the street were too much for them. We "joked" about certain addicts "being on Dr. Harvey's payroll" because they kept being readmitted to hospital, needing medical care, and seemingly participating in the "training" of generations of house staff and students—until they disappeared, succumbing sometime in the decade of their fifties to overdoses, getting murdered, getting long-term jail sentences, or "burning out their addiction," whatever that meant. Leaving residency, I was sick of the cycle of addiction. I was burned out, whatever that meant.

During my Indian Health Service time in Albuquerque, there was blessed relief from heroin. OK, Las Vegas, New Mexico, was known as "Smack City," and by rumor small planes flew into private airstrips in the Penitente countryside with their cargoes from Mexican cartels, but the Pueblo people and Checkerboard area Navajos we served seemed mainly free from the scourge of opioids. When I moved subsequently to the University of Washington's health system and assumed responsibility for the General Internal Medicine Division, however, the nightmare recurred. First in the Veterans Administration Medical Center, then in the public hospital, I had a substantial number of patients who had been exposed to narcotics, either in Vietnam or on the streets of Seattle. Once again, they were my demanding, angry patients. One of them, who was unsatisfied with my response to his need for prescription refills, sent his brother to the front door of my home to remind me of my obligations to provide more controlled substances. Thereafter, whether coincidentally or not, the back window of our car was broken out on two occasions, making it clear that it needed to be parked somewhere other than in front of our house. I was angry.

Later that year, one of the general internal medicine physicians moved away from Seattle and left the weekly clinic sessions at the King Country Drug Treatment Center uncovered. I had no one else to fill this need, so I took on this responsibility myself. It was a hassle just to get there. The drug treatment center was on a "campus" well outside Seattle. When I asked for directions, the center nurse said: "It's easy. Just follow the signs and trucks to the county landfill. The road to the treatment center branches off to the right just before you get to the dump." Patients were committed to the drug treatment center by order of civil courts as an alternative to jail time and could not leave the campus for the duration of their sentence, usually a minimum of six weeks. I imagined them reading the signs as they were transported to the center and noticing that they were almost deposited as garbage before—at the last minute—being taken to the treatment center. Once there, they were compelled to complete detoxification. There were group sessions in the morning and afternoon. Smoking was permitted outside the dorms. Meals were provided. The water from the taps in the clinic and the dorms was tested from time to time because it was never clear—sometimes cloudy, usually somewhat yellow-green. The massive landfill up the valley on some days contributed a bouquet to the air we all breathed. Methane?

In clinic, I saw more patients than I could thoughtfully assess. Mostly they came with complaints of pain. Everything hurt—heads, backs, arms, hands. They wanted pain relief, and I could offer NSAIDs (nonsteroidal anti-inflammatory drugs) and acetaminophen. They loudly and angrily despised what I could offer. They demanded that I order x-rays and/or referrals to specialists in the hospital. The nurse told me that I could authorize transport for such visits, but that there would be a great risk of patients arranging contacts with suppliers who would arrange to meet them in hospital toilets. I leaned on my physical exam and communication skills and held the line, getting even more flaming anger from the patients. "Enough already with this crap! Aren't you a real doctor?"

Finally, I began to understand the time course of withdrawal and detoxification in the treatment center patient population. Fresh out of jail and on our campus, *they hurt.* Everything hurt—their bodies, their loss of usual life circumstances, the absence of their friends and family, their loss of independence and freedom, having to sit through the stupid group sessions. Nothing I said made sense. It differed from one patient to another, but sometime about two to three weeks after admission, their pain began to abate, the sessions began to be better, the food more acceptable. I discovered that until detoxification was truly complete, they didn't have dreams they could describe to me when I asked: "Are you having any dreams?" After about three weeks, I could sensibly ask other questions. "Do you have any children? How old are they? With whom are they living? When did you last see that third-grader of yours? Do you know how she's doing in school? What kind of work have you done? Could you think about doing that again when you finish up here? Where are you actually *from*? Where would you like to live? Have you got any plans?" The patients kept coming to clinic, not for pain complaints but for conversations. If anything, there were even more patients on my afternoon schedule than at first, but I loved seeing people make progress. I was able to see through the ravages of their addiction and husks of their ruined lives to the *persons* they were.

I had detoxed and rehabbed myself.

After reading this story, try using an exegesis method to explore its content.

1. Who in this story can I see as myself?
2. From the point of view of whomever you have chosen, what do you bring to the situation that makes these events possible?
3. Who else in this story (or its organizational or cultural context) influences this story?
4. Where/what in this story is "the good," the value, the virtue, the "North Star," or the principle we might seek to preserve?
5. What, then, ought I do?

PART D

ORGANIZATIONAL PROFESSIONALISM AT THE INTERFACE BETWEEN PHYSICIANS AND ADMINISTRATORS

27

Organizational Professionalism

A Healthcare Organization's Ethical Responsibilities

Kelly N. Michelson, Joshua M. M. Faber, and Chad M. Teven

Key Points

- Healthcare organizations have responsibilities to numerous stakeholders, including patients, employees, other organizations, and the community. Many of these responsibilities rest on fundamental ethical considerations and medical professionalism.
- An organization must recognize, understand, and serve as a steward of these responsibilities in order to deliver effective and equitable care.
- Moving forward, as novel technology, staffing and patient care models, and healthcare discovery and delivery continue to evolve, healthcare organizations must leverage not only the foundational underpinnings of organizational ethics and professionalism but also identify and consider new issues that will arise.
- Through concerted efforts toward fulfilling responsibilities of improved healthcare on a wider scale (i.e., public healthcare), healthcare organizations will optimize the health of patients on an individual level.

Tying Medical Professionalism to Organizational Ethics

Administrators of healthcare organizations now play a bigger role in patient care than ever before. They distribute scarce healthcare resources, set clinical policies, and direct research priorities through funding allocations. All of these functions were once managed primarily by clinicians or clinician researchers bound to a code of professional ethics in which patient primacy is highlighted. Healthcare organizations, however, which are largely administrator led, do not have the same time-tested relationship to medical ethics and professionalism.

This chapter outlines the implications of this shift in responsibilities by addressing three central questions. First, to whom are healthcare organizations obligated? Second, what are those obligations? Finally, what happens when different obligations come into conflict with one another?

We start by framing the relationship between professionalism and organizational ethics. Next, we explore the unique responsibilities of the medical profession as well as organizations that deliver care to patients, such as hospitals. Here we also discuss the relationship between professional ethics and bioethics. The final and largest aspect of the chapter highlights the professional and ethical relationship between healthcare organizations and five key stakeholders: patients, employees, communities, partner organizations, and innovators.

Professional Ethics

Professional ethics specify the obligations of a given profession to individuals and institutions. Professions are distinct from other occupations in that professions require academic training and direct their members to serve a social good.[1] These characteristics also tend to elevate professions to a higher social status than other occupations. Traditional examples of professions in the United States include medicine, law, and education.

The social power that professions enjoy, coupled with their service obligations, has led to the development of professional ethics. These ethical considerations are frequently articulated as principles or virtues; principles are behavioral or decision-making guidelines, while virtues are character traits to which to aspire.[2] In either case, professional ethics ultimately derive their power from consensus, which typically takes the form of professional association guidelines or licensing rules. While different professions adhere to distinct ethical codes, ethicists have endeavored to highlight a subset of ethics that are accepted across all professions. Common professional virtues include variations on benevolence, integrity, respect, trustworthiness, and a good work ethic.[2,3] Though a cross-profession set of principles has yet to be specified, principlism is an indispensable component of medical professional ethics.

Medical professional ethics specify the obligations of clinicians to patients, communities, and clinical innovation. Without medical professional ethics, the medical community risks violating patient trust. Without trust, patients may not share pertinent clinical information, act on medical advice, or seek help when they are ill. As a result, adherence to professional ethics is essential for the practice of good medicine.

While the origin of medical professional ethics is multifactorial, the American Medical Association (AMA) has regularly updated a consensus code applicable to all specialties since 1847.[4,5] The code currently consists of nine principles that fall into three categories[6]:

1. **Patient care:** Care must be delivered competently, respectfully, confidentially, and honestly.
2. **Clinical innovation**: Physicians "shall continue to study, apply, and advance scientific knowledge."[(p1)]
3. **Health policy**: Physicians should support access to care for all patients and work toward changing laws that are not in patients' best interests

The AMA obligation to patient care is critical but difficult to implement because it is expressed as a set of virtues, not a set of principles. Instead, medical professionals commonly operationalize this obligation through the principles of biomedical ethics (Table 27.1). These principles—beneficence, nonmaleficence, justice, and autonomy—help clinicians navigate the ethically challenging facets of clinical decision-making.[7]

Table 27.1 Summary of the Core Principles of Biomedical Ethics

Principle	Summary
Beneficence	Act in the patient's benefit
Nonmaleficence	Avoid patient harm
Justice	Ensure fair distribution of the benefits and harms of care
Autonomy	Respect patient decision-making

Distinct medical specialties have tailored professional ethics to their particular needs.[6,8] Nurses have also developed their own professional ethics codes.[9] These more bespoke ethical codes supplement the virtues and principles highlighted by the AMA.

Organizational Ethics

Organizational ethics specify the obligations of organizations to their stakeholders. Organizational ethics may be developed in multiple ways. While some companies internally define their own unique set of values, others may choose to align themselves to a code of ethics generated by a third party (e.g., a business association code of ethics). Like professional ethics, organizational ethics frequently involve a virtue ethics approach or a principlist approach.

Healthcare organizations are obligated to serve patients, employees, the community, the profession of healthcare leadership, and the organization itself.[10,11] To achieve these ends, organizations must promote professional medical ethics and bioethics.[12,13] Promoting professional medical ethics is required for healthcare organizations to serve clinical employees. Similarly, implementing bioethics is necessary for organizations to serve patients. In addition to these ethical frameworks, the American College of Healthcare Executives (ACHE) regularly publishes a code of ethics that lists virtues, principles, and operational rules that healthcare organizations ought to adopt to faithfully fulfill their obligations.[10]

Unfortunately, even when the leaders of healthcare organizations are confident in their ethics, they may struggle to turn vision into practice. Administrators are the primary stewards of organizational ethics, but, at a large organization, operationalizing organizational ethics may require tens of thousands of people to align themselves to controversial policies. Businesses have many tools at their disposal—hiring screens, employee trainings, compensation structures, public communications, and others—that they may leverage to produce ethical outcomes.[11,14,15] This entire arsenal is necessary to address the ethical challenges that healthcare organizations must face.

Organizational ethics in healthcare are essential for facilitating good medical care and public health. Ethical healthcare organizations help medical professionals adhere to professional ethics and ensure patients are treated appropriately, thus building patient trust and strengthening the therapeutic relationship. Healthcare organizations also have additional obligations beyond their medical staff and patient care. They have responsibilities to their communities, the profession, and various business interests. Below, we explore how healthcare organizations can negotiate these varied obligations.

Organizational Responsibilities to Patients

Administrators at healthcare organizations must "lead the organization in prioritizing patient care above other considerations."[10] To that end, we believe that prioritizing patient care requires administrators to commit to bioethical principles. We reject the notion that bioethics should only guide clinical behaviors. We also recognize that prioritizing patient care is empirically difficult. It can be impossible to predict, for example, how certain administrative decisions impact patient care. Nonetheless, administrators must demonstrate that their decisions are aligned with patient interests before moving forward.

Implicit Obligations of Organizations to Patients

Healthcare organizations have explicit and implicit obligations to patients. Explicit obligations are articulated in the law and the ACHE code of ethics. Examples include delivering an adequate standard of care, obtaining informed consent, and protecting patient privacy.[16–18] Implicit obligations are implied by explicit obligations. The most important implicit obligation is organizational commitment to bioethics principles.

Healthcare organizations cannot fulfill their explicit responsibilities to patients without committing to bioethics principles. Organizations are explicitly obligated to[10]

- "Work to provide a process that ensures the autonomy and self-determination of patients"
- "Work to ensure the existence of a process to evaluate the safety, quality, and equity of care or service rendered"
- "Build trust with all patients"

The principles of bioethics are the best tools for achieving these goals. First, autonomy is itself a principle to which organizations have an explicit obligation. Second, balancing safety, quality, and equity is akin to balancing the three remaining principles—beneficence, nonmaleficence, and justice. Finally, the principles of bioethics are routinely and effectively applied to build and maintain patient trust.

Balancing Patient Obligations

Organizations may have obligations that compete with patient obligations or impair alignment with patient care goals. For example, healthcare organizations must maintain revenue flows and profit margins to operate. One way to pursue this goal is through consolidation, which involves acquiring competing care providers, and may potentially lead to anticompetitive behavior, including price gouging. At best, the organization's administrators may generate increased revenue that may be reinvested in new clinical capabilities and technology. Unfortunately, the patient may subsequently see a more than 60% rate increase without a commensurate increase in care quality.[19]

The impacts of consolidation may be directly opposed to organizations' obligations to patients.[20] Patients may receive worse care, violating the principle of beneficence. Financially strained patients may be unable to afford care, violating the justice principle.

Also, patients may have less control over care decisions due to fewer providers from which to choose, affecting autonomy. In contrast, administrators might argue the opposite case, that consolidation is not only ethically permissible but is required. Patients in a consolidated system may have access to greater specialized technologies and services, facilitating beneficence. Additionally, consolidated systems may have more resources to invest in services like in-person translators, which improves social influencers of health (nonmedical factors that influence health outcomes[21]) and satisfies justice.

When making decisions with unclear implications for patient care, administrators must reduce the risk that patients will suffer negative consequences. This may involve a two-step process:

1. Evaluate whether a decision will inherently benefit or harm patients.
2. Impose restrictions on decisions with uncertain outcomes to improve the probability that they benefit patients and reduce the probability that they harm patients.

The government enforces this process in extreme circumstances. When Chicago's Advocate and Northshore health systems attempted to merge in 2016, the Federal Trade Commission (FTC) blocked the arrangement on the grounds that it would reduce market competition.[22] Decreased competition may result in negative consumer effects (to payers and patients), particularly increased prices or decreased quality.[23] The FTC focused primarily on pricing. In prior cases, the FTC was able to retrospectively demonstrate that prices increased more than expected after a merger had already gone through. In other words, the merger was associated with unexpectedly large price increases. This finding was construed as economic harm to consumers, and it resulted in substantial postmerger regulatory requirements. In the 2016 case, the FTC prospectively demonstrated that prices would increase more than expected. They showed that, even though patients would not directly see an increase in prices, payers would. Moreover, since payers may pass off cost increases to patients through charges like premiums and copays, multiple consumer groups would be harmed by this outcome. In this way, the FTC did not need the merger to occur before demonstrating that a merger would harm consumers through price increases.

The Affordable Care Act medical loss ratio (MLR) rule addresses step 2 in this process by requiring that health insurers spend a prespecified percentage of premium revenue on patient services.[24] Thus, while insurer price increases may harm patients by restricting their purchasing power, the rule increases the probability that price hikes also yield some patient benefit. For instance, imagine an insurer raises premium prices to generate an extra $1 million in revenue every year. Before the MLR, 100% of that extra revenue could be returned to executives through end of year bonuses. Due to the MLR, some of that revenue may still be returned to executives, but a large component must also be invested in programs that benefit patients, like care management services or provider network expansion.

Government intervention is not sufficient, however. Organizations need to consistently regulate themselves. One approach is the establishment of an ethics task force or ethics committee charged with incorporating patient-centered ethics into administrative decisions.[25] Ideally, these committees would have veto power over decisions misaligned with organizational obligations to patients. This is not common, however. One study of 600 American hospitals found that while 97% of hospitals have healthcare ethics programs, only 26% had programs that address business ethics with variable authority.

Healthcare organizations have explicit and implicit ethical obligations to patients. Following through on these principles can be challenging in the face of competing obligations. One way to ensure ethical behavior is to intentionally incorporate patient-centered ethical reasoning into business decisions. We recommend healthcare organizations empower task forces to fulfill this duty.

Organizational Responsibilities to Employees

Arguably the most important duty of a healthcare organization relates to its primary responsibility to provide safe, equitable, and effective patient care. A key component of a healthcare organization's ability to provide for such care requires creating and nurturing an environment where the organization's clinical staff (i.e., physicians and other healthcare practitioners) can carry out this mission. A healthcare organization, therefore, also has an essential duty toward its providers.[26] This obligation of a healthcare organization to its providers is not solely concerned with optimizing patient care, however. Indeed, a healthcare organization has responsibilities and obligations to its professionals that are both related to and independent of patient care.

Similar to a hospital's obligation to patients and visitors, a fundamental responsibility that a hospital has to its employees is, in effect, to provide protection (i.e., a safe and healthy working environment). The work environment should also be free from harassment, discrimination, and other illegal activity. Like other employers, healthcare organizations must also ensure that basic daily needs are met (e.g., food and bathroom services), adhere to employment laws and regulations, honor contracts between employer and employees, and take reasonable action—proactive and in response—to reduce the risk of a hostile work environment.[27] These responsibilities are apparent, however, and not unique to healthcare organizations.

Healthcare organizations, in our opinion, have additional duties to their employees that may not be required of nonclinical organizations. While many different duties and responsibilities exist, the remainder of this section focuses on the ethical responsibilities of healthcare organizations to their clinically oriented medical staff and to any staff with exposure to patients and their families (Table 27.2). To that end, healthcare organizations ought to facilitate a psychologically safe environment for staff to perform their duties, including caring for patients and acting professionally. This requires a culture of transparency, communication, and open discussion. For example, reporting never-events, near-misses, and other potentially harmful clinical occurrences should be encouraged, and the employee who made a report should be protected from retaliation. Additionally,

Table 27.2 Examples of Responsibilities of Healthcare Organizations to Employees With Clinical Responsibilities

- Provision of a psychologically safe environment
- Culture of transparency, communication, and open discussion
- Encouragement of reporting of adverse events
- Protection from retaliation
- Resources to combat moral distress
- Resources to combat burnout
- Promotion of wellness

there has been an increasing recognition that moral distress is a significant cause of burnout among healthcare workers. Moral distress and maladaptive coping behaviors have been exacerbated recently, brought out by the COVID-19 pandemic.[28] Exposure to secondary trauma can also have lasting emotional impacts on any staff members who interact with patients and families.

An important question arises regarding whether and with which mechanisms hospitals should provide emotional support to providers who desire and would benefit from it. Hospitals must recognize that a one-size-fits-all approach is suboptimal because different people are likely to feel supported by different actions. Support for mental and emotional well-being through multiple alternative channels is therefore beneficial. Peer support is essential, via both formal and informal means, and should be reinforced by institutional leadership. An example is the Resilience in Stressful Events (RISE) program at Johns Hopkins Hospital, an integrated mental health support program that leverages existing hospital programs, including psychiatry and spiritual care.[29] Similarly, programs geared toward the promotion of wellness have demonstrated success. An advantage of these programs is the empowerment of workers to utilize resources to help themselves, which becomes particularly important in cases where employees are uncomfortable with or choose against seeking help once a problem has arisen.[30]

One area that may serve as a strong pillar of support for patients and clinicians, as well as in promoting an environment of medical professionalism, is a hospital medical ethics body. These bodies can take on many forms and structures and vary in function around the United States and globally.[31] However, clinical ethics services (e.g., consultants and ethics committees) in general serve many vital roles, including offering guidance in cases of moral or ethical dilemmas, protecting the rights and well-being of patients, ensuring that clinical studies are conducted in accordance with ethical standards for human-based research, and training and education of clinical staff.[32] Moreover, these bodies provide support to health personnel concerning individual cases and general.

Medical ethics and professionalism have for many years been closely linked. The seventh edition of the American College of Physicians Ethics Manual notes that practicing medicine professionally rests on the profession's ethical foundations.[33,34] These ethical foundations, which entail the concepts of the patient-physician relationship, autonomy, and consent, must be considered dutifully. To that end, we believe that healthcare organizations are responsible for providing clinical ethics services for patients and employees.

In addition to ethics services, healthcare organizations can promote medical professionalism in several ways. In 2017, Egener et al. produced a charter on professionalism for healthcare organizations, an interdisciplinary effort supported by five organizations, including the American Hospital Association, the Federation of American Hospitals, the Commonwealth Fund, the American Board of Internal Medicine Foundation, and North Shore Long Island Jewish Health System.[35,36] This charter described the values and actions necessary to facilitate a culture of professionalism in the hospital setting.[34] Key domains highlighted by the charter included patient partnerships, organizational culture, community partnerships, and operations and business practices (Table 27.3). Healthcare organizations have a moral responsibility—to patients, to employees, to the community, to society—to develop standards and practices that promote medical professionalism and sustain a culture of professionalism. Indeed, these behaviors serve many important objectives of hospital systems, including the promotion of patient

Table 27.3 Key Domains Highlighted by the Charter on Professionalism for Healthcare Organizations[35]

• Patient partnerships • Organizational culture • Community partnerships • Operations and business practices

safety, the performance of ethical research, a positive work environment for employees, and fair and appropriate education for trainees and other learners.[37]

Ethical and Professional Innovation in Healthcare Organizations

In recent years, the field of medicine has advanced substantially and rapidly from the degree of technological innovation aimed at improving clinical outcomes. One key area of innovation has been in the field of artificial intelligence (AI). Machine learning, deep learning, big data, and natural language processing are examples of AI already in use in clinical practice.[38] Another emerging area of innovation is precision medicine. Precision medicine, catalyzed by the convergence of multiple disciplines, including genetics, metabolomics, imaging, and informatics, has important implications for disease diagnosis, treatment, and prognostication specific to an individual patient.[39] The development and implementation of novel technologies and therapeutics to improve patient care are exciting, often offering new hope for patients with untreatable conditions. However, healthcare innovation can also be problematic, especially if it is not developed using a thoughtful approach. For example, myriad potential ethical (e.g., potential bias, patient autonomy, etc.) and professional (e.g., patient welfare, integrity, sensitivity to diverse patient groups, impact on workflow, etc.) concerns are associated with healthcare innovation, which should be proactively managed whenever possible. To that end, academic medical centers, hospital systems, and healthcare organizations that employ novel treatment and technology or support innovation research (i.e., by providing funding, personnel, and resources) have a responsibility to ensure that implementation and investigation meet standards for appropriate, ethical, and professional use.

To illustrate the point, we consider using AI-based digital technologies to facilitate the collection, storage, and analysis of massive quantities of clinical data. Large data sets (i.e., big data) and machine learning techniques can be utilized to develop algorithms and models that predict a patient's risk of developing a pathologic condition (e.g., cardiovascular risk score). Physicians can use this previously unobtainable information to inform clinical decision-making and make recommendations.[40] Though this may fundamentally improve patient care and delivery, several concerns must be considered, namely, that issues regarding patient privacy, confidentiality, and appropriate use of collected data are present.[41] Additionally, if the data or underlying assumptions on which an algorithm or model was derived were biased or otherwise flawed, the output of that algorithm or model may also be biased. Indeed, algorithmic bias has important implications for healthcare systems, including the potential to negatively impact patient care, exacerbate social inequalities, and yield uninterpretable results.[42,43]

Clinical organizations that investigate and employ emerging therapeutic modalities and technologies in clinical care have an ethical obligation to minimize attendant risks to patients. This includes, for example, a responsibility to protect the fundamental right of patient privacy by ensuring that collected data are protected and confidential. To do so may require adopting validated measures and safeguards to promote data security.[44] In the case of model development, actions that reduce the risk of algorithmic bias ought to be employed. Examples include training algorithm developers and data scientists to recognize potential bias, the use of diverse and underrepresented patient populations in model development, algorithmic transparency and explainability, and careful examination of potential bias after algorithmic development (i.e., before clinical implementation).[42,45]

We expect that as technological innovation continues to increase, so will the list of potential concerns and challenges associated with novel technologies. Healthcare organizations and their employees, particularly the scientists and clinicians researching and implementing emerging technology, must stay vigilant to these possible pitfalls. Hospital systems ought to develop processes that facilitate recognition and, ideally, prevent adverse effects associated with innovation. Additionally, efforts for quality improvement at both the research and clinical stages of development are essential.

Moving forward, ethical innovation will continue to be heavily informed by foundational ethical principles (e.g., the right to privacy). However, applying conventional frameworks of ethical analysis alone may be insufficient in managing novel ethical concerns that may arise.[43] Such problems, which are often first identified empirically, have led to the development of novel strategies of ethical analysis. McCradden et al. recently proposed an ethical framework for the clinical translation of healthcare machine learning.[46] The framework consists of three phases: (1) an exploratory research phase (to obtain and clean the data, develop a model, and train the data); (2) a silent period evaluation (to test the model in a live environment without directly impacting patient care); and (3) a prospective clinical evaluation (to test the model's impact on patient care and outcomes). In an accompanying editorial, Blumenthal-Barby et al. recommended extending this thoughtful framework with the addition of a fourth stage, namely, continual reevaluation of the model over time.[47] Healthcare organizations interested in innovation must be aware of not only the potential unintended consequences of emerging technologies but also how to mitigate these adverse effects. Similar to medicine in general, a fundamental obligation of clinical organizations participating in healthcare innovation is to first, do no harm.

Responsibilities of Healthcare Organizations to Communities

Beyond responsibilities to patients and employees, we believe that healthcare organizations have responsibilities to support efforts within the community that enhance the health of the population broadly. This public health obligation is described in the 2017 Charter on Professionalism for Health Care Organizations.[35,36] Efforts to enhance community health supports organizations' obligation to adhere to the principles of beneficence and justice. By helping to address the root causes of illness in the community, organizations can positively impact the health of both their patients and the entire community while simultaneously reducing disparities. Some define these efforts as professional competencies related to service and fairness.[48]

We know that approximately 10% to 20% of an individual's health is attributable to clinical services and approximately 20% to 30% to genetics. The remaining 50% to 70% of health is attributable to social influencers.[49] The Centers for Disease Control and Prevention identifies five domains that impact social influencers of health: economic stability, education, healthcare access, neighborhoods and built environment, and social and community context.[21] Given the profound impact of these nonmedical and often community-based factors, promoting the health of individuals requires efforts that engage communities. The Charter on Professionalism for Health Care Organizations suggests that this obligation can be met by an organization's commitment to addressing social influencers of health, partnering with communities, advocating for access to high-quality healthcare, and committing to the community through innovative and strategic community investments. These suggestions have been amplified by the National Academies of Sciences, Engineering, and Medicine in a 2019 statement that describes five ways that healthcare organizations can address social influencers of health (Table 27.4).[50,51]

The importance of healthcare organizations' engagement with the community to advance population health and address social influencers of health has been further emphasized by delivery and payment reform initiatives implemented within organizations such as Medicaid. While it is generally prohibited to use federal Medicaid funds to support costs of nonmedical services, states can design programs, benefits, and services that seek to improve population health using nonmedically based strategies.[52] For example in a January 7, 2021, letter describing opportunities in Medicaid and Children's Health Insurance Program (CHIP) to address social influencers of health, the Centers for Medicare and Medicaid Services noted that states can use Medicaid for housing-related services, nonmedical transportation, home-delivered meals, educational services, employment, community integration and social supports, and case management.[53] Such programs not only offer a pathway for healthcare organizations to fulfill their obligations to the community, they also underscore that any organization seeking to advance the health of individuals and populations has an obligation to engage in such work.

Responsibilities of Organizations to Other Organizations

Part of an organization's responsibility to the community extends to their responsibilities to other healthcare organizations within their immediate and extended community.

Table 27.4 Opportunities for Healthcare Organizations to Address Social Influencers of Health

Awareness	Increase awareness about social risks and community assets that impact health
Adjust	Adjust care delivery to meet the specific needs of the community
Assist	Help patients with social needs access existing community resources that support their health
Align	Align organizational assets with community assets to produce synergy
Advocate	Leverage political, social, and economic influence to advocate for community-based improvements that impact health

This may seem somewhat counterintuitive during times when even not-for-profit healthcare organizations are vying for patients to remain economically competitive. But in the same way individual clinicians have an obligation to support public health through their practice and advocacy, so do organizations have an obligation to support public health through their engagement with other organizations. Resource scarcities particularly highlight the importance of interreliance among organizations and the ethical obligation for organizations to be good stewards of all resources.

The United States Food and Drug Administration 2021 report to congress about drug shortages noted that shortages continue to pose a challenge to public health.[54] During times of scarcity, whether of medications, technology, or even space, organizations have an ethical obligation to collaborate with one another to ensure fair distribution within the community (i.e., justice). This can occur at the level of single patients. For example, one hospital may share a cancer medication with another hospital so the second hospital can provide life-saving therapies in a timely manner, a practice that exists today. Sharing of scarce resources became a particularly relevant issue during the COVID-19 pandemic. At the onset of the COVID-19 pandemic, some organizations, such as pediatric hospitals, were overstaffed and overresourced, while other organizations, such as those with adult intensive care units, struggled to find equipment like ventilators or dialysis machines, and clinicians had to work extended hours to address the massive influx of patients. In such circumstances, many have argued that organizations have ethical obligations to work together for the sake of the public good.[55] We agree with that contention.

References

1. Larson MS. *The Rise of Professionalism: Monopolies of Competence and Sheltered Markets.* Routledge; 2017.
2. Airaksinen T. Professional ethics. In: Chadwick R, ed. *Encyclopedia of Applied Ethics.* 2nd ed. Elsevier Scientific Publishing; 2012:612–623. https://doi.org/10.1016/B978-0-12-373932-2.00080-6
3. May WF. The virtues in a professional setting. *Annu Soc Christ Ethics.* 1984;4:71–91.
4. Davis M. What can we learn by looking for the first code of professional ethics? *Theor Med Bioeth.* 2003;24(5):433–454. doi:10.1023/b:meta.0000006831.28435.38
5. Code of medical ethics overview. American Medical Association. Accessed July 20, 2022. https://www.ama-assn.org/delivering-care/ethics/code-medical-ethics-overview
6. McCullough L, Coverdate J, Chervenak F. *Professional Ethics in Obstetrics and Gynecology.* Cambridge University Press; 2019.
7. Beauchamp TL, Childress JF. *Principles of Biomedical Ethics.* Oxford University Press; 2019.
8. Adams J, Schmidt T, Sanders A, Larkin GL, Knopp R. Professionalism in emergency medicine. SAEM Ethics Committee. Society for Academic Emergency Medicine. *Acad Emerg Med.* 1998;5(12):1193–1199. doi:10.1111/j.1553-2712.1998.tb02695.x
9. Olson LL, Stokes F. The ANA code of ethics for nurses with interpretive statements: resource for nursing regulation. *J Nurs Regul.* 2016;7(2):9–20.
10. ACHE code of ethics. American College of Healthcare Executives. Accessed July 20, 2022. https://www.ache.org/about-ache/our-story/our-commitments/ethics/ache-code-of-ethics

11. Gibson JL. Organizational ethics and the management of health care organizations. *Healthc Manage Forum.* 2007;20(1):32–34, 38–41. doi:10.1016/S0840-4704(10)60257-8
12. Bishop LJ, Cherry MN, Darragh M. Organizational ethics and health care: expanding bioethics to the institutional arena. *Kennedy Inst Ethics J.* 1999;9(2):189–208. doi:10.1353/ken.1999.0009
13. Schyve PM. Patient rights and organization ethics: the Joint Commission perspective. *Bioethics Forum.* 1996;12(2):13–20.
14. Martinez C, Skeet AG, Sasia PM. Managing organizational ethics: how ethics becomes pervasive within organizations. *Bus Horiz.* 2021;64(1):83–92. doi:https://doi.org/10.1016/j.bushor.2020.09.008
15. Sims RR. The institutionalization of organizational ethics. *J Bus Ethics.* 1991;10(7):493–506.
16. Health information privacy beyond HIPAA: a 2018 environmental scan of major trends and challenges. National Committee on Vital and Health Statistics. Accessed January 11, 2022. https://ncvhs.hhs.gov/wp-content/uploads/2018/05/NCVHS-Beyond-HIPAA_Report-Final-02-08-18.pdf
17. Moffett P, Moore G. The standard of care: legal history and definitions: the bad and good news. *West J Emerg Med.* 2011;12(1):109–112.
18. Spatz ES, Krumholz HM, Moulton BW. The new era of informed consent: getting to a reasonable-patient standard through shared decision making. *JAMA.* 2016;315(19):2063–2064. doi:10.1001/jama.2016.3070
19. Gudiksen KL, Montague Ad, King JS. Mitigating the price impacts of health care provider consolidation. Milbank Memorial Fund. September 2021. https://www.milbank.org/wp-content/uploads/2021/09/Mitigating-the-Price-Impacts-of-Health-Care-Provider-Consolidation_2. pdf. Accessed June 11, 2024.
20. Xu T, Wu AW, Makary MA. The potential hazards of hospital consolidation: implications for quality, access, and price. *JAMA.* 2015;314(13):1337–1338. doi:10.1001/jama.2015.7492
21. Social determinants of health. World Health Organization. Accessed July 14, 2022. https://www.who.int/health-topics/social-determinants-of-health#tab=tab_1
22. Tenn S, Vandergrift S. Geographic market definition in urban hospital mergers: lessons from the Advocate-NorthShore litigation. *Antitrust Source.* 2017;17(3):1–10.
23. Oldale A, Schrag J, Taylor C. The 2010 horizontal merger guidelines at ten: a view from the FTC's Bureau of Economics. *Rev Indust Org.* 2021;58(1):33–50.
24. Hall MA, McCue MJ. How the ACA's medical loss ratio rule protects consumers and insurers against ongoing uncertainty. Commonwealth Fund. July 2, 2019. Accessed August 8, 2022. https://www.commonwealthfund.org/publications/issue-briefs/2019/jul/how-aca-medical-loss-ratio-rule-protects-consumers-insurers#:~:text=The%20rule%20protects%20consumers%20by,a%20three%2Dyear%20rolling%20average
25. Nelson WA, Taylor E, Walsh T. Building an ethical organizational culture. *Health Care Manag (Frederick).* 2020;39(4):168–174. doi:10.1097/HCM.0000000000000304
26. Obligations to protect health care professionals. American Medical Association. Accessed June 10, 2022. https://www.ama-assn.org/delivering-care/ethics/obligations-protect-health-care-professionals
27. Bagley CE. *Managers and the Legal Environment.* 9th ed. Cengage Learning; 2018.
28. Wilson CA, Metwally H, Heavner S, Kennedy AB, Britt TW. Chronicling moral distress among healthcare providers during the COVID-19 pandemic: a longitudinal analysis of mental health strain, burnout, and maladaptive coping behaviours. *Int J Ment Health Nurs.* 2022;31(1):111–127. doi:10.1111/inm.12942

29. Edrees H, Connors C, Paine L, Norvell M, Taylor H, Wu AW. Implementing the RISE second victim support programme at the Johns Hopkins Hospital: a case study. *BMJ Open.* 2016;6(9):e011708. doi:10.1136/bmjopen-2016-011708

30. Wu AW, Buckle P, Haut ER, et al. Supporting the well-being of health care providers during the COVID-19 pandemic: the CopeColumbia response. *Gen Hosp Psychiatry.* 2020;67:62–69. doi:https://doi.org/10.1177/2516043520931971

31. Slowther A, Bunch C, Woolnough B, Hope T. Clinical ethics support services in the UK: an investigation of the current provision of ethics support to health professionals in the UK. *J Med Ethics.* 2001;27(suppl 1):i2–i8. doi:10.1136/jme.27.suppl_1.i2

32. Rasoal D, Skovdahl K, Gifford M, Kihlgren A. Clinical ethics support for healthcare personnel: an integrative literature review. *HEC Forum.* 2017;29(4):313–346. doi:10.1007/s10730-017-9325-4

33. Sulmasy LS, Bledsoe TA, Acp Ethics P, Human Rights C. American College of Physicians Ethics Manual: Seventh Edition (Spanish version). *Ann Intern Med.* 2019;170(12 suppl 2):S1–S32. doi:10.7326/IsTranslatedFrom_M18-2160_Spanish

34. Doukas DJ, Kirch DG, Brigham TP, et al. Transforming educational accountability in medical ethics and humanities education toward professionalism. *Acad Med.* 2015;90(6):738–743.

35. Egener BE, Mason DJ, McDonald WJ, et al. The Charter on Professionalism for Health Care Organizations. *Acad Med.* 2017;92(8):1091–1099. doi:10.1097/ACM.0000000000001561

36. Andresen ML, Mason DJ. A new charter on professionalism and health care organizations. *Am J Nurs.* 2017;117(9):11. doi:10.1097/01.NAJ.0000524522.42427.09

37. Warnock GL. Reflecting on principles of professionalism. *Can J Surg.* 2008;51(2):84–87.

38. Jarvis T, Thornburg D, Rebecca AM, Teven CM. Artificial intelligence in plastic surgery: current applications, future directions, and ethical implications. *Plast Reconstr Surg Glob Open.* 2020;8(10):e3200. doi:10.1097/GOX.0000000000003200

39. Jameson JL, Longo DL. Precision medicine—personalized, problematic, and promising. *N Engl J Med.* 2015;372(23):2229–2234. doi:10.1056/NEJMsb1503104

40. Beam AL, Kohane IS. Big data and machine learning in health care. *JAMA.* 2018;319(13):1317–1318. doi:10.1001/jama.2017.18391

41. Pyrrho M, Cambraia L, de Vasconcelos VF. Privacy and health practices in the digital age. *Am J Bioeth.* 2022;22(7):50–59. doi:10.1080/15265161.2022.2040648

42. Panch T, Mattie H, Atun R. Artificial intelligence and algorithmic bias: implications for health systems. *J Glob Health.* 2019;9(2):010318. doi:10.7189/jogh.09.020318

43. Smit JR, Mostert M, van Delden JJM. Protecting privacy while optimizing the use of (health)data: the importance of measures and safeguards. *Am J Bioeth.* 2022;22(7):79–81. doi:10.1080/15265161.2022.2075973

44. Spector-Bagdady K, Rahimzadeh V, Jaffe K, Moreno J. Promoting ethical deployment of artificial intelligence and machine learning in healthcare. *Am J Bioeth.* 2022;22(5):4–7. doi:10.1080/15265161.2022.2059206

45. Wachter S, Mittelstadt B, Russell C. Counterfactual explanations without opening the black box: automated decisions and the GDPR. *Harv J Law Technol.* 2018;31(2):841–887.

46. McCradden MD, Anderson JA, Stephenson EA, et al. A research ethics framework for the clinical translation of healthcare machine learning. *Am J Bioeth.* 2022;22(5):8–22. doi:10.1080/15265161.2021.2013977

47. Blumenthal-Barby J, Lang B, Dorfman N, Kaplan H, Hooper WB, Kostick-Quenet K. Research on the clinical translation of health care machine learning: ethicists experiences on lessons learned. *Am J Bioeth.* 2022;22(5):1–3. doi:10.1080/15265161.2022.2059199

48. Egener B, McDonald W, Rosof B, Gullen D. Perspective: organizational professionalism: relevant competencies and behaviors. *Acad Med.* 2012;87(5):668–674. doi:10.1097/ACM.0b013e31824d4b67

49. McGovern L, Miller G, Hughes-Cromwick P. Health policy brief: the relative contribution of multiple determinants to health outcomes. *Health Affairs.* August 21, 2014. Accessed July 13, 2022, https://www.healthaffairs.org/do/10.1377/hpb20140821.404487/full/healthpolicybrief_123.pdf

50. Committee on Integrating Social Needs Care into the Delivery of Health Care to Improve the Nation's Health. *Integrating Social Care into the Delivery of Health Care: Moving Upstream to Improve the Nation's Health.* National Academies Press; 2019 .

51. Cheney C. 5 ways healthcare organizations can address social determinants of health. Healthleaders. Accessed July 14, 2022. https://www.healthleadersmedia.com/clinical-care/5-ways-healthcare-organizations-can-address-social-determinants-health

52. Hinton E, Stolyar L. Medicaid authorities and options to address social determinants of health (SDOH). Kaiser Family Foundation. Accessed July 14, 2022. https://www.kff.org/medicaid/issue-brief/medicaid-authorities-and-options-to-address-social-determinants-of-health-sdoh/

53. Opportunities in Medicaid and CHIP to address social determinants of health (SDOH). Centers for Medicare and Medicaid Services. Accessed July 14, 2022. https://www.medicaid.gov/federal-policy-guidance/downloads/sho21001.pdf

54. Report to Congress drug shortages for calendar year 2021. US Food and Drug Administration. Accessed July 14, 2022. https://www.fda.gov/media/159302/download

55. Paquette ET, Derrington S, Fry JT, et al. Shifting duties of children's hospitals during the COVID-19 pandemic. *J Hosp Med.* 2020;15(10):631–633. doi:10.12788/jhm.3490

28
Professionalism and Employment Issues

Thomas D. Harter

Key Points

- Professions are demarcated from other types of employment by virtue of the level of expertise required to practice in a field, the monopoly professionals have over the right to practice, that the work itself intends to serve a public good, and that professions are permitted to self-regulate.
- All physicians are employees of some sort, even those who are self-employed. Physicians are unique among all professions given their effect on the human experience.
- Physician obligations to employers involve commitments that overlap with their obligations to patients and are based on what they are expected to provide in their role as an employee, including competence, collegiality, a broad scope of care, and a commitment to fairness and justice in the provision of care.
- Healthcare employers (HCEs) have commitments to physicians that also overlap with patient care obligations. At a minimum, they owe physicians safe working spaces (including proper equipment and staffing), sound financial stewardship to ensure they can remain stalwarts within the communities they serve, and investment in the well-being of physicians.
- The growing demand for physicians is outpacing supply. Many physicians have turned to locums' practices rather than commit themselves to a single employer. HCEs have also begun to increase their utilization of advanced practice clinicians toward meeting healthcare demands. Both pose threats to professionalism and physician employment.

Physicians as Employees

One of the areas of medical professionalism that is underexplored is physician employment and the challenges that can arise from being both independent practitioners *and* employees. Most of the literature on medical professionalism focuses on the independent practices of physicians and what it means—or should mean—to be a medical professional at the interface of patient care. Explorations of this sort consider things such as assessing and maintaining proficiencies, how to navigate the transition from being a student to an independently practicing physician, how physicians should integrate and interact within the societies in which they practice, or what it means for physicians to be patient care advocates.

What are largely missing from this literature are assessments of medical professionalism in terms of employment. All working physicians are employees, whether they are self-employed or members of a group practice or clinic, hospital, health system, or some other entity that provides patient care. This chapter focuses on the concept of medical professionalism in terms of physicians as employees, not as physicians qua physicians.

There are three specific aims of this chapter. First, it explores what it means to be an employee and why physicians are unique professionals and thus constitute a different kind of employee. It then addresses what physicians and their employers owe—or should owe—one another in terms of their employment relationships. From there, the chapter identifies the core concepts and values that support the obligatory commitments that physicians and their employers owe one another. Last, the chapter addresses two specific employment issues that physicians currently face that stretch and challenge their medical professionalism and physician employment: locum work and the growing use of advance practice clinicians.

Employment and Physicians

A full exploration of the ties between human activity, work, employment, and compensation is far beyond the scope of this chapter. However, in terms of understanding medical professionalism regarding physician employment, some philosophical context is necessary. Humans are unique from other animals in that not only they are contemplative and can create meaning and value about their lives, but also they can act in ways that are reflective and demonstrative of those values. Work and labor are distinct forms of human activity that attempt to produce goods and services that help sustain, as well as enhance the quality of, our individual lives and the lives of others.[1,2]

Work that is considered valuable (i.e., the work produces goods or services toward bettering the lives of others) is also compensated in some way. Ancient human civilizations often used bartering systems to provide food or shelter for work. In the modern world, work is compensated primarily through monetary currency.[3] During the Commercial Revolution, compensation changed to allow for payment in the production of goods or for periods of time people spent working.[3] Those who work and are compensated are thus considered employees. Two other essential features of being an employee—and what truly distinguishes employment from slavery—is that persons who work as employees freely enter and exit from their work; they are not themselves property—they retain their autonomy and can choose for themselves whether and when they wish to work.

Of course, not all employment is thought of or treated the same by society. Specifically, professions are considered a category of employment different from all other types of jobs or occupations. This is because of four basic attributes that are applied to professions that are not wholly applied to other types of job or occupations. These attributes are expertise, monopoly, public interest, and self-regulation.

> Expertise is special knowledge of a theoretic, academic nature. One distinguishing feature of the expertise is that it requires the exercise of professional judgment, not just the application of technical rules. The monopoly status is usually a license

> granted by the state that restricts practice of the expertise to licensees. The public interest is essentially a promise made by the profession to society that its members will benefit, not harm, society. The promise to act in the public interest is at the heart of every profession and is typically codified in their code of ethics. Codes of ethics, therefore, serve to identify how members of a particular profession must conduct themselves if the public interest is to be preserved. Self-regulation is a privilege granted to a profession to regulate its members. The profession, therefore, has a duty to self-regulate.[4(p146)]

While all jobs or occupations require some education or training to develop and utilize job-related skills, may serve the public interest in some way, or even require some forms of certification or licensure, only professional employment requires all these attributes of individual members. Perhaps the most important aspect that distinguishes professional employment from other nonprofessional occupations is the need to make value judgments that extend beyond the mere application of one's training.

Why Physicians Are Unique Employees

Medicine is just one of many professions. However, being a physician is commonly considered a unique type of profession that stands apart from all others.[5] Many chapters in this textbook tap into the whys and hows of the medical profession and medical professionalism across the continuum of physician training and practice. But saying that the medical profession is important and unpacking and elucidating the many issues regarding medical professionalism does not fully tell us why being a physician is, itself, a unique type of profession.

While it may be tempting to say that the social contract between physicians and society or the specialness of patient-physician relationships is sufficient to explain why the medical profession constitutes unique employment, this is not the case. All professions are relationship based and have nuanced expectations for how members of that profession should act in their professional roles among clients and society in general. However, if we turn to humanities literature, we begin to understand why being a physician is different from nearly all other kinds of professions.

Kalanithi, in particular, helps us appreciate the distinction I make here between the medical profession and all others. In *When Breath Becomes Air*, Kalanithi reflects on his decision to become a neurosurgeon by recalling a conversation between one of his mentors and the parents of a child about to undergo neurosurgery. He muses: "As I sat there, I realized that the questions intersecting life, death, and meaning, questions that *all* people face at some point, usually arise in a medical context. In the actual situations where one encounters these questions, it becomes a necessarily philosophical and biological exercise" (emphasis mine).[6]

Simply, there is no other profession that affects the lived human experience in the same way as being a physician. To be a physician requires more than expertise in biological human processes and professional judgment in the application of technical training. To be a physician also requires helping individuals navigate inherently value-laden questions about the impacts of medical care on one's quality and quantity of life. No other profession requires that level of understanding, commitment, and care among its members. When a physician errs or acts in ways unbecoming of the profession, trust in that physician—and the medical profession in general—can be threatened and negatively affect the health and well-being of individuals and communities. This same threat does not exist with any other profession. I might get upset with my lawyer or accountant if I think their work has resulted in me being treated unfairly, but their professional actions do not potentially affect the very nature of my existence in ways physicians can and do through the practice of medicine.

Given this idea about physicians constituting a unique profession different from others, it follows that they are unique types of employees. As noted by Doukas and Fins, the basis of medical professionalism is rooted in antiquity, in which being a physician involves being committed to the primacy of patient welfare.[7] Physicians are expected to balance their personal needs and the needs of their employers against the needs of their patients. When these needs conflict with one another, the guiding question is not "What is in the best interest of the physician or employer?" but rather "What is in the best interest of the patient?"

What Physicians and Employers Owe One Another

Physicians and their healthcare employers (HCEs) have an interdependent relationship. Obviously HCEs could not exist without physicians to care for patients, but physicians also rely on HCEs since HCEs provide resources—such as equipment, medicines, physical space, and staff—necessary for physicians to function as patient care providers. The interdependence of the relationship between physicians and HCEs results in both having unique obligations to one another that are tied to and motivated by, yet different from, the obligations of physicians toward their professional development and patient care (Table 28.1).

What Physicians Owe HCEs

Professionalism development sets the foundation for understanding and thinking about what physicians owe HCEs. HCEs exist to meet the medical needs of the communities in which—and for which—they operate. As such, HCEs are extensions of the services and care provided by physicians. It makes sense, therefore, to imagine that physicians, as employees of HCEs, owe HCEs a commitment to provide care in alignment with the tenets of medical professionalism, in terms of both professional identity formation and the practice of medicine.

Levinson et al. have established a framework for thinking about what aspects of medical professionalism translate in physician obligations to employers, the medical professional itself, and the patients for which they serve.[8] Rather than unpack and elucidate professionalism solely in terms of values or commitments, this framework takes the additional step of conceptualizing professionalism in terms of specific behaviors. For example, in thinking about the professional obligation to provide patient-centered care at the individual level, Levinson et al. highlight the need of physicians to learn how to communicate empathetically and compassionately toward building rapport with patients and families and learning to work collaboratively with other care team members to maximize the care team's effectiveness. In thinking about patient-centered care at the

Table 28.1 Commitments and Obligations That Physicians Owe to Their Employers and That Employers Owe to Physicians

Physician Commitments to Healthcare Employers (HCEs)	**HCE Commitments to Physicians**
Competence: Physicians are obliged to dutifully meet and maintain all necessary institutional, state, federal licensing and credentialing certifications.	*Safe Work Environments*: HCEs owe physicians workspaces and resources that allow them to practice medicine according to medical standards of care.
Collegiality: Physicians should dutifully maintain good working relationships with colleagues and other professional staff toward providing high-level patient care.	*Resource Stewardship*: HCEs owe physicians (and the communities they serve) sound financial planning and execution that allow HCEs to remain economically viable and solvent.
Care: To patients: Physicians are obligated to provide care consistent with the Physician Charter and in accord with applicable ethical codes of conduct. To colleagues: Physicians should consider the impact of personal decisions on colleagues, such as transferring a patient or changes to their practice availability. To oneself: Physicians are obligated to care for themselves to avoid existential distress and workplace exhaustion.	*Investment in Physician Well-being*: HCEs owe physicians: - Fair compensation relative to the services provided, size of the organization, and geographic location of the HCE. - Compensated and protected opportunities for continuing medical education. - Protected time to engage in personal development outside of work. - Mechanisms for addressing moral or existential distress. - Organizational or legal support in the event a lawsuit from a patient or patient family.
Fairness and Justice: Physicians are obligated to be good resource stewards and not subject their patients or employers to medically unsupported treatment decisions that potentially expose patients to unnecessary harms and contribute to medical waste and other unnecessary expenditures.	

organizational level, Levinson et al. highlight the need of physicians to help develop institutional policies regarding things such as timely access to care or compensation that supports clinician time with patients.[8]

What this means is that, at the most basic level of employment, physicians owe their employers some development of professionalism behaviors or—at the least—a commitment to the continued cultivation of those behaviors. However, the development and cultivation of oneself in terms of medical professionalism does not cover the full breadth of obligations physicians owe HCEs. Given that physicians are expected to use their training in practice—although, of course, there is no strict societal obligation that demands medical doctors practice medicine on completion of their training—there are other basic, subsequent obligations that physicians own HCEs, some of which are directed by practice standards, law, and other licensure obligations. For example, physicians as employees are expected to report to their scheduled shifts prepared to care for their designated patients in both hospital and clinical environments, as well as practice only within the scope of their training and refer patients to other medical experts as indicated.

Levinson et al. also highlight the importance of physicians being advocates for their patients in terms of justice and the provision of equitable care. In alignment with this aspect of professionalism development, there emerges a concurrent obligation of physicians to their HCEs to be good financial stewards; to refrain from providing nonessential medical care and focus on reduction of financial waste by identifying practice variations that result in subjecting patients to unnecessary tests or procedures, developing and following medically sound organizational practice standards, as well as avoid making solitary or rogue resource decisions.[8,9]

In gross sum, there are at least four basic commitments physicians owe their employers: competence; collegiality; care (to patients, colleagues, and oneself); and fairness and justice. Each of these commitments clearly has roots in professionalism development and is the basis of subsequent obligatory behaviors. Whether there are other commitments physicians owe their employers is taken up further in the chapter.

What HCEs Owe Physicians

Just as physicians are unique types of employees, so are HCEs unique types of employers. In thinking about healthcare organizations, these often are major employers in their communities and often contribute directly or indirectly to a community tax base, enabling other social services to be funded. In rural areas, smaller healthcare organizations or hospitals may be the only access point for persons to receive healthcare.[9] Additionally, like physicians, healthcare organizations—which are commonly led by physicians—operate within the historical social contract between society and healthcare, leading them to have many of the same obligations physicians do toward the patients and communities they serve. In this same way, smaller HCEs—those characterized here as group practices' or self-employed physicians—share the same obligations to benefit and care for the patients and communities they serve.

One way to understand the unique difference between HCEs and other types of employers is to consider what happens when the business closes. Most businesses literally stop operating for periods of time throughout a 24-hour period, and while their closure might be an inconvenience for patrons, it generally is not detrimental to their overall health or well-being. Likewise, if those businesses permanently close, there can be negative effects on the local economy and the employees who lose their jobs and negative impacts on the people who frequented that business, but there is no underlying social contract or covenant that is violated by their closure. However, the temporary or permanent closure of an HCE is potentially devastating to the health of the community. HCEs—notably hospitals—must always remain open to ensure access to emergency-level care.[9,10]

That HCEs have patient-directed obligations, there are duties imposed on them that affect physician practices and that overlap with what they specifically owe physicians as their employers. HCEs, for example, have a duty to function in economically sustainable ways to ensure they remain open and treat those needing care and avoid making solitary or rogue resource allocation decisions so that they can remain solvent. They also have a duty to ensure the safety of patients and staff alike while working with patients and physicians to equitably serve as many patients as possible. Regarding both these points,

HCEs have a duty to create policies and practice standards that are medically sound, culturally competent, and contextually relevant to their patient and staff populations.[9]

Given this overarching understanding of the role of HCEs in the provision of healthcare within communities and their subsequent obligations to patients that overlap with physician obligations as employees, what emerges are several obligations and commitments that HCEs owe specifically to physicians. These include:

Safe work environments: HCEs owe physicians resources that allow them to practice medicine according to the standards of care physicians are expected to provide to their patients. This includes adequate space, equipment, and staff.

Sound stewardship of resources: HCEs owe physicians (although not exclusively, as this obligation overlaps with HCEs' obligations to the communities they serve) financial plans that allow the HCEs to remain economically viable and solvent. This includes making sound financial investments and purchasing decisions toward fulfilling their duty to have the resources needed for physicians in their practices.[11]

Investment in physician well-being: The work in lifestyle medicine, moral distress, and moral resilience all lead to the important understanding that physicians must take care of themselves and have their personal needs met for them to fulfill their patient-directed obligations. HCEs thus owe a commitment to the well-being and growth of physicians as both professionals and individuals. This includes ensuring physicians are fairly compensated for their work; that they have the financial resources necessary for continuing medical education, as well as blocked time for them to engage in those educational endeavors; that physicians have enough free time to cultivate their personal interests toward becoming morally resilient individuals; and that HCEs provide some mechanism for supporting physicians who are experiencing moral distress or potentially lapses in professionalism, particularly when those physicians may be practicing in ways that are noticeably placing patients in harm's way, including offers of legal support for when patients sue physicians.[12–17]

Bidirectional Guiding Values

Given these commitments of physicians to HCEs and HCEs to physicians, what principles ground them?

Fairness and Justice

The concepts of fairness and justice are interesting here because of how they typically are treated in medical ethics and professionalism literature specifically as applying to patient care. Additionally, I noted fairness and justice as a commitment that physicians owe HCEs. However, both concepts can be guiding values that specifically apply to the employment relationship that exists between physicians and HCEs. With employers, fairness and justice are values that can guide decisions that affect physicians as employees differently from how they commonly are applied to patient care. For example, the values of fairness and justice might help guide employment decisions about compensation, benefits packages, or hiring to minimize the impacts of implicit or explicit bias. With physicians as employees, justice and fairness are values that might guide employee decisions about their service availability or negotiations about benefits and compensation, retirement plans, or other reasons for possibly leaving an employer.

Honesty and Transparency

The commitments of physicians to HCEs and HCEs to physicians are also grounded by the values of honesty and transparency. At a minimum, for physicians to meet their commitments to HCEs, they must be forthright and honest about their skills and potential deficiencies, as well as known employment issues that potentially negatively affect their HCE (e.g., new conflicts with other employees or threats of legal action to a physician by a patient). There is an open question here about how honest and transparent physicians should be with employers that is rooted in business ethics literature, which is not taken up in this chapter but might also apply to otherwise private information about the physician that could affect their patient care, such as, for example, disclosure of conscientious objections to certain treatments.[18]

Likewise, HCEs should be honest and transparent with physicians about any number of decisions that could affect physicians' abilities to practice medicine and provide patient care. For example, during the early stages of the COVID-19 pandemic, in order for HCEs to meet their commitments to physicians, it was argued that HCEs should have open conversations with physicians about the current financial state of the organization in order to create realistic expectations for physicians about their financial stressors toward creating plans to effectively manage reductions in available resources.[9,19]

Voice and Respect for Persons

Perhaps the ultimate binding pair of values that drive the commitments of physicians to HCEs and HCEs to physicians are voice and respect for persons. Even if one were to argue that HCEs—and other organizations—do not qualify as unique persons worthy of respect, the fact remains that HCEs themselves are led by individuals. What marks the difference between flourishing and nonflourishing employment relationships is the ability for employees and employers to respect one another and hear the relevant concerns of the other toward identifying and creating viable and sustainable solutions to those problems that aim to help patients.[16,20–22]

The concept of voice is unique here. HCEs typically have no issue with voicing organizational perspectives, changes, or decisions on their employees. However, in order for physicians to meet their commitments to HCEs as employees, HCEs should be intentional about creating a culture and opportunities to hear the voice of physicians.[9] Since physicians are the primary providers of patient care through their expertise and licensure, the failure to hear physician voice in organizational decision-making jeopardizes HCEs' abilities to meet obligations to patients and the communities they serve.

Loyalty

Physicians and HCEs have ethical and professional obligations to patients and the communities they serve. Given this, it is perhaps tempting to think that loyalty is a commitment physicians and HCEs owe one another. However, this is not the case. Physicians have no obligation to be loyal to their HCEs. If they did, they never would leave an employer when they are dissatisfied or a better job offer comes along. Likewise, an HCE has no obligation to keep a physician as an employee if that physician violates the HCE's work expectations. Likewise, as we see in the literature on whistleblowing, the concept of loyalty—or disloyalty—can be used to harm an employee who publicly discloses information about potentially unethical practices by their employer.[23]

However, despite not rising to the level of a commitment physicians and HCEs owe one another, the concept of loyalty still can be seen as an important value that helps ground the ability of physicians and HCEs to fulfill their other commitments to one another. Loyalty can engender a feeling of security and trust, which in turn can give individuals—whether employees or employers—the opportunity to meet or address gaps in their commitments to one another without triggering a worry or fear of retaliation. This is especially vital for physicians who are expected to constantly make value-laden treatment decisions that almost always carry some risk of potential negative outcome for patients.[24]

Specific Employment Issues

It would be remiss and naïve to write a chapter on physicians as employees through the lens of medical professionalism without addressing the elephant in the room: the growing demand for physicians far outpacing supply and the subsequent impacts on physician employment. As noted in a 2021 report by the Association of American Medical Colleges (AAMC), the United States alone is facing an unsustainable situation by which the US population is expected to grow from approximately 328 million persons to 363 million between 2019 and 2034, with approximately 42.5% of that number over retirement age, which is concurrent with the number of physicians expected to reach retirement age by 2034.[25] Per the AAMC report, the estimated shortfall in physicians to meet the growing US population between by 2034 will be about 38,000–124,000.[25] Despite remaining one of the most highly compensated professions,[26] the demands on physicians—such as workloads, bureaucratic regulations and time spent on required documentation of patient care, and liability concerns—diminish the impact of compensation on the desire to enter the medical profession.[27,28] There are two notable consequences of this predicted shortfall that challenge the commitments of physicians as employees to HCEs.

Locum Tenens

The COVID-19 pandemic appears to have accelerated the exodus of physicians from full-time employment. According to a 2022 survey conducted by AMN Healthcare of healthcare executives across the United States, 88% of respondents ($n = 202$) used locums at some point in the prior 12 months to address staff shortages, with anesthesiologists and hospitalists being the most utilized.[29] A locum tenens is a physician working temporarily in another practice who, because of their temporary status, is not offered or entitled to the benefits and organizational protections offered to full staff members.

For our purposes here, the central question is do—or should—locums have the same commitments or expectations of other physicians to HCEs? In short, the answer is yes. Locums, although not full employees of an HCE, are still employees of some sort whether they are self-employed or employed (or represent) some organization that staffs physician locums. When we look at the four employment commitments of physicians as employees—competence, collegiality, care, and fairness and justice—there is nothing about being a locum that excuses them from these commitments. Even if one were to question locums being obliged to collegiality, it does not change the fact that locums as physicians are still expected to follow the same standards of medical professionalism as other full physician employees. That is, locums should still act in ways befitting of all physicians engaged in patient care.

Utilization of Advanced Practice Clinicians

One way to address the outpacing of demand with supply of physicians is to fill the gap with advanced practice clinicians (APCs). APCs—defined here as those with physician assistant or advanced nursing degrees—are now considered vital in the provision of healthcare.[30,31] While their utilization creates important opportunities for HCEs to meet patient care demands, their growing employment also creates some potential threats for physicians in ways that challenge their professionalism and commitments to HCEs.

Two primary concerns for physicians with the increased use of APCs are their (1) scope of training and (2) scope of practice. Regarding scope of training, APC degree programs simply require far less education, training, and clinical practice exposure than physician degree program.[31] Regarding scope of practice, there are ongoing moves by professional organizations and legislative bodies to increase the professional rights and responsibilities of APCs toward becoming independent practitioners.[32] In 2019, for example, Wisconsin passed Act 90, permitting APCs to make clinical determinations of treatment decision-making capacity for patients, a new legislative privilege previously reserved only for physicians or licensed psychologists.[33] One reason Act 90 is potentially concerning in the realm of patient care is that determinations of treatment decision-making capacity are ethically and legally significant, yet often involve clinically relevant nuances that can be difficult to detect even for seasoned physicians or psychologists with specialized training.[33, 34,35]

From an HCE perspective, use of APCs makes sense to cover the growing physician shortage. APC practitioner pathways are presently more abundant than MD pathways, and they are cheaper to recruit and employ.[30] From a physician perspective, though, APCs still require physician oversight, which does not actually help alleviate work stresses, but potentially increases them, especially in cases in which physicians disagree with APC treatment decisions and feel compelled to correct them.

When professionalism conflicts arise between APCs and physicians, there is a question of whose professionalism standards ought to apply. An examination of the similarities and differences between APCs and physicians is beyond the scope of this chapter. However, at a quick glance, it is clear that many of the professionalism and ethical standards guiding APC practices overlap with the professionalism and ethical standards of physicians.[36,37] Still, it remains the case that physicians—as the mostly highly trained and experienced medical providers—are charged with and expected to be fully responsible for any treatment decisions affecting patient care and, ultimately, remain accountable for those decisions regardless of their employment environment. As noted in business ethics literature, when there are questions about what ethical and legal standards ought to apply with international business dealings, the standards that offer the broadest scope of ethical practice and protection of individuals ought to apply.[38] The same reasoning holds in patient care; the professionalism standards of those with the greatest scope of responsibility and authority—that is, physicians—ought to apply in the care of patients.

The commitments of physicians to HCEs and HCEs to physicians outlined in this chapter, as well as the underlying values that guide those commitments, support the idea that physicians and HCEs should attempt to resolve those conflicts in ways that do not jeopardize or compromise patient care. Should physicians find themselves in a position in which they can no longer meet their commitments to HCEs—or, alternatively, find themselves violating their professional and ethical obligations to patients—the commitments and values physicians are expected to follow as employees would then support them changing practices and finding employment elsewhere. A full re-evaluation of the commitments, values, and potential threats to physicians as employees also will be necessary in the event of healthcare reform that changes physician employment structures and practices in the United States.

References

1. Arendt H. *The Human Condition*. 2nd ed. University of Chicago Press; 1998.
2. Koehn D. Ethical issues in human resources. In: Bowie N, ed. *The Blackwell Guide to Business Ethics*. Blackwell Publishers; 2002:225–243.
3. Paycom. From salt to stipends: the history of the salary. Accessed May 8, 2023. https://www.paycom.com/resources/blog/from-salt-to-stipends-the-history-of-the-salary/
4. Armstrong MB. Ethical issues in accounting. In: Bowie N, ed. *The Blackwell Guide to Business Ethics*. Blackwell Publishers; 2002:145–164.
5. Collier R. Professionalism: the historical contract. *CMAJ*. 2012;184(11):1233–1234.
6. Kalanithi P. *When Breath Becomes Air*. Random House; 2016:70.
7. Doukas D, Fins J. The evolution and symbiosis of medical ethics and professionalism. In: Merlo G, Harter TD, eds. *Medical Professionalism: Theory, Education, and Practice*. Oxford University Press; 2024.
8. Levinson W, Ginsburg S, Hafferty FW, et al. A practical approach to "professionalism." In: Levinson W, Ginsburg S, Hafferty FW, et al. *Understanding Medical Professionalism*. McGraw-Hill Education; 2014:1–16.
9. Harter TD, Iltis A, Clay MC, et al. COVID-19 and financial vulnerability: what health care organizations and society owe each other. *Am J Bioeth*. 2020;20(7):139–141.
10. Ozar D, Berg J, Werhane, PH, et al. *Organizational Ethics in Health Care*. American Medical Association; 2000.
11. Repenshek M. Stewardship and organizational ethics. *Health Progress*. 2004;85(3):31–35, 56.
12. Merlo G. *Principles of Medical Professionalism*. Oxford University Press; 2021.
13. Rosenzweig S. Compassion and professional formation. In: Merlo G, Harter TD, eds. *Medical Professionalism: Theory, Education, and Practice*. Oxford University Press; 2024.
14. Schindler B, Novack DH, Cohen DG, et al. The impact of the changing health care environment on the health and well-being of faculty at four medical schools. *Acad Med*. 2006;81(1):27–34.
15. Rorty M, Werhane P, Mills A. The third face of medicine: ethics, business and challenges to professionalism. In: Arnold DG, ed. *Ethics and the Business of Biomedicine*. Cambridge University Press; 2009:198–219.
16. Bowie N. Treating employees with respect. In: Arnold DG, Beauchamp TL, Bowie NE, eds. *Ethical Theory and Business*. 10th ed. Cambridge University Press; 2020:45–48.
17. Gawande A. When good doctors go bad. *New Yorker*. 2000. Accessed May 8, 2023. https://www.newyorker.com/magazine/2000/08/07/when-good-doctors-go-bad
18. Harter TD. Toward accommodating physicians' conscientious objections: an argument for public disclosure. *J Med Ethics*. 2015;41(3):224–228.
19. McGuire A, Aulisio MP, Davis D, et al. Ethical challenges arising in the COVID-19 pandemic: an overview from the Association of Bioethics Program Directors (ABPD) task force. *Am J Bioeth*. 2020;20(7):15–27.
20. Bowie N. *Business Ethics: A Kantian Perspective*. Blackwell Publishers; 1999.
21. Freeman RE. Managing for stakeholders. In: Arnold DG, Beauchamp TL, Bowie NE, eds. *Ethical Theory and Business*. 10th ed. Cambridge University Press; 2020:220–228.

22. Hartman EM. *Organizational Ethics and the Good Life.* Oxford University Press; 1996.
23. Duska R. Whistleblowing and employee loyalty. In: Arnold DG, Beauchamp TL, Bowie NE, eds. *Ethical Theory and Business.* 10th ed. Cambridge University Press; 2020:124–127.
24. Thompson J. *Lead True.* Forbes Books; 2017.
25. Association of American Medical Colleges. AAMC report reinforces mounting physician shortage. Accessed May 8, 2023. https://www.aamc.org/news/press-releases/aamc-report-reinforces-mounting-physician-shortage
26. US News. How much does a physician make. June 11, 2021. Accessed May 8, 2023. https://money.usnews.com/careers/best-jobs/physician/salary
27. Rand Health. Factors affecting physician professional satisfaction and their implications for patient care, health systems, and health policy. October 24, 2018. Accessed May 8, 2023. file:///C:/Users/TDHarter/Downloads/RAND_RR439.pdf
28. Rand Health. Effects of health care payment models on physician practice in the United States. Accessed May 8, 2023. https://www.rand.org/pubs/research_reports/RR2667.html
29. AMN Healthcare. 2022 survey of locum tenens staffing trends. 2022. Accessed May 8, 2023. https://www.amnhealthcare.com/siteassets/amn-insights/surveys/amn-survey-locum-tenens-2022.pdf
30. Martsolf GR, Barnes H, Richards MR, et al. Employment of advanced practice clinicians in physician practices. *JAMA Intern Med.* 2018;178(7):988–990.
31. Chekijian SA, Elia TR, Horton JL, et al. A review of interprofessional variation in education: challenges and considerations in the growth of advanced practice providers in emergency medicine. *AEM Educ Train.* 2020;5(2):e10469. doi:10.1002/aet2.10469
32. American Medical Association. AMA successfully fights scope of practice expansions that threaten patient safety. Accessed May 8, 2023. https://www.ama-assn.org/practice-management/scope-practice/ama-successfully-fights-scope-practice-expansions-threaten
33. A.B. 287, 2019-2020 Legislature, Reg. Sess. (Wis. 2019). February 5, 2020. https://docs.legis.wisconsin.gov/2019/related/acts/90
34. Appelbaum PS. Assessment of patients' competence to consent to treatment. *N Engl J Med.* 2007;357(18):1834–1840.
35. Grisso T. *Evaluating Competencies: Forensic Assessment and Instruments.* 2nd ed. Kluwer Academic; 2003.
36. Cassidy BA, Blessing JD. *Ethics and Professionalism: A Guide for the Physician Assistant.* F. A. Davis Company; 2008.
37. Blair KA. *Advanced Practice Nursing Roles: Core Concepts for Professional Development.* 6th ed. Springer Publishing Company; 2019.
38. Bowie N. Relativism and the moral obligations of multinational corporations. In: Arnold DG, Beauchamp TL, Bowie NE, eds. *Ethical Theory and Business.* 10th ed. Cambridge University Press; 2020:436–439.

29
Supporting the Safe Practice of Physicians as They Age

Thomas H. Gallagher and Andrew A. White

Key Points

- Growing evidence suggests that traditional approaches to medical professionalism are failing to support the safe practice of physicians as they age.
- Increasing physician age is clearly a risk factor for worse patient outcomes. In response, several organizations are adopting late career practitioner (LCP) programs that assess the physical and cognitive well-being of all physicians over a certain age.
- Published literature suggests such programs identify at least 10% of screened physicians as having impairments likely to affect their ability to provide safe patient care.
- More proactive approaches are needed to support physicians in practicing safely across the entirety of their careers.

Introduction

You are on a hospital's credentialing committee and have been asked to evaluate the performance of a colleague who is a prominent surgeon in his mid-70s. The surgeon specializes in a difficult operation and has performed it hundreds of times over his career, making him the most experienced surgeon of his type in the region. However, the hospital's risk manager has grown concerned over a string of unanticipated adverse outcomes and asks you to determine if the surgeon should continue to operate. Although the surgeon asserts his competence, you have noticed the surgeon has a resting tremor and begin to wonder if his dexterity and technical performance have deteriorated with age. The hospital relies on reporting oneself or colleagues with declining skills to identify unsafe physicians, but this mechanism is almost never employed. His colleagues concur that it is time for the surgeon to retire, but value his experience, hesitate to take steps that would anger him, and assume he will recognize his limitations. The department chief adds that the hospital would struggle to recruit a surgeon to replace him.

Few issues highlight the challenges of turning the principles of medical professionalism into practice as dramatically as ensuring the safe practice of physicians as they age. The hallmark of medical professionalism is self-regulation, which involves both setting standards associated with entry into the profession and ensuring the ongoing ability of practitioners to meet these standards over the course of their career.

However, there are good reasons to believe that relying on typical mechanisms for overseeing the safe practice of physicians, such as credentialing, peer review, continuing education, and maintenance of certification, may not be well suited for identifying physicians who are struggling to provide safe patient care as they age.[1] Age is the single biggest risk for cognitive impairment in physicians.[2] Other safety conscious industries such as aviation assess operators' performance more frequently as they age, and several include mandatory retirement ages.[1] Yet medicine has largely ignored accumulating evidence linking physician age to worse patient outcomes and has relied mostly on calls for physicians to monitor their practice and their colleagues' performance more closely as they age, despite evidence that these strategies are likely to be ineffective. Distorted notions of what being a good colleague means, coupled with complex power dynamics and financial pressures, often lead physicians to look the other way when they notice older clinicians struggling to practice effectively. A growing number of organizations are recognizing that applying principles of professionalism requires adopting new approaches to support the safe practice of late career late career practitioners (LCPs).

The Relationship of Physician Age to Safe Practice

The potential for older physicians to have worse patient outcomes is supported by a robust literature detailing the impact of age on physicians' knowledge and on their abilities in technical, cognitive, and physical domains.[3] While no single study establishes a definitive link between older physician age and a particular outcome, cumulatively this literature suggests that the risk that physicians older than age 65 pose to patient safety justifies new approaches to ensuring satisfactory physician performance after this age.

The Demographic of the Physician Workforce Is Changing, With a Significant and Rising Proportion of Physicians Continuing to Practice Late in Their Career

Per the American Medical Association (AMA) Masterfile (an authoritative source on US physician practice patterns), as of July 2021, of physicians in direct patient care 19% were age 65 or older, an increase of over 300% since 1975.[4] In addition, recent economic and policy forces have catalyzed a widespread migration of US physicians from self-employment in smaller physician groups toward employment in large, vertically integrated health systems.[5,6] As the number of employed physicians grows, it provides both new opportunities and responsibilities to rethink how notions of professionalism, peer review, and self-regulation are implemented.

Increasing Physician Age Is an Important Risk Factor for Poor Patient Outcomes

The most important line of evidence regarding the need for programs to assess the competence of physicians more closely as they age is data suggesting that older physicians in both surgical and nonsurgical settings are at increased risk of having worse patient outcomes. This is a complex literature, given that physicians often change the volume and complexity of patients for whom they provide care as they approach the latter stages of their career. Exemplar studies addressing this topic are provided in Table 29.1.

Table 29.1 Exemplar Studies on Relationship Between Physician Age and Patient Outcomes

Physicians Studied	Primary Outcomes	Principle Findings	Notes
275 cardiac surgeons[27]	Patient mortality in 83,547 cardiac surgeries	Increased surgeon age correlated with higher patient mortality ratio	Relationship between surgeon age and mortality remained after multivariate analysis
532 surgeons[28]	Mortality and morbidity in 12,275 carotid endarterectomies	Mortality rate 2–3 times higher for surgeons older than 65	20 years since licensure remained predictor of patient mortality in multivariate analysis, adjusting for surgeon volume and patient characteristics
86 surgeons[29]	Hernia repair outcomes among 1,629 operations	Odds of having a hernia recurrence were higher for surgeons older than age 45	Relationship between surgeon age and outcome present among both experienced and inexperienced surgeons
Surgeons performing 1 of 8 operative procedures in Medicare patients[30]	Operative mortality as identified in Medicare data from 460,000 patients	Surgeons > 60 years had higher mortality rates with pancreatectomy, coronary artery bypass grafting (CABG), and carotid endarterectomy compared with surgeons ages 41–50 years	
206 congenital heart surgeons[31]	Morbidity and mortality in 62,851 congenital heart surgeries	Odds of major morbidity/mortality were ~ 25% higher for operations performed by very senior surgeons (35–55 years from medical school, ~ 60–80 years old)	
59 internal medicine physicians at a New York teaching hospital[32]	In-hospital and 30-day mortality in 6,572 inpatient admissions	Patients cared for by physicians with more than 20 years in practice had 1.7 times higher in-hospital mortality and 1.5 times higher 30-day mortality compared with physicians with 0–5 years in practice.	Increased mortality risk especially pronounced among medically complex admissions
18,854 hospitalists[33]	Mortality among 736,537 Medicare admission	Patients treated by older physicians had higher mortality	Relationship between physician age and outcome not found for older physicians treating high volume of patients

It is important to note that interpreting studies of the relationship between physician age and patient outcomes is complex, especially because many physicians treat fewer and less complex patients toward the latter part of their career. However, the studies in this table included statistical methods to control for patient volume and complexity, and the relationship between increasing physician age and worse patient outcomes persisted.

Studies Linking Physician Age to Factors Associated With Lower Quality Care

Supplementing the above studies is a literature that describes the relationship between physician age and other outcomes associated with lower quality of care. Multiple studies suggest that older physicians are

- *More likely to be the subject of patient complaints.* For example, in their review of over 18,000 complaints against physicians in Australia, Bismark and colleagues found physicians aged 55–65 were 1.43 times as likely to have multiple complaints filed against them by patients compared with colleagues 35 years old or younger.[7]
- *More likely to be disciplined by state medical boards.* Morrison and colleagues found that in California, physicians who had been in practice more than 20 years were twice as likely to be disciplined by the Medical Board of California.[8] In the Canadian province of Ontario, the Peer Assessment Committee of the College of Physicians and Surgeons of Ontario conducted peer assessments of the office practices by reviewing records of 918 physicians.[9] In this study, 35% of physicians older than 75 were found to have grossly deficient records or unsatisfactory level of patient care (or both) compared with 9% of physicians younger than 50.

The literature suggesting an increased risk of poor patient outcomes as physicians age is further supported by multiple studies regarding the impact of physicians' age on performance. Several outstanding review articles have summarized the robust literature on how age affects physicians' physical, cognitive, and psychomotor skills. The most comprehensive review synthesized over 900 published articles to determine the current state of the science as it pertains to factors known to support or inhibit physician performance.[10] Their key findings include the following:

- *"Physical and cognitive performance decline with age*
- *Problems with psychological wellness increase with age*
- *Aging negatively impacts patient outcomes*
- *Younger doctors perform better on knowledge tests/practice assessments*
- *Younger physicians better adhere to guidelines"*

None of these findings likely come as a surprise to practicing physicians, given their experience with the impact of age on their patients' abilities and the challenges of staying up to date as more time elapses since their formal training.

The Inadequacy of Existing Approaches to Professional Self-Regulation to Address the Issue of LCPs

There are some arguments that new strategies for ensuring the safe practice of LCPs might not be as necessary if physicians could accurately identify declining competence in themselves or their colleagues and were willing to report their concerns to organizational leaders for investigation. Unfortunately, the evidence is clear that none of these mechanisms is likely to be effective. In a 2006 systematic review, Davis and colleagues published a study exploring "how accurately physicians self-assess compared with external observations of their competence."[11] While noting that the evidence was suboptimal in quality, they concluded: "The preponderance of evidence suggest that physicians have a limited ability to accurately self-assess." Similarly, there is a lack of association between a surgeon's self-perception of cognitive change and objective measures of such change. In their report, the Society of Surgical Chairs (SCC) noted: "Thus, the self-imposed plans of surgeons to transition from active practice seems to be an ill-founded solution to the issue of age-associated functional impairments in surgeons."[12] Unfortunately, the limitations of physicians' abilities to self-assess suggests that those physicians most in need of support to practice safely as they age may be the least likely to recognize these deficits on their own and highlights the importance of mandatory organizational programs to screen LCPs.

The strategy of relying on physicians to report concerns they have about a colleague's declining competence is also flawed. In a large survey of physicians in 2010, Desroches and colleagues found that only 64% of physicians report feeling prepared to effectively deal with an incompetent colleague.[13] Of physicians with knowledge of an incompetent colleague, 33% had not reported this concern to the relevant authority. Similarly, a survey of 1,800 interns and residents by Martinez and colleagues found that during their most recent inpatient month, 49% reported observing a patient safety breach, and 75% reported observing unprofessional behavior.[14] However, only 71% reported speaking up about the observed patient safety breach, and 46% reported speaking up about the unprofessional behavior. Over time, the profession will need to reexamine whether our reticence to speak up with concerns about our peers' performance is actually the type of collegial behavior to which we should aspire.

Finally, while patients frequently observed problems in their care (including concerns that physicians might not be practicing appropriately as they age), they also hesitate to share their concerns. In one research study conducted with cancer patients, only 13% of patients who thought something serious and harmful had gone wrong in the care had reported their concern to their providers or the organization. The most common barrier to speaking up for these patients was fear of disrupting their relationship with their treatment team.[15] Physicians are in the ideal position to let patients know it is fine to share any concerns they may have about their care, which would lessen patients' worries about adversely affecting their ongoing relationship with that provider.

How Should the Medical Profession Oversee the Practice of LCPs?

There are a host of open questions facing healthcare organizations about their role in overseeing LCPs' scope of practice and retirement decisions: Who should evaluate an

LCP's performance and how? Should organizations make adaptations for LCPs with declining performance or force retirement? How can we promote LCP career longevity without sacrificing patient safety?

In some nations, these challenges are not left solely to the medical profession and employers. For example, regulatory agencies in Australia and Canada have developed age-based peer review and health assessments for LCPs.[16,17] Mandatory retirement ages for surgeons apply in India, Japan, China, and Finland.[12] However, it would be challenging for US state licensing boards to institute similar requirements and do so in a uniform way across the fifty states. An aging physician workforce, rising physician employment, and growing public expectations for safe care have pushed healthcare leaders to seek better institutional approaches to assessing and supporting employed LCPs.[18]

The strength of the evidence above has prompted the influential US SCC to recommend mandatory LCP screening and some countries to implement LCP programs. In 2019 the SCC published a report that both summarized the risks that older surgeons could pose to patients and recommended a much more proactive approach to the problem, including mandatory cognitive and psychomotor testing of surgeons by at least age sixty-five.[12] The conclusion of their recommendations is as follows: "The recommendations of the SSC are for health care organizations to engage in orderly long-term planning and discussions with senior surgeons for their transitioning into meaningful nonclinical roles and for chairs to advocate at their local institutions and with their national societies for mandatory cognitive and psychomotor testing beginning by at least 65 years of age."

In response to these and other calls to address the issue of LCPs more explicitly, some institutions have developed programs that require LCPs to undergo age-based cognitive and physical health screening before renewing hospital credentials.[12,19,20] These programs typically begin screening around age 70 and make participation mandatory for all practitioners. Most programs screen for age-related decline with a combination of a brief cognitive test, basic health and vision exams, and review of practice performance data. If concerns arise on screening, comprehensive assessment follows, including extended neuropsychiatric testing or intensive peer review. When in-depth testing needs exceed the resources and expertise within a health system, a handful of referral centers offers comprehensive testing processes.[21] Because physicians may raise concerns about the relevance of some tests to their clinical performance, programs typically tailor assessments and performance expectations to the LCP's specialty and practice requirements.

Among cognitive screening tests, the MicroCog stands out for reliability, tolerability, sensitivity, affordability, and the availability of normative data for physicians.[12] The MicroCog has important limitations, however. It requires specific software and a trained individual to administer the in-person exam. Furthermore, all screening tests involve some risk of false-positive or false-negative results that must be discussed with LCPs. At present, there are no screening methods that can replace the key function of cognitive testing. Although patient complaint narratives[22] or other health system data may provide hints about LCP cognitive decline, we are unaware of robust methods for screening physicians' practice data with adequate sensitivity and specificity.

Once in-depth testing confirms concerns about an LCP's practice performance, employers face a choice between terminating employment and adjusting staff privileges to allow a more limited practice. While policies and procedures must provide consistency and due process, each circumstance requires considerable individualization and collaboration with the LCP involved. A professional challenge for both the physician and medical staff leaders is to maximize fairness to the LCP, access to care, and physician autonomy while making patient safety the ultimate guiding value. Although institutional leaders seeking promptness and certainty might urge retirement in all cases, we believe employers have an obligation to consider adaptions to the work environment that allow safe and ongoing work, such as shifting to a low-volume, focused practice. This approach requires frequent monitoring and may not be possible in all situations. Yet, a more nuanced approach supports a culture of trust and provider wellness. Adapting the work environment for ongoing practice engenders trust by demonstrating a commitment for LCPs to have a safe and rewarding late career. Without this trust, physicians may see screening programs as exclusionary or biased tools and resist their adoption.

Historically, many conversations with LCPs about practice restriction or retirement occurred belatedly, after medical harm, generating an atmosphere of shame or conflict. To foster mutually agreeable retirement decisions, employers must take steps to build trust with physicians earlier in their career. First, investment in lifelong career development will help mid- and late-career physicians to feel that their employer reliably helps them to achieve their potential.[23] Second, LCP programs should consider ways to affordably adopt periodic screening tests at younger ages, aligning medicine with a paradigm used in aviation. Establishing baseline performance during an individual's fifties or sixties would contextualize changes during their seventies. Crucially, it would also destigmatize screening health and cognitive function, casting it as a career-wide patient safety behavior, rather than a punishment for LCPs. Third, employers should expand ways for retiring physicians to maintain their sense of professional identity. For example, pathways for phased retirement, succession planning in clinical programs, and the development of robust emeritus roles allow LCPs ways to plan for a graceful and gratifying retirement.[24]

Experiences and Outcomes With Current LCP Programs

Emerging data about LCP program outcomes offer guidance for employers considering adopting this approach. Yale New Haven Hospital and Hartford Hospital have published comprehensive accounts of their procedures and aggregate outcomes.[19,25] The findings are congruent and validate the need for LCP programs to be used more widely. Both organizations applied a two-step process consisting of screening with brief cognitive and physical tests, followed by in-depth testing if concerns were found.

Researchers at Hartford Hospital tracked reappointment outcomes during a 23-month period for 160 individuals aged seventy or older. Among those, 118 sought reappointment and underwent MicroCog testing as part of initial screening. Of those 118 providers screened, nineteen were requested to complete a full cognitive exam based on concerning findings. At this stage, two providers elected to retire rather than completing a comprehensive evaluation. Of the seventeen who completed a full neurocognitive evaluation, thirteen met criteria for mild cognitive impairment (MCI). While one of the LCPs diagnosed with MCI elected to retire, the other twelve continued to practice with practice modifications and close monitoring organized by a Focused Professional Practice Evaluation (FPPE). Ultimately, the testing found that 14.4% of LCPs over seventy had MCI, but many could continue to work in patient care with increased oversight.

LCP program administrators at Yale utilized a similar approach to screen 141 clinicians over seventy during a three-year period. To prevent clinicians from preparing for tests, they did not identify the precise battery of cognitive screening tests used, but described the exam as taking fifty to ninety minutes and having components similar to a MicroCog. Individuals with normal scores and no other health or performance concerns proceeded to recredentialing; those with borderline findings performed repeat screening in one year; and those with weaknesses relevant to their practice area underwent full neurocognitive screening. Among 141 clinicians screened, eighteen (12.7%) were ultimately found to have deficits likely to impair their practice of medicine. Of note, none of these had come to the attention of medical staff leadership, highlighting the inadequacy of typical peer review and monitoring practices in the oversight of LCPs. All eighteen LCPs voluntarily elected to either retire or make practice modifications. The authors concluded that the success of their program hinged on the selection of a skilled neuropsychologist and a review committee with the trust of the practitioner community. Although such neuropsychologists may not be accessible in rural areas, LCP programs can be established in rural hospitals through collaboration with larger urban centers.

There is also evidence that participants in LCP programs find them to be helpful and not overly burdensome. Bazzo and colleagues, who lead the Physician Assessment and Clinical Education (PACE) program in San Diego, California, recently published results of a pilot study of a screening process for senior physicians age fifty and older.[26] Thirty senior physicians volunteered to participate in the program. Of these, 27% were found to "require/may require" further evaluation after cognitive assessment, though no physicians were found to have physical or mental health issues that would prevent them from practicing competently. Participants described the screening process as a positive experience that was effective, acceptable, efficient, and relevant to their practice. This aligns with reports from other LCP programs. Leaders at the University of Virginia and LifeBridge health found that efforts to contextualize the program as part of a broader safety initiative and to personalize the intake and review process facilitated LCP acceptance.[18] Similarly, program leaders at Intermountain Health found that LCPs welcomed the process when it was framed as a constructive opportunity to identify strengths and opportunities for growth.

LCP programs have not been universally embraced to date. At Stanford, California, adoption of an LCP program that included cognitive testing prompted such an outcry from physicians that this element of the program was dropped. The LCP landscape was further complicated when the US Equal Opportunity Employment Commission (EEOC), the arm of the federal government that is responsible for enforcing federal laws that make it illegal to discriminate against an applicant or employee for a variety of reasons, including age (40 or older), filed a lawsuit in 2020 against Yale New Haven Hospital alleging their LCP program constituted age discrimination and also was in violation of the Americans With Disability Act. The EEOC-Yale New Haven Hospital lawsuit is ongoing. In January 2021, Hennepin Healthcare in Minnesota resolved a similar complaint with the EEOC by agreeing to stop screening physicians and nurse practitioners aged seventy and older for cognitive decline. While the Yale New Haven LCP program continues to operate as the EEOC litigation progresses, many organizations who were on the verge of launching an LCP program when the lawsuit was filed have put these plans on hold pending resolution of this litigation.

Looking to the Future

Historically, cases such as the one at the beginning of this chapter have laid bare the challenges associated with reliably implementing principles of professional self-regulation. The medical profession has traditionally deeply valued deferential treatment of colleagues. There are several other factors that might make it hard for an individual physician or nurse to come forward with their concerns, such as the surgeon's seniority and prominence. The hospital might hesitate to take action against the surgeon due to concern about the financial impact losing the surgeon might have on the organization.

Yet while there are some circumstances in which age-related changes in cognition, physical skills, or knowledge currency might mean that continued practice for a given physician is no longer possible, there are often opportunities to support LCPs in continued safe practice with accommodations or greater oversight. Modifications in practice allow the profession to continue to benefit from the wisdom and experience of our senior colleagues while ensuring patient safety. Ultimately, adapting our peer review and credentialing processes to monitor the physical and mental well-being across the continuum of their careers could supplant age-based screening regimens. But until that time arrives, LCP programs will play an important role in ensuring the safe practice of physicians as they age.

References

1. Dellinger EP, Pellegrini CA, Gallagher TH. The aging physician and the medical profession: a review. *JAMA Surg.* 2017;152(10):967–971. doi:10.1001/jamasurg.2017.2342
2. Devi G, Gitelman DR, Press D, Daffner KR. Cognitive impairment in aging physicians: current challenges and possible solutions. *Neurol Clin Pract.* 2021;11(2):167–174. doi:10.1212/CPJ.0000000000000829
3. Choudhry NK, Fletcher RH, Soumerai SB. Systematic review: the relationship between clinical experience and quality of health care. *Ann Intern Med.* 2005;142(4):260–273. doi:10.7326/0003-4819-142-4-200502150-00008
4. American Medical Association. US physicians and students workforce statistics. Accessed March 17, 2022. https://www.ama-assn.org/system/files/2020-04/physicians-students-workforce-stats.pdf
5. Furukawa MF, Kimmey L, Jones DJ, Machta RM, Guo J, Rich EC. Consolidation of providers into health systems increased substantially, 2016–18. *Health Aff (Millwood).* 2020;39(8):1321–1325. doi:10.1377/hlthaff.2020.00017
6. Kane CK. Recent changes in physician practice arrangements: private practice dropped to less than 50 percent of physicians in 2020. 2021. https://www.ama-assn.org/system/files/2021-05/2020-prp-physician-practice-arrangements. pdf
7. Bismark MM, Spittal MJ, Gurrin LC, Ward M, Studdert DM. Identification of doctors at risk of recurrent complaints: a national study of healthcare complaints in Australia. *BMJ Qual Saf.* 2013;22(7):532–540. doi:10.1136/bmjqs-2012-001691
8. Morrison J, Wickersham P. Physicians disciplined by a state medical board. *JAMA.* 1998;279(23):1889–1893. doi:10.1001/jama.279.23.1889

9. McAuley RG, Paul WM, Morrison GH, Beckett RF, Goldsmith CH. Five-year results of the peer assessment program of the College of Physicians and Surgeons of Ontario. *CMAJ.* 1990;143(11):1193–1199.
10. Yen W, Niels T. State of the science on risk and support factors to physician performance: a report from the Pan-Canadian physician factors collaboration. *J Med Regul.* 2019;105(1):6–21.
11. Davis DA, Mazmanian PE, Fordis M, Van Harrison R, Thorpe KE, Perrier L. Accuracy of physician self-assessment compared with observed measures of competence: a systematic review. *JAMA.* 2006;296(9):1094–1102. doi:10.1001/jama.296.9.1094
12. Rosengart TK, Doherty G, Higgins R, Kibbe MR, Mosenthal AC. Transition planning for the senior surgeon: guidance and recommendations from the Society of Surgical Chairs. *JAMA Surg.* 2019;154(7):647–653. doi:10.1001/jamasurg.2019.1159
13. DesRoches CM, Rao SR, Fromson JA, et al. Physicians' perceptions, preparedness for reporting, and experiences related to impaired and incompetent colleagues. *JAMA.* 2010;304(2):187–193. doi:10.1001/jama.2010.921
14. Martinez W, Lehmann LS, Thomas EJ, et al. Speaking up about traditional and professionalism-related patient safety threats: a national survey of interns and residents. *BMJ Qual Saf.* 2017;26(11):869–880. doi:10.1136/bmjqs-2016-006284
15. Mazor KM, Roblin DW, Greene SM, et al. Toward patient-centered cancer care: patient perceptions of problematic events, impact, and response. *J Clin Oncol.* 2012;30(15):1784–1790. doi:10.1200/JCO.2011.38.1384
16. Medical Board of Australia. Expert advisory group on revalidation: Final report. August 2017. http://www.medicalboard.gov.au/documents/default.aspx?record=WD17%2F24295&dbid=AP&chksum=Txmn8C7v%2BC53Wjsz3sXn2w%3D% 3D
17. College of Physicians and Surgeons of Manitoba. Annual report. 2017. 2017. Accessed July 29. http://www.cpsm.mb.ca/assets/Annual%20Reports/CPSMAnnRep2017.pdf
18. White AA, Sage WM, Mazor KM, Gallagher TH. Assessing and supporting late career practitioners: four key questions. *Jt Comm J Qual Patient Saf.* 2020;46(10):591–595. doi:10.1016/j.jcjq.2020.07.001
19. Cooney L, Balcezak T. Cognitive testing of older clinicians prior to recredentialing. *JAMA.* 2020;323(2):179–180. doi:10.1001/jama.2019.18665
20. White AA, Sage WM, Osinska PH, Salgaonkar MJ, Gallagher TH. Patient safety and the ageing physician: a qualitative study of key stakeholder attitudes and experiences. *BMJ Qual Saf.* 2019;28(6):468–475. doi:10.1136/bmjqs-2018-008276
21. Katlic MR, Coleman J. The aging surgeon. *Ann Surg.* 2014;260(2):199–201. doi:10.1097/SLA.0000000000000667
22. Cooper WO, Martinez W, Domenico HJ, et al. Unsolicited patient complaints identify physicians with evidence of neurocognitive disorders. *Am J Geriatr Psychiatry.* 2018;26(9):927–936. doi:10.1016/j.jagp.2018.04.005
23. Collins RT 2nd, Sanford R. The importance of formalized, lifelong physician career development: making the case for a paradigm shift. *Acad Med.* 2021;96(10):1383–1388. doi:10.1097/ACM.0000000000004191
24. Baumgartner W, Ziminski C, Van Beek J, Rand C. Everyone wins when retiring faculty of health professions schools are supported. *Acad Med.* 2021;96(10):1375–1376. doi:10.1097/ACM.0000000000004147

25. Young KP, Robinson KJ, Dicks RS, Kumar A, Orlando R. Assessing late career practitioners for cognitive decline: an evidence-based approach. *NEJM Catalyst.* 2021;2(2). https://catalyst.nejm.org/doi/abs/10.1056/CAT.20.0215

26. Bazzo DEJ, Smith P, Wenghofer EF. A pilot study of a screening process for evaluating the physical, mental, and cognitive health of senior physicians. *J Med Regul.* 2021;107(2):33–40.

27. Hartz AJ, Kuhn EM, Pulido J. Prestige of training programs and experience of bypass surgeons as factors in adjusted patient mortality rates. *Med Care.* 1999;37(1):93–103. doi:10.1097/00005650-199901000-00013

28. O'Neill L, Lanska DJ, Hartz A. Surgeon characteristics associated with mortality and morbidity following carotid endarterectomy. *Neurology.* 2000;55(6):773–781. doi:10.1212/wnl.55.6.773

29. Neumayer LA, Gawande AA, Wang J, et al. Proficiency of surgeons in inguinal hernia repair: effect of experience and age. *Ann Surg.* 2005;242(3):344–348; discussion 348–352. doi:10.1097/01.sla.0000179644.02187.ea

30. Waljee JF, Greenfield LJ, Dimick JB, Birkmeyer JD. Surgeon age and operative mortality in the United States. *Ann Surg.* 2006;244(3):353–362. doi:10.1097/01.sla.0000234803.11991.6d

31. Anderson BR, Wallace AS, Hill KD, et al. Association of surgeon age and experience with congenital heart surgery outcomes. *Circ Cardiovasc Qual Outcomes.* 2017;10(7). https://www.ahajournals.org/doi/10.1161/CIRCOUTCOMES.117.003533

32. Southern WN, Bellin EY, Arnsten JH. Longer lengths of stay and higher risk of mortality among inpatients of physicians with more years in practice. *Am J Med.* 2011;124(9):868–874. doi:10.1016/j.amjmed.2011.04.011

33. Tsugawa Y, Newhouse JP, Zaslavsky AM, Blumenthal DM, Jena AB. Physician age and outcomes in elderly patients in hospital in the US: observational study. *BMJ.* 2017;357:j1797. doi:10.1136/bmj.j1797

30
Resilience and Medical Professionalism

Henry J. Michtalik and Albert W. Wu

Key Points

- Clinician resilience can be supported or challenged by properties of the organization in which they work and is associated with medical professionalism.
- Burnout, resulting from unmanaged chronic workplace stress, can make it difficult for clinicians to uphold the standards of professionalism.
- Professionalism is strengthened by job satisfaction and employee motivation, which in turn can be strengthened by job enrichment.
- Stressful work-related events can be traumatic for clinicians, who can benefit from timely, confidential peer support.
- Fixing the workplace and practice environment may be more successful than fixing the worker at promoting clinician resilience and well-being.

Tying Resiliency to Medical Professionalism

A general definition of resilience is "the ability to recover from or adjust easily to misfortune or change."[1] Resilience is defined in the *American Psychological Association* (APA) *Dictionary of Psychology* as "the ability to successfully adapt to challenging experiences, especially through mental, emotional, and behavioral flexibility and adjustment to external and internal demand."[2] In the classic paper by Connor and Davidson on developing new resilience scale, resilience is defined as "the personal qualities that enable one to thrive in the face of adversity."[3(p76)] In medicine, resilience is associated in both direct and indirect ways with medical professionalism.

It is easy to characterize resilience as an individual trait. However, it is important to recognize the distinction between individual and organizational resilience. When referring to a larger system, resilience can be defined as the ability to prepare for and adapt to changing conditions and withstand and recover rapidly from disruptions.[4] Organizational resilience refers to their ability to carry out their mission in the face of adversity. In addition, there are important interactions between individual and organizational resilience. In particular, an individual's resilience can be supported or challenged by properties of the organization where they work.

Medical professionalism is the ideal that attracts many to the field of medicine. For the American Board of Medical Specialties, professionalism is a belief system and behaviors that support trustworthy relationships between patients and their physicians.[5] The American Board of Internal Medicine defines medical professionalism as the daily expression of the desire to help people and society as a whole by providing quality healthcare to those in need.[6] The American Board of Internal Medicine (ABIM) describes six elements of professionalism: altruism, accountability, excellence, duty, honor/integrity, and respect. In addition to physicians, these standards apply to other healthcare professionals who work directly with patients, including nurses, pharmacists, and others.

The failure of resilience—the failure to recover quickly or easily from difficulties—makes it more difficult for a clinician to uphold the expression of professionalism. As defined in the *International Classification of Diseases, Eleventh Revision* (*ICD-11*): "Burn-out is a syndrome conceptualized as resulting from chronic workplace stress that has not been successfully managed. It is characterized by three dimensions: feelings of energy depletion or exhaustion; increased mental distance from one's job, or feelings of negativism or cynicism related to one's job; and reduced professional efficacy."[7] The World Health Organization (WHO) classifies burnout as an occupational phenomenon, rather than as a medical condition. Burnout can lead to a lack of professionalism. It can erode the trust and trustworthiness of physicians and challenge their ability to practice the elements of professionalism. It also poses a threat to the quality of care and patient safety by harming teamwork and impairing decision-making.

Job Satisfaction and Motivation

Professionalism is strengthened by job satisfaction and employee motivation, yet what leads to satisfaction and dissatisfaction can vary both by individual and with time. In a classic paper published in 1968 in the *Harvard Business Review*, Herzberg examined how to motivate employees.[8] In twelve different investigations with over two thousand employees across various industries, the article describes the importance of "dissatisfiers" (which it refers to as hygiene factors), which maintain the status quo, such as company policy and administration, supervision, work conditions, and salary. In contrast, "satisfiers" (intrinsic motivators) motivate employees for greater productivity, such as achievement, recognition, the work itself, responsibility, achievement, and growth. The opposite of a satisfier is not a dissatisfier; the opposite of dissatisfaction is no dissatisfaction, and the opposite of satisfaction is the lack of satisfaction. Although these concepts originated in 1968, they remain relevant today to work in healthcare. Workload, the electronic medical record (EMR) and pay are examples of hygiene factors that maintain the status quo. In contrast, autonomy, task variety, and recognition are intrinsic motivators that foster professionalism and mitigate burnout by strengthening the sense of personal achievement and reducing the sense of emotional exhaustion. The concept of job enrichment, allowing for less supervision, more opportunities for achievement, and vertical job loading, further strengthens motivation. In contrast, horizontal job loading, which is focused on a "product," such as the number of patients seen or shorter length of hospital stay, does not necessarily further the sense of job enrichment. With the expanded focus in the clinical environment on productivity, we must not forget about job enrichment and explicitly address this with professional development opportunities, recognition, and fostering achievement in what is important to healthcare employees.

Factors That Influence Well-Being

There are many factors that influence healthcare worker well-being. The National Academy of Medicine has developed a conceptual model of factors affecting clinician

This conceptual model depicts the factors associated with clinician well-being and resilience; applies these factors across all health care professions, specialities, settings, and career stages; and emphasizes the link between clinician well-being and outcomes for clinicians, patients, and the health system. The model should be used to understand well-being, rather than as a diagnostic or assessment tool. In electronic form, the external and individual factors of the conceptual model are hyperlinked to corresponding landing pages on the Clinician Well-Being Knowledge Hub. The Clinician Well-Being Knowledge Hub provides additional information and resources. The conceptual model will be revised as the field develops and more information becomes available.

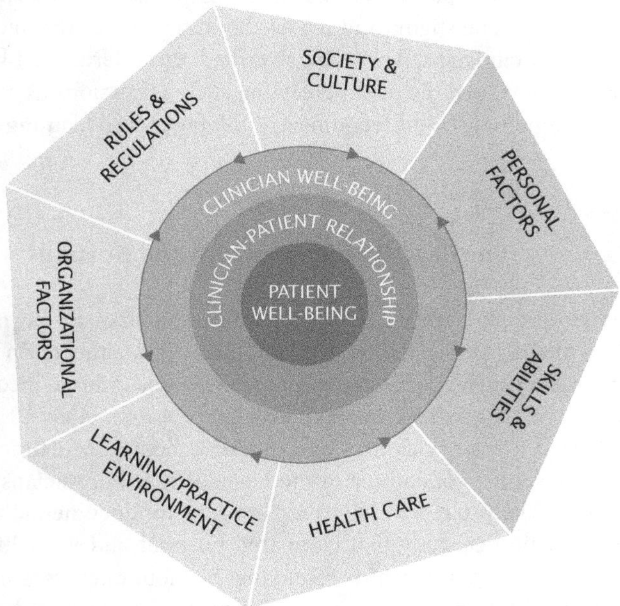

Figure 30.1 Factors affecting clinician well-being and resilience—conceptual model.

well-being and resilience (Figure 30.1).[9] This model illustrates the many interrelated factors that affect clinician well-being and burnout. It emphasizes relationships between clinician well-being, the clinician-patient relationship, and patient well-being.

Seven factors affect clinician well-being: personal factors, skills and abilities, healthcare responsibilities, learning/practice environment, organizational factor, rules and regulations, and society and culture all play a role. Personal factors directly influence clinician well-being. Individual characteristics, such as younger age and female gender, and personal traits, such as learning style, may increase risk for burnout. Personal, social, and family circumstances, such as family dynamics and financial stresses can also contribute to risk, as can unbalanced work-life integration. Clinician skills and abilities, including coping strategies and mindfulness can also directly influence clinician well-being. However, these two individual categories represent a minority of influential factors relative to factors that lie outside of the individual's control. Organizational leadership, culture, policies, and healthcare responsibilities can be important to individual burnout and well-being. Skilled and effective leadership can have a positive influence on well-being. Organizational culture, specifically an emphasis on quality of care and work-life balance, is associated with increased satisfaction, whereas an emphasis on productivity is associated with decreased satisfaction. Effective teamwork, supportive professional relationships, fairness, and opportunity can protect against burnout, whereas discrimination and marginalization erode that protection. Professional policies, licensure requirements, insurance requirements, reimbursement policies, and risk of litigation all contribute to burnout. The requirements by state medical boards and accrediting bodies for physicians to report mental health conditions discourage many from seeking needed treatment. A heavy burden of administrative tasks required to be reimbursed for care or obtain treatment for patients can be oppressive and draining. Reporting requirements for quality measures and "pay for performance" also consume clinician time. Unrealistic expectations and societal stigma and biases about mental health conditions have many harmful effects on clinicians. These are absorbed and internalized by clinicians, who avoid reporting their own distress, perceiving such admissions as a sign of weakness. Instead, they compensate by perfectionism, intolerance, and blaming of themselves and others.

The Practice Environment and Burnout

The work environment is often cited as an important factor for burnout, for example, inpatient (hospitalist) versus outpatient (ambulatory) healthcare. In a study by Linzer et al. in 2016 evaluating work-life and wellness in general internal medicine, the authors found 67% reported high stress, burnout averaged approximately 40%, and half of participants reported low work control and excessive home EMR time.[10] When directly comparing the responses of ambulatory to hospital-based physicians, ambulatory providers were more likely to report job stress, less time for documentation, and decreased team efficiency. Another study that compared burnout and work-life balance among hospitalists and outpatient internists found that burnout rates were similar, 52% versus 55%, respectively.[11] However, hospitalists were more likely to score low on the personal accomplishment subscale for burnout, despite better ratings on schedule flexibility. Professional development opportunities and recognition remain important for both clinical settings to foster professionalism and collegial relationships.

Within these clinical environments, and especially for hospitalists, there can be multiple practice models which can also affect job satisfaction, burnout, and professionalism. In a survey of over 3,000 hospitalists within different practice models, including multistate hospitalist companies, the authors found differences in clinical and nonclinical responsibilities as well as the factors that were most important to job satisfaction across the practice models.[12] For example, for "local hospitalist-only groups" optimal autonomy and organizational fairness were more important; in contrast, for university or medical school employees task variety, patient relationships, and recognition by leadership had more significance. Global job satisfaction and burnout, however, were similar across the different models. This finding emphasizes the concept of job fit. A practice model may emphasize particular features, such as autonomy, that may be more important to some individuals. By working within a practice model that aligns with the employee's own values, it provides a more conducive environment to provide quality healthcare to those in need.

Stresses in Healthcare

There are many stresses in healthcare. Healthcare is a high-risk occupation for the emotional health of healthcare workers. The death of patients is unavoidable in hospital care and can be even more stressful if it is unexpected, if it befalls a child or favorite patient, or if a health worker has not witnessed it before. Unexpected adverse events, and even routine complications, are disappointments for all. Difficult decisions, particularly around contested end-of-life decisions with staff and family members are particularly stressful. These may contribute to the helpless feelings that are part of moral distress, which occurs when one knows the ethically correct action to take but feels powerless to take that action. In recent years, the incidence of workplace violence has increased to the point that it is one of the most frequent stresses in some organizations.

In the last few years, the COVID-19 pandemic has added a host of unaccustomed stresses. As in other large-scale disasters, health worker distress became a secondary pandemic that in retrospect was largely predictable.[13–15]

Additional stressors included the personal risk of infection and worry about spreading infection to loved ones, high demand, and extreme workloads. Many were redeployed and required to perform unfamiliar tasks, separated from their accustomed team members. They were exposed to difficult decisions and uncertainty, and high levels of patient suffering and death, with many dying alone, away from their families.[16]

The Second-Victim Syndrome

An exceptionally stressful incident can be traumatic for a health worker. The term *second victim* was introduced in 2000 to describe the near-universal experience of healthcare workers who are traumatized by making a medical error that harms a patient.[17] Both hazards and adverse events and patient safety are caused by systems of care that contain a multitude of flaws and latent errors. Thus, although patients and their families are the first and obvious victims of medical mistakes, physicians can be psychologically harmed by the same errors and can be considered to be second victims.

Attention to this experience has increased, along with recognition that types of concerned incidents are much broader than errors and adverse events. It is now understood that anyone working with patients in healthcare can be affected by patient adverse events. In addition, initial thinking about the second victim experience focused on extremely stressful, one-time events. However, the day-to-day stresses attendant to work life in healthcare are much more common. Some of the stresses involve incidents in which a patient is harmed. However, a larger proportion include disappointing outcomes that may not have been prevented, difficult decisions, and conflicts with patients, family members, or other workers. Not all stresses are associated with bad outcomes, such as harrowing events like a prolonged successful resuscitation. Workplace violence against health workers has also become disturbingly common.[18]

The term has also provoked controversy. There has been discontent with the term, particularly among patients who have been harmed and treated poorly by the system, patient advocates, and some physicians.[19,20] However, no satisfactory replacement has been found, and the term has come into widespread use.

A more recent definition defines a second victim as "any health care worker, directly or indirectly involved in an unanticipated adverse patient event, unintentional healthcare error, or patient injury and who becomes victimized in the sense that they are also negatively impacted."[21]

The acute and longer term symptoms of the second victim experience represent the repertoire of how humans react to stress. Within minutes of a stressful event, the symptoms of an acute stress response may develop. First described by Walter Cannon in 1915, these can include tunnel vision, loss of hearing, and shaking, anxiety, aggressive or freezing behavior, and negative thoughts.[22,23] People may experience dissociative symptoms such as a sense of numbing, detachment, or lack of emotional responsiveness; a reduction in awareness of their surroundings; a feeling of detachment from their surroundings; depersonalization; or amnesia.

Healthcare workers commonly feel responsible for the adverse outcome, feeling as though they have failed, and question their knowledge and competence. They may lose confidence in their own ability.[24] A meta-analysis found that the most common symptoms were troubling memories, anger toward oneself, regret and remorse, distress, fear of making future errors, embarrassment, guilt, and sleep disturbance.[25]

Some people develop an acute stress disorder, also referred to as acute stress reaction.[26] This can develop within hours to days or weeks and includes marked symptoms of anxiety or increased arousal, which includes sleep disturbance, irritability, poor concentration, hypervigilance, and restlessness. The person may also report headaches and gastrointestinal and rheumatologic symptoms. They have persistent flashbacks or other reexperiences of the incident and may avoid things that prompt those recollections. The person also has impaired social or work functioning.

People with acute stress disorder are at increased risk of developing post-traumatic stress disorder (PTSD), defined as a constellation of symptoms that persist for more than a month, including intrusive memories, avoidance, negative changes in thinking and mood, and changes in arousal. The latter can include maladaptive coping behavior, like consuming alcohol or substances; difficulty concentrating; irritability; and angry outburst.

In the short and longer term, there are negative consequences for both the affected individual and the healthcare team. Individuals are more likely to make medical errors or deliver lower quality care and are also at greater risk for burnout.[27] In addition, they may be unable to provide the degree of compassion and caring that benefit their patients.

Both absenteeism and presenteeism can be a problem. Individuals may call out sick. An individual experiencing the aforementioned symptoms and behaviors is likely to detract from team functioning and morale. Both of these increase workload for team members and can accelerate team turnover. As demonstrated during the COVID-19 pandemic, the impact can extend to posing a threat to the institutional mission.[15]

Resilient Zone Model

The resilient zone model has been used to conceptualize an individual's emotional self-regulation in response to stress.[28] The resilient zone represents a space in which a person is in a physical and mental state of well-being. The body is usually able to handle day-to-day stresses and maintain homeostasis. However, excessive stress can bump a person out of their resilient zone into a dysregulated state. This may be a zone of hyperarousal in which the person feels anxious, agitated, irritable, and even manic. They may also land in a zone of hypoarousal in which they feel sad, depressed, exhausted, or unmotivated. In either state, it is difficult to concentrate, learn, make decisions, and perform optimally.[29]

Psychological first aid (PFA) has been proposed as a strategy to help individuals subjected to overwhelming stress. Originally developed in the 1950s, PFA has been used primarily in developing countries after large-scale crisis events. The WHO's 2011 *Guide for*

Field Workers describes it as "humane, supportive, and practical help to support fellow human beings" in the immediate aftermath of serious crisis events.[30]

Psychological first aid has received empirical support for providing five essential elements for restoring social and behavior function these include promoting a sense of safety, calm, and self and collective efficacy, connectedness, and instilling hope.[31–33] PFA can be adapted and applied to healthcare settings and has been recommended for the treatment of acute stress disorder.[33–35] It has also been proposed for widespread training for all healthcare workers analogous to cardiopulmonary resuscitation (CPR) training.[36]

The RISE (Resilience in Stressful Events) Peer Support Program

At Johns Hopkins, the Resilience in Stressful Events (RISE) program was created in 2011 to help health workers deal with the psychological effects of patient adverse events.[37,38] The program was based on providing timely PFA and emotional support, delivered by peer volunteers who work in the same institution. As a brief intervention, the goal is to ease the person back into their resilient zone so that their normal homeostatic mechanisms can resume.

The intervention is delivered by a multidisciplinary team of volunteers who work at the hospital and dedicate a portion of their time to supporting their colleagues. The RISE program is accessible to all hospital workers twenty-four hours a day, 365 days a year via a secure messaging system. Responders call back within thirty minutes and arrange to meet confidentially with individuals or with groups. During the COVID-19 pandemic, there was a dramatic increase in the number of calls for support. To accommodate this, the Johns Hopkins RISE team expanded its membership and added proactive rounding to units where there were reports of stress, collaborated systematically with other supportive resources, and participated in the COVID-19 incident command center.[38,39]

Burnout Interventions

Interventions to reduce burnout have been implemented with some success. However, many interventions have focused narrowly on the impact of duty hour restrictions for providers in training.[40] Similarly, interventions have varied in type, scope, and duration, making individual interventions difficult to directly compare or implement. A systematic review of controlled interventions to reduce burnout in physicians found these interventions reduce burnout, with a stronger effect for interventions directed at the organizational level versus those directed at the physician.[41] Organizational interventions include structural changes (e.g., varying the intensity or operations); fostering communication (e.g., transparency of changes and rationale); teamwork; and job control (e.g., front-line workers being involved in management decisions); reducing workload; and optimizing schedules. Physician-directed interventions focused on mindfulness, communication, education, and resiliency. However, only four interventions had confidence intervals that did not cross into equivalence, three of which were organizational. Effective organizational interventions included providing separate night coverage for intensive care unit physicians (in contrast to continuous coverage), a system-directed intervention on quality improvement and workflow with improvements in communication, and a two- versus four-week rotation model for the general internal medicine inpatient service. The only significant physician-directed intervention used a two-month mindfulness-contemplation exercises program focused on being present in the moment, contemplation, and breathing. This intervention required a 2.5-hour session each week. As part of professionalism, these types of interventions should be included within the workday or similarly accounted for as part of work. Requiring these types of interventions on personal time adds stress to the work hours problem they aim to mitigate.

The Impact of COVID-19 Pandemic on Well-Being

The COVID-19 pandemic further stressed the healthcare system. In a national study of healthcare providers in the United States of over 20,000 respondents representing forty-two organizations, 49% were burnt out, 43% were overloaded with work, and 38% were anxious or depressed; nearly two-thirds feared being exposed to COVID-19 or transmitting the virus.[15] Stress scores were highest among nursing and medical assistants and social workers, inpatient providers, women, and Black and Latinx workers. Feeling valued by their organization reduced the odds of burnout by 40%. Similarly, a national registry of US healthcare workers found that 41% experienced burnout, with over half reporting feeling tired "a lot of the day" or stressed. Again, women were more likely to report burnout or distressed experiences (fatigue, stress, insomnia, worry, sadness, pain, or anger). Participants over the age of 30 years were less likely to report burnout.

These findings were not isolated to the United States. In an international systematic review of general practitioner well-being, burnout varied greatly, from 25% to 46%, with female practitioners reporting higher stress levels, greater burden, and more anxiety and burnout.[42] Regarding practitioner age, some studies showed older participants have less burnout, whereas others did not. A thematic analysis of the stressors and moderators of well-being included emotional support, interdisciplinary communication (e.g., consultations), national and organizational preparedness, conflicting and diverse sources of information, competition for personal protective equipment (PPE), and the changing nature of work (e.g., telemedicine). Another study conducted in the United States asked healthcare professionals what they were most concerned about during the pandemic, what leadership messaging and behaviors were needed, and helpful sources of support during the pandemic.[43] The study identified five main themes, which can be summarized as "hear me" (listen and act), "protect me" (decrease risk of infection), "prepare me" (training and support), "support me" (acknowledge human limitations), and "care for me" (if I am infected or quarantined). Addressing these areas is important for maintaining professionalism and collegiality by caring for the individual provider with a focus on their concerns. Some interventions implemented at our own site that addressed these themes included town halls and weekly scheduled update meetings (hear me); PPE training and safety monitors for proper don/doff of PPE (protect me); specific training sessions and champions (prepare me); hydration and respite stations (support me); and sick leave and backup providers in case of COVID-19 infection (care for me). Addressing these themes is important for maintaining professionalism and collegiality by caring for the individual provider, with a focus on their concerns.

Future Directions

A number of solutions have been proposed to support healthcare workers and to promote resilience and professionalism in the workforce.[44]

The Coping with COVID survey included a stepwise conceptual model for promoting resilience and well-being.[15] Although this model used burnout as a final outcome, it also includes mediators such as fear, anxiety/depression, work overload, feeling valued, and meaning/purpose as well as an intermediate outcome called a "stress score." This score included self-reported stress, anxiety/depression, and work overload. This model explained over half of the variance in burnout, with stress highly correlated with burnout. By focusing on these intermediary variables, it may be possible to both detect and prevent burnout before it occurs in its more terminal stages. Similarly, this approach can help to protect medical professionalism and remediate potential challenges. Individual strategies (e.g., self-check-ins, meeting basic needs, staying connected) as well as leadership strategies (e.g., monitor well-being, centralized point of information, supportive environment) are both needed.[45]

The National Academy of Medicine discusses interventions that focus on fixing the workplace rather than fixing the worker.[46] Their goal is to improve clinician well-being and the resilience of the organization. The workgroup postulates that a resilient organization is one that has matched job demands with resources provided to its workers and created a culture of well-being. Such an organization is better able to achieve their organizational objectives and to withstand challenges during crises.

Conclusion

Working in healthcare exposes clinicians to significant stresses. The failure of resilience threatens both clinician well-being and their ability to uphold the ideals of professionalism. Preservation of the physical and mental health of clinicians and other health workers is essential to the delivery of safe, compassionate, and high-quality care.[47–49] An organizational culture of safety and access to confidential mental well-being and social support services can have a positive impact on worker well-being. This in turn can help to support medical professionalism.

References

1. *Miriam Webster Dictionary*. Home page. Accessed May 29, 2023. https://www.merriam-webster.com/dictionary
2. American Psychological Association. Resilience. Accessed May 29, 2023. https://www.apa.org/topics/resilience
3. Connor KM, Davidson JRT. Development of a new resilience scale: the Connor-Davidson Resilience Scale (CD-RISC). *Depress Anxiety*. 2003;18:76–82. http://dx.doi.org/10.1002/da.10113
4. National Institute of Standards and Technology, US Department of Commerce. Information system resilience. Accessed May 29, 2023. https://csrc.nist.gov/glossary/term/information_system_resilience

5. American Board of Medical Specialties. ABMS member boards promote professionalism. September 12, 2022. Accessed May 29, 2023. https://www.abms.org/newsroom/abms-member-boards-promote-professionalism/
6. ABIM Foundation. Medical professionalism. Accessed May 29, 2023. https://abimfoundation.org/what-we-do/medical-professionalism
7. Burn-out an "occupational phenomenon": *International Classification of Diseases*. World Health Organization. May 28, 2019. Accessed May 29, 2023. https://www.who.int/news/item/28-05-2019-burn-out-an-occupational-phenomenon-international-classification-of-diseases
8. Herzberg F. One more time: how do you motivate employees? 1968. *Harv Bus Rev*. 2003;81(1):87–96.
9. Factors affecting clinician well-being and resilience—conceptual model. National Academy of Medicine. 2018. Accessed May 29, 2023. https://nam.edu/clinicianwellbeing/resources/factors-affecting-clinician-well-being-and-resilience-conceptual-model/
10. Linzer M, Poplau S, Babbott S, et al. Worklife and wellness in academic general internal medicine: results from a national survey. *J Gen Intern Med*. 2016;31(9):1004–1010.
11. Roberts DL, Shanafelt TD, Dyrbye LN, West CP. A national comparison of burnout and work-life balance among internal medicine hospitalists and outpatient general internists. *J Hosp Med*. 2014;9(3):176–181.
12. Hinami K, Whelan CT, Miller JA, Wolosin RJ, Wetterneck TB. Job characteristics, satisfaction, and burnout across hospitalist practice models. *J Hosp Med*. 2012;7(5):402–410.
13. Everly GS, Wu AW, Potash JB. Phases of psychological response in COVID-19: a preliminary heuristic. *Am J Disaster Med*. 2021;16(1):5–12. doi:10.5055/ajdm.2021.0381
14. Busch IM, Moretti F, Mazzi M, Wu AW, Rimondini M. What we have learned from two decades of epidemics and pandemics: a systematic review and meta-analysis of the psychological burden of frontline healthcare workers. *Psychother Psychosom*. 2021;90(3):178–190. doi:10.1159/000513733
15. Prasad K, McLoughlin C, Stillman M. Prevalence and correlates of stress and burnout among US healthcare workers during the COVID-19 pandemic: a national cross-sectional survey study. *eClin Med*. 2021;35:100879. https://www.thelancet.com/journals/eclinm/article/PIIS2589-5370(21)00159-0/fulltext
16. World Health Organization. Implications of the COVID-19 pandemic for patient safety: a rapid review. 2022. https://www.who.int/publications/i/item/9789240055094. Accessed June 11, 2024.
17. Wu AW. Medical error: the second victim. The doctor who makes the mistake needs help too. *BMJ*. 2000;320(7237):726–727. doi:10.1136/bmj.320.7237.726
18. Busch IM, Scott SD, Connors C, Story AR, Acharya B, Wu AW. The role of institution-based peer support for health care workers emotionally affected by workplace violence. *Jt Comm J Qual Patient Saf*. 2021;47(3):146–156. doi:10.1016/j.jcjq.2020.11.005
19. Clarkson MD, Haskell H, Hemmelgarn C, Skolnik PJ. Abandon the term "second victim." *BMJ*. 2019;364:l1233.doi:10.1136/bmj.l1233
20. Wu AW, Shapiro J, Harrison R, et al. The impact of adverse events on clinicians: what's in a name? *J Patient Saf*. 2020;16(1):65–72. doi:10.1097/PTS.0000000000000256
21. Vanhaecht K, Seys D, Russotto S, et al; European Researchers' Network Working on Second Victims (ERNST). An evidence and consensus-based definition of second victim: a strategic topic in healthcare quality, patient safety, person-centeredness and

human resource management. *Int J Environ Res Public Health.* 2022;19(24):16869. doi:10.3390/ijerph192416869

22. Cannon WB. *Bodily Changes in Pain, Hunger, Fear and Rage.* D. Appleton & Company; 1915.
23. Brown TM, Fee E. Walter Bradford Cannon: pioneer physiologist of human emotions. *Am J Public Health.* 2002;92(10):1594–1595.
24. Scott SD, et al. The natural history of recovery for the health care provider "second victim" after adverse patient events. *Qual Saf Health Care.* 2009;18:325–330.
25. Busch IM, Moretti F, Purgato M, Barbui C, Wu AW, Rimondini M. Psychological and psychosomatic symptoms of second victims of adverse events: a systematic review and meta-analysis. *J Patient Saf.* 2020;16(2):e61–e74. Erratum in: *J Patient Saf.* 2020;*16*(3):e211. doi:10.1097/PTS.0000000000000589
26. Acute stress reaction F43.0. *ICD-10 Version:2019.* Accessed May 29, 2023. https://icd.who.int/browse10/2019/en#/F43.0
27. West CP, Tan AD, Habermann TM, Sloan JA, Shanafelt TD. Association of resident fatigue and distress with perceived medical errors. *JAMA.* 2009;302(12):1294–1300. doi:10.1001/jama.2009.1389
28. Trauma Resource Institute. Resilient zone model. Accessed May 29, 2023. http://traumaresourceinstitute.com (
29. Miller-Karas E. Building resilience to trauma. In: *The Trauma and Community Resilience Models.* 2nd ed. New York, NY. Routledge; 2023.
30. Snider L, Van Ommeren M, Schafer A. *Psychological First Aid: Guide for Field Workers.* World Health Organization; 2011.
31. Hobfoll SE, Watson P, Bell CC, et al. Five essential elements of immediate and mid-term mass trauma intervention: empirical evidence. *Psychiatry.* 2007;70:283–315; discussion, 316–369.
32. McNally RJ, Bryant RA, Ehlers A. Does early psychological intervention promote recovery from posttraumatic stress? *Psychol Sci Public Interest.* 2003;4(2):45–79.
33. US Department of Veterans Affairs, U.S. Department of Defense. *VA/DoD Clinical Practice Guideline: Management of Post-traumatic Stress.* 2010. Accessed February 14, 2023. http://www.healthquality.va.gov/PTSD-FULL-2010c.pdf
34. Everly GS, Lee McCabe O, Semon NL, et al. The development of a model of psychological first aid for non–mental health trained public health personnel: the Johns Hopkins RAPID-PFA. *J Public Health Manag Pract.* 2014;20:S24–S29.
35. Kavan MG, Elsasser GN, Barone EJ. The physician's role in managing acute stress disorder. *Am Fam Physician.* 2012;*86*(7):643–649.
36. Gispen F, Wu AW. Psychological first aid: CPR for mental health crises in healthcare. *J Patient Saf Risk Manag.* 2018;23(2):51–53.
37. Edrees H, Connors C, Paine L, Norvell M, Taylor H, Wu AW. Implementing the RISE second victim support programme at the Johns Hopkins Hospital: a case study. *BMJ Open.* 2016;6(9):e011708. doi:10.1136/bmjopen-2016-011708
38. Wu AW, Connors CA, Norvell M. Adapting RISE: meeting the needs of healthcare workers during the COVID-19 pandemic. *Int Rev Psychiatry.* 2021;33(8):711–717. doi:10.1080/09540261.2021.2013783
39. Wu AW, Connors C, Everly GS Jr. COVID-19: peer support and crisis communication strategies to promote institutional resilience. *Ann Intern Med.* 2020;172(12):822–823. doi:10.7326/M20-1236

40. West CP, Dyrbye LN, Erwin PJ, Shanafelt TD. Interventions to prevent and reduce physician burnout: a systematic review and meta-analysis. *Lancet.* 2016;388(10057):2272–2281.
41. Panagioti M, Panagopoulou E, Bower P, et al. Controlled interventions to reduce burnout in physicians: a systematic review and meta-analysis. *JAMA Intern Med.* 2017;177(2):195–205.
42. Jefferson L, Golder S, Heathcote C, et al. GP wellbeing during the COVID-19 pandemic: a systematic review. *Br J Gen Pract.* 2022;72(718):e325–e333.: doi:10.3399/BJGP.2021.0680
43. Shanafelt T, Ripp J, Trockel M. Understanding and addressing sources of anxiety among health care professionals during the COVID-19 pandemic. *JAMA.* 2020;323(21):2133–2134.
44. West CP, Dyrbye LN, Erwin PJ, Shanafelt TD. Interventions to prevent and reduce physician burnout: a systematic review and meta-analysis. *Lancet.* 2016;388(10057):2272–2281. https://doi.org/10.1016/S0140-6736(16)31279-X
45. National Academy of Medicine. Strategies to support the health and well-being of clinicians during the COVID-19 outbreak. Accessed May 29, 2023. https://nam.edu/initiatives/clinician-resilience-and-well-being/clinician-well-being-strategies-during-covid-19
46. Sinsky CA, Daugherty Biddison L, et al. 2020. Organizational evidence-based and promising practices for improving clinician well-being. Discussion Paper. *NAM Perspect.* Accessed May 29, 2023. National Academy of Medicine. https://doi.org/10.31478/202011a
47. World Health Organization. Critical preparedness, readiness and response actions for COVID-19: interim guidance. 2021;2(27):1–3. Accessed May 29, 2023. https://www.who.int/publications-detail/critical-preparedness-readiness-and-response-actions-for-covid-19
48. Jarosińska A, Walicka A, Jarosińska D, Miecznikowska D, Cuchí P. Operational considerations for case management of COVID-19 in health facility and community. *Pediatria i Medycyna Rodzinna.* 2020;16(1):27–32.
49. Clancy C, Goodrich K, Moody-Williams J, et al. Quality, safety, and standards organizations COVID-19 impact assessment: lessons learned and compelling needs. *NAM Perspect.* 2021;2021:10.31478/202107d. Accessed May 29, 2023. https://pubmed.ncbi.nlm.nih.gov/34611603/

31

Remediating Unprofessionalism Among Trainees

Theory, Method, and Practice

Jason Adam Wasserman, Michael J. Redinger, and Tyler S Gibb

Key Points

- Effective remediation of unprofessional behavior by medical educators is challenging, in part because there is no consensus about specific remediation strategies.
- A just culture approach allows for educators to offer effective remediation by following the nuances of context, intent, and developmental stage respective to the unprofessional behavior.
- Developing effective remediation practices and culture is essential to ensure high-quality professionalism education and continued excellence in teaching medical trainees.

Professionalism in Academic Medicine

Professionalism is widely recognized as a core competency in medicine. While sometimes misconstrued as a set of behavioral pleasantries and good bedside manner, professionalism is a highly nuanced, complex, multilayered concept. This complexity has given rise to a wealth of literature attempting to define professionalism in medicine and how it might be taught in the classroom and clinic.[1,2] However, the increased attention to professionalism has only amplified its complexity as this discourse has laid bare its many facets and ambiguities. While different authors have variously focused on professionalism as a virtue, an identity, a behavior, or a skill, in reality it is all of those things.

In this multifaceted view of professionalism, responding to unprofessionalism by trainees simultaneously represents legal, psychological, spiritual, epistemic, philosophical, and practical challenges. Unsurprisingly, strategies for addressing lapses in professionalism remain varied and difficult to assess and validate.[7,22] Insofar as medical education aims to shape not only the knowledge, but also the attitudes and skills of students, much more attention should be placed on best practices for responding to professionalism lapses by trainees. While there are some clear kinds of unprofessionalism that entail serious consequences and around which there is usually significant consensus (e.g., cheating on an exam, inappropriate relationships with patients), addressing less egregious lapses in professionalism can be ambiguous and raise considerable disagreement. While there is consensus that addressing nonegregious lapses is a critical part of professional development, it can be difficult to unpack all of the dimensions of a particular case and strike the proper balance between formative feedback and disciplinary action.

Lucey mentions that we should "consider professionalism lapses to be either analogous to or a form of medical error" and to create "a 'just environment' in which people are encouraged to report professionalism challenges, lapses, and near misses."[14(p14),15] Insightfully, scholars suggest that the lens of medical error can focus us on understanding professionalism as a learned set of skills that require psychologically safe learning environments in which to develop.[12]

In this chapter, we unpack and extend the idea of addressing professionalism through a lens of medical error, drawing on just culture principles that are already familiar to healthcare systems.[16,23] Our previous work highlights how repurposing these concepts helps clarify the ambiguous terrain of professionalism remediation in medical education by providing an architecture for institutional discourse that (1) promotes formative learning environments and (2) fairly and rigorously addresses situations where individuals fall short of expectations. While this chapter begins with describing the ongoing challenges of professionalism remediation and the application of a just culture framework in the remediation of unprofessionalism, we undertake a more thorough discussion of the nuances of this approach, as well as show more practical considerations related to directly addressing these issues with trainees. In particular, we illustrate how a just culture approach sets a foundation for best practices that can be employed in a remediation process. This is critical for academic medicine as it wrestles with how to calibrate expectations of emerging professionals and ensure accountability that is fair, reflexive, and rigorous. It also fulfills its primary aim of thoroughly preparing future physicians for clinical practice.

Challenges of Professionalism Remediation

Professionalism has been recognized as critical for medicine since its origins. Indeed, much of the attention to "ethics" among premodern philosophers of medicine centered on the character of physicians, the manifestation of appropriate humility in providing care, and their interprofessional relationships with each other. Additionally, the sociological contours of professional work highlight the importance of setting standards of professionalism and facilitating adherence to them. Medicine should embody and reflect the "community of profession" where physicians retain a high degree of collective and individual autonomy even in the face of greater external regulation. They, therefore, remain collectively responsible for regulating their disciplinary terrain, including setting and enforcing professional norms within it.[10]

The complexity of medicine also means that professionalism can never be fully captured by a set of rules but will inevitably rely on value-based commitments from each professional.[9] Over the last four decades, the different yet complementary ways of conceptualizing medical professionalism (as a virtue, identity, behavior, and skill) have only increased its ambiguity. Yet, paradoxically, the incursion of external regulation in medicine suggests cultivating a robust and widely endorsed sense of the concept is more important than ever. Ultimately, professionalism is simultaneously a virtue, an identity, a perspective, a skill, and a behavior. Promoting professionalism in medical education, therefore, means identifying and recruiting students with appropriate value orientations but then also fostering their sense of professional self, their understanding of professional norms, their ability to self-regulate their actions under pressure, and their internalization of those norms and values through the habituation of professional practices over time. In the middle of this complex process sits the question of how to identify, evaluate, and respond to lapses in professionalism by trainees.

How to comprehensively evaluate whether trainees meet expectations, whatever those might be, is daunting. As a result, faculty often fall back on, at least implicitly, an attitude of "we'll know it when we see it." They often suggest that while professionalism is not something that experts can easily define in the abstract, lapses in professionalism are comparatively obvious. However, this usually only works to identify outlier behaviors that are strikingly good or bad, leaving more commonplace instances of unprofessionalism unaddressed.[14] This is problematic. Suppose we intend to include professionalism among the core competencies of medical education. In that case, we cannot only address grievous failures but must foster their growth and development among all our students. Indeed, the confounding nature of evaluating and addressing unprofessionalism is made all the more daunting because our students are "in development."

Understanding accountability is critically important, in terms of not only responding appropriately to individual trainees on their developmental path but also cultivating a learning environment that fosters rather than impedes professionalism. The multiple problematics of addressing lapses in professionalism have a common epicenter in their ambiguity. We struggle to clearly define when there has been a lapse and to evaluate its degree of severity in the context of trainee development. Before we can adequately remediate a lapse in professionalism, we have to make sense of what happened and all of the contributory factors involved, individual and systemic. In the next section, we identify a framework for doing this, which will motivate the balance of the chapter focused on best practices for remediation.

Evaluating Professionalism Lapses: A "Just Culture" Approach

Understanding lapses in professionalism as a form of medical error presents an opportunity to utilize the extensive work of healthcare systems that, for more than 20 years, have attempted to address high rates of medical error by drawing on best practices from other high-stakes, high-performance industries such as aviation. This has led to a focus on systemic solutions that both focus on error-proofing processes (e.g., employing forcing functions that make error impossible, such as pin index systems for anesthetic gas hoses) and create institutional cultures that promote safety. In particular, addressing medical errors requires a "culture of psychological safety" that can allow for open dialogue and dissent and facilitate transparent reporting.[8,13]

Among many attempts to promote responses to an error that centrally focus on improving systems and developing personnel rather than on punishment, Marx has articulated a popular procedural approach that recognizes the qualitative differences between inadvertent human error, at-risk behavior, and reckless behavior.[16] In Marx's schema, inadvertent human error results from suboptimal individual functioning, but where a person has not intended or even known they were committing an error or engaging in error-prone behavior (e.g., forgetting to do a regularly scheduled patient repositioning). According to Marx, the proper response is to console the person and reflect on ways that the system in which the person was operating could be made less susceptible to error. At-risk behavior is when an actor knowingly does something wrong or inappropriate but genuinely believes such behavior is inconsequential (e.g., a surgeon who skips a preoperative timeout because she is busy reviewing imaging). In response, it is essential to coach the person who committed the error to raise awareness about the purpose and significance of particular rules and procedures. Finally, reckless behavior refers to a conscious disregard for protocols and processes (e.g., knowingly looking at the medical records of a personal acquaintance). In response, it is vital to institute disciplinary actions as a deterrent.[13] A series of questions posed by Pedroja can further help in classifying an error and therefore identifying the most appropriate way to respond, including

- Did the staff have appropriate skills and relevant training?
- Were the risks were known?
- Were the rules known, or should they have been known?
- Were the expectations clear?
- Were there were relevant exceptional circumstances that justify or mitigate the violation? [21]

We have proposed corresponding categories for lapses in professionalism, where "no-fault suboptimality" (akin to inadvertent human error) calls for affirmation, support, and advising; non-egregious unprofessionalism (akin to at-risk behavior) calls for remediation; and egregious unprofessionalism (akin to reckless behavior) calls for disciplinary action. While perhaps not perfectly analogous to the context of professionalism, these definitions and responses can offer needed clarity about understanding kinds of professionalism lapses and how to respond appropriately without being overly prescriptive.[23] As with the medical error above, we can adapt Pedroja's interrogatives for the context of trainee unprofessionalism to assist us in understanding how best to respond

- Was the expectation clear to the trainee?
- Were there factors beyond the trainee's control?
- What were the trainees' intentions with respect to the behavior?
- Did the trainee have a good faith belief that the violation of the expectation was inconsequential?

The answers to these lead us to a continuum between formative and punitive responses. With this adapted just culture framework in place, we can identify the best general strategy for responding to lapses in professionalism.[23] The following section elaborates best practices for responding to these events. We then conclude by turning a case example to highlight the utility of this model and these more granular best practices for evaluating and responding to professionalism lapses among medical trainees.

Best Practices for Professionalism Remediation

The modified just culture framework described in our previous work,[23] and reviewed in brief above, helps calibrate an overall conception of a lapse in professionalism by a trainee. Depending on how much is known about the lapse, this may help in advance to establish the goals of the conversation and orient the person or group designated to address the incident toward the appropriate balance of formative and punitive consequences. In other cases, mentors and faculty members may partly direct the initial discussions with the student toward exploring the serial interrogatives described above to evaluate what happened and calibrate a response. In such cases, throughout the initial conversations, the person or group designated to address the issues should address the questions above to the trainee to gather the information needed. However, professionalism remediation entails an overall conceptualization of the situation and a complex interaction between the trainee and those leading the remediation. The interactive nature of professionalism remediation can be even more complicated, though in different ways, than evaluating and classifying an incident. This section discusses best practices for engaging in remediation with a trainee following a lapse in professionalism. Here, we take "remediation" to encompass all the ways one might address the incident to improve performance in the future. For clarity, we center much of the discussion on the initial conversation with the trainee about the incident. The best practices described next are then exemplified with the case application in the subsequent section.

Take Your Own Pulse

There are a number of factors that can impede the productivity of a remediation, but in our experience, the foremost modifiable factor is the discomfort of the person tasked with addressing it. Remediation conversations can become highly emotional. Trainees who have had a professionalism lapse may feel shame and guilt, which can often be expressed as anger, defensiveness, or sadness. These can interfere with the productive, forward-looking goals of the remediation. Despite the best practices for destigmatizing the situation described below, one cannot control how a trainee will respond. However, we can manage our own level of emotion and manage our discomfort, which in turn will help level the otherwise emotional nature of the moment.[17]

Along with the discursive strategies below, which help mitigate the uncomfortable nature of the discussion, it can be helpful to acknowledge to oneself that such conversations are difficult and sometimes awkward. We perform poorly and make bad decisions under stress, so it is important to maintain an even temperament both externally and internally throughout the process. For most, it is human nature to avoid conflict, and no matter how much one tries to excise the posture of conflict from the encounter, it may remain an undercurrent of the remediation. Acknowledging the resulting discomfort is helpful at the outset, as is self-monitoring whether one is feeling flustered or uncomfortable throughout the conversation.

Set the Tone

Along with monitoring one's emotional state and discomfort, setting up an environment that contributes to the goals and desired tone of the meeting is vital. Generally, it is appropriate to let the trainee know about the general nature of the meeting in advance. However, it is also important not to engage in extensive discussion or to allow the student to try to "litigate" the issue over email. Instead, identifying the problem that has been raised in general terms is sufficient, and if the student demands more information, it is appropriate to defer to the forthcoming meeting. If the trainee seeks an impromptu discussion about the issue (e.g., unexpectedly stopping by one's office), they are likely to have an emotional response. In such situations, it will be essential to de-escalate at the moment and defer the conversation to the scheduled time.

If possible, conducting the meeting in a private but "neutral" space is advisable (e.g., a conference room rather than an office). Sitting adjacent to the trainee rather than across a desk or table also conveys a sentiment of collaborating on an issue rather than reflecting opposing sides or an adversarial setting.[20] Finally, where appropriate, starting the meeting with some small talk unrelated to the professionalism lapse can help ease everyone into a conversational mode and help build trust.

Establish Parameters and Goals

As the conversation begins, it can be helpful to communicate the institution's view of professionalism to the trainee. Institutional views of professionalism might entail a description of how professionalism is part of the core competencies within the academic program (rather than as a topic separate from or ancillary to the core educational program), as well as acknowledging the view of professionalism as a behavioral event rather than a function of character. For example, one might begin by saying

> At the school, we only admit students that we believe have the right values and commitments. We define a professionalism lapse simply as an event that was suboptimal and for which there were modifiable factors under the student's control. Thus, when professionalism issues come up, we try to identify what factors caused those and how we can provide support and education so that they don't happen again.

Emphasizing that the purpose of the meeting is intended to be formative instead of punitive from the outset may increase the willingness of the student to engage in self-reflective and honest conversation. This brief introduction helps shift the focus away from the trainee's character or sense of self, which would make them more prone to perceiving the remediation as an existential threat or an indictment of their core character and toward an objective review of what occurred. Ultimately, one goal is to externalize the professionalism lapse, rendering the action an object of legitimate critical evaluation by all involved, including the trainee, rather than an accusation of a character defect, which may precipitate unhelpful defensiveness.

Elicit Narrative

After setting the stage to promote dialogue, limit defensiveness, and destigmatize the remediation process, it is essential to conduct the conversation in ways that maximize information sharing, insight and reflection, and openness to improvement. The strategies here parallel best practices for empathic interviewing in the clinical context, including using open-ended questions and eliciting narrative with minimal encouragers.[3] This approach often begins by asking the student what happened and allowing them time to fully articulate their view of the situation. In the best situations, the student will have already reflected on what happened, which would include critically examining the action and the context of the lapse, having insights about its root causes, and plans to improve performance in the future. In other situations, the trainee may not have engaged in much reflection and may not be as forthcoming with their narrative and thoughts. In that case, the use of minimal encouragers can help spur the conversation further. Simply remaining silent when the trainee pauses while talking can communicate that you want them to continue. Other times, short, nondirective statements such as "uh huh" and "yes" will encourage the trainee to continue their narrative. Still, in different situations, one may request that they provide more detail and description straightforwardly. In some situations, trainees may have significantly limited insights into their behavior. While this will require a more directive posture, questions should still be sufficiently open ended to elicit a narrative: "What would you do differently next time?"; "How do you think the faculty member perceived what you said?"; "If you saw a colleague doing the same thing, what advice would you give them?"

The overall goal at this point in the conversation is to elicit the trainee's perspective with as little input or direction as possible by soliciting the trainee's view of the situation, their conceptualization of the event, and their professional identity more generally. This undisturbed view is essential for calibrating the response and providing the student with the most appropriate education and support. It is endemic to the role of the educator to share our insights and lessons with learners. However, consistent with the more general push toward self-directed inquiry, doing so too early in the conversation can obviate the trainee's reflections about the lapse and, more importantly, the opportunity for them to practice this kind of self-reflection, which is a crucial skill of the profession. Instead, observing them as they engage in this kind of reflection gives the remediator the opportunity to address the need to improve performance around the particular issue and to affirm and guide their emerging capacity for self-assessment.

Conclude With Empathy and Action Items

After the student's insights and reflections have been fully elicited, it is then appropriate for the person or group conducting the remediation to share their thoughts and observations about the lapse in professionalism. Certainly, these can be corrective. Trainees sometimes fail to fully appreciate the gravity of their actions or why those actions have been perceived as unprofessional. Or they may not have as many ideas about improving their performance in these areas as those with more experience navigating various professional challenges. Thus, sharing one's expertise, insights, and experiences remains a critical part of the remediation. It is important to preface this part of the discussion with a demonstration of genuine concern for the trainee, reiterating that the goal of the remediation is to improve performance and noting that this is a natural part of professional development. It should be clear to the trainee that, in all but the most egregious of cases, such as criminal behavior that puts patients at risk, the sincere hope of the faculty is to see the student improve, grow, and succeed.

The conclusion of the conversation should center on the next steps. Here also the trainee's insights are essential. Opening this part of the conversation with an open-ended question is advisable (e.g., "What do you think your next steps should be?"). Eliciting the trainee's ideas is helpful because the trainee will naturally have greater buy-in for any viable ideas they can generate. Of course, in many cases, the trainee will not be able to sufficiently articulate a remediation plan, or at least not entirely. As mentioned above, the insights and experience of the faculty will be vital as they propose action items that the trainee themselves may not have articulated. It is, of course, essential that the remediation plan be proportional to the lapse that occurred. Often, remediation plans involve changes that the trainee makes on their own rather than requiring the ongoing involvement of faculty or mentors.

In other cases, a more robust plan may require multiple meetings, monitoring, or the assignment of a designated professionalism mentor. In choosing such a mentor, suggestions from the trainee can help identify individuals with whom they already have rapport and whom they may already respect.

At the same time, the nature of professionalism mentorship requires a mentor that holds high professionalism standards, understands the significance of professionalism as a core competency, and is able and willing to engage in difficult conversations with the trainee and give direct and honest feedback.

The closing of the meeting should involve clear articulation of the identified next steps, who is responsible for each, and a timeline about when each individual should accomplish them. Of note, this may involve the trainee or faculty member taking responsibility for action items related to the remediation of the student and the faculty member pursuing identified issues within the learning environment or institution that may have played a critical contributing role. Following up with the trainee about these issues conveys sincerity about the holistic and formative view of professionalism inherent in the just culture framework. For students concerned that any minor professionalism lapse and need for brief remediation may result in long-term professional harm, it may be helpful to reiterate, at least whenever it is accurate, that the process is formative, time limited, and information sharing constrained to only those considered to have a "need to know." For other students who struggle to buy into the process, it may be necessary to inform them that failure to participate in the process's formative aspects could be interpreted as egregious unprofessionalism and result in punitive action.

Applying the Just Culture Framework and Remediation Best Practices

In this section, we examine a case of relatively commonplace unprofessionalism. We provide a sample dialogue to elaborate on the best practices for remediation, including a remediation plan, and then briefly apply the just culture framework to calibrate the appropriate remediation plan. Importantly, nothing about our just culture framework or the strategies for remediation are meant to be definitive. Reasonable people can disagree about the seriousness of a particular action or the best strategies for addressing it. Moreover, the idiosyncrasies of any real-world situation have to be navigated with nuance and adjustment. The analysis and sample discussions that follow are intended only as sample approaches to the best practices mentioned above while recognizing that there might be many variations or reasons to deviate from those best practices in particular cases.

Given the static and brief nature of cases presented in text format, readers will inevitably find themselves unsure about particular claims or the answers to particular questions. In a real-life case, these ambiguities suggest matters that warrant further inquiry. We necessarily make assumptions for this text, while other issues may remain undetermined. The critical point is to exemplify how the just culture framework can be employed to assess the accusation of a lapse in professionalism.

A Case of Commonplace Unprofessionalism

GN is an internal medicine (IM) PGY-3 with plans to apply for an infectious disease fellowship. Their evaluations have generally been "meets expectations," but narrative comments have raised several concerns about professionalism. In particular, GN rarely attends the biweekly case review sessions led by the IM Fellows, which address challenging or unique cases. When asked about this, they noted that these were "optional, not required sessions." At the same time, GN struggled to differentiate necrotizing fasciitis from cellulitis in a recent patient case, which was a condition covered at these case review sessions. At other meetings and events, they often text on their phone during presentations and discussions. Several times, GN belatedly called to notify the coordinator, rather than the residency director, that they would be late because of child care issues. The late and inappropriately directed notification caused problems with clinical coverage because the program director did not know where GN was.

> One clinical faculty, Dr. S., pulled GN aside to address some of these issues. Dr. S. reported that GN became very angry and tearful, and Dr. S. did not think GN "heard the message." There were no noticeable changes to GN's behavior after the conversation with Dr. S.

The Talk—A Model Conversation

As the professionalism advisor for graduate medical education at your institution, you are tasked with mentoring GN. You schedule a meeting with GN in a conference room. Your email request for a meeting is brief:

> Dear GN,
>
> I received a concern related to some recent absences, attentiveness, and communication. I'd like to meet with you to discuss these. Please let me know if you can meet at noon on Wednesday.
>
> Sincerely, Dr. BR

GN's reply was also brief, but reasonably courteous:

> Dear Dr. BR,
>
> I'm concerned to hear this. I wish someone would have spoken to me directly before raising it to you. I'm happy to meet with you at noon on Wednesday.

Prior to GN's arrival, you take a couple of minutes to review the concerns and jot down key questions that you have, particularly those related to GN's understanding of the expectations, perception of barriers to meeting those expectations, intentions when engaging in some of the observed behaviors, and GN's perception of these alleged professionalism lapses (see "Take Your Own Pulse").

GN arrives and is polite, but there is a clear undertone of frustration. You begin by establishing the parameters of the conversation:

BR: As you may know, one of my roles here is as professionalism advisor. In that role, I often explore issues with residents where things are happening that are suboptimal, and we look for ways to make it better. Sometimes that involves things that program can do to remove barriers for trainees so they can better meet expectations, and it involves helping trainees identify things they need to work on in order to improve.

GN: Okay. I mean, like I said, I don't know why whoever is concerned about me couldn't have just said something to me themselves.

BR: Why don't you tell me what's been going on from your perspective?

GN: I don't really know. I've missed some shifts, but I've always called in. I have a two-year-old son and his babysitter has canceled on me at the last minute four times over the last three weeks. There's just nothing I can do about that. But I don't know why it's a problem because I've always called in.

BR: [*nods and waits*]

GN: And, I guess that's really it. I guess that's why I'm here. . . . I mean Dr. S. got mad at me for being on my phone during our prerounding meeting, but honestly, we had been going round and round about the same patient for like 20 minutes and my babysitter was having trouble getting my son to eat anything for lunch, so I was having to send her things he likes to eat.

BR: Before you said that no one had addressed these issues with you, but it sounds like Dr. S. at least tried to do that.

GN: I wouldn't say they *tried*. They pulled me over to the side, but several other residents could still hear and just told me that I needed to shape up and there was no excuse for missing shifts and that they hadn't missed a single shift in over ten years. I was so embarrassed I just started crying. And then Dr. S. said I had a deficit in clinical knowledge, but I haven't had a single issue with my patients except that I mixed up two skin conditions. But that's what my attending is there for, to catch my mistakes and help me learn from them.

BR: Dr. S's conversation with you aside, how do you think that's being perceived by your colleagues and faculty?

GN: [*with a perturbed tone*]

I mean, clearly not well. But I'm an adult and I have other responsibilities outside of here.

BR: [*nodding slightly*]

mm hmm

GN: I mean, I guess I understand why they'd be annoyed with me too. But I feel like I can't do as much as the other residents, or prepare as hard, or be as focused as they are because I have my son.

BR: If you could roll back time about 6 months and do it over again, what would you change?

GN: I'd definitely have a backup babysitter on call. Maybe a few of them just in case. And I guess I could get my mother to be available by phone if there are questions or concerns from the sitter. She lives far away, but she knows him really well and she could answer those kinds of questions.

BR: It sounds to me like those would both be good ideas going forward.

GN: I guess so.

BR: We all have lots of demands on us and sometimes genuine emergencies come up. But your work here, both in terms of taking care of patients and in terms of learning as much as you can for your future patients, is important too. I think everyone just wants you to be present, both physically and mentally, so that you can make the most out of your experience here and so that you can make the best contributions to your team.

GN: I can appreciate that.

BR: [*waiting for a few seconds, but realizing GN won't continue speaking*]

But also, I'm a bit concerned by something you said before about "going round and round about a patient and getting nowhere."

GN: Uh huh.

BR: Well, as you know, sometimes we have patients with tricky conditions and figuring out how best to care for them can be really challenging. Rather than seeing that conversation as boring or fruitless, I wonder whether you might be missing an opportunity to contribute to your knowledge and expertise about a difficult case, and whether you might also be missing an important learning opportunity that might help you with future patients in a similar situation.

GN: I guess.

BR: [*wondering whether GN's last statement was fully sincere or just intended to placate*]

Why don't you work on those things over the next couple of weeks and let me know how it's going over email. And then, let's plan to meet again on the 31st? In the meantime, I'm going to inquire about the process for reporting unexpected absences and get you clear information about that. If we need to talk sooner to work through any barriers, just let me know.

GN: Okay.

Using the adapted series of interrogatives, we can assess this case through a lens of just culture, helping to focus us on improving performance at both the individual and systemic levels (See Table 31.1). First, we would ask *whether the expectations were clear to the trainee.* Zimbardo (1969) first coined the phrase "hidden curriculum" to describe the "the unspoken or implicit academic and social rules, values, and expectations that are taught to medical students."[11,24] Ambiguous or unclear expectations lead to frustration. In this case, the implicit expectation of attending the IM fellow case review sessions may not have been sufficiently clear to GN given that these are explicitly described as optional. In fact, GN cited this as a justification for not attending. Unclear or unspoken expectations are an opportunity for systemic improvement across medical education. GN's residency program leadership may consider whether attending the IM fellow sessions should be required or, perhaps, only required for those with particular knowledge deficits. Either way, the expectation should be clear. In any event, if the sessions are described as *optional*, then it would be difficult to say someone who does not attend has acted unprofessionally.

Additionally, all trainees should be aware of clinical competence expectations. GN should know whether accurately differentiating necrotizing fasciitis and cellulitis is a reasonable clinical competency at this stage in their training. Further investigation might be necessary, but based on the conversation with Dr. BR, GN perceives her difficulty in distinguishing those two conditions as a learning opportunity rather than something she should already know. Gaining greater clarity on this may involve examining the residency's curriculum and learning objectives. Finally, it does seem clear that GN

Table 31.1 Just Culture Assessment

Interogative	Summary Assessment	Action
Were the expectations clear to the trainee?	Expectations of Attendance at Session: Unclear Expectations of Clinical Knowledge : Potentially unclear (needs further investigation) Expectations about Behavior at Educational Sessions (e.g., texting): Clear	Give feedback to the program on clarifying these expectations Investigate how expectations of clinical knowledge are communicated; give feedback as appropriate Establish with trainee that expectations were clear; explore other factors below.
Were there factors beyond the trainee's control?	Potentially, but the chronic nature of these incidents suggests they have not been adequately responded to by the trainee	Evaluate systemic processes that have aggravated the situation (e.g., notification process for trainee absence) Give trainee feedback on need to resolve external factors that are persistently interfering with performance; assist as able in helping resolve those
What were the trainee's intentions?	Nonmalicious, but inconsiderate of impact on the learning environment	Acknowledge that trainee did not have malicious intentions but is still responsible for impact of actions (see below)
Did trainee have a good faith (but incorrect) belief that this unprofessionalism was justified or inconsequential?	Yes: trainee appears to believe that external factors justify behavior Yes: trainee appears to believe that behavior is inconsequential	Provide feedback related to permissibility of emergency situations, but persistent, recurring issues need to be addressed and are not justified Give feedback to trainee about the consequences of this behavior on both trainee's own learning and career and on others

knows that texting during those educational sessions contravenes the expectation of engagement in meetings and presentations.

Second, we explore whether *factors beyond the trainee's control made it impossible to meet the expectation.* Certainly, emergencies with child care sometimes can render it impossible to make it to a shift or may require the attention of a working parent during work hours. These factors can be beyond the control of a trainee. However, at a minimum, the frequency of absences and the continued personal phone use during educational events raises the question of whether GN has made a reasonable effort to anticipate and proactively address these issues. The chronic nature of these professionalism concerns suggests that GN has not made an adequate effort. Indeed, when asked about what might have been done differently, GN quickly identified several viable steps that may help. Here also, however, there are systemic issues that may also need to be addressed. In particular, GN notified the program coordinator of her child care situation, but due to no fault of GN, there seems to be a communication gap that resulted in the program director not being notified. There may be program-level improvements that could attenuate the burdens and irritations associated with unexpected trainee absences, including a better or at least clearer notification system and expectations.

Third, we should explore *the trainee's intentions.* Though intentions can be hard to discern and impossible to verify, conversations with the trainee about why these behaviors are continuing may elicit information that helps identify what kind of remediation may be appropriate and effective. For example, a trainee who suggests texting and being disengaged during an educational session because they found it boring and unimportant requires a different response than when a trainee believes media multitasking during a presentation does not impede learning. In the example case, GN seems to understand that texting during meetings and presentations is distracting but fails to appreciate its impact on the team, the patient, or her own learning.

Finally, we want to investigate whether the trainee *had a good faith belief that the alleged violations of professional expectations were justified or inconsequential.* As with the notion of intention, it can be challenging to assess and impossible to verify whether one's claims about the justification for a professionalism lapse are genuinely made in good faith. Nevertheless, the information provided in the conversation suggests that GN had a good faith, although mistaken, belief that their efforts in the program were sufficient and that the need to attend to personal obligations provided sufficient justification for times when GN fell short.

In the conversation with GN, BR utilizes many of the best practices articulated above. GN seems to begin the conversation frustrated and exhibits some defensiveness and hostility at other points. However, by continuing to explore her thoughts, BR minimized conflict and kept the conversation focused on assessing what happened and determining how GN can improve. Indeed, BR allows GN space to formulate a strategy for improvement, which inevitably engenders greater buy-in than if BR had taken a paternalistic or directive approach.

At the same time, BR does not let GN "off the hook" on things about which GN appears to lack insight (e.g., the notion of going "round and round" about a patient). Because GN did not appear sufficiently reflective about this incident, BR stepped in to offer some insights, but only after GN had the opportunity.

Remediation Plan

Based on the information learned from the conversation with GN, we would classify the behavior as "nonegregious unprofessionalism." She does not seem wantonly dismissive of the expectations but instead appears to justify her actions to herself primarily by appealing to the importance of her child care challenges. GN's behavior should not be excused or tolerated, but at the same time, the impediments and failures to meet the program's expectations should be appropriately addressed. Of course, if GN's problematic behavior continued, there could no longer be a good faith belief that these lapses were inconsequential or justified. At that point, the approach to GN's remediation should escalate.

The conclusion of the conversation between GN and BR does not constitute a formal remediation plan of the sort we might expect in serious or egregious unprofessionalism. There are, however, clear next steps and a plan to follow up. Notably, there will be an opportunity to evaluate GN's attempts to resolve these issues over the next couple of weeks. Preplanning the follow-up meeting also helps mitigate the perception that the second meeting is related to continued shortcomings in her performance rather than an inherent part of the process. Depending on how successful GN is at implementing changes, that meeting can be used to provide additional feedback or affirmation of success (or sometimes both). Perhaps most important, while GN's attitude and lack of insight may be frustrating, BR does not lose focus on the goal of educating and mentoring the trainee. It would be easy for BR to become frustrated, but this likely would only exacerbate conflict and cause GN to become even more defensive.

While it is clear that GN needed feedback about the questionable behavior, systemic issues have also been uncovered. For one, there does not appear to be a clear absence policy or a straightforward or effective process for reporting unexpected absences. The residency coordinator appears to receive notices from GN but may not reliably forward them to the residency director. Additionally, the list of clinical knowledge expectations may need to be more explicitly articulated to trainees so they can be aware of deficits. Frustration with a trainee not attending optional instructional sessions also signals a gap between departmental norms and explicit expectations, which may need to be addressed. Finally, it may be worth following up with Dr. S. about the conversation with GN. Certainly, GN may be overreacting to or misremembering Dr. S.'s feedback, but aspects of that conversation likely could have been improved (e.g., not having an impromptu conversation and not discussing professionalism concerns in front of others). More broadly, training faculty in best practices for giving effective feedback, particularly regarding potentially sensitive professionalism issues, may improve the learning environment.

Navigating Around Land Mines in the Conversation

Conversations about unprofessionalism and unmet professional expectations can be challenging for everyone involved. Sensitivity to potential land mines that are unique to professionalism remediation can help improve the process, reduce stress and anxiety, and encourage the receptiveness of the trainee. These land mines include unknown or disputed facts, high emotions, defensiveness or argumentativeness, and lack of insight or self-reflection.

Unknown or Disputed Facts

Important facts about what happened and the context of the alleged unprofessional behavior, may be unknown to the remediator. Regardless of the diligence of inquiry beforehand, the faculty mentor will simply lack some facts and much of the nuance until they have an initial conversation with the trainee. Epistemological humility is thus important for faculty members as they engage in remediation conversations. Similarly, the trainee accused of unprofessionalism may disagree with or refute some of the facts as understood by the faculty member. For example, in the case above, the facts related to the conversation between GN and Dr. S. may be disputed. However, other aspects of unprofessionalism are not. Focusing on lessons derived from points of agreement is, therefore, essential for effective remediation.

High Emotions

Emotions are likely to run high during these conversations. Trainees accused of unprofessionalism can be emotionally triggered, regardless of the validity of the concerns.

Medical trainees are often highly accomplished individuals who are accustomed to being successful and respected by their peers and mentors. Accusations of unprofessionalism can be shocking, disorienting, or demoralizing and can trigger feelings of inadequacy, self-doubt, and imposter syndrome. In some situations, these conversations can rekindle past experiences that were difficult or traumatic. Although it is nearly impossible to predict how a trainee will be emotionally impacted, faculty mentors should be aware of the potential for disproportionate or extreme emotional reactions. In the case above, GN responded reasonably well. Had GN exhibited a more extreme, disproportionate emotional reaction, however, it may have been necessary for BR to step back and unpack that reaction and its causes first, before attempting to address the professionalism lapse itself. Including other faculty or staff with competence and training in dealing with emotional dysregulation may be helpful as well.

Defensiveness or Argumentativeness

Some trainees will react to accusations of unprofessionalism with high emotions and a high degree of defensiveness or argumentativeness. This response may reflect an automatic immature defense mechanism where they intellectualize or deny when faced with a perceived "attack." Intellectualization and denial allow the trainee to unconsciously shield themselves from the natural painful feelings that result from being made aware of their shortcomings. Faculty mentors may need to respond by acknowledging the trainee's emotions and asking them to purposely reflect on these emotions as part of the remediation process.

Suppose the trainee consistently tries to reorient the conversation away from their actions. In that case, the faculty member may need to remind the trainee that while the systemic failures that contributed to the situation should and will be addressed, the purpose of the meeting is also to try to problem-solve how the trainee might have responded more appropriately.

Lack of Insight or Self-Reflection

Trainees accused of unprofessionalism may demonstrate a lack of self-reflection or an appreciation of the concerns of unprofessional behavior or poor insight. Beyond providing education not only about professional and ethical standards broadly, it may also be helpful to share with the trainee those studies demonstrating that professionalism concerns identified early in the course of training are predictive of future professional misconduct. Highlighting the stark consequences of malpractice litigation or citation by the state board of medicine, including case studies, may improve the trainee's understanding of the importance of professionalism training and remediation.

Institutional Concerns

The remediation process and policies should proactively address institutional legal considerations. Professionalism remediation efforts should not inadvertently create legal issues for the institution or the faculty mentors. Professionalism remediation approaches must be sensitive to legal liability, which may implicate federally protected learner information privacy standards.[6] Privacy protections are equally important in the inquiry stage of remediation, as in the intervention and follow-up stages of the process. Given the sensitivity surrounding professionalism conversations and the potential for escalation to punitive consequences that the trainee could challenge via litigation, documentation and procedural soundness are essential. Having staff or faculty uninvolved with the trainee's evaluations (e.g., colleagues from human resources or employee relations) act as witnesses to the conversation may be prudent in some cases. The professionalism mentor might consider audio recording the conversation for their records. However, states vary regarding whether or not both parties must consent to the recording of the meeting. Consultation with institutional legal counsel before creating a formal professionalism remediation process is recommended to address these kinds of concerns.

Four additional land mines prevalent to professionalism remediation deserve further exploration and study: the dynamic nature of professionalism in healthcare; the impact of professionalism remediation on underrepresented in medicine and minority trainees; choosing appropriate mentors; and sensitively assessing the impact of student mental health on professionalism lapses and as a barrier to remediation.

Dynamic Understandings of Professionalism

Standards of professionalism will inevitably change as cultural norms and expectations of physician behavior change over time. For example, visible tattooing that may have been considered unprofessional decades prior may now pass entirely unnoticed if not encouraged as an expression of individuality. Professional guidelines in social media use also have varied over time as social media has become increasingly ubiquitous, generations of new physicians grew up as digital "natives," and the distinction between personal and professional online identities becomes blurred. Professional societies, teaching institutions, regulatory bodies, and the public play a valuable role in an ongoing dialogue exploring which behaviors constitute unprofessionalism.

The Impact on Underrepresented Minority (URM) Trainees

Because of that fluctuation in professional standards, those charged with developing, teaching, and enforcing professional standards must ensure that those standards are not implicitly or explicitly biased against marginalized communities. For example, professionalism standards have been rightly criticized for penalizing trainees with natural hairstyles more common in the African American community and disproportionately policing female attire. Moreover, accusations of unprofessionalism land disproportionately on minority trainees and faculty members, as well as those who are underrepresented in medicine.[19] Remediation efforts must be sensitive to the dynamic nature of professionalism and the growing recognition that professionalism standards may unjustly be used as tools to exclude members of marginalized communities from the medical profession. The just culture framework presented in this chapter helps to create an unbiased, dynamic, transparent, and repeatable approach to addressing accusations of unprofessionalism in healthcare. These characteristics will help mitigate the nefarious influence of unconscious and conscious bias and the hidden curriculum, which may disproportionately impact minority trainees.

Choosing the Right Mentor

Appropriate reflection on the experiences of individual students and the intersectional factors that may contribute to trainee marginalization help ensure that the faculty mentors have the appropriate resources and skills for success. The choice of a faculty member is critical but complex. A mentorship model of remediation turns significantly on the mentor's quality, ability, availability, and skills necessary to engage effectively with and help a struggling trainee. Many institutions will be able to readily identify a handful of exceptional faculty members to be effective, positive, life-changing mentors. However, these faculty mentors will likely have many other time and resource commitments. Faculty development is critical to equitably sharing the mentoring load, ensuring high quality mentorship, and that trainees receive consistent coaching that reflects a shared institutional philosophy. Moreover, properly accounting for and crediting the work of these mentors is incumbent on the institution to ensure that the work is valued and appropriately compensated.

Because the quality of mentorship is so essential, poor mentors must be identified, and if development and mentoring are unsuccessful, their interactions with trainees who need excellent mentorship should be restricted or eliminated. Additionally, mentors should demonstrate professionalism in their own practices. Poor mentors can undermine the utility of any approach to professionalism remediation, both when they do not engage in remediation best practices and when they are more generally poor role models. The literature has long discussed these aspects of both beneficial and harmful hidden curriculum in medical training.[18]

Assessing the Impact of Mental Health on Professional Lapses

In explaining their professionalism lapses, students may share their belief that mental health issues contributed to the situation. A study examining physicians referred for unprofessional conduct found that while over 70% were fit for duty, a majority met the criteria for at least one psychiatric diagnosis. It also found that alleged disruptive behavior was correlated with abnormal personality diagnoses and a history of childhood abuse, trauma, depression, and substance abuse.[26] Another study of serious ethical violations in medicine found that more than half of cases involved a wrongdoer with suspected cluster B personality disorder or substance use disorder.[5] Finally, a study of student misconduct found a strong association between subjective burnout and professionalism lapses.[4]

The potential intersection of mental illness and unprofessionalism raises challenges for those charged with remediation. While mental illness has been shown to correlate with unprofessional behavior, in many cases, a direct causative explanation is less clear-cut. Those charged with professionalism remediation may need to mandate a fitness for duty evaluation, especially if the professionalism lapses are repetitive or place patients or others at risk of harm. Erratic behavior may suggest the need for substance use disorder assessment and drug screening. Sensitive questioning may reveal trainee depression or suicidal ideation and provide an opportunity to intervene. Addressing systematic causes of trainee burnout may decrease the risk of unprofessional conduct in the trainee population as a whole. While many medical schools have utilized these and other strategies for remediation of professionalism lapses, consistent success remains elusive.[25]

Conclusion

Effective remediation of unprofessional behavior by trainees will continue to be challenging for medical educators. A consensus on specific remediation strategies is unlikely to materialize since a precise definition of what professionalism entails is dynamic and responsive to cultural, generational, and societal shifts. Nonetheless, utilizing a just culture approach offers a great deal of potential utility and allows for the nuances of context, intent, and developmental stage to be considered.

Despite the complexity of professionalism remediation, identifying unprofessionalism, addressing it, and giving trainees every opportunity to develop into excellent healthcare providers is the burden and privilege of medical educators. If medicine continues to be one of the most respected professions in society, trainees must continue to develop professionalism worthy of that respect. A just culture framework for professionalism remediation may be the best approach to ensuring excellence in clinical skills and professionalism in future physicians.

References

1. Birden H, Glass N, Wilson I, Harrison M, Usherwood T, Nass D. Teaching professionalism in medical education: a best evidence medical education (BEME) systematic review. BEME guide no. 25. *Med Teach.* 2013;35(7):e1252–e1266. doi:10.3109/0142159x.2013.789132
2. Birden H, Glass N, Wilson I, Harrison M, Usherwood T, Nass D. Defining professionalism in medical education: a systematic review. *Med Teach.* 2014;36(1):47–61. doi:10.3109/0142159x.2014.850154
3. Cole SA, Bird J. *The Medical Interview.* 3rd ed. Saunders; 2014.
4. Dyrbye LN, Massie FS, Eacker A, Harper W, Power D, Durning SJ, et al. Relationship between burnout and professional conduct and attitudes among US medical students. *JAMA.* 2010;304(11):1173–1180.
5. DuBois JM, Anderson EE, Chibnall JT, Mozersky J, Walsh HA. Serious ethical violations in medicine: a statistical and ethical analysis of 280 cases in the United States from 2008–2016. *Am J Bioeth.* 2019;19(1):16–34.
6. Family Education Privacy Rights [FERPA], 20 U.S.C. § 1232g (1974).
7. Frankel RM. Remediating professional lapses of medical students: each school an island? In: Byyny RL, Papadakis MA, Paauw DS, eds. Medical professionalism: best practices. Alpha Omega Alpha Honor Medical Society; 2015:115–133.
8. Gawande A. *The Checklist Manifesto: How to Get Things Right.* Metropolitan Books; 2009.
9. Gibb TS, Redinger MJ, Crutchfield PA, Minser J. Ethical and Professional considerations in integrated behavioral health. *Pediatr Clin North Am.* 2021.;68(3):607–619.
10. Goode WJ. Community within a community: the professions. *Am Sociol Rev.* 1957;22(2):194–200.
11. Hafferty FW. Beyond curriculum reform. *Acad Med.* 1998;73:403.
12. Herron P. A calling to professionalism. *MedEdPublish.* 2017;6(4):49.
13. Khatri N, Brown GD, Hicks LL. From a blame culture to a just culture in health care. *Health Care Manage Rev.* 2009;34(4):312–322.

14. Lucey CR. The problem with professionalism. In: Byyny RL, Papadakis MA, Paauw DS, eds. *Medical Professionalism: Best Practices.* Alpha Omega Alpha Honor Medical Society; 2015:9–21.

15. Lucey C, Souba W. Perspective: the problem with the problem of professionalism. *Acad Med.* 2010;85:1018–1024.

16. Marx D. *Whack-a-Mole: The Price We Pay for Expecting Perfection.* By Your Side Studios; 2009.

17. Mischel W, DeSmet AL, Kross E. Self-regulation in the service of conflict resolution. In: Deutsch M, Coleman PT, Marcus EC. *The Handbook of Conflict Resolution: Theory and Practice.* 2nd ed. Jossey-Bass; 2006:294–313.

18. Michalec B, Hafferty FW. Stunting professionalism: the potency and durability of the hidden curriculum within medical education. *Soc Theory Health.* 2013;11:338–406.

19. Osseo-Asare A, Balasuriya L, Huot SJ, Keene D, Berg D, Nunez-Smith M, et al. Minority resident physicians' views on the role of race/ethnicity in their training experiences in the workplace. *JAMA Netw Open.* 2018;1(5):e182723.

20. Parker T, Lambert RJ. *Is That Your Hand in My Pocket? The Sales Professional's Guide to Negotiating.* Thomas Nelson; 2008.

21. Pedroja ATA. The culture of safety. In: Agrawal A, ed. *Patient Safety: A Case-Based Comprehensive Guide.* Springer; 2019:341–353.

22. Pfeil SA, Paauw DS. Review of current models for remediation of professionalism lapses. In: Byyny RL, Papadakis MA, Paauw DS, eds. *Medical Professionalism: Best Practices.* Alpha Omega Alpha Honor Medical Society; 2015:51–57.

23. Wasserman JA, Redinger M, Gibb T. Responding to unprofessional behavior by trainees—a "just culture." *Framework.* 2020;382:773–777. doi:10.1056/nejmms1912591

24. Zimbardo P. The hidden curriculum and its role in education. *School Rev.* 1969;77:561.

25. Ziring D, et al. How do medical schools identify and remediate professionalism lapses in medical students? A study of US and Canadian medical schools. *Acad Med*: 2015;90(7):913–920.

26. Finlayson AJ, Dietrich MS, Neufeld R, et al. Restoring professionalism: the physician fitness-for-duty evaluation. *Gen Hosp Psychiatry.* 2013;35(6):659–663.

32

Advocating for Diversity, Equity, Inclusion, and Social Justice

A Reimagined Professionalism

Carlos S. Smith, Saleem Razack, and P. Preston Reynolds

Key Points

- Structural and social justice consciousness needs to be a focus of medical professionalism and medical professionalism education.
- A focus on increasing diversity within healthcare is important but will fail unless the healthcare environment is, itself, structured to accommodate and support individuals from diverse backgrounds.
- An antioppressive framework is a promising means by which to attain an organizational structure able to accommodate and support diversity among its medical professionals.

Introduction—Structural Discrimination and the Professionalization of Medicine and Healthcare

Medicine in North America grew on the foundation of structural discrimination that permeated every aspect of the health professions and patient care. In this chapter, we focus on the United States and Canada since both have initiatives to reframe professionalism around diversity, equity, inclusion, belonging, and justice. To be clear, there is a need to bring structural and social justice consciousness into professionalism—this is the crux of the chapter, what is lacking is that most models of professionalism are relational, minus context. We propose the context as key, particularly given the vast health inequities and disparities that remain globally today.[1] Additionally, understanding the historic narratives that align with today's zeal for eliminating and mitigating current health inequities and disparities is key. Worth noting is a specific attention to expanding the typical notions of diversity, equity, and inclusion, to also include belonging and justice. Increasing diversity is frequently the focus of our academic medical systems and individual institutions, but little consideration is given to whether the environment supports diverse individuals' well-being and satisfies the basic human need to feel secure, respected, and engaged,[2,3] let alone moving toward a true understanding of health justice, not simply an implied fairness as medical and health ethics typically suggest. Justice fully embraces the idea that need should be a major factor in determining how resources are allocated for health, combined with the idea of a professional duty to optimize the well-being of those who are least fortunate.[4,5]

The historic nature of structural discrimination and its widespread effects is not exclusive to medicine, but inclusive of all health professions. Thus, a professionalism of inclusion must embrace a focus on diversity across the health professions. In fact, the greater focus on medicine alone may present as a bias since there is an ethical responsibility for interprofessional education and practice. While there may be differences in the learning environments of various health professions, what unites is stronger than what divides. And unfortunately, historic and structural discrimination is a tie that binds. Structural discrimination refers to the laws and policies that maintained a system of oppression against minority persons, which included African Americans, Native Americans, Indigenous persons, immigrants, and ethnic and religious minorities, such as Catholics and Jews.[6–11] Widespread application of Jim Crow racism in American medicine with its denial of access to minorities fueled the creation of parallel systems of healthcare, health professions schools, and professional organizations designed to meet the health, educational, and professional needs of Blacks and whites. Hospitals opened to care for Blacks during slavery and did not close until the 1970s–1990s. In hospitals that did admit Black patients, these individuals were segregated into basements, attics, and separate "colored" wards. Denied access to white educational institutions, Black medical and dental schools opened to educate minority students. Nursing schools for Black students took root within the Black hospital system. Professional organizations representing Black physicians, dentists, pharmacists, and nurses were the last element in the construction of separate worlds of professionalization in America.[12,13]

Maintenance of structural discrimination required an accreditation system first established by the all-white American Medical Association, American College of Surgeons, Association of American Medical Colleges, American Dental Association, and National League of Nurse Educators.[12–14] The Flexner Report of 1910, with a review of all North American medical schools, reinforced segregated health professions education and clinical care for decades. Subsequent accreditation standards exposed the extreme challenges Black institutions faced satisfying strenuous requirements with limited resources and even less access to the white medical power structure. Sources of financial support expanded the built landscapes of segregated healthcare and health professions education. In doing so, American philanthropy and the US federal and state governments reinforced structural discrimination and validated a medical ethos of white medical privilege.[12–15]

In response, health activists exposed the injustice of medical racism, spotlighting the inequity in the organization of medicine and health of different populations. Their efforts culminated in a movement that racially integrated hospitals and opened the doors for Black trainees and physicians, dentists, and nurses into historically predominantly white hospitals and professional schools of higher education.[13,15,16]

When we consider the imperative to transform health professions education with a focus on equity, diversity, and inclusion, we must know this history of structural discrimination and its persistence into the twenty-first century in all aspects of health professions education. We see this pattern of oppression today in our learning environments—classrooms, ambulatory clinics, and hospital wards, as well as in our healthcare financing systems. Minorities and socially disadvantaged persons continue to be segregated into academic dental and medical teaching clinics, safety net and teaching hospitals, federally qualified health centers and free clinics, where they remain far removed from private offices, hospitals, and specialty clinics.

Health disparities that persist in all disease categories and among all ethnic groups confirm the ongoing impact of structural discrimination. Implicit and explicit bias shapes the professional formation of learners and the delivery of clinical care itself.[17–19] With global initiatives focused on sustainable development and health as a human right, professionalism must be grounded in a framework that transforms learning and clinical spaces that ensure diversity, equity and inclusion, and the professional formation of students as global citizens.

Professionalism and the Learning Environment

Conditioning is often thought of as an athletic process, strengthening the body, even building muscle memory for future action and injury prevention. Academically, conditioning has been described as a process that leads to a higher level of function with the goal of optimizing performance.[20] In the same way, professionalism is the manner in which health professionals are conditioned into their chosen pathways. Paralleling athletic conditioning, the active learning that takes place across the health professional journey should be one that strengthens and maximizes health outcomes of patients, as well as clinician and provider well-being. Central to the concept of conditioning is creation of learning environments that intentionally minimize risk.

Do we use professionalism to strengthen the profession, patient, and provider? Likewise, do we use professionalism to minimize risk for the profession, patient, and provider? Does the learning environment itself strengthen, protect, or actually harm patients, clinicians, and learners?

Learning environments across the health professions are not simply locations of learning, research, and professional practice. They, in and of themselves, are a primary actor in the professional development of students, residents, and faculty as well in the delivery of healthcare to patients. The organizational culture of health professions schools impacts how students and residents learn, the quality of care patients receive, and the satisfaction that faculty and staff have in their work.[21,22] While often designated administrative functions, organizational development, diversity and inclusion initiatives, human resources and compliance, quality assurance, and so forth are aspects of the learning environment that influence each health professions' ability to fulfill its particular social contract. The social contract speaks to the fundamental idea of describing the relationship between the health professions and the society they serve.[23–25] Professionalism has come to serve as the cornerstone of this social contract because society has used the idea of the profession to organize the services delivered by health professionals. Thus, what it means to be a health professional in today's culture greatly influences what is expected of said health professional, physician, dentists, pharmacist, nurse, and more. Vast studies show that diverse professionals serve diverse populations well, the fervor of which is engrained within the fact that the social contract guarantees access to quality healthcare and standards. This makes clear the necessity of incorporating the concepts of diversity, equity, inclusion, belonging, and justice throughout professionalism as a construct for both clinical practice and learning.

Recent studies examining professional identity formation (PIF) in dental students have drawn attention to the dental education learning environment. While educators can positively influence students, emerging scholarship demonstrates that students can be negatively influenced if the environment is hostile and exclusionary or if there are many individuals who model unprofessional behaviors.[26,27] Similarly, medical educators emphasize the need for intentional improvements in the learning environment. A qualitative study among underrepresented minority (URM) medical students found that these students negotiated invisible forces that shaped and influenced their professional identity, and that URM physicians' also felt invisible and isolated, leading to an overall lack of immediate belongingness to the profession.[28] These educators place responsibility on institutional leadership for creating—or not creating—inclusive environments that positively influence student, resident, and faculty behavior.

Role Modeling and the Learning Environment

A multifaceted approach is recommended, including surveys on the climate of professionalism, to truly assess an organization's culture.[29] All accrediting organizations for medical education in the United States require teaching hospitals to ensure the learning environment fosters professionalism behaviors of trainees and faculty. A key element of learning environment professionalism is role modeling; however, a major challenge persists in that more than half of 2016 medical school graduates said that they experienced disconnects between what they were taught about professional behaviors/attitudes and what they saw being demonstrated by faculty. [30] In a study of residents' perspectives on professionalism, they rated their personal commitment as significantly higher than the commitment of their residency program. They also stated that poor role modeling impacted their attitudes about the importance of professionalism. Even with accreditation requirements for learning environments, evolving curricula, and faculty development programs to promote professionalism and belonging, it remains clear that residents perceive their commitment to professionalism greater than that of the institution in which they find themselves working and learning.

Role modeling remains the primary method of professionalism instruction throughout student, resident, and fellowship training because it is available and because it is fundamental to professional formation. It is important to remember that most faculty in the United States and Canada trained well before ethics and professionalism were formally introduced into undergraduate and graduate medical or dental education. Furthermore, there remain today faculty who trained in institutions that had only recently racially integrated.[31] While role modeling is a primary method of cultivating professionalism, it has long been established that poor role modeling of professionalism in the clinical learning environment is a key aspect of the hidden curriculum.[32,33] The hidden curriculum can be one that fosters positive attributes such as when faculty model empathy, engage in bystander intervention training, and advocate for cultural change, cultivating not only more inclusive learning environments, but also ones with a dedicated antiracist lens. An antiracist learning environment requires intentional self-awareness, embedding antiracism education into practice, dismantling oppressive structures, and regularly measuring progress. [34]

Studies abound documenting implicit bias of students, residents, and faculty—in medicine, dentistry, and nursing—toward minority patients, those with Medicaid, and other socially and medically disadvantaged groups.[35] Given the history of structural racism across the professions, one should not be surprised that discriminatory attitudes persist generation to generation. If the health professions are to meet their social contract—to provide care to all persons with respect and without discrimination and maintain their commitment to excellence, issues of stigma, and more expressly, social hierarchy, who is worthy of care, lies at the center of professionalism and what behavior is modeled by learners and their faculty. What does it say about the learning environment and role modeling that learners' empathy and attitudes about treating underserved populations actually decline as they progressed through school?[36–39]

Well-Being and the Learning Environment

Working as a healthcare professional is a demanding and stressful occupation. Clinician anxiety, burnout, depression, and even suicide are increasing.[40] The World Health Organization included burnout in the eleventh revision of the *International Classification of Diseases* (*ICD-11*), conceptualizing it as an occupational phenomenon resulting from chronic workplace stress that has not been successfully managed.[23] Burnout can be characterized using three dimensions: (1) feelings of energy depletion or exhaustion, (2) increased mental distance or cynicism from one's job, and (3) reduced professional efficacy.[41] Research suggests burnout is more prevalent in healthcare professionals relative to the general population, and that the learning environment is critical to mitigation of stress and burnout.

Among resident physicians, symptoms of burnout have been associated with greater explicit and implicit racial biases. Given the high prevalence of burnout and the negative implications of bias for healthcare, symptoms of burnout may be factors in racial disparities in healthcare.[42] Clinician well-being is linked to patient well-being and improved patient outcomes and person-centered care.[43,44] Even the National Academy of Medicine explicitly centered the learning and practice environment as one of myriad factors ultimately influencing patient well-being and outcomes.[44]

Current trends in burnout research document the prevalence of burnout, explore ways to prevent it, and study the influence it has on patient outcomes. Higher levels of burnout have been associated with lower empathy scores.[29] Scores indicative of higher burnout showed a significant negative correlation with professionalism climate scores. Though studies have found a strong negative correlation, the direction of the relationship has not been determined. It could be that students who are burned out have a more negative view and are more likely to think poorly of the professionalism of their fellow students, residents, and faculty within the learning environment; this perception can also have a negative impact on what students learn.[29] Yet, it could also indicate that burnout leads to less desirable professional behaviors or that less professional learning environments may contribute to medical student burnout.

In pharmacy education, studies have shown that well-being often declines as students progress, with higher rates of student stress, anxiety, and depression reported later in the curriculum.[45] In fact, scholars have proposed well-being as the missing component of professionalism in pharmacy education.[45] Women who belong to underrepresented racial or ethnic groups and have intersectional identities (immigrant family of origin, religious/ethnic minority, student, wife, mother) may face additional and even exponential discrimination, which can impact their sense of well-being, belonging, and perception of workplace stress. If health systems and health professions educational institutions do not begin to recognize these factors and effectively address them, women physicians, as well as all gender identities of underrepresented and systematically excluded backgrounds, will continue to be at high risk for burnout.[46,47]

Resilience is one of few proven protective factors for combating burnout and increasing provider wellness.[48,49] Keys to successful resilience and well-being programs emphasize change of both learning environments and organizational culture. Well-being as a component of professionalism can no longer be targeted toward individual efforts (chair yoga, mindfulness at the desk station, etc.), but must be designed and implemented at a systems level with engagement of all health professionals at all levels of learning and among all team members.

Equity and Combating Racism in the Learning Environment

In light of the COVID-19 pandemic and global racial reckoning surrounding Black Lives Matter and anti-Asian hate protests, the reframing of professionalism must speak to societal issues, including health inequities that reflect long-standing structural discrimination. Key to that reframing is an expansion of previous definitions of professionalism to allow for interventions and transformed systems and practices—not simply refraining from doing harm but actively interfering or taking action if wrong is being witnessed.[50,51] Health professions education ought to take seriously this realigned understanding of professionalism, particularly given the history of bias associated with a history of white medical supremacy that imposed professionalism standards leading to expectations and rules that heavily emphasized appearance, grooming, hairstyles, or cultural attire, which communicated preference as opposed to professional action.[52] One of the authors was required to wear pressed whites (short jacket, skirt, or pant) every day throughout residency training, even in the intensive care units. The highly staged white coat ceremony where students throughout the world receive their first symbol of doctorhood and badge of professional status reinforces the whiteness of medicine, rather than its cultural diversity and inclusiveness. What would this ceremony look like if after donning a white coat, students then put on a coat that reflected their unique personality, background, and culture—coats of various colors, fabrics, and styles? For professionalism to be relevant to future generations of students, clinicians, and our patients, we must embrace the radiance and complexity of a multicultural world we share with people around the world.

The American College of Physicians (ACP), in its recommendations for optimizing clinical learning environments expressly states: "The learning environment should foster respect, inquiry, and honesty and empower every individual, including learners, to raise concerns about ethics, professionalism, and care delivery."[53(p507)] Furthermore, teamwork and respect for colleagues must be both taught and demonstrated. The ACP calls for leaders to "create and sustain a strong ethical culture by encouraging discussion of ethical concerns, making values in everyday decision-making explicit, and embodying expectations of professionalism in which patient well-being is a core value."[53(p507)]

Likewise, a multilevel professionalism framework for remediating unprofessional behavior delineates a model comprising six levels, one of which speaks to the learning environment. It defines the environment level as

> the diverse contexts in which the medical student lives, works and learns, and which influence his or her behavior. Within the realm of medical education, it describes the academic learning environment: both the hidden and the formal curriculum, as well as the clinical, patient-related environment. The personal environment of the student

refers to his or her personal life and circumstances, such as problems at home, physical or mental illness and personal history.[54(p305)]

In reality, personal lives are rarely separated from the person who shows up for work, and thus our personal lives continuously influence professional performance, with the learning environment shaping the expression of both personal and professional values, attitudes, and behaviors of learners and of faculty.

An ideal learning environment is one that is safe—physically, intellectually, and emotionally. A safe environment means that everyone must consistently demonstrate respect for patients and for each other through role modeling, establishing expectations, and providing mechanisms that promote these behaviors.[55] If one member of a team or component of an organization fails to assume responsibility, the entire system may fail. The Charter on Professionalism for Healthcare Organizations (HCOs) echoes this sentiment, with explicit commitments to creating a healthy workplace that embraces inclusion and diversity within the organizational culture. To nurture professionalism, encourage the pursuit of employee excellence, and achieve outstanding healthcare with the broader community, creation of workplace environments that are physically and psychologically safe is paramount.[56]

New models of professionalism, similar to well-being initiatives, must be both institutionally and individually based. An ideal organizational professionalism model embodies sustainable governance policies and procedures that address workplace climate, harassment, explicit and implicit biases, cultural sensitivity, organizational well-being, and workforce equity (including gender equity).[47] A learning environment that fosters respect and antiracism is one that no longer allows for gender and minority biases in salary and career advancement. Many of our academic health centers and health professions schools are so steeped in systemically oppressive behaviors and origins that simply naming the occurrence and possibility of racism and misogyny within healthcare is often received as a declaration of disloyalty and outright fabrication. Most often, the absence of "seeing" racism in our learning and practice environment is due to the privileged position of not having to see or experience it. Unfortunately, those clinicians and patients from historically oppressed, systemically excluded, and continually marginalized see and feel the negative anti-inclusive elements all too well and regularly. In fact, workforce disparities have negatively impacted the training and career advancement of many people, including but not limited to individuals who identify with underrepresented racial and ethnic minority groups, women, people with disabilities, and the lesbian, gay, bisexual, transgender, and queer or questioning + community.[56]

Transformation of learning and clinical spaces is at the crux of reimagining a professionalism that truly upholds the social contract embedded within all health professions. A reimagined professionalism is one that ceases to ask: "How can we increase workforce diversity, how can we make our fields more attractive to historically underrepresented minorities, why are Black residents more likely to receive negative feedback from attendings, or why are patients fearful or distrustful of those who can offer them the care they are seeking?" These questions, and many more like them, put the responsibility on the very people for whom the systems (higher education, professional education, healthcare systems delivery, etc.) have not been designed. Instead, a reimagined professionalism asks: "Why are predominantly white spaces so difficult to navigate and integrate, why are heterosexual relationships and family dynamics considered so normative at the exclusion of other dynamics, why are Anglo-Saxon and American nationalistic Christian holidays still deemed as normative within the traditional calendar, what barriers and policies contribute to higher proportions of Black residents failing or receiving negative feedback, why are residency and fellowship programs so hostile to the Black mind and body, or what have health systems and providers done to earn the distrust of systemically excluded and historically oppressed populations—they altruistically claim to serve?

Professionalism, and a reimagining of its ideals, mission, and aims, could have a profound effect across healthcare delivery and its participants. The learning environment is central to creating a professionalism that ensures equitable healthcare for all.

Transformed Learning: An Antioppressive Professionalism of Inclusion

Scenario: You are a new staff member in adolescent psychiatry. You have discovered that the intake form for families is 35 pages long, written in English at the grade 11 level. Filling out the form is an absolute requirement to even be placed on a waiting list for an appointment. About 35%–40% of the parents in your city are not able to complete such a form by virtue of English being a second language, and for those with capacity in English, the grade 11 level is for most parents too high.

The above scenario is an example of a structural inequity. As a staff member in adolescent psychiatry, what is your professional responsibility in this case? How can this issue first be analyzed and addressed, but then also used as a teachable moment for the psychiatry residents under your supervision?

In English translations of Greek versions of the Hippocratic oath, there is one part of the sermon that is often used to give the idea that health equity has always been part of the social formulation of "medical professionalism":

> Into whatever homes I go, I will enter them for the benefit of the sick, avoiding any voluntary act of impropriety or corruption, including the seduction of women or men, *whether they are free men or slaves.*[57]

If we put the above statement into plain English, it says something to the effect that if a physician makes a house call, he or she will avoid improper behaviors such as seducing any of the people in the household, whether those people be enslaved, otherwise indentured, or not. To draw a modern analogy, this could extend to undocumented populations, who are without status and therefore lacking power. This seems like a noncontroversial rallying point about the boundaries of professional behavior for physicians, which most, if not all, could see as worthy of being upheld.

It gets trickier when the following is considered: In addition to refraining from acts of impropriety, what is the professional obligation to question and work to dismantle the very institution of slavery or indenture, which places the bound people in the house at risk of becoming victims of sexual impropriety and thus affects their mental and physical health? To be clear, notions of biologic racism and the desire for creation of a human hierarchy have their foundation in ancient Greek philosophy and society.[58–60] Perhaps the physician, as a member of the unjust society in which he or she lives also benefits directly from the enslavement or indenture of persons. Must the physician reflect on his or her position in society and the obligations to work for greater social justice that that position brings? When that physician is training an apprentice, is providing opportunities to reflect on societal injustices including the experiences of enslaved or indentured peoples in medical care part of the professional obligation of training the next generation?

In the scenario above, the structural inequity has to do with the clinic's implicit demand for a command of written English, which many families cannot meet, as a prerequisite for access to much needed mental health expertise. It is likely that command of written English is much more than a skill that some have and others do not, but rather a proxy of many well-known forms of marginalization within society—immigrant or refugee status, racialization, socioeconomic status, and the like.[61] If the new adolescent medicine faculty member was motivated to address the structural inequity, what attitudes, skills, and knowledge would the member need to have to do so? How would this member model and teach these knowledge, skills, and attitudes to the learners under his or her supervision? Could this be considered the skillset for a professionalism of inclusion and anti-oppression?

There are three major educational objectives in the skill set of a professionalism of inclusion and anti-oppression[62]:

1. Attitudinal: An explicit formulation of the construct of professionalism to include social justice/health equity and antioppression as explicit goals of the medical profession and individual physician toward both the patients in front of them and the more distant concept of populations of (potential) patients.[50]
2. Skills based: This objective includes analytical skills in the apprehension and analysis of forms of structural inequity, whether these factors are more "downstream" (i.e., within systems of healthcare) or "upstream" (societal injustices, e.g., discriminatory rental practices).[63] It also includes analytical skills in working toward change in ways that are co-created with persons from the directly affected populations of any particular unjust societal or healthcare structure.
3. Knowledge based: This objective includes the ability to name and define important concepts, such as structural racism, antioppressive and decolonized practices, and to understand the evidentiary basis that links these issues to relevant health outcomes within a particular context of practice.[64]

What does an attitudinal formulation toward social equity and antioppression look like in an inclusive construct of professionalism? In most statements today that link social justice/health equity with professionalism, the verb phrases used include examples such as "committing to health equity" or "promoting health equity" as professional obligations. We posit that these are the wrong verbs of an antioppressive professionalism of inclusion.[65,66]

In addition to building and supporting structural racism, the medical profession has a long history of contributing to social injustices and health inequities while claiming not to. An antioppressive professionalism of inclusion must recognize this fact and that the structures of learning within medical schools and clinical training may actually perpetuate such injustices. For instance, within most jurisdictions in Canada, there is a legacy of sterilization of Indigenous women against their will or in ways not meeting past standards of informed consent.[67] This practice was widespread, legal, and indeed ordered and structured by the state. In 1928, the Canadian province of Alberta, followed shortly thereafter by British Columbia, passed sexual sterilization acts that disproportionately and with a thinly veiled eugenic philosophy targeted Indigenous women.[68] While the act was repealed in 1972, there have been cases of alleged sterilization of Indigenous women against their will right up to 2018 in Canada.[69,70] In the United States, it is estimated that over 70,000 persons were sterilized, many after the US Supreme Court voted in 1927 in support of legalized sterilization as a way for states to manage the mentally ill, illiterate, poor, sexually promiscuous, and rural populations as well as minority populations of African Americans and Native Americans.[69,71,72]

These are some of many graphic examples, which have included the infamous Tuskegee trials where African American men were not treated for syphilis to study its natural history, and there were starvation studies in Indigenous children.[73] From the perspective of medicine's social contract, returning to the clinical example of forced sterilizations, we must remember that physicians, including surgery residents, performed the operations, presumably obligated under the professional expectation to act "ethically" and "in the best interests" of their patients with society condoning these acts. How they formulated "best interests" can only be guessed at, but must have come from a social position of profound othering and paternalism.

These legacies are with us today and must be owned and understood in any reformulation of professionalism for greater social justice moving forward. With respect to the appropriate verb phrase to express the attitude sought for in an antioppressive professionalism of inclusion, <u>understanding</u> the health care system as a tool of discrimination and injustice (in addition to working toward helping patients improve their health, <u>living</u> in this muddiness of this contradiction, and <u>aligning</u> practices with those that <u>disrupt</u> and/or <u>dismantle</u> unjust structures from within.

Moving now to consider the aptitudes of an antioppressive and inclusive professional, what are the skills that ought to be developed and how should they be taught? We suggest that in teaching this new construct of professionalism the focus must be on moving from professionalism as a pedagogy of privilege to one much less hierarchical and elitist. We have drawn inspiration from Brazilian educator Paulo Freire, whose book chapter "Pedagogy of the Oppressed" describes what such learning might encompass.[74]

Freire's pedagogy was born to combat power asymmetries brought by the social inequality that marks Latin American countries. According to Freire, education is a political enterprise toward full citizenship and freedom that starts from concrete experiences and is fueled by curiosity and the desire to move one's reality toward social justice. This education for freedom, or "liberation," aims to develop a critical consciousness, a capacity to analyze reality and identify its oppressive elements to change them. Liberation came to replace what Freire called "banking education," a process to deliver pacified individuals capable of following the rules dictated by an elite not interested in sharing power.[75] Liberation is a continuum of understanding that promotes the necessary empowerment of people to transform their realities. Once engaged in the liberation process, it becomes one`s responsibility to help other people to go through the same process. Although Freire's ideas were published forty years ago, they are still relevant for the professionalism conversation.

Liberation does not understand reality as a fixed entity, and the transformations of individuals and society are considered essential outcomes of the education process. In this context, the relationship between teachers and students is horizontal, democratic, and dialogical.[76] Students are not passive receptacles of knowledge but active agents with opinions, wills, responsibilities, and contributions to give. Real learning only occurs when both realities, teachers' and students', are transformed after the learning encounter. Welcoming students' participation and voice is relevant because the initial power asymmetry between teachers and students parallels the asymmetry between health professionals and patients. If students learn from their teachers how to use power with the individuals and not over them, they will have learned an important lesson of humility. Moreover, when teachers facilitate students' liberation, they are role modeling how students may support their future patients in a similar process.

The concept of liberation and critical consciousness becomes even more relevant when applied to health professional-patient relationships. Liberation of patients conceptually is the achievement of the WHO model of health, facilitating the ability of patients to live vibrant and fulfilling lives.[77] The liberation of patients demands supporting them to become empowered to join the conversation about what is good professionalism, the relevant health outcomes, and how the healthcare system and professionals allocate scarce resources. Liberated patients feel empowered to speak up against injustice. Liberated health professionals welcome patients' voices in a democratic dialogue and share power and responsibilities to act with patients to transform their realities. This democratic dialogue based on mutual respect gives birth to a professionalism of critical consciousness, which is participatory and based on democratic solidarity and shared social responsibility.[50]

Instructionally, students are encouraged to develop a critical reflective practice around their day-to-day cases, uncovering social contradictions and analyzing how social structures impact on health. In the opening case, learners would analyze the power dynamics that helped create the original policy as well as all of the agents involved in the decision-making. Was the voice of potentially marginalized patients brought into the discussion? Is resource allocation an issue? Such analytic skills have been termed "structural competence"; this new competence along with an attitude to work toward change for greater social justice encompass the concept of critical consciousness.

What forms of knowledge underpin the skills and attitudes that must be developed? In order to develop an inclusive and antioppressive professionalism, practitioners and learners must explicitly add another "agent" to the traditional relational formulation of the doctor-patient relationship—the sociopolitical context in which the interaction occurs. This formulation of caring within the doctor-patient relationship is often termed the cultural safety paradigm. Cultural safety was originated by Maori nursing educator Irihapeti Ramsden as a means to formulate the best way to approach the care of Maori patients in New Zealand by explicit consideration of the institutions of care as key elements in the brutal colonization experience of Maori people within the modern state of New Zealand.[78] Such a model has found widespread application in the realm of Indigenous health in multiple contexts and is an excellent way to incorporate power analyses and their importance in healthcare into the basic unit of interaction—the doctor or healthcare worker—patient interaction. Viewed through the lens of cultural safety, key concepts such as systemic discrimination/oppression/marginalization and privilege emerge.

Tomorrow's clinicians will live in a global world where health as a human right is understood as a mandate, not a luxury, and a core component of sustainable development. They will face issues such as the impact of the climate crisis on health, migration of populations, and the emergence of new and old infections. Our professionalism of the twenty-first century must prepare our learners to be comfortable with complexity and cultural diversity as the norm, a fluidity to navigate across settings and care for all persons.

Throughout this section, we have referred to a professionalism that is antioppressive and inclusive as the way forward for greater social justice. Just whom, then, are to be "included"? It is clear that greater voice and deliberate power sharing with patients from groups marginalized with society is needed and must be the primary focus. We also draw the reader's attention to the needs of the diverse learners who are served within educational programs in medicine, dentistry, nursing, and pharmacy. When teaching about past or present injustices, it must be clear that within the audience or classroom there are likely to be learners with direct experience of the issues being discussed and that recognition of systemic injustices and skills in trauma-informed teaching will be required.

References

1. Royal CD. Science, society, and dismantling racism. *Health Equity*. 2023;7(1):38–44.
2. Rossi AL, Wyatt TR, Huggett KN, Blanco MA. When I say . . . diversity, equity and inclusion (DEI). *Med Educ*. 2022:56(7):701–702.
3. Huang S. *Why Does Belonging Matter at Work? The Society for Human Resource Management (SHRM)*. 2020 .
4. Braveman PA, Kumanyika S, Fielding J, et al. Health disparities and health equity: the issue is justice. *Am J Public Health*. 2011;101(S1):S149–S155.
5. Daniels N. Democratic equality: Rawls' complex egalitarianism. In: Freeman S, ed. *The Cambridge Companion to Rawls*. Cambridge University Press; 2003:241–276.
6. Clarfield AM, Paltiel O. A 56-year-old medical calendar from McGill opens a fascinating window on medicine's past. *CMAJ*. 1995;153(9):1343.
7. Stevens R. *In Sickness and in Wealth* . Basic Books; 1989.
8. Duffin J. The Queen's Jews: religion, race, and change in twentieth-century Canada. *Can J Hist*. 2014;49(3):369–394.
9. Frank JW, Wang EA, Nunez-Smith M, Lee H, Comfort M. Discrimination based on criminal record and healthcare utilization among men recently released from prison: a descriptive study. *Health Justice*. 2014;2:1–8.
10. Nardone A, Chiang J, Corburn J. Historic redlining and urban health today in US cities. *Environ Justice*. 2020;13(4):109–119.
11. Harris AP, Pamukcu A. 2020). The civil rights of health: a new approach to challenging structural inequality. *UCLA L Rev*. 2020;67:758.
12. Byrd WM, Clayton LA. *An American Health Dilemma, Vol 1: Race, Medicine and Health Care in the United States, Beginnings to 1900*. Routledge; 2000*; Vol 2: Race, Medicine and Health Care in the United States, 1900–2000*. Routledge; 2002.
13. Hine DC. *Black Women in White: Racial Conflict and Cooperation in the Nursing Profession, 1890–1950*. Indiana University Press; 1989.
14. Ward TJ Jr. *Black Physicians in the Jim Crow South*. University of Arkansas Press; 2003.
15. Beardsley EH. *A History of Neglect: Health Care for Blacks and Mill Workers in the Twentieth Century South*. University of Tennessee Press; 1989.
16. Reynolds PP. Dr. Louis T. Wright and the NAACP: pioneers in hospital integration. *Am J Public Health*. 2000;90:883–892.
17. Bavli I, Jones DS. Race correction and the X-ray machine—the controversy over increased radiation doses for Black Americans in 1968. *N Engl J Med*. 2022;387(10):947–952.

18. Neighbors HW, Mattingly DT, Johnson J, Morse K. The contribution of research to racial health equity? Blame and responsibility in navigating the status quo of anti-Black systemic racism. *Soc Sci Med.* 2023;316:115209.

19. Li A, Deyrup AT, Graves JL, Ross LF. Race in the Reading: A Study of Problematic Uses of Race and Ethnicity in a Prominent Pediatrics Textbook. *Acad Med.* 2022;97(10):1521–1527.

20. American Academy of Family Physicians, American Academy of Orthopaedic Surgeons, American College of Sports Medicine, American Orthopaedic Society for Sports Medicine, American Osteopathic Academy of Sports Medicine, & American Medical Society for Sports Medicine. The team physician and conditioning of athletes for sports: a consensus statement. *Med Sci Sports Exerc.* 2001;33(10):1789–1793.

21. Fleming E, Smith CS, Ware TK, Gordon NB. Can academic dentistry become an anti-racist institution? Addressing racial battle fatigue and building belonging. *J Dent Educ.* 2022;86(9):1075–1082.

22. Ester TV, Tucker-Lively FL, Smith C, Taylor GW, Ware TK, Inglehart MR. The status of climate studies in the United States and Canadian dental schools: deans' perspectives. *J Dent Educ.* 2021;85(10):1616–1626.

23. Manca A, Gormley GJ, Johnston JL, Hart ND. Honoring medicine's social contract: a scoping review of critical consciousness in medical education. *Acad Med.* 2020;95(6):958–967.

24. Wasylenki D, Byrne N, McRobb B. The social contract challenge in medical education. *Med Educ.* 1997;31(4):250–258.

25. Cruess SR, Cruess RL. Professionalism and medicine's social contract with society. *AMA J Ethics.* 2004;6(4):185–188.

26. Kwon JH, Shuler CF, von Bergmann H. Professional identity formation: the key contributors and dental students' concerns. *J Dent Educ.* 2022;86(3):288–297.

27. Smith CS, Stilianoudakis SC, Carrico CK. Professionalism and professional identity formation in dental students: revisiting the professional role orientation inventory (PROI). *J Dent Educ.* 2022;87(5):646–653.

28. Wyatt TR, Rockich-Winston N, Taylor TR, White D. What does context have to do with anything? A study of professional identity formation in physician-trainees considered underrepresented in medicine. *Acad Med.* 2020;95(10):1587–1593.

29. Brazeau CM, Schroeder R, Rovi S, Boyd L. Relationships between medical student burnout, empathy, and professionalism climate. *Acad Med.* 2010;85(10):S33–S36.

30. Association of American Medical Colleges. Medical school graduation questionnaire: 2016 all schools summary report. July 2016. Accessed September 4, 2022. https://www.aamc.org/download/464412/data/2016gqallschoolssummaryreport.pdf

31. Reynolds PP, White C, Martindale JR. Residents' perspective on professionalism in the learning environment. *Curr Probl Pediatr Adolesc Health Care.* 2019;49(4):84–91.

32. Hafferty FW. 1998. Beyond curriculum reform: confronting medicine's hidden curriculum. *Acad Med.* 1998;73(4):403–407.

33. Smith KL, Saavedra R, Raeke JL, O'Donell AA. The journey to creating a campus-wide culture of professionalism. *Acad Med.* 2007;82(11):1015–1021.

34. Sotto-Santiago S, Poll-Hunter N, Trice T, et al. A framework for developing antiracist medical educators and practitioner–scholars. *Acad Med.* 2021;97(1):41–47.

35. Habibian M, Seirawan H, Mulligan R. Dental students' attitudes toward underserved populations across four years of dental school. *J Dent Educ.* 2011;75(8):1020–1029.

36. Ward J, Cody J, Schaal M, Hojat M. The empathy enigma: an empirical study of decline in empathy among undergraduate nursing students. *J Prof Nurs*. 2012;28(1):34–40.

37. Hojat M, Vergare MJ, Maxwell K, et al. The devil is in the third year: a longitudinal study of erosion of empathy in medical school. *Acad Med*. 2009;84(9):1182–1191.

38. Sherman JJ, Cramer A. Measurement of changes in empathy during dental school. *J Dent Educ*. 2005;69(3):338–345.

39. Crandall SJ, Reboussin BA, Michielutte R, et al. Medical students' attitudes toward underserved patients: a longitudinal comparison of problem-based and traditional medical curricula. *Adv Health Sci Educ Theory Pract*. 2007;12(1):71–86.

40. Calvo JM, Kwatra J, Yansane A, Tokede O, Gorter RC, Kalenderian E. Burnout and work engagement among US dentists. *J Patient Saf*. 2021;17(5), 398–404.

41. World Health Organization. Burn-out an "occupational phenomenon": *International Classification of Diseases*. 2019. Accessed March 19, 2022. https://www.who.int/news/item/28-05-2019-burnout-an-occupational-phenomenon-internationalclassification-of-diseases. Accessed June 12, 2024.

42. Dyrbye L, Herrin J, West CP, et al. Association of racial bias with burnout among resident physicians. *JAMA Netw Open*. 2019;2(7):e197457–e197457.

43. Shanafelt T, Goh J, Sinsky C. The business case for investing in physician well-being. *JAMA Intern Med*. 2017;177(12):1826–1832.

44. National Academies of Sciences, Engineering, and Medicine. *Taking Action Against Clinician Burnout: A Systems Approach to Professional Well-Being*. The National Academies Press. Washington, DC; 2019.

45. Thurston MM, Hammer D. Well-being may be the missing component of professionalism in pharmacy education. *Am J Pharm Educ*. 86(5):391–394.

46. Shanafelt TD, Noseworthy JH. Executive leadership and physician well-being: nine organizational strategies to promote engagement and reduce burnout. *Mayo Clin Proc*. 2017; 92:129–146.

47. Chin EL, Britto VM, Parekh R. Diversity and medical professionalism. *Health Aff (Millwood)*. 2020;39: 722.

48. Alsharif A. The protective role of resilience in emotional exhaustion among dental students at clinical levels. *Psychol Res Behav Manag*. 2020;13:989.

49. Smith CS, Carrico CK, Goolsby S, Hampton AC. An analysis of resilience in dental students using the resilience scale for adults. *J Dent Educ*. 2020;84(5):566–577.

50. Razack S, de Carvalho Filho MA, Merlo G, Agbor-Baiyee W, de Groot J, Reynolds PP. Privilege, social justice and the goals of medicine: towards a critically conscious professionalism of solidarity. *Perspect Med Educ*. 2022;11(2):67–69.

51. Zaidi Z, Razack S, Kumagai AK. Professionalism revisited during the pandemics of our time: COVID-19 and racism. *Perspect Med Educ*. 2021;10(4):238–244.

52. Gray A. *The Bias of "Professionalism" Standards*. Stanford Social Innovation Review; 2019.

53. Lehmann LS, Sulmasy LS, Desai S, ACP Ethics, Professionalism and Human Rights Committee. Hidden curricula, ethics, and professionalism: optimizing clinical learning environments in becoming and being a physician: a position paper of the American College of Physicians. *Ann Intern Med*. 2018;168(7):506–508.

54. Barnhoorn PC, Houtlosser M, Ottenhoff-de Jonge MW, Essers GT, Numans ME, Kramer AW. A practical framework for remediating unprofessional behavior and for

developing professionalism competencies and a professional identity. *Med Teach.* 2019;41(3):303–308.

55. Goldstein EA, Maestas RR, Fryer-Edwards K, et al. Professionalism in medical education: an institutional challenge. *Acad Med.* 2006;81(10):871–876.
56. Liu HY, Larson AR, Strong SA, et al. Workforce diversity, equity, and inclusion: a crucial component of professionalism in psychiatry. *Psychiatr Clin.* 2022;45(2):243–258.
57. Greek Medecine. Hippocrates. Rationality and medicine. Accessed September 18, 2022. https://www.nlm.nih.gov/hmd/greek/greek_oath.html
58. Sullivan S. *The Physiology of Sexist and Racist Oppression.* Oxford University Press; 2015.
59. Graves Jr JL, Goodman AH. *Racism, Not Race: Answers to Frequently Asked Questions.* Columbia University Press; 2021.
60. Ward JK, Lott TL (eds.). *Philosophers on Race: Critical Essays.* John Wiley & Sons; 2008.
61. Sentell T, Shumway M, Snowden L. Access to mental health treatment by English language proficiency and race/ethnicity. *J Gen Intern Med.* 2007;22(2):289–293.
62. Swanwick T. *Understanding Medical Education: Evidence, Theory, and Practice.* Wiley-Blackwell; 2018:1–6.
63. Metzl JM, Hansen H. Structural competency: theorizing a new medical engagement with stigma and inequality. *Soc Sci Med.* 2014;103:126–133.
64. Aqil AR, Malik M, Jacques KA, et al. Engaging in anti-oppressive public health teaching: challenges and recommendations. *Pedagogy Health Promot.* 2021;7(4):344–353.
65. Project MP. Medical professionalism in the new millennium: a physicians' charter. *Lancet.* 2002;359(9305):520–522.
66. Ing EB. Equity, diversity and inclusion and the CanMEDS framework. *Can Med Educ J.* 2021;12(5):75.
67. Stote K. The coercive sterilization of aboriginal women in Canada. *Am Indian Cult Res J.* 2012;36(3):117–150.
68. Clarke E. Indigenous women and the risk of reproductive healthcare: forced sterilization, genocide, and contemporary population control. *J Hum Rights Soc Work.* 2021;6(2):144–147.
69. Leason J. Forced and coerced sterilization of Indigenous women: strengths to build upon. *Can Fam Physician.* 2021;67(7):525–527.
70. Dhaliwal RK. Settler Colonialism and the contemporary coerced sterilizations of Indigenous women. *Polit Sci Undergrad Rev.* 2019;4(1):29–39.
71. Rutecki GW. Forced sterilization of native Americans: later twentieth century physician cooperation with national eugenic policies? *Ethics Med.* 2011;27(1):33.
72. Fofana MO. Time and time again: the reincarnations of coerced sterilisation. *J Med Ethics.* 2021;48(11):805–809.
73. Lowenstein PR, Lowenstein ED, Castro MG. Challenges in the evaluation, consent, ethics and history of early clinical trials–Implications of the Tuskegee "trial" for safer and more ethical clinical trials. *Curr Opin Mol Ther.* 2009;11(5):481.
74. Freire P. Pedagogy of the oppressed. In: John Beck, Chris Jenks, Neil Keddie and Michael F.D. Young, eds. *Toward a Sociology of Education.*Routledge; 2020:374–386.
75. Blackburn J. Understanding Paulo Freire: reflections on the origins, concepts, and possible pitfalls of his educational approach. *Commun Dev J.* 2000;35(1):3–15.

76. Shor I, Freire P. *A Pedagogy for Liberation: Dialogues on Transforming Education.* Greenwood Publishing Group; 1987.

77. World Health Organization (WHO). *World Health Organisation Definition of Health;* 2011.

78. Ramsden I. *Cultural Safety and Nursing Education in Aotearoa and Te Waipounamu.* Doctoral dissertation. Victoria University of Wellington.

33

The Unbearable Whiteness of Professionalism

Marginalized Identities, Authenticity, and Building Inclusive Ways of Being

Saleem Razack

Key Points

- Building an inclusive medical community relies on recognizing the community is an ecosystem that aims to promote human flourishing among its members. Adopting the concept of solidarity helps achieve this aim.
- Patient care is enhanced when medical professionals are valued for their diversity and individuality.
- The purpose of the socialization process of professional identity formation is to forge an embodied and enduring way of being for the person undergoing it, manifested through behaviors and other forms of signaling, of which hairstyle is one. As members of a collectivity, for physicians there are going to be understandings of norms—including communication styles, dress, and the boundaries of permissible behaviors within collegial and doctor-patient relationships.

Expanding Our Understanding of Medical Professionalism

Opening Scenario: After 30 years as a respected medical educator in a professional identity formation course in a "top" medical school, Dr. Farhana Khan, a racialized medical educator, feels she just can't teach "this stuff, this way anymore." The course, which consists of monthly seminars and reflective practice sessions with a group of six medical students across the four years of medical school, provides an opportunity to connect with students as they negotiate the development of their professional identities. Recently, in a seminar on Indigenous health and professionalism, the speakers (both of whom are white males) spoke about the importance of committing to improve the health of "our" Indigenous people through positive engagement in relationship building between the doctor and "his" patients. A student in the seminar asked about addressing systemic racism in healthcare as also a professional imperative of social justice. The speakers stated that the purposes of medicine are to remain neutral and to avoid becoming politicized. "We should stay in our lane," they opine authoritatively.

Something snapped in Dr. Khan that day, and she knew that she could no longer be a preceptor and mentor in this prestigious course. One of her students, present at the seminar, is from an Indigenous nation, and Dr. Khan could see the troubled reaction she was having to the way the topic was being discussed.

"I have been a fraud all these years. It all feels so inauthentic, 'white,' and 'male,'" she said to herself. She wondered if we are fostering the development of professional identities that will care for diverse populations well in the future. She wonders if she is even a part of the "we" in the question that she just posed to herself.

There are many implicit agreements that candidates make in the process of internalizing a medical education and joining a profession, such that membership in that profession ends up being experienced as a vocation rather than a job—that one has been "called to do it" rather than having it "just happen."[1] Here are a few agreements germane to the discussion of this chapter:

1. **To join medicine is to agree to place value on thinking and reasoning through problems a certain way.** I refer here to the notion that scientific thinking through the empiric observation of the behaviors of populations can be applied to individuals who share traits with the individuals within the populations of study through reasoning a practice, as a way of understanding and treating health problems.
2. **To join medicine is to agree to be reviewed forever and henceforth by peers.** All processes of self-regulation, from disciplinary action, to grant review, to practice assessment depend on the notion that practice or knowledge is made better through review by peers, and that a standard of care can be defined and upheld. Medical education can be seen as a process of progressive developmental peer review.
3. **To join medicine is to agree to be socialized with your cohort and by your teachers and preceptors into a group with behavioral norms, ideologies, and ways of being.** It is a movement from distal to proximal participation within a community of practice. To define norms is also to define ways in which such norms may be transgressed or not met.

In this chapter, we explore these concepts with respect to learners who join medicine and who may not see themselves easily within the way it is taught, how they are being socialized, and what they are learning. I refer here to students whose social characteristics (race, gender, sexuality, [dis]ability status, social class, among many socially important forms of difference) are either numerically underrepresented within the body of medical practitioners or epistemically underrepresented in what is being learned. Such learners join medicine with a greater social distance to traverse as they are progressively invited into the community of practice, and their experiences of the socialization often contain elements disturbing to them and that may cause them to act in ways that they experience as inauthentic.

As the reader engages in the chapter, I ask that he or she keep the opening scenario in mind. We return to it at the end.

For the purposes of discussion, a few operational definitions are required. I define "professionalism" operationally as a social construct, a "thing" that exists not in the observable natural world, but in the social world, because the players within society have agreed that it exists.[2] As such, it defines behavioral norms and relationship parameters (between a doctor and patients, and between the collectivity of physicians and society) and carves out a unique space for its practitioners in the labor of caring for sick people (diagnosing disease and ordering treatments, i.e.). The process by which the role of the physician is internalized and embodied within a specific individual can be defined as professional identity formation. Professionalism can and has been reduced to a series of behaviors ("ways of doing"),[3] or knowledge systems ("ways of knowing"),[4] but for the purposes of understanding diverse learners' experiences of the socialization process of professional identity formation,[5] it is best to consider the calling into the "vocation" as a pervasive and embodied "way of being and acting" in the world.

In an expansive sense, we consider three broad questions:

1. In what ways might the very construct of professionalism be intersected by notions of social hierarchy—whiteness, maleness, and hegemony, for example—and what is the evidence for this?
2. How is the socialization process of becoming a physician—often referred to as professional identity formation—experienced by persons from social groups whose individuals and knowledge systems are underrepresented in medicine?
3. How might inclusive forms of professionalism and professional identity formation be built and how might this serve both learners and patients better in the future?

Professionalism as a Social Construct and Hegemonically Intersected Knowledge System

Illustrative Scenario 1: In an event commemorating Queer Pride month at a medical school, a history of medicine lecture is arranged. In this lecture, the presenters review the history of the delisting of homosexuality from the *Diagnostic and Statistical Manual of Mental Disorders,* which occurred in 1973. The advocacy stories of psychiatrists who were also homosexual are featured. The presenters draw parallels to contemporary discussions about diagnostic categories for gender diverse and trans individuals as well as access to gender-affirming care. One learner, who identifies himself as gay, comments that it seems evident that the profession "really let down" gay and gender diverse people in the past with respect to the social contract, with its support and active participation in conversion therapies, for instance. A senior emeritus professor of psychiatry raises his hand and says that he was part of the discussions at the time, and people should not judge what they do not know. "We did the best we could at the time, and we helped people."

Professionalism in medicine has been defined as a social contract between society and physicians.[6] In exchange for the discharge of unique expertise, within the confines of certain professional ethical obligations, physicians are given a monopoly over practice and a prestigious and influential role within society. Ethically, they are expected to operate within the values of altruism, placing patients' best interests first, justly (treating patients equitably), and obeying the "prime directive" of primum non nocere. In short, they are upholders, gatekeepers, and primary agents within health-care systems, which are themselves seen as designed to act benignly in patients' best interests.

There is an inherent elitism in such a formulation of professionalism. It recalls days of yore, and its rallying motto might be *noblesse oblige* (French, translated as nobility obliges), a term used to state that with nobility comes not only privilege, but also responsibility to those in one's "charge."[7] When applied to nobility, or to persons with a higher station in life than others, such a social contractual formulation has been criticized as providing those occupying that higher station with a convenient justification for their privilege.

Professionalism as a social construct has been analyzed critically through discourse analysis, for inherent knowledge power relations.[8] In the formulation of the preceding paragraph, who gains or loses power? It can be argued that the deal of the "contract" is a sweet one for physicians, whose prestigious roles as agents of medical acts, with a monopoly that virtually guarantees excellent financial compensation, are winners in the deal. Conversely, through rigorous autonomously regulated standards, the public or "society" can place their trust in the quality of those acts. Through the prestige awarded to the profession, physicians, while simultaneously principal agents of systems of healthcare, are also definers and interpreters of its "truths"—efficacy, equity, and excellence.

If professionalism is a discourse that has created a social contract that fosters a stance of elitism and privilege, then how might this social construct formulation affect the professional socialization experiences of diverse learners?

Case Analysis Through an Equity Lens

In the illustrative scenario of the Queer Pride event described in Scenario 1, we could see the issue as one of generational misunderstanding, but that would be an incomplete analysis. In looking to a past when gay men were pathologized as having a disease and "treated" for it through disproven approaches such as conversion and electroshock therapy, the presenters provide food for thought as to how constructs of professionalism at the time allowed such approaches to proceed "ethically" (i.e., what paternalistic approaches allowed such practices to be seen as acceptable). If we permitted ourselves the opportunity, we could ask how power and representation within the profession at the time may have served to not meet the needs of homosexual-identifying patients and how the very knowledge systems accessed to create the medicine (e.g., the construction of homosexuality as an illness, with treatments) might have been biased and intersected with heteronormative versions of "ideal" masculine ways of being. In drawing the parallel of the present-day discussions of gender-affirming care, the presenters likely sought to show that the past inequities echo strongly into the present and provide an opportunity to examine contemporary professionalism for its openness to gender diverse individuals.

The emeritus professor's explanation of the professional thinking of the time with respect to homosexuality was a missed opportunity for a critical discussion of professional obligations and would have had relevance to contemporary issues. For the gay-identified learner, such a discussion might have given the message of an inclusive professionalism where the history of people like him would be honored. If we situated the social constructs of professionalism within a history of evolving social contingencies that require constant renegotiation and reinterpretation of relevance, as well as recognizing that the profession itself was and is part of past and contemporary injustices, such a learner might be able to bring his whole authentic self into the journey from distal to proximal participation in the community of practice that is the medical profession. In short, he might be able to "see"' himself and "his kind" as having a legitimate place within the construct.

To recognize past injustices perpetrated through notions of professional behavior and to accept that current injustices might require a reformulation of the social construct in the here and now requires a cultivated stance of humility, diminished hierarchy and elitism, and acceptance that the profession of medicine is of society, not apart from it. In previous work, I and coauthors have referred to this stance as a "professionalism of solidarity" rather than the "noblesse oblige" version where the hierarchy and prestige are seen as "natural" consequences of medical expertise.[9,10] A professionalism of solidarity embraces social justice for all as a key component of health and seeks to align inclusively with all struggles against marginalization and oppression while recognizing the need for specificities of struggles as well.

In translations of old Greek versions of the Hippocratic oath, there is one article that is often used to make the case that health equity has been a concern of physicians from the beginning: "Into whatever homes I go, for the benefit of the sick, I shall refrain from inappropriate relationships with the men and women in the household, whether they be bond or free."[11] In plain language, this article of the oath essentially states that, as a physician, if one makes a house call, one should not engage in sexual relations with anyone in the house *even if they be slaves*. From a traditional professionalism perspective, there seems to be little to argue with here! However, from a professionalism of solidarity perspective, we might be asked, as a professional obligation, to question and act against the very institution of slavery as a major determinant of health through its perpetuation of injustice. Thinking of contemporary issues in professionalism curricula, one can think of learning examples such as discussions of the sociopolitical dimensions of "diagnosis" in mental health or discussions about physicians' roles in addressing the structural determinant roots of the common illnesses they treat.

The basic skill, or habit of mind, of a professionalism of solidarity is critical consciousness, as elaborated by Brazilian educator Paulo Freire. Critical consciousness seeks to develop within individuals the ability to recognize structures of inequity (structural competency) and then to act to change them (social justice orientation).[12]

Freire's pedagogy was born to combat power asymmetries brought by the social inequality that marks Latin American countries. According to Freire, education is a political enterprise toward full citizenship and freedom that starts from concrete experiences and is fueled by curiosity and the desire to move one's reality toward social justice. This education for freedom, or "liberation," aims to develop a critical consciousness, a capacity to analyze reality, and identify its oppressive elements to change them. Liberation came to replace what Freire called "banking education," a process to deliver pacified individuals capable of following the rules dictated by an elite not interested in sharing power. In many ways, traditional medical education can be considered as a pedagogy of privilege based on the "banking education model."[13] Liberation is a continuum of understanding that promotes the necessary empowerment of people to transform their realities. Once engaged in the liberation process, it becomes one's responsibility to help other people to go through the same process.

A professionalism of solidarity that has critical consciousness as a key skill and that fosters the development of structural competence within its holders has the capacity to integrate and include diverse learners more authentically because their histories become part of the professionalism conversation and subsequently their professional identity formation. A fundamental shift in how the doctor-patient relationship is conceptualized is required, however. The relationship must be seen as a dyad between not only doctor and patient, but also one occurring within specific sociopolitical and historical contexts. In short we are called on to ask not "What is the problem and why is it happening?" but rather "Why this problem at this time, to this degree, in this specific patient, with his/her specific life experiences?"—in short an ecological model of disease causation. The paradigm described here has been labeled as a "cultural safety" model and was first elaborated by Maori nursing educator Irihapeti Ramsden[14] when describing approaches to healthcare for Indigenous people in New Zealand. It has found widespread acceptance in multiple settings of Indigenous health and has application across the continuum of forms of structural marginalization and injustice.

Returning to the scenario, we would need to ask how structural heteronormativity operated within the profession of psychiatry that required the activism to dismantle homosexuality as a disease in 1973 and what has lived on and continues to be perpetuated in the profession currently. We would then be asked to commit to dismantling current inequities as well—through small actions in the clinical encounter, to more meso actions perhaps within our institutions or programs, and finally to larger scale collective actions through professional societies and more. In this way, a professionalism committed to including the voices of gender and sexuality diverse patients and learners and ready to be judged for its cultural safety by them and not by internal standards would become manifest.

Professional Identity Formation and Diverse Learners

Illustrative Scenario 2: A Black female student is reprimanded on her internal medicine rotation for coming to the wards with dreadlocks, worn flowing down her neck and back, and she is wearing a modest pantsuit under her lab coat. Her supervisor states that her hair should be done differently, and that families may feel threatened by her hairstyle. On another rotation the same day, this time in social pediatrics, where medical students work at a clinic for children in foster care, a supervisor assesses what a white female medical student is wearing ($300 Converse shoes, expensive jewelry, and designer label top and pants), and while wondering if this will be off-putting for the families cared for in the clinic, says nothing. Several families point out the expensive clothing worn by the medical student throughout the day.

The purpose of the socialization process of professional identity formation is to forge an embodied and enduring way of being for the person undergoing it, manifested through behaviors and other forms of signaling, of which hairstyle is one. As members of a collectivity, for physicians there are going to be understandings of norms—including communication styles, dress, and the boundaries of permissible behaviors within collegial and doctor-patient relationships.

Great injustice and inequity can manifest within groups. In the second illustrative case, who gets to decide what is appropriate dress or hairstyle and by what standards should this be judged? How did the norms develop—did they come about through Eurocentric understandings of respectful dress and hairstyle? What of the patient perspective here? How do patients perceive the different forms of dress and hairstyle? Is there space for more inclusive ways of being in the conceptualization of professional behaviors and dress code norms?

From the perspective of an inclusive professionalism, it is easy to appreciate that for a policy as mundane as hairstyle codes, attempts should be made to understand different cultural norms and to accommodate them wherever possible. There likely will not be one "norm" but many. Such inclusivity might manifest in other ways as well—communication styles, accommodation of forms of religious dress, and more.

The second illustrative scenario presents a fairly superficial manifestation of professionalism (hairstyle and dress codes), as well as showing how, through norms, judging standards might be inequitable. There are deeper issues, however, with the goal of seeking inclusive professionalisms. Within the medical literature there are many poignant examples where learners and professionals from diverse racial, gender, and sexuality groups[15–17] have felt that they are forced to enact norms of professional behavior that needlessly ask them to act in ways that are experienced as inauthentic. Should the LGBTQ2SIA* student change her gender atypical communication style when acting as a professional? Should the Northern England resident on rotation in London train herself to speak in "BBC" English? These are difficult questions to answer and require a complex calculation between patient expectations (which themselves may be the result of the noninclusivity and injustices of general society), learner expectations, and the profession's capacity to adapt to changing demographics and expectations on the part of its members.

The second big issue with inclusive professionalism has to do not with the manifestation of norms, but rather with the representation and gaze on difference contained within the knowledge systems of professionalism. A professionalism that is blind to its ability to be part of oppressive structures (as described with the case of the depathologizing of homosexuality) is unlikely to be inclusive to learners from the groups in question. They will experience this blindness as a manifestation of privilege that commits on them a form of epistemic violence. Epistemic violence is defined as domination committed through knowledge—silencing, denial, undervaluing, and nonrecognition of contributions and the value of different forms of knowledge. An example of this related to the scenario of dress codes would be nonrecognition of the inherent Eurocentrism of the standards of dress and hairstyle—applying a so-called white gaze[18] on determining the legitimacy of forms of knowledge and the practices they give rise to.

What does it mean to feel forced to act or behave in ways that are not authentic? Authenticity is defined as the subjective alignment between one's internal experiences and external expressions.[19] Fundamentally, it deals with the alignment between symbolic representation in its various forms (communication styles, words said, dress and body adornment as forms of symbolic representation) and how the subject sees those aligned with "who they are." It is an act of constructing meaning. Simply put, a professional who is acting authentically is able to bring their "whole self" to the work that they do and to feel psychologically safe doing so.

Misalignment occurs when the symbols that are manifest externally do not jive with internal subjective experience. For instance, for the resident wearing dreadlocks, that may be a way to connect with a past of oppression and ultimate emancipation or may have religious significance. Understood this way, to be told to change the hairstyle could be seen as a threat to personhood. Moreover, symbols often have multiple meanings. A white coat might signify authority and belonging for some, but unnecessary hierarchy and social distance for others.

Authenticity is a key component of relationship building, and there are many data that show that the professional relationship between a doctor and a patient has therapeutic aspects to it.[20,21] The literature generally supports positive effects on the professional's well-being, greater behavioral consistency as experienced by the patient, and more open communications.[22] Therefore, from the perspective of promoting efficacious professional relationships, there is a justification to work at nurturing inclusive forms of professionalism structurally.

To regulate behavior also has the potential to be a form of oppression. The literature is replete with narratives and studies that repeatedly show that minoritized professionals are more likely to receive disciplinary regulation for issues of professionalism.[23] For instance, those that call out discriminatory comments of colleagues (racism, sexism, and the like) are far more likely to be labeled as "unprofessional" than those who said the discriminatory statements in the first place. We must ask ourselves whether the behaviors are the problem or the narrowness of the definition of what is acceptable or not, as well as if there are structural inequities that should not be there in who gets regulated.

Building Inclusive Professionalisms of Solidarity

Illustrative Scenario 3: An amendment to the second-year medical school white coat ceremony is proposed. In this ceremony, students receive their white coats as a rite of passage toward the more clinical part of the program. White coats are always uniform and unvarying. The committee overseeing the ceremony is approached by a group of students to consider changing it. The students have come on behalf of their classmate, who is the first Indigenous candidate to be in the program in many years. They ask if she may embroider a meaningful symbolic portrayal to represent her community of origin on the left breast pocket of her white coat. The committee agrees and actually makes this option available to all students. This year's white coat ceremony is a resounding success, with much discussion between students and faculty about the meaning behind the representation choices made. Many faculty members express that they wish they could have done it this way in the past and that the discussions have allowed everyone to know each other much better.

Institutions, and professionalism can be considered as an institution because it is an organized set of socially regulated practices, can be said to be inclusive if through their policies and procedures they simultaneously promote a sense of belonging in individuals and show a high value in the uniqueness that individuals bring to the institution. In the white coat ceremony just mentioned, the fact that the collectivity receives a white coat as a rite of passage shows an attempt to promote everyone's belonging. The modification, where students have a place to express their individuality, is an example of a practice that shows valuing of uniqueness.

Inclusive professionalisms do well when they understand the collectivity of practitioners as an ecosystem, who will be called on to do many tasks different from each other and who yet will be part of the same profession. In a biologic ecosystem, life forms are interconnected but they play different roles. Similarly, this is the case with the community of physicians. Some will work in community practice and will need the individuality of skills and background for that. Others may work in laboratory practice. To be inclusive in the approach to professionalism would be to identify the core that everyone shares and the other parts that benefit from individualism—the ability and invitation to bring one's whole self to work. In this paradigm solidarity is manifest through a recognition of the profound interdependence of the collectivity of practitioners in their common task to care for populations.

Much of this sounds easy, but the cultivation of a profound epistemological humility is required in teachers and regulators. Respect for different knowledge and meaning systems as valuable in and of themselves, as well as being able to see our own meaning and knowledge systems as having limitations and rootedness in the promotion of inequities, results in a series of teaching skills and styles that need to be developed. There are many, but they all share the crucial aspect that they are dialogic in nature—listening to stories in order to understand better the subjects (i.e., learners) engaged with and to even risk one's own subjective transformation through the exchange. Dialogism, simply put, is the exploration of meaning through conversation.[24] Its focus is on the subjects of the conversation and how they change through it and are understood better by the other subject. It is contrasted by other forms of communication, such as dialectic exchange. Dialectic exchange focuses less on the subjects and more on the objects of conversation (information exchanged).[25] Classic dialectics views conversations as being a series of advancements of theses, which abut against subsequent antitheses, and which ultimately resolve through synthesis. A story or narrative is dialogic. A medical history can be understood as dialectic.

The best approach to the development of inclusive professionalisms of solidarity is to do so co-creatively, with learners, and ideally patients, in ways that consciously seek to diminish hierarchies and that demonstrate to participants that they are seen and valued. Co-creation is a collaborative and dialogic process in which input from all groups is sought in nonhierarchical ways in design, including social innovations such as "professionalism." Within discussions of professionalism, such an approach serves to constantly remind those engaging within it that the negotiations that have produced the set of behaviors known as professionalism are socially contingent. Healthy questioning of these social contingencies results, such that professionalism is not seen as a monolith received "from high." The willingness to question the social contingencies helps formulate professionalisms of solidarity.

Conclusions

Let's return to the opening case of Dr. Khan. Clearly Dr. Khan experienced a moment of clarity that led to not only distress, but also a reframing of her understanding of professionalism. In hearing the presenters' words and seeing the reaction of the Indigenous student in her group, she appreciated the structural inequities and racism built into the very way professionalism was being constructed in that moment. Perhaps she had similar concerns in the past that were preverbal and difficult to articulate.

How was this moment dystonic for her with respect to the three implicit agreements outlined above, which everyone who enters the profession is asked at the very least to acknowledge:

1. **To Join Medicine Is to Agree to Think a Certain Way:** We can argue that in joining the profession, one's professionalism is about seeking to assert the primacy of objective scientific understandings in driving diagnosis and treatment, enacted through the heart of humanism and relational connection with patients. What Dr. Khan glimpsed in the seminar session was that that this seemingly objective knowledge has within it a baggage of societal injustices and that objectivity is not ensured. It can only be elaborated through a process of critical reflexivity. An inclusive professionalism of solidarity is able to see and value perspectives from socially diverse individuals in strengthening understanding collectively and helping give objectivity a sturdier table on which to rest.
2. **To Join Medicine Is to Agree to be Reviewed by Peers:** In the scenario, Dr. Khan is certainly judging her peers' statements. But did she speak up? Was she psychologically safe to do so? Is there a way she could have done it in which issue could have been taken with the ideas and not with the people expounding them to invite everyone to grow through the interaction? Inclusive professionalisms of solidarity

must be enacted in not only safe spaces, but also brave spaces, where difficult conversations can be discussed collegially and all voices can be heard, with a recognition of structural discrimination as a present "third party" in the encounter.

3. **To Join Medicine Is to Agree to be Socialized in a Professional Identity:** In the scenario, Dr. Khan wondered whether this was being done in the best ways to serve the needs of diverse populations well. The key element for teachers is to always treat teaching interactions with learners as always having the potential to have students in the audience who may have direct experience with the topic at hand, and because of this a trauma-informed teaching approach is required. Ways that minimize hierarchy and allow for dialogic discussions between learners in which knowledge is co-created rather than transmitted are much more likely to be favorable to inclusive professionalisms of solidarity.

The ultimate goal of building inclusive professionalisms of solidarity is to promote diverse human flourishing. A diverse profession, where persons with many different experiences of society, including structural marginalization and oppression, is a strong one. The medical community is an ecosystem. Some of us are the trees, and we need to be tree-like. Some of us are the insects, and we need to be insect-like. And so on and so on. Yet we are all part of the ecosystem. Inclusive professionalisms of solidarity, through their teaching and socialization processes, show us that the ecosystem is home to all of us, and we must hold solidarity for each other so all of us can bring our true selves to our roles as professionals, to the benefit of the patients we serve, safely and with the understanding that what we show is valued by the collectivity.

References

1. Tweedie J, Hordern J, Dacre J. *Advancing Medical Professionalism.* Royal College of Physicians; 2018.
2. Martimianakis MA, Maniate JM, Hodges BD. Sociological interpretations of professionalism. *Med Educ.* 2009;43(9):829–837.
3. Lesser CS, Lucey CR, Egener B, Braddock CH, Linas SL, Levinson W. A behavioral and systems view of professionalism. *JAMA.* 2010;304(24):2732–2737.
4. Plochg T, Klazinga NS, Starfield B. Transforming medical professionalism to fit changing health needs. *BMC Med.* 2009;7(1):1–7.
5. Cruess RL, Cruess SR, Boudreau JD, Snell L, Steinert Y. Reframing medical education to support professional identity formation. *Acad Med.* 2014;89(11):1446–1451.
6. Cruess RL, Cruess SR. Expectations and obligations: professionalism and medicine's social contract with society. *Perspect Biol Med.* 2008;51(4):579–598.
7. Razack S, Maguire M, Hodges B, Steinert Y. What might we be saying to potential applicants to medical school? Discourses of excellence, equity, and diversity on the web sites of Canada's 17 medical schools. *Acad Med.* 2012;87(10):1323–1329.
8. Castellani B, Hafferty FW. The complexities of medical professionalism. In: *Professionalism in Medicine.* Springer; 2006:3–23.
9. Razack S, de Carvalho Filho MA, Merlo G, Agbor-Baiyee W, de Groot J, Reynolds PP. Privilege, social justice and the goals of medicine: towards a critically conscious professionalism of solidarity. *Perspect Med Educ.* 2022;11(2):67–69.

10. Zaidi Z, Razack S, Kumagai AK. Professionalism revisited during the pandemics of our time: COVID-19 and racism. *Perspect Med Educ.* 2021;10(4):238–244.
11. Marks JW. Definition of Hippocratic oath. n.d. Accessed May 31, 2022. https://www.medicinenet.com/hippocratic_oath/definition.htm
12. Freire P. *Education for Critical Consciousness.* Bloomsbury Publishing; 2021, May 20.
13. de Carvalho Filho MA, Ledubino A, Frutuoso L, da Silva Wanderlei J, Jaarsma D, Helmich E, Strazzacappa M. Medical education empowered by theater (MEET). *Academic Medicine.* 2020 Aug 1;95(8):1191–200.
14. Ramsden I. *Cultural Safety and Nursing Education in Aotearoa and Te Waipounamu* Doctoral dissertation. Victoria University of Wellington ; 2002.
15. Frost HD, Regehr G. "I am a doctor": negotiating the discourses of standardization and diversity in professional identity construction. *Acad Med.* 2013;88(10):1570–1577.
16. Wyatt TR, Rockich-Winston N, White D, Taylor TR. "Changing the narrative": a study on professional identity formation among Black/African American physicians in the US. *Adv Health Sci Educ.* 2021;26(1):183–198.
17. Volpe RL, Hopkins M, Haidet P, Wolpaw DR, Adams NE. Is research on professional identity formation biased? Early insights from a scoping review and metasynthesis. *Med Educ.* 2019;53(2):119–132.
18. Stewart KD, Gachago D. Step into the discomfort: (Re)orienting the White gaze and strategies to disrupt Whiteness in educational spaces. *Whiteness Educ.* 2022;7(1):18–31.
19. Veen M. Wrestling with (in)authenticity. *Perspect Med Educ.* 2021;10(3):141–144.
20. Burks DJ, Robbins R. Psychologists' authenticity: implications for work in professional and therapeutic settings. *J Humanist Psychol.* 2012;52(1):75–104.
21. Jongman-Sereno KP, Leary MR. The enigma of being yourself: a critical examination of the concept of authenticity. *Rev Gen Psychol.* 2019;23(1):133–142.
22. Arnason V. Towards authentic conversations. Authenticity in the patient-professional relationship. *Theor Med.* 1994;15(3):227–242.
23. Adewumi T, Delgado P, Carr M, Sowah E, Vassar M. The main themes and experiences shared with the hashtag# BlackintheIvory: a qualitative analysis. *bioRxiv.* 2022 Jan 1 .
24. Bakhtin MM. *The Dialogic Imagination: Four Essays.* University of Texas Press; 2010 Mar 1.
25. Wegerif R. From dialectic to dialogic. In: Timothy Koschmann, ed. *Theories of Learning and Studies of Instructional Practice.* Springer; 2011:201–221.

34
Health Law and Organizational Professionalism

Julie L. Agris

Key Points

- Consider the concept of organizational professionalism and the way in which it has the potential to bolster deteriorated and deteriorating trust in the US health sector.
- Discuss potential dividends of championing organizational professionalism in multiple sectors and dimensions of the US health system.
- Analyze the latitude provided within health law that facilitates opportunities to bolster organizational professionalism, improve healthcare delivery, and support the restoration of trust in the health sector

Introduction and Overview

Myriad circumstances have illuminated concerns regarding the ability to trust individuals and organizations associated with the US health sector. For example, the COVID-19 pandemic brought about varying degrees of skepticism related to the soundness of science, the credibility of its propagators, and the institutions with which they are affiliated. Working to restore lost trust and bolster confidence in the health system has become a focus to combat this problematic change. One effort to bolster a collective restoration of trust in the health sector is a focus on professionalism and professional behavior. Professionalism is critical at both the individual and organizational levels in the health sector. While professionalism at the individual level is critically important, so too is professionalism at the organizational level.

An evolving concept, called organizational professionalism (OP), is a critical component of any effort to model or achieve professionalism in the health sector. Individuals within the health system at every level may offer laudable efforts to enhance professional behavior and strengthen professionalism; however, those efforts may be impossible to realize without supportive healthcare organizations that champion professional and supportive environments and recognize the importance of professionalism at the organizational level or OP. As efforts to demonstrate and strengthen OP have evolved, laws and regulations are often identified as potential impediments or untapped assets to support these important efforts. This chapter aims to establish a framework for exploring the ways in which the law, particularly elements of health law (HL), may intersect with and ultimately strengthen these critical endeavors. To organize this scaffold and enable deeper analyses, this chapter provides a brief overview of OP domains, identifies of areas on which OP domains intersect with specific HL topics and acknowledges the potential to impede OP efforts, then concludes with a case study of using privacy law as an example to identify ways in which the law may be leveraged to support OP. The chapter also suggests preliminary strategies and recommendations for improving identified obstacles and ways in which the law can serve to support efforts to prioritize OP and bolster trust and trust-building in the health sector.

Ultimately, this chapter serves as a tool for healthcare leaders who hope to leverage implementation of HL in a manner that is supportive of achieving OP in their organizations. This work is also meant as an impetus to spur a larger discussion that is needed to thoroughly strategize about best practices in the implementation of HLs to ensure that the law supports, rather than impedes, efforts to implement professionalism in healthcare organizations. Application of OP principles in any number of areas of HL subjects will illuminate endless possibilities in which the law has the potential to support professionalism at the individual and organizational levels in the health sector.

Overview of the Organizational Professionalism and HL Frameworks

An Organizational Professionalism Framework

The Charter on Professionalism for Health Care Organizations [1] ("Charter") offers an aspirational framework for healthcare organizations to structure their analysis of OP. The charter domains include Patient Partnerships, Organizational Culture, Community Partnerships, and Operations and Business Practices.

Patient Partnerships

The charter domain of Patient Partnerships identifies healthcare organizations that prioritize a patient-centered approach that collaborates with patients to ensure outcomes consistent with their goals and values. Such organizations are likely to value patient feedback and continuously strive to improve their delivery of care through responsiveness to that feedback. In turn, these organizations are presumed to enjoy enhanced patient trust and loyalty. For example, a healthcare organization that demonstrates the value of patient feedback by responding to patient experience surveys, whether positive or negative, is more likely to gain or retain patient loyalty from individuals who feel heard and involved in the patient improvement process.

Organizational Culture

The charter domain of Organizational Culture identifies healthcare organizations that enjoy the benefit of effective leadership that prioritizes the delivery of high-quality care through shared beliefs and behaviors reflecting the priorities of patients and staff. Leaders of such organizations model, establish, and support a culture of professionalism and accountability in which these priorities are lived on a daily basis. For example, leaders who model professional behavior, such as greeting one another as they pass in the hall, with the expectation that all individuals within the organization will do the same, aim to encourage, if not mandate, a culture of professionalism.

Community Partnerships

The charter domain of Community Partnerships identifies healthcare organizations that support the establishment of healthy communities by collaborating with entities in the community, including policymakers and businesses. Such an approach requires an understanding of the social factors and needs at play in the surrounding community coupled with partnerships aiming to improve the community's health. To achieve this, organizational leaders collect tangible quantitative and qualitative feedback from the community, strategize to incorporate such feedback to make improvements, and consistently provide explanations of decision-making to the community to keep the lines of communication open.

Operations and Business Practices

The charter domain of Operations and Business Practices identifies healthcare organizations adhering to their noneconomically driven mission, vision, and values that promote individual professionalism and OP. These organizations prioritize a fiduciary commitment to patients and ethical business practices by placing evidence-based care and patient and staff safety at the center of care. Healthcare leaders of these organizations acknowledge that behaving in a patient-centered, ethically grounded manner enhances patient loyalty, staff morale, and the organization's brand. Organizations that prioritize financial gain over patients' best interests run the risk of eroding the public trust.

To facilitate further analysis of the intersection between the law and OP, the next section outlines a HL framework. This framework suggests a way to organize legal concepts in the HL space to facilitate further analysis of potential opportunities to enhance OP using varied areas of the law.

On establishing a commitment to achieve OP in healthcare organizations, leaders examine current activities and behaviors occurring within their organization. Ongoing organizational operations are often undertaken because they are mandated by the law. Implementation of legal requirements often includes latitude and flexibility. The elasticity with which certain regulations may be operationalized creates opportunities for OP domain enhancement. To identify these prospects requires an examination of untapped potential embedded in the HL field. Therefore, the following section sets out a HL framework to facilitate further analysis and opportunities for supporting the achievement of OP within healthcare organizations.

A Health Law Framework

Legal scholars have suggested that a distinct field of law should include "commonality" within the field and "distinctiveness" from other fields of law.[2] The importance of carving a specialty within the law is beyond the scope of this chapter; however, establishing HL as a subfield of the greater field of law is helpful to frame the remaining discussion. Legal scholars agree that the field of HL is established, but its particular scope is vast and without a consensus-based definition. Literature suggests HL as a field that requires understanding of antitrust, tax, corporations, torts, Employee Retirement Income Security Act (ERISA), and insurance law in addition to specialized subjects such as Medicare, Medicaid, certificate of need regulations, and the corporate practice

Table 34.1 Proposed Divisions of the Health Law Subfield

The Law of Health Care Finance
The Law of Health Care Organizations
The Law of Health Care Quality, Patient Safety, and Liability
The Law of Health Care Ethics and Bioethics

of medicine law.[3] In other words, the field of HL is extensive. To make the topic approachable for interested learners of HL, one approach is to divide the field into sections (see Table 34.1).

Each of these areas of law is vast and includes a multitude of opportunities for contribution to the analysis and improvement of OP domains. In the area of "Law of Healthcare Finance," individuals would consider topics including the innerworkings of Medicare and Medicaid laws, the Affordable Care Act and its legal and political challenges, and the ways in which healthcare financing laws may perpetuate discrimination and unequal treatment in the health system. In the area of "Law of Healthcare Organizations," individuals would consider topics including laws that support the delivery of healthcare through the behaviors of organizations engaged in legal transactions, laws addressing the legal relationships between and among differing entities within the healthcare enterprise, and corporate law to leverage optimal organizational structures. In the area of "Law of Healthcare Quality, Patient Safety, and Liability," individuals would consider topics including laws requiring the intersection of private and public entities to ensure the delivery of high-quality healthcare, and the implications of medical malpractice laws on the delivery of care to patients. Finally, in the area of "Law of Healthcare Ethics and Bioethics," individuals would consider areas of law protecting human rights of those interacting with the healthcare delivery system as patients or participants in medical research. Each application of OP principles to specific areas of HL requires context-specific evaluation. We use the delineations outlined to suggest specific areas for future consideration.

Intersection of the OP and HL Frameworks

There are many ways to structure a strategy to position HL as a supportive mechanism to improve OP endeavors. Meshing the two aforementioned frameworks allows our analysis to proceed by connecting the domains of OP that might obviously intersect with the law. Beyond this identified approach or the scope of this chapter, there are myriad alternative approaches that we may consider to leverage law to support achieving OP in the future.

For purposes of this initial exploration, we proceed with identifying several potential areas for examination in which the outlined HL sections herein lend themselves to an analysis using the specified OP domains (see Table 34.2).

Table 34.2 illustrates one method of analysis that is the application of each OP domain to each identified HL section and the resulting identification of opportunities for improvement in the health sector. To initiate this analysis, an OP domain is identified in column 1, a corresponding HL framework is identified in column 2, and the intersection of OP and the specific HL topics that are ripe for further exploration are identified in

Table 34.2 Identification of Topics Ripe for Initial Exploration at the Intersection of Organizational Professionalism and HL*

Column 1	Column 2	Column 3
Organizational Professionalism Framework	**Health Law (HL) Framework**	**Suggested Health Law (HL) Topics to Serve as Vehicles for Organizational Professionalism (OP) in Health Care Organizations**
Patient Partnership Domain	The Law of Health Care Ethics and Bioethics	• Physician-Patient Relationship Formation • Patient Abandonment • Informed Consent • Confidentiality and Disclosure of Protected Health information • Conflicts of Interest Disclosure • Interdisciplinary Definitions of Professionalism to Enhance Understanding across Professions • Reproductive Health Decision-making • Abortion • Contraception • Sterilization • Assisted Reproductive Technology (ART) • Life & Death Decision-making • Determination of Death • Organ Transplantation • Adults with Decision-making Capacity • Adults without Decision-making Capacity • Children • Futile Treatment • Medically Assisted Dying • Regulation of Research Involving Human Subjects

(*continued*)

Table 34.2 Continued

Column 1	Column 2	Column 3
Organizational Culture Domain	The Law of Health Care Organizations	• Physician/Staff Contracts, Labor, & Employment • Emergency Medical Treatment and Labor Act (EMTALA) • Equal Access to Health Care • Antidiscrimination Law • Race, Color, & National Origin • Sex & Gender • Disability • Genetic Information • Mental Health & Addiction • Health Reform • Access • Cost • Quality • Choice
Community Partnership Domain	The Law of Health Care Quality, Patient Safety, and Liability	• Medical Licensure and Discipline • Medical Privileges & Credentialing • Scope of Practice • Unlicensed Providers • Complementary and Alternative Medicine • Hospital Regulations • Nursing Home Regulation • Private Accreditation • Provider & Health Care Organization Negligence, Liability, & Vicarious Liability • Health Plan Liability • Accountable Care Organization (ACO) Liability • Tort Reform for Medical Injuries

Operations and Business Practices Domain	The Law of Health Care Finance	• Health Insurance Regulation • Employee Retirement Income Security Act (ERISA) • Patient Protection and Affordable Care Act (ACA) • HIPAA & COBRA • Medicare Law • Medicaid Law • State Laws • Payment Incentives • Price Transparency • Legal Action for Unpaid Medical Bills • Population Health & Public HL • Social Determinants of Health and the Law • Health Care Organizational Structures & Corporate Law • Antitrust in Health Care • Taxation in Health Care • Health Care Compliance • Privacy and Confidentiality • Fraud and Abuse • False Claims Act • Anti-kickback Statute • Stark Law

*Identified topics may be addressed in myriad settings, including educational environments, academic medical centers, private health services organizations, or system-level policies, depending on the focus of the matter on which the individual healthcare entity is working to improve.

column 3. Column 3 identifies potential opportunities for improvement in intersecting areas in which the laws surrounding the topics identifies could be revised, evaluated, or enhanced to improve the way in which they support OP goals. The sections in this part of the chapter delve more deeply into examples of the ways in which the areas identified in column 3 of Table 34.2 may facilitate discussion and efforts to improve professionalism, specifically OP, in healthcare organizations.

For example, as outlined in Table 34.2 areas within the Law of Healthcare Ethics and Bioethics section include many opportunities to enhance the Patient Partnership OP domain. Column 3 identifies multiple areas of the law in which the current status and implementation may not fully support OP goals. A deeper examination of each using the domains of OP would inevitably reveal opportunities for improvement. Similarly, materials found within casebooks, such as the Law of Healthcare Organizations (Casebook for citation: https://www.westacademic.com/Health-Law-Cases-Materials-and-Problems_4) includes many opportunities to enhance the Organizational Culture OP domain. The Law of Healthcare Quality, Patient Safety, and Liability (Casebook for citation: https://www.westacademic.com/Law-and-Health-Care-Quality-Patient-Safety-and-Liability_4) includes many opportunities to enhance the Community Partnership OP domain. The Law of Healthcare Organization and Finance (Casebook for citation: https://www.westacademic.com/The-Law-of-Health-Care-Organization-and-Finance_9781685612498) includes many opportunities to enhance the Operations and Business Practices OP domain. The sections following Table 34.2 use these resources to develop an initial framework and explore these intersecting areas by identifying the potential for them, but a deeper exploration of the potential within each area of the law is beyond the scope of this chapter, but ripe for further exploration, research, and recommendations for improvement.

Intersection of the Patient Partnership Domain and the Law of Healthcare Ethics and Bioethics

As indicated in Table 34.2, an initial analysis of the ways in which the OP domain of Patient Partnerships overlaps with the Law of Healthcare Ethics and Bioethics unveils myriad areas of the law that are ripe for exploration. Although not an exhaustive list, the initially identified areas of law at this intersection include

1. Physician-patient relationship formation
2. Patient abandonment
3. Informed consent
4. Confidentiality and disclosure of protected health information (PHI)
5. Conflicts of interest disclosure
6. Interdisciplinary definitions of professionalism to enhance understanding across professions
7. Reproductive health decision-making
    a. Abortion
    b. Contraception
    c. Sterilization
    d. Assisted reproductive technology (ART)

8. Life and death decision-making
    a. Determination of death
    b. Organ transplantation
    c. Adults with decision-making capacity
    d. Adults without decision-making capacity
    e. Children
    f. Futile treatment
    g. Medically assisted dying
9. Regulation of research involving human subjects

As a reminder, the charter domain of Patient Partnerships identifies healthcare organizations that prioritize a patient-centered approach that collaborates with patients to ensure outcomes consistent with their goals and values. Such organizations are likely to value patient feedback and continuously strive to improve their delivery of care through responsiveness to that feedback. In turn, these organizations are presumed to enjoy enhanced patient trust and loyalty.

Each of the identified areas of law includes opportunities to enhance the domain of Patient Partnerships on implementation. For example, a healthcare organization with a goal of enhancing or achieving OP will inevitably confront questions about best practices related to Confidentiality and Disclosure of Patient Health Information. One analysis of this intersection would proceed as discussed next.

Healthcare organizations enjoy flexibility when implementing laws governing this area of medical practice. For example, the law requires healthcare organizations to develop, implement, and maintain detailed local policies related to this area of the law. Therefore, healthcare organizations have the flexibility to implement policies supportive of establishing and maintaining healthcare organizations that keep patients at the center of care when implementing policies related to protecting health information. A healthcare organization could choose the most restrictive path of releasing patient information in order to avoid as much liability as possible, even if the law allows for greater flexibility. Alternatively, a healthcare organization could choose to develop, implement, and maintain policies that are protective of patient information while also being cognizant of the potential adverse impact of reading the law too strictly and implementing policies that thwart a patient's ability to receive the highest possible quality of care because there was a delay in disclosing medical information for fear of organizational liability.

These decisions are referred to herein as decisions of the organization. However, the reality is these decisions are actually being made on behalf of the organization by individuals within the organization who have been deemed to have the requisite knowledge to competently analyze and implement the law in a way that benefits and protects the organization. Therefore, the questions in each of these analyses are as follows: Who is making the decision on policy development and if the organization is committed to promoting OP? How have the parameters of OP been disseminated and indoctrinated into the organization? Without purposeful education on the principles and domains of OP, implementation of legal requirements through the lens of OP will be difficult, if not impossible, to achieve. A case study of this topic with an analysis of each OP domain appears herein. For teaching and learning purposes, case studies to facilitate the analysis of each intersecting area appearing in Column 3 of Table 34.2 are currently under development. The remaining sections give a brief overview of these intersection areas that are critical to any effort to leverage law, specifically HL, as a tool to bolster OP.

Intersection of the Organizational Culture Domain and the Law of Healthcare Organizations

Similar to the section above, Table 34.2 illustrates several topics at the intersection of Organizational Culture and the Law of Healthcare Organizations. Although not an exhaustive list, the initially identified areas of law at this intersection include

1. Physician/staff contracts, labor, and employment
2. Emergency Medical Treatment and Labor Act (EMTALA)
3. Equal access to healthcare
4. Antidiscrimination law
    a. Race, color, and national origin
    b. Sex and gender
    c. Disability
    d. Genetic information
    e. Mental health and addiction
5. Health reform
    a. Access
    b. Cost
    c. Quality
    d. Choice

Recall that the charter domain of Organizational Culture identifies healthcare organizations that enjoy the benefit of effective leadership that prioritizes the delivery of high-quality care through shared beliefs and behaviors that reflect the priorities of patients and staff. Leaders of such organizations model, establish, and support a culture of professionalism and accountability in which these priorities are lived on a daily basis. For example, leaders who model professional behavior, such as greeting one another as they pass in the hall, with the expectation that all individuals within the organization will do the same, aim to encourage, if not mandate, a culture of professionalism.

To reiterate, healthcare organizations enjoy the benefit of determining how they will implement certain laws. In the case of implementation of laws that could have a direct impact on the Organizational Culture domain, healthcare organizations enjoy flexibility on the way in which they conduct their physician and staff contracting in their organizations. While every healthcare organization is required to provide high-quality patient care that embeds accountability throughout this process, the manner in which healthcare organizations choose to do so can have a significant impact on Organizational Culture. For example, in the case of physician contracting, if a healthcare organization employs a punitive approach to contract negotiations as a result of a medical error that did not rise to the level of medical negligence, the impact may severely deteriorate morale and exacerbate moral injury. Therefore, this flexibility provides opportunities in not only this particular example, but also the areas of the law identified in the list above and in Table 34.2, to give healthcare organizations the potential to leverage the flexibility provided in mandated laws to implement policies, procedures, and the tenor of their organization with an aim toward achieving and enhancing OP. Similar analyses should be conducted in each of the identified legal areas included herein and will unearth further opportunities for law to serve as a vehicle toward OP.

Intersection of the Community Partnership Domain and the Law of Healthcare Quality, Patient Safety, and Liability

Areas of the law at the intersection of Community Partnerships and the Law of Healthcare Quality, Patient Safety, and Liability include

1. Medical licensure and discipline
2. Medical privileges and credentialing
3. Scope of practice
4. Unlicensed providers
5. Complementary and alternative medicine
6. Hospital regulations
7. Nursing home regulation
8. Private accreditation
9. Provider and healthcare organization negligence, liability, and vicarious liability
10. Health plan liability
11. Accountable care organization (ACO) liability
12. Tort reform for medical injuries

Recall that the charter domain of Community Partnerships identifies healthcare organizations that support the establishment of healthy communities by collaborating with entities in the community, including policymakers and businesses. Such an approach requires an understanding of the social factors and needs at play in the surrounding community coupled with partnerships aiming to improve the community's health. To achieve this, organizational leaders collect tangible quantitative and qualitative feedback from the community, strategize to incorporate such feedback to make improvements, and consistently provide explanations of decision-making to the community to keep the lines of communication open.

To leverage the flexibility in their determination of the way in which they will implement laws within their entities, leaders of healthcare organizations must analyze the law, understand their mandate, and appreciate the way in which they are capable of implementing the law while simultaneously promoting OP principles. For example, similar to the analysis in the previous section, if a healthcare organization chooses to implement policies in which a medical error that does not rise to the level of negligence impacts the privileging and credentialing process, such an approach may severely deteriorate morale and exacerbate moral injury.

Therefore, implementation of privileging and credentialing requirements must include the consideration of whether the approach balances promoting the trust of the community through the provision of high-quality care using a no or low-tolerance, rigorous vetting process versus one that promotes a "just culture" in which providers and staff are encouraged to admit mistakes when they occur in order to improve the quality of care provided within the healthcare organization. This arguably harsh approach has the potential to bolster important community partnerships by demonstrating that communities can trust the healthcare organization as a result of the rigorous vetting process and removal of providers that fall below the standard of care, but it also has the potential to severely deteriorate morale, exacerbate moral injury, and ultimately weaken organizational culture. Similar analyses could be conducted in each of the legal areas included herein.

Intersection of the Operations and Business Practices Domains and the Law of Healthcare Finance

The intersection of the OP Operations and Business Practice Charter domain and the Law of Healthcare Finance present multiple areas of law for consideration, including

1. Health insurance regulation
   a. ERISA
   b. Patient Protection and Affordable Care Act (ACA)
   c. Health Insurance Portability and Accountability Act (HIPAA)
   d. Consolidated Omnibus Budget Reconciliation Act (COBRA)
   e. Medicare law
   f. Medicaid law
   g. State laws
   h. Payment incentives
   i. Price transparency
   j. Legal action for unpaid medical bills
2. Population health and public health law
   a. Social determinants of health and the law
3. Healthcare organizational structures and corporate law
4. Antitrust in healthcare
5. Taxation in healthcare
6. Healthcare compliance
   a. Privacy and confidentiality
   b. Fraud and abuse
      i. False Claims Act
      ii. Antikickback statute
      iii. Stark Law

Recall that the charter domain of Operations and Business Practices identifies healthcare organizations adhering to their noneconomically driven mission, vision, and values that promote individual and OP. These organizations prioritize a fiduciary commitment to patients and ethical business practices by placing evidence-based care and patient and staff safety at the center of care. Healthcare leaders of these organizations acknowledge that behaving in a patient-centered, ethically grounded manner enhances patient loyalty, staff morale, and the organization's brand. Organizations that prioritize financial gain over patients' best interests run the risk of eroding the public trust.

One example in this area is the degree to which healthcare organizations pursue patients for unpaid medical bills. Healthcare organizations are free to choose to conduct their coding and billing practices in compliance with all legal requirements. However, the extent to which they will pursue patients, in court, to recoup bad debt for care provided is a business decision. This means a healthcare organization could position themselves to argue that the mission of their organization is to provide care to their patient population, and while patients are required to and should pay the reasonable costs for their medical care, if they reasonably prove that they are not able to do so, the healthcare organization could resolve to call that free care provided for charitable purposes, rather than an unpaid medical debt requiring legal action, including but not limited to, a healthcare provider suing their patient for a debt owed. This serves as another example of an area of the law in which flexibility exists to allow for implementation of local policies that incorporate OP principles in the areas of Operations and Business Practices. Similar analyses should be conducted in each of the legal areas included herein.

Additional Opportunities for Analyses

The method of analysis outlined herein reveals areas of the law for initial exploration. A deeper consideration of OP domains applied to any one of these areas of HL reveals the opportunity to apply all OP domains to that particular area of law. In other words, these initial analyses of one OP lens being applied to one area of HL are meant to encourage a deeper, multifaceted analysis in which all OP domains are applied to each identified HL area. For your consideration, an application of all four OP domains to one identified area of HL appears in Table 34.3. This is meant to encourage deeper exploration and research on each of these initially identified areas of law with an aim toward developing multifaceted recommendations and opportunities for HL to support the achievement of OP in healthcare organizations.

Recommendations

Recommendation to Establish Commonly Understood Terms of HL and OP Across Healthcare Disciplines

Current definitions throughout the fields of HL, OP, and their intersections are varied and disparate. To improve our ability to communicate with one another, health lawyers, and those they advise, including healthcare executives, providers, and their designees, must have a better understanding of basic terms using common definitions. For example, to lead the charge toward OP in a healthcare organization, a healthcare executive must understand the importance of implementing specific legal requirements with an eye toward simultaneously improving OP within a healthcare organization. They must first understand the existence of OP and the domains within. In other words, our individual professions and the professionals within are well aware of the general term *professionalism*. We collectively understand that each of our professions have embedded responsibilities and specific requirements to demonstrate achievement of those responsibilities

Table 34.3 Sample Application of OP Domains to Specific Legal Provisions of the Health Insurance Portability and Accountability Act (HIPAA)

Organizational Professionalism Domain Framework	Health Law (HL) Provision	Recommendations for HCOP to use Health Law (HL) as the Vehicle to Improve Organizational Professionalism
Patient Partnership Domain	45 CFR § 164.520 Notice of Privacy Practices for Protected Health Information	• Consistent with the OP domain of Patient Partnerships, health care organizations (HCOs) should evaluate the degree of health literacy of their Notice of Privacy Practices (NPP). In the post-breach notification status of any HCO, demonstrating to the public that the organization understands and values the rights of its patients can be recuperative. The NPP is an opportunity to partner with patients to understand their rights and for health care providers to build trust with their patients and the larger community they serve. HCOs should establish a way in which the content of the NPP is communicated in a reasonably understandable fashion to patients and use this document as an opportunity to open dialogue with patients about the degree to which they value the privacy of their patients and the confidentiality of PHI. Such an approach has the potential to improve trust in the health care sector while simultaneously promoting the free flow of information between patients and providers with an aim toward improving the quality of care delivered to patients.
Organizational Culture Domain	45 CFR § 164.530(b)(1) Administrative Requirements Standard: Training	• Consistent with the OP domain of Organizational Culture, HCOs should embrace the training requirement as an opportunity to engage with every dimension of its workforce. The law requires periodic training, but rather than making this dreaded compliance training, the mandate to educate every member of the workforce should be leveraged as an opportunity to educate each person on the seriousness with which the organization treats privacy and confidentiality of PHI. Embedded within the training of each member of its workforce is the opportunity to communicate the importance of individual and organizational professionalism and the domains outlined within.
Community Partnership Domain	45 CFR § 164.404(a)(1) Notification to Individuals Standard: General Rule	• Consistent with the OP domain of Community Partnership, HCO's leadership should approach unauthorized disclosures of PHY as breaches and comply with the breach notification requirements. Notification of any breach should be communicated openly and honestly to the community. HCOs should provide explanations for the misstep, openly and honestly. Further, HCOs should prepare to explain decision-making that led to the breach and acknowledge the ways in which those decisions could have been made differently if the facts support this outcome. HCOs should comply readily and diligently with all legal requirements of the breach notification rule with professionalism. To support the Community Partnership Domain, lines of communication should remain open between HCOs and the community. Further, HCOs should prepare to comply readily with all investigatory inquiries from government inquires with professionalism, demonstrated by their responsiveness, attention to detail, and transparency. Each of these efforts will support HCOs goal of being a model health care organization in the community which aims to achieve the domains of OP as it promotes the restoration of trust in its organization.
Operations and Business Practices Domain	45 CFR § 164.502 Uses and Disclosures of Protected Health Information: General Rules	• Consistent with the OP Domain of Operations and Business Practices, HCOs should recognize their fiduciary commitment to patients and ethical business practices. When using and disclosing PHI, standard operating practices should consider the principles of OP, specifically as they relate to Operations and Business Practices. Decisions surrounding how, when, and to what extent PHI may be used and disclosed should hold patients' best interest as a core value. The decision to administer Operations and Business Practices in such a patient-centered, ethical manner will lead to patient loyalty, increased staff morale, and improvement of HCOs brand as it recovers from the publicity surrounding any breach of PHI.

at the individual level. However, healthcare leaders are less aware of the concepts of OP, the articulated domains within, or the importance of paying attention to them in order to ensure that individuals might achieve their desired level of professionalism at the individual level.

On establishing commonly understood definitions of OP and its domains, an interprofessional, collective commitment to achieve and maintain OP will be critical. Ultimately, a pledge to uphold the values of an environment that strives to achieve OP will support demonstrated professionalism at the individual level and enhance an organization's ability to provide high-quality patient care.

Recommendations for Enhancing Education and Scholarship Research at the Intersection of HL and OP

Education is at the root of any attempt to shift commonly understood definitions and behaviors. Literature is developing in the areas of HL and OP separately, but little has been written at the intersection of these fields. As outlined herein, there are myriad opportunities for discovering intersections that have the potential to compliment goals aimed toward enhancing professionalism and trust in the health sector.

To add this important subject to the curriculum, scholars must commit to exploring these topics and expanding scholarly literature comprehensively. In addition, individuals developing curriculum for the health professions must understand and prioritize OP as a subject requiring competency. Incorporating HL and OP competencies are a natural progression to already established curricula. Most areas of study in the health sector currently include an examination of professionalism, ethics, or bioethics. Implementation of law using OP principles would be a natural enhancement to any of the established curricula in these areas. An example of one way to implement this subject into the health professions curriculum through a case study format may be found in further in the chapter.

Recommendations for Implementing HL to Support OP in Practice

The practice of medicine and delivery of healthcare services are critical components of any society. In the post-COVID-19 US health system, an ongoing recovery continues to evolve. While trust in the health system and the professionals who practice within have been questioned by some in recent years, remaining consistent in our commitment to science, data, and professionalism has the potential to shift the tides. Increasing and maintaining professionalism in the health sector has the potential to move healthcare delivery into a more functional and improved direction.

Healthcare organizations are currently required to implement innumerable statutes, regulations, polices, and procedures. This chapter outlines several areas of the law that are already in existence as avenues on which to layer the work of professionalism, specifically OP (see Table 35.2). This initial identification of potential areas for consideration are meant to spur healthcare leaders to think about ways in which they might consider modifying their approaches to implementation of already mandated legal requirements. As outlined in the case study herein, implementation of regulations, such as 45 CFR §

164.530(b)(1), have been required for many years and are not likely to change in the years to come, but how we implement such legal provisions has the potential to positively impact healthcare organizations and their work, without creating new administrative burdens. In other words, the law serves as the vehicle, while OP serves as the fuel to implement it. Finding collective agreement on the definition of OP among healthcare professionals, then implementing those agreed on values into the already existing, legally compliant systems has the potential to shift and improve current mindsets and improve trust among stakeholders in the health sector without any additional mandate.

Conclusion

One approach to bolster deteriorated and deteriorating trust in the US health sector is to enhance OP in healthcare organizations. US medical education and broader healthcare education have focused on professionalism at the individual level for decades; however, acknowledging professionalism at the organizational level is a newer concept. Although the health sector continues its pursuit of consensus on the components of OP, the currently articulated charter domains serve as a sound framework. Due to the complexity of the health system and the healthcare delivery entities within, additional unfunded mandates to implement, monitor, and measure new metrics are rarely well received by healthcare leaders. However, an understanding of the importance and potential dividends of championing a professional organization that proactively supports professional behavior and individual professionalism is likely to gain momentum if healthcare leaders are encouraged that it is possible to accomplish these laudable efforts by enhancing the way in which business practices already occur in the health sector. The latitude permitted by certain laws and regulations provides an opportunity for the law to support and bolster OP domains, improve healthcare delivery, and support the restoration of trust in the health sector.

Case Study Application

Case Study: Implementation of the HIPAA Privacy Rule: A Vehicle to Enhance Organizational Professionalism in the Health Sector

Please read the fact pattern below and for each OP domain (Patient Partnership, Organizational Culture, Community Partnership, and Operations and Business Practices); identify at least one example of a way in which remediation from the event could support a healthcare organization's effort to improve and maintain OP.

> In a series of articles published by the local *Herald Tribune* reports bring attention to a spree of robberies in a private office building that houses multiple businesses, including one of the outsourced billing departments of the Healthcare Organization for the People (HCOP). The department is housed in this external facility because the main hospital ran out of office space and needed to find an alternate location for these billing offices that did not require direct access to patients for patient care, so being housed in an alternate location was the decision of the corporate entity ultimately responsible for HCOP.

The most recent reports bring to light the fact that one of the computers stolen included a workstation from HCOPs business offices. A review of business documents determine that PHI was likely housed on the stolen hard drive within the workstation. A new privacy officer has been hired by the organization and quickly realizes that several policies (including the policy guiding Notice of Privacy Practices and Training requirements) to implement HIPAA were drafted using an online template when the law went into effect over a decade ago, and some necessary policies were never established or implemented. As the newly hired chief organizational professionalism officer, it is your job to advise the new privacy officer on your recommended best approach to close the current gaps on HCOP's policy implementation quandary and be ready to defend the impending investigation from the Office for Civil Rights (OCR), which is likely to arrive any day.

Questions for Discussion

1. Identify and analyze the dimensions of the *Patient Partnership* domain that may be a focus to establish, promote, and maintain OP in HCOP.
2. Identify and analyze the dimensions of the *Organizational Culture* domain that may be a focus to establish, promote, and maintain OP in HCOP.
3. Identify and analyze the dimensions of the *Community Partnership* domain that may be a focus to establish, promote, and maintain OP in HCOP.
4. Identify and analyze the dimensions of the *Operations and Business Practices* domain that may be a focus to establish, promote, and maintain OP in HCOP.

Teacher's Manual to Guide Discussion

All healthcare organizations, as healthcare providers under the law, are required to implement certain legal provisions to protect the confidentiality of their patients' healthcare information. The laws governing this area of any healthcare organizations provision of healthcare services is inevitably complex. Each healthcare organization has its own legal and operational structure in addition to its own organizational culture and political dynamics. Therefore, the law governing the confidentiality of PHI purposefully incorporates a great deal of flexibility for healthcare organizations to ensure that the law is implemented in a way that is functional for each individual organization while simultaneously meeting the intended purpose of the law.

In the case study fact pattern herein, the chief organizational professionalism officer should advise the chief privacy officer that there are ways to leverage the flexibility of the law while simultaneously rectifying the potential misstep of failing to regularly update the HCOP's HIPAA policies. There are innumerable examples of ways in which specific provisions of the law could be implemented to facilitate this goal. Table 34.4 provides examples for guidance and promoting class discussion.

In summary, this case study serves as an example of the way in which HL legal provisions may be analyzed through a lens of OP domains. The law is often not overly prescriptive. This provides great flexibility and creativity when considering how to implement legal provisions. To consider OP domains in the implementation and local policymaking process within healthcare organizations is an opportunity to leverage law as a

Table 34.4 Case Study Identifying Opportunities for HL to Support Achieving Organizational Professionalism

Organizational Professionalism Domain Framework	Health Law (HL) Provision	Recommendations for HCOP to use Health Law (HL) as the Vehicle to Improve Organizational Professionalism
Patient Partnership Domain	45 CFR § 164.520 Notice of Privacy Practices for Protected Health Information	Consistent with the OP domain of Patient Partnerships, HCOP should evaluate the degree of health literacy of their Notice of Privacy Practices (NPP). In the post-breach notification status of any health care organization, demonstrating to the public that the organization understands and values the rights of its patients can be recuperative. The NPP is an opportunity to partner with patients to understand their rights and for health care providers to build trust with their patients and the larger community they serve. HCOP should establish a way in which the content of the NPP is communicated in a reasonably understandable fashion to patients and use this document as an opportunity to open dialogue with patients about the degree to which they value the privacy of their patients and the confidentiality of PHI. Such an approach has the potential to improve trust in the health care sector while simultaneously promoting the free flow of information between patients and providers with an aim toward improving the quality of care delivered to patients.
Organizational Culture Domain	45 CFR § 164.530(b)(1) Administrative Requirements Standard: Training	Consistent with the OP domain of Organizational Culture, HCOP should embrace the training requirement as an opportunity to engage with every dimension of its workforce. The law requires periodic training, but rather than making this dreaded compliance training, the mandate to educate every member of the workforce should be leveraged as an opportunity to educate each person on the seriousness with which the organization treats privacy and confidentiality of PHI. Embedded within the training of each member of its workforce is the opportunity to communicate the importance of individual and organizational professionalism and the domains outlined within.
Community Partnership Domain	45 CFR § 164.404(a)(1) Notification to Individuals Standard: General Rule	Consistent with the OP domain of Community Partnership, HCOP's leadership should approach the situation as a breach of PHI. This should be communicated openly and honestly to the community. HCOP should provide explanations for the misstep, openly and honestly. Further, HCOP should prepare to explain decision-making that led to the breach and acknowledge the ways in which those decisions could have been made differently if the facts support this outcome. HCOP should comply readily and diligently with all legal requirements of the breach notification rule with professionalism. To support the Community Partnership Domain, lines of communication should remain open between HCOP and the community. Further, HCOP should prepare to comply readily with all investigatory inquiries from government inquires with professionalism, demonstrated by their responsiveness, attention to detail, and transparency. Each of these efforts will support HCOP's goal of being a model health care organization in the community which aims to achieve the domains of OP as it promotes the restoration of trust in its organization.
Operations and Business Practices Domain	45 CFR § 164.502 Uses and Disclosures of Protected Health Information: General Rules	Consistent with the OP Domain of Operations and Business Practices, HCOP should recognize its fiduciary commitment to patients and ethical business practices. When using and disclosing PHI, standard operating practices should consider the principles of OP, specifically as they relate to Operations and Business Practices. Decisions surrounding how, when, and to what extent PHI may be used and disclosed should hold patients' best interest as a core value. The decision to administer Operations and Business Practices in such a patient-centered, ethical manner will lead to patient loyalty, increased staff morale, and improvement of the HCOP brand as it recovers from the publicity surrounding the breach of PHI.

tool, rather than an impediment, toward achieving OP. Using these strategies to bolster the existence of OP in healthcare organizations will better support the establishment and perpetuation of healthcare organizations in which providers and support staff can mirror professional behavior as the delivery of high-quality patient care remains everyone's collective goal.

References

1. Egener B, Mason D, McDonald W, et al. The charter on professionalism for health care organizations. *Acad Med.* 2017;92(8):1091–1099.
2. Aagaard TS. Environmental law as a legal field: an inquiry in legal taxonomy. *Cornell Law Rev.* 2010;95:221, 242.
3. Elhauge ER. Can health law become a coherent field of law. *Wake Forest Law Rev.* 2006;95:365, 368.

35
Maintaining Ethical Physician-Industry Relationships

Armaan Singh, Eric A. Singer, and Parth K. Modi

> **Key Points**
>
> - Physicians are often at the center of marketing campaigns by industry, and evidence demonstrates marketing to physicians is effective in modifying their prescribing behaviors.
> - The Open Payments registry is a valuable tool for researchers and policymakers to better understand physician-industry relationships and their ties to medical research.
> - Physician-industry relationships are both necessary and not inherently unethical or unprofessional but are at risk of being unethical and unprofessional. Transparency and other mitigation strategies can help ensure physician-industry relationships adhere to the basic tenets of medical professionalism.

Introduction

> Patients and the public benefit when physicians and researchers collaborate with pharmaceutical, medical device, and biotechnology companies to develop products that benefit individual and public health. At the same time, concerns are growing that wide-ranging financial ties to industry may unduly influence professional judgments involving the primary interests and goals of medicine. Such conflicts of interest threaten the integrity of scientific investigations, the objectivity of professional education, the quality of patient care, and the public's trust in medicine.[p1]

This opening paragraph from the National Academy of Medicine's 2009 report *Conflict of Interest in Medical Research, Education, and Practice* concisely summarizes the fundamental tension in the philosophically distinct but often intertwined enterprises of medical care and the healthcare industry.[1] This report signaled to the US public and policymakers that conflicts (COIs) of interest between healthcare providers and the medical industry were an essential concern and, in large part, prompted the development of federal policy to address this issue. The authors of this report reached several general conclusions (Box 35.1).

While physicians and nurses are often portrayed as the face of healthcare in popular culture and media, modern medicine requires multiple parties, including individual healthcare providers, facilities, public and private payers, and commercial entities (e.g.,

Box 35.1 Broad Conclusions of the 2009 National Academy of Medicine Committee on Conflict of Interest

- The goals of conflict of interest policies in medicine are primarily to protect the integrity of professional judgment and to preserve public trust rather than to try to remediate bias or mistrust after they occur.
- The disclosure of individual and institutional financial relationships is a critical but limited first step in the process of identifying and responding to conflicts of interest.
- Conflict of interest policies and procedures can be strengthened by engaging physicians, researchers, and medical institutions in developing conflict of interest policies and consensus standards.
- A range of supporting organizations—public and private—can promote the adoption and implementation of conflict of interest policies and help create a culture of accountability that sustains professional norms and public confidence in professional judgments.
- Research on conflicts of interest and conflict of interest policies can provide a stronger evidence base for policy design and implementation.
- If medical institutions do not act voluntarily to strengthen their conflict of interest policies and procedures, the pressure for external regulation is likely to increase.

drug and device manufacturers), among others. Together, these groups contribute to an American health system whose spending exceeded of $4.1 trillion in 2020 and whose costs are mainly sponsored by the federal government (36% of total healthcare spending) and households (26%).[2] The spending on pharmaceutical drugs alone in 2021 was estimated to be more than $570 billion.[3] Thus, although nearly all entities engaged in the delivery of healthcare include patient care as part of their mission, the growing impact of the economics of the healthcare industry cannot be understated. As healthcare spending in the United States now comprises almost 20% of the gross domestic product, it is essential to understand how commercial entities use their influence and money to interact with physicians and other healthcare providers.[4] At the root of this scrutiny is the public concern that the professionalism and impartial judgment of physicians may be compromised by their relationships with industry and influence the quality of patient care, research, and the public health.

Before exploring the potential breaches of professionalism that may result from COIs, we must first understand the ethical obligations of physicians and how they differ from those of the pharmaceutical and medical device manufacturers. The physician-scholar Edmund Pellegrino argues that as part of a physician's claim to the "profession" of practicing medicine, there is a corresponding commitment to the suppression of self-interest, when necessary, for the welfare of the patient.[5] Consequently, a member of the profession of medicine not only has the knowledge and skill to help a patient, but also commits to using that knowledge in the best interests of the patient rather than their own self-interest. This commitment to patient beneficence is what allows physicians the privilege to probe deeply in their patients' lives and provide meaningful care.

Although it is established that the profession of medicine is based on trust and patient preeminence, the same cannot be said about the drug and device industries. As healthcare companies, they have the obligation to be in accordance with US federal and state laws. But as for-profit corporations, these manufacturers also have a fiduciary responsibility to their shareholders to be profitable. The famed economist Milton Friedman's shareholder theory, also known as the Friedman doctrine, is a series of corporate principles that is nearly ubiquitous across corporate America. The Friedman doctrine states that an entity does not have any social responsibility to the society around it, but rather has the sole responsibility to abide by its shareholders.[6] Consequently, social responsibility is a responsibility of the shareholders rather than of company executives or employees. This doctrine has had deep influence across business schools and publicly owned corporations in the United States.[7] Thus, it should be expected and not necessarily condemned that healthcare companies will market their products as aggressively as any other industry, within the bounds of the law.[6]

The aim of this chapter is to provide physicians and other healthcare professionals with a framework to understand and manage their role in physician-industry relationships. We first highlight the prevalence of marketing to physicians and its effects on physician behavior and then provide some practical strategies to help physicians manage their relationships with industry. We hope that it will become clear that physicians cannot afford to deny or ignore the influence of relationships with industry and should remain proactive in managing these to minimize undue influence, improve their clinical decision-making, and foster a patient-physician relationship based in trust.

The Ubiquitous Nature of Pharmaceutical and Device Marketing to Physicians

The issue of physician-industry relations is far from a new topic: As far back as 1980, concerns around this issue have been raised in preeminent journals such as the *New England Journal of Medicine*.[7] Unlike other salespeople, drug industry representatives do not promote their products directly to end consumers (i.e., patients), but instead aim to influence physician prescribing habits. Early studies confirmed that financial interactions between industry and physicians were common. In 2000, more than $4.8 billion was spent on promotion of pharmaceuticals to doctors by drug industry representatives, while $15.7 billion was spent on pharmaceutical marketing overall.[8] A 2009 national survey found that 84% of physicians had some form of financial interaction with industry manufacturers.[9]

Most physicians in the United States are familiar with the most common of industry relationships, interactions with pharmaceutic sales representatives (or "drug reps"), which often start with seemingly innocuous experiences, such as brief conversations or presentations of new data. Drug reps are selected for their outgoing and personable natures and are then trained to assess physicians' personalities and preferences.[10] They remember details of a physician's family life, favorite cuisine, or recreational pursuits. Drug reps have a repertoire of finely tuned playbooks to build relationships with all types of physicians, from "high prescribers" to "mercenary" doctors who expect gifts in exchange for prescriptions.[10,11] The best drug reps will constantly tailor messages according to their physician's response, using gifts to create both expectation and obligation. These gifts, which have become widespread throughout the United States, range from free meals and drinks to cash payments. Some physicians will be recruited as "thought leaders" to speak at local conferences and get-togethers on behalf of a new drug or device, all while being rewarded with lavish dinners and travel.[10]

For decades, drug companies have been able to monitor the return on investment of these promotional efforts by tracking prescriptions. Health information companies, such as IMS Health, Dendrite, Verispan, and Wolters Kluwer, purchase prescription records.[12] These records do not contain private patient information but contain the prescribing physicians' unique ID, which can be linked to the Physician Masterfile of the Centers for Medicare and Medicaid Services (CMS), which itself contains demographic information regarding all US physicians. Reps and their data science teams can use these files to create research reports at the level of a single physician, allowing them to pinpoint and track even minor changes in prescribing behavior. All this research is used to identify physicians who are the most susceptible to marketing efforts as well as gauge the success of various marketing strategies.[12]

The Open Payments Registry and Increased Transparency

In response to increasing concerns of financial COIs for physicians, the US Congress passed the Physician Payments Sunshine Act in 2010.[13] This act included the creation of the Open Payments registry, which publicly reports all payments greater than $10 from drug and device manufacturers to US physicians, nurse practitioners, physician assistants, and CRNAs (certified registered nurse anesthetists). The payment data are segmented into three data sets: (1) general payments not in connection with a research agreement or protocol, (2) research payments in connection with a research agreement or protocol, and (3) physician ownership or investment interest information about physicians or their immediate family members who hold an ownership or investment interest in an applicable manufacturer (Table 35.1). Each observation in the data set includes the payment amount in US dollars; the form of the payment (e.g., cash, stock, etc.); and the nature of the payment (e.g., food and beverage, consulting fee, etc.).[14]

Table 35.1 Overview of the Content in Each of the Major Data Sets Within the Open Payments Registry

Payment Data Set	Data Available Within Set	2021 Totals[14]
General payments not in connection with a research agreement or protocol	• Payment amount (US dollars) • Form of the payment (e.g., cash, stock, etc.) • Nature of the payment (e.g., food and beverage, consulting fee, etc.)	• $2.55 billion • 11.42 million payments
Research payments in connection with a research agreement or protocol		• $7.09 billion • 672,000 payments
Physician ownership or investment interest information about physicians or their immediate family members who hold an ownership or investment interest in an applicable manufacturer		• $1.26 billion • 3,100 payments

Although there had been prior registries with information regarding physician-industry relationships, the Open Payments registry has been a uniquely valuable tool for researchers and policymakers. It has provided a national, centralized database with mandatory reporting that has enabled researchers to assess industry payments across a broad range of medical specialties and product classes.

Since the first reported data from the Open Payments registry in 2014, research in the topic of financial COIs has grown considerably in volume and quality. From 2015 to 2021, industry payments to physicians and teaching hospitals totaled over $14.7 billion and $5.1 billion, respectively.[14] Studies using these data have established the association between industry payments and clinical research,[15] clinical practice guidelines recommendations,[16] and even physician formulary recommendations[17] (Table 35.2). Financial relationships between the pharmaceutical industry and physicians have consistently shown that payments can influence provider prescribing habits: A meta-analysis of thirty-six studies of industry payments noted that *every single included study found some positive association between payments and prescribing.*[18] These results spanned a broad range of physician specialties and drug classes. The authors also found strong evidence that this relationship was causal; nine of the included studies did time series analyses that demonstrated a temporal association between receipt of industry payments and increased prescribing. Twenty-five included studies found evidence of a dose-response relationship, with increasing number or value of payments associated with greater increases in prescriptions. While most studies have focused on pharmaceutical company payments, medical device companies are even more aggressive: Marketing payments from device manufacturers are seven times as large as those from pharmaceutical manufacturers as a proportion of industry revenues.[19]

While these studies suggest that industry marketing efforts are generally successful in influencing physician prescribing behavior, one might ask: Might this be in the service of good quality care? It is possible that in cases where patients would benefit from a new, high-value drug, these industry payments may benefit patient health. But research shows that industry spending on pharmaceutical marketing disproportionally targets drugs that are considered less effective or that offer little therapeutic advancement.[20,21] Another review found that the receipt of information from pharmaceutical companies was associated with lower quality prescribing.[22]

Despite the preponderance of research highlighting the influence of industry payments to physicians, these payments have remained common. Barriers to reform remain, often due to physician resistance. There has been a long-standing belief among many physicians that physicians are trained experts whose practice won't be affected by gifts or in-kind payments from drug and device reps.[11,18] Furthermore, these physician-industry interactions often go undisclosed—a recent study demonstrated that 80% of urologist authors writing editorials about new surgical devices who received payments related to those devices failed to disclose these payments in published editorial pieces.[25] Another 2018 study demonstrated that of 225 publications from the 100 doctors receiving the greatest compensation from ten device manufacturers, only 37.3% included disclosure of those payments.[27] It could be argued that this failure to disclose has far-reaching impacts beyond their own patients, as these editorials may influence practicing physicians around the world. It is critical for physicians to realize that, as human beings, they are susceptible to the psychological heuristics and reciprocity norms that make these industry payments effective marketing tools.

Table 35.2 Overview of Several Categories of Physician-Industry Interactions, With Illustrative Research Findings

Category	Illustrative Article, Journal, Year	Summarized Findings
Physician Pharmaceutical Prescribing Patterns	Mitchell et al., *Annals of Internal Medicine*, 2021[18]	• Meta-analysis of 36 studies comprising 101 analyses. • Of 101 individual analyses, 89 identified a positive association. • Payments were associated with increased prescribing of the paying company's drug, increased prescribing costs, and increased prescribing of branded drugs.
Physician Medical Device Selection	Annapureddy et al., *JAMA*, 2020[23]	• Cross-sectional study examining patients who received a first-time ICD or CRT- D device from any of the 4 major manufacturers. • Patients more often received an ICD made by the manufacturer that provided the largest payments to the physicians than to each of the other manufacturers individually (absolute differences in proportional range = 14.5%–30.6%).
Pharmaceutical Involvement in Clinical Trials	Peppercorn et al., *Cancer*, 2007[15]	• Retrospective study to examine shift in funding from public to private sponsors for breast cancer clinical research. • Studies that reported pharmaceutical involvement were more likely to be positive (84% vs. 54%; $P = .02$), to be single-arm studies (66% vs. 33%; $P = .03$), and to evaluate metastatic disease (72% vs. 46%; $P = .06$)
Industry Associations With Practice Guideline Authors	Mitchell et al., *JAMA Oncol.*, 2016[24]	• Cross-sectional study to quantify conflicts of interest with industry among authors of the National Comprehensive Cancer Network (NCCN) guidelines. • 86% of NCCN authors had financial conflicts of interest, including 84% who accepted general payments and 47% who accepted research payments.
Physician Formulary Recommendations	Chren et al., *JAMA*, 1994[17]	• Nested case-control study to examine whether industry relationships influence physician requests to add drugs to a hospital formulary. • Physicians were more likely to have requested formulary additions made by the companies whose pharmaceutical representatives they had met (OR 4.9; 95% CI 3.2 to 7.4) or from whom they had accepted money (OR 1.7; 95% CI 1.0 to 2.7) than they were to have requested drugs made by other companies.
Medical Device Editorials	Singh et al., *Urology*, 2022[25]	• Retrospective study to examine the impact of physician payments on editorial reviews of new devices • Authors of at least one favorable article were more likely to have received payments from the device manufacturers than authors of neutral articles ($P = .014$) • Most (80%) authors with payments did not report a relevant conflict of interest within any of their articles.
Breadth of Physician Interaction	Modi et al., *Urology Practice*, 2017[26]	• Retrospective study to describe both research and nonresearch payments to urologists in the United States. • An estimated 8,600 urologists (>65% of the US total) had nonresearch financial relationships with industry. • 93% of urology-directed research funding was provided to nonteaching institutions.

CRT-D, cardiac resynchronization therapy defibrillator; ICD, implantable cardioverter defibrillator.

Guidance from Professional Organizations

Several professional organizations have developed guidance regarding ethical interactions with industry. The American Medical Association (AMA) states, in its code of medical ethics: "A physician shall uphold the standards of professionalism" and "shall . . . regard responsibility to the patient as paramount." This ethos is reflected in the mandates of many societies, including the American College of Surgeons and the American Society of Clinical Oncology (ASCO). While these principles provide a framework for considering issues of financial COIs, they do not provide specific guidance. Going further, the code of medical ethics opinion on "financial relationships with industry in continuing medical education [CME]" provides further specificity in stating "physicians must ensure that the profession independently defines the goals of physician education, determines educational needs, and sets its own priorities for CME." This statement from the AMA recommends:

1. Being transparent about financial relationships that could potentially influence educational activities.
2. Providing information about the source and nature of commercial support and individual financial relationships with industry as well as steps that have been taken to reduce the influence of these relationships.
3. Avoiding faculty that have financial COIs unless necessary for the success of the educational activity.

Similarly, the Council of Medical Specialty Societies (CMSS) has published a "Code for Interactions With Companies." [28] This council, which includes more than thirty medical specialty society organizations, adopted principles to provide guidance on issues of independence, transparency, industry charitable contributions, corporate sponsorships, society meetings, satellite continuing medical education symposia, company educational programs, exhibits, research grants, clinical practice guidelines, and society journals. However, the CMSS does not require member societies to adopt this code and allows for individual groups to vary in their interpretation and implementation of these principles.

In general, both sets of guidelines encompass two broad strategies: disclosure of financial relationships with industry and divestment from (i.e., avoidance of) industry-sponsored events and speakers, where possible. ASCO, one of the CMSS member societies that has adopted the Code for Interactions With Companies, has implemented strict COI policies that encompass both disclosure and divestment. In 2013, ASCO adopted a COI policy that not only required general disclosure of all relationships with commercial healthcare companies but also restricted the presentation and publication of research that included first, last, or corresponding authors who had been employed, invested in, or served as a paid speaker for a healthcare company.[29] However, after concerns from their membership, the restriction on authors with company ties was put on hold, and this aspect of the policy further investigated. After gathering data for two years, ASCO published a revised policy that eliminated the restriction on research by authors with close industry ties.[30] In this document, they cite reduced federal funding for biomedical research and the important and valuable work being performed by private genomics and health informatics companies with proprietary data as part of the rationale for this change. Ultimately, the ASCO policy concluded "continued disclosure of commercial relationships, rigorous peer review, and management of potential COIs" would be sufficient.

Another important professional organization providing guidance on this issue is the Pharmaceutical Research and Manufacturers of America (PhRMA). This organization has released a report, "Code on Interactions With Health Care Professionals," which outlines principles set forth for industry organizations to maintain ethical relationships with healthcare professionals (Table 35.3).[31]

Disclosure Versus Divestment

The example of ASCO's COI policy above highlights the challenges of implementing a policy of divestment. While we have described the progress made in transparency and disclosure, many argue that this is not enough. Indeed, while disclosure of financial COI in medicine has increased globally in the last decade, there is little evidence that the Sunshine Act and other such policies have had any meaningful impact on industry or physician behavior. Data from the Sunshine Act suggests that total payments have increased from 2014 to the present. Further, the twenty highest-spending medical technology companies have more than tripled their payments to physicians in this time period.[32] Moreover, there is evidence from the social sciences that disclosure may lead to a "moral license" among those providing disclosure to exaggerate their claims.[33] In addition, people receiving information after a disclosure do not sufficiently discount the claims made in light of the disclosure and, indeed, may feel a greater sense of trust as a result of the disclosure. These data have led many commentators to call for less focus on disclosure and further steps toward divestment from industry financial ties.[34]

However, as the ASCO example demonstrates, this move toward divestment will not be easy. Brems and colleagues analyzed the COI policies of organizations that publish clinical practice guidelines. Of forty-six organizations, thirty-six (78%) had a COI policy. Among these organizations, only two (6%) met their standard of requiring divestment of financial COI. On the other hand, disclosure of financial COI was the most commonly met standard (33/36; 92%).[35] This study suggests that while disclosure has been embraced by the biomedical field, divestment may be harder to accomplish.

Lexchin and Fugh-Berman argue that, ultimately, we should eliminate industry relationships from the practice of medicine.[34] However, given the interconnectedness of medical practice and the healthcare industry, this will be extremely challenging to achieve and may generate significant costs in terms of lost collaborations and stalled development of innovative drugs, devices, and delivery systems. However, there are some achievable opportunities with regard to divestment from industry financial relationships.

Recommendations for Divestment

A fundamental duty of a profession is to be responsible for the education and training of its members. In the United States, CME is required in most states and is accredited by the Accreditation Council for CME (ACCME), which established policies to ensure unbiased content. Nonetheless, much of CME is funded, directly or indirectly, by the pharmaceutical and medical device industries,[36] who use this as another route for marketing

Table 35.3 Summarized Elements of PhRMA Code on Interactions With Healthcare Professionals

1. Basis of interactions	Interactions should be focused on informing healthcare professionals about products, providing scientific and educational information, and supporting medical education. Promotional materials should be (a) accurate and not misleading, (b) make claims only when properly substantiated, (c) reflect the balance between risks and benefits, (d) be consistent with Food and Drug Administration (FDA) requirements governing such communications.
2. Informational presentations by pharmaceutical company representatives and accompanying meals	Company representatives may present information during healthcare professionals' workday, including mealtimes. In this context it is appropriate for occasional, incidental meals to be offered as a business courtesy to the healthcare professionals and members of their staff. The meal must be (a) modest by local standards, (b) not part of entertainment or recreational event, (c) provided in a manner conducive to informational communication.
3. Prohibition on entertainment and recreation	Companies should not provide any entertainment or recreational items to any healthcare professional who is not a salaried employee of the company. These items should not be offered regardless of (1) the value of these items, (2) whether the company engages the professional as a speaker or consultant, (3) whether the entertainment or recreation is secondary to an educational purpose.
4. Pharmaceutical company support for continuing medical education (CME)	Support for CME is not intended to promote a specific medication. Companies should separate CME grant-making functions from sales and marketing departments. The company should not provide any advice or guidance to the CME provider regarding the content or faculty for a program funded by the company. Financial support should not be offered for the costs of travel, lodging, or other personal expenses of nonfaculty healthcare professionals attending CME.
5. Pharmaceutical company support for third-party educational or professional meetings	Any financial support should be given to the conference's sponsor and not directly to a healthcare professional. Financial support should not be offered for the costs of travel, lodging, or other personal expenses of nonfaculty healthcare professionals attending these conferences or meetings.
6. Consultants	It is appropriate for consultants to be offered reasonable compensation and reimbursement for reasonable travel, lodging, and meal expenses. Any compensation or reimbursement. should be reasonable and based on fair market value and should not take into account the volume or value of past or potential future business. These factors support the existence of a true consulting relationship: (1) written contract; (2) legitimate need for consulting services has been identified in advance; (3) criteria for selecting consultants are directly related to the purpose; (4) the number of professionals retained is not greater than the number reasonably necessary to achieve the purpose; (5) the company maintains records and makes use of the services provided by consultants; (6) the venue of any meeting with consultants is conducive to the service. Luxury resorts, high-end restaurants, and entertainment or other recreational venues are not appropriate.
7. Speaker programs and speaker training meetings	Speaker programs can offer important educational opportunities but are distinct from CME programs. The speakers and material should clearly identify the company and be compliant with FDA guidelines.

(continued)

Table 35.3 Continued

8. Healthcare professionals who are members of committees that set formularies or develop clinical practice guidelines	These professionals often have significant experience in their fields and may be valuable as speakers or consultants. Companies should require any professional to disclose to their committee the existence and nature of their relationship with the company. Professionals serving as speakers or consultants should be required to follow the procedures set forth by the committee, including recusing themselves from decisions relating to the medicine for which they have provided services.
9. Scholarships and educational funds	Financial assistance for students and trainees may be offered as long as the selection of individuals who will receive the funds is made by the academic or training institution.
10. Prohibition of noneducational and practice-related items	Providing items that do not advance disease or treatment education, even minimal value items, should not be offered to professionals or members of their staff.
11. Educational items	Educational items that are valued at $100 or less may be offered if they do not have value outside of their professional responsibilities. These should not be offered on more than an occasional basis.
12. Prescriber data	Companies may use nonpatient identified prescriber data to facilitate communications with healthcare professionals. They should (a) respect the confidential nature of this data; (b) develop policies regarding the use of these data; (c) educate employees and agents about those policies; (d) maintain an internal contact person for questions about use of these data; (e) identify disciplinary actions for misuse of the data. Additionally companies should respect the wishes of professionals who request that their prescriber data not be made available to company sales representatives.
13. Independence and decision-making	No items, grants, or financial support should be offered to a healthcare professional in exchange for prescribing products or a commitment to do so.
14. Training and conduct of company representatives	Companies should ensure that all representatives who visit healthcare professionals receive training about the laws, regulations, and industry codes of practice.
15. Adherence to code	All companies that interact with healthcare professionals about pharmaceuticals should adopt procedures to comply with this code.

to physicians.[37,38] Thus, eliminating industry sponsorship of CME activities and professional conferences and meetings is one important step toward ensuring independent and unbiased educational material for medical professionals.

Second, physicians and scientists in leadership, editorial, and guideline development roles should be free of financial COIs with industry. It is clear that interactions between physicians and industry are necessary and valuable for the development of drugs, devices, and other medical innovations. However, the same individuals who participate closely with industry should not be called on to lead professional organizations, develop educational materials, oversee research publication, or develop clinical guidelines. This last example is especially important, as contributions to clinical guidelines are potentially the most far-reaching contributions of any individual physician. Such an exclusion should not be seen as an implication that those who have financial COI are in any way morally corrupt, but an acknowledgment that we are all human and vulnerable to deeply held psychological heuristics and biases. Safeguarding the scientific neutrality of important institutions (e.g., journal editors, professional society leaders, guidelines committee members) can be accomplished by establishing strict requirements for divestment of financial COI for these select leaders.

Finally, individual physicians should—independent of policies established by governments, hospitals, or professional organizations—aim to avoid financial entanglements with industry. As outlined by Fugh-Berman and Ahari, industry representatives use a number of strategies to influence the behaviors of physicians.[12] Simply avoiding interactions with industry representatives (i.e., free samples, meals in the office, trinkets) can serve to preserve unbiased and independent practice and prevent often subtle manipulation. While the many challenges of practicing modern medicine (i.e., onerous billing and documentation requirements, declining reimbursement, the perception of reduced prestige) can lead to a feeling of nihilism or sense that one deserves more, physicians should not trade the ability to come to an unbiased judgment of the best medical care for patients for small validations from industry sources.

Conclusions

Physician interactions with the healthcare industry are a common and necessary component of the delivery of modern medical care. However, there is a preponderance of evidence suggesting that financial relationships, even with low-value transactions, can influence physician behavior in a number of important domains. In light of these data, it is important the physicians thoughtfully assess their own financial relationships with industry and, where appropriate, restrict these. Similarly, professional organizations should maintain careful safeguards to maintain administrative and scientific leadership that is free of financial relationships with industry. These steps are needed to maintain the trust that the profession of medicine has enjoyed and that is invaluable to our work caring for patients.

References

1. Lo B, Field MJ, eds.; Institute of Medicine (US) Committee on Conflict of Interest in Medical Research, Education, and Practice. *Conflict of Interest in Medical Research, Education, and Practice.* (National Academies Press; 2009. Accessed September 20, 2022. http://www.ncbi.nlm.nih.gov/books/NBK22942/

2. Hartman M, Martin AB, Washington B, Catlin A, The National Health Expenditure Accounts Team. National health care spending in 2020: growth driven by federal spending in response to the COVID-19 pandemic: national health expenditures study examines US health care spending in 2020. *Health Aff (Millwood).* 2022;41(1):13–25. doi:10.1377/hlthaff.2021.01763
3. The use of medicines in the US. 2022. IQVIA. Accessed September 20, 2022. https://www.iqvia.com/insights/the-iqvia-institute/reports/the-use-of-medicines-in-the-us-2022
4. NHE Fact Sheet. CMS. Accessed September 13, 2022. https://www.cms.gov/Research-Statistics-Data-and-Systems/Statistics-Trends-and-Reports/NationalHealthExpendData/NHE-Fact-Sheet
5. Pellegrino ED. Professionalism, profession and the virtues of the good physician. *Mt Sinai J Med N Y.* 2002;69(6):378–384.
6. Friedman M. A Friedman doctrine—The social responsibility of business is to increase its profits. *New York Times.* September 13, 1970. Accessed November 15, 2022. https://www.nytimes.com/1970/09/13/archives/a-friedman-doctrine-the-social-responsibility-of-business-is-to.html
7. Bower JL, Paine LS. The error at the heart of corporate leadership. *Harv Bus Rev.* May 1, 2017. Accessed November 15, 2022. https://hbr.org/2017/05/the-error-at-the-heart-of-corporate-leadership
8. Relman AS. The new medical-industrial complex. *N Engl J Med.* 1980;303(17):963–970. doi:10.1056/NEJM198010233031703
9. Rosenthal MB, Berndt ER, Donohue JM, Epstein AM, Frank RG. Demand effects of recent changes in prescription drug promotion. *Forum Health Econ Policy.* 2003;6(1):1–26. doi:10.2202/1558-9544.1044
10. Campbell EG, Gruen RL, Mountford J, Miller LG, Cleary PD, Blumenthal D. A national survey of physician–industry relationships. *N Engl J Med.* 2007;356(17):1742–1750. doi:10.1056/NEJMsa06450811.
11. Brody H. *Hooked: Ethics, the Medical Profession, and the Pharmaceutical Industry.* Rowman & Littlefield Publishers; 2007.
12. Fugh-Berman A, Ahari S. Following the script: how drug reps make friends and influence doctors. *PLoS Med.* 2007;4(4):e150. doi:10.1371/journal.pmed.0040150
13. The physician payments sunshine act. *Health Aff.* Accessed June 14, 2021. https://www.healthaffairs.org/do/10.1377/hpb20141002.272302/full/
14. OpenPayment Facts. CMS.gov. Accessed July 6, 2022. https://openpaymentsdata.cms.gov/summary
15. Peppercorn J, Blood E, Winer E, Partridge A. Association between pharmaceutical involvement and outcomes in breast cancer clinical trials. *Cancer.* 2007;109(7):1239–1246. doi:10.1002/cncr.22528
16. Tibau A, Bedard PL, Srikanthan A, et al. Author financial conflicts of interest, industry funding, and clinical practice guidelines for anticancer drugs. *J Clin Oncol.* 2015;33(1):100–106. doi:10.1200/JCO.2014.57.8898
17. Chren MM, Landefeld CS. Physicians' behavior and their interactions with drug companies. A controlled study of physicians who requested additions to a hospital drug formulary. *JAMA.* 1994;271(9):684–689.

18. Mitchell AP, Trivedi NU, Gennarelli RL, et al. Are financial payments from the pharmaceutical industry associated with physician prescribing? A systematic review. *Ann Intern Med.* 2021;174(3):353–361. doi:10.7326/M20-5665

19. Bergman A, Grennan M, Swanson A. Medical device firm payments to physicians exceed what drug companies pay physicians, target surgical specialists. *Health Aff (Millwood).* 2021;40(4):603–612. doi:10.1377/hlthaff.2020.01785

20. Greenway T, Ross JS. US drug marketing: how does promotion correspond with health value? *BMJ.* 2017;357:j1855. doi:10.1136/bmj.j1855

21. Lexchin J. The relation between promotional spending on drugs and their therapeutic gain: a cohort analysis. *CMAJ Open.* 2017;5(3):E724–E728. doi:10.9778/cmajo.20170089

22. Spurling GK, Mansfield PR, Montgomery BD, et al. Information from pharmaceutical companies and the quality, quantity, and cost of physicians' prescribing: a systematic review. *PLoS Med.* 2010;7(10):e1000352. doi:10.1371/journal.pmed.1000352

23. Annapureddy AR, Henien S, Wang Y, et al. Association between industry payments to physicians and device selection in ICD implantation. *JAMA.* 2020;324(17):1755–1764. doi:10.1001/jama.2020.17436

24. Mitchell AP, Basch EM, Dusetzina SB. Financial relationships with industry among national comprehensive cancer network guideline authors. *JAMA Oncol.* 2016;2(12):1628–1631. doi:10.1001/jamaoncol.2016.2710

25. Singh A, Faris S, Agarwal P, Reynolds LF, Modi PK. Association between industry payments and published position on use of devices for the treatment of lower urinary tract symptoms. *Urology.* 2022;159:87–92. doi:10.1016/j.urology.2021.10.025

26. Modi PK, Farber NJ, Zavaski ME, Jang TL, Singer EA, Chang SL. Industry payments to urologists in 2014: an analysis of the Open Payments Program. *Urol Pract.* 2017;4(4):342–347.

27. Ziai K, Pigazzi A, Smith BR, et al. Association of compensation from the surgical and medical device industry to physicians and self-declared conflict of interest. *JAMA Surg.* 2018;153(11):997–1002. doi:10.1001/jamasurg.2018.2576

28. Kahn NB, Lichter AS. The new CMSS code for interactions with companies managing relationships to minimize conflicts. *J Vasc Surg.* 2011;54(3, supplement):34S–40S. doi:10.1016/j.jvs.2011.05.109

29. American Society of Clinical Oncology. American Society of Clinical Oncology policy for relationships with companies: background and rationale. *J Clin Oncol.* 2013;31(16):2037–2042. doi:10.1200/JCO.2013.49.4997

30. American Society of Clinical Oncology. Modification of authorship restrictions for research studies in the American Society of Clinical Oncology conflict of interest policy. *J Clin Oncol.* 2017;35(7):799–800. doi:10.1200/JCO.2016.71.8528

31. PHrMA. Code on interactions with health care professionals. Codes and guidelines. Accessed November 20, 2022. https://phrma.org/-/media/Project/PhRMA/PhRMA-Org/PhRMA-Org/PDF/P-R/PhRMA-Code---Final.pdf

32. Sunlight doesn't dent industry funding to doctors over half-decade. MedTech Dive. Accessed September 13, 2022. https://www.medtechdive.com/news/sunlight-doesnt-dent-industry-funding-to-doctors-over-half-decade/568228/

33. Cain DM, Loewenstein G, Moore DA. The dirt on coming clean: perverse effects of disclosing conflicts of interest. *J Leg Stud.* 2005;34(1):1–25. doi:10.1086/426699

34. Lexchin J, Fugh-Berman A. A ray of sunshine: transparency in physician-industry relationships is not enough. *J Gen Intern Med.* 2021;36(10):3194–3198. doi:10.1007/s11606-021-06657-0

35. Brems JH, Davis AE, Clayton EW. Analysis of conflict of interest policies among organizations producing clinical practice guidelines. *PLoS One.* 2021;16(4):e0249267. doi:10.1371/journal.pone.0249267

36. Fugh-Berman A. Industry-funded medical education is always promotion—an essay by Adriane Fugh-Berman. *BMJ.* 2021;373:n1273. doi:10.1136/bmj.n1273

37. Steinman MA, Bero LA, Chren MM, Landefeld CS. Narrative review: the promotion of gabapentin: an analysis of internal industry documents. *Ann Intern Med.* 2006;145(4):284–293. doi:10.7326/0003-4819-145-4-200608150-00008

38. Kesselheim AS, Mello MM, Studdert DM. Strategies and practices in off-label marketing of pharmaceuticals: a retrospective analysis of whistleblower complaints. *PLoS Med.* 2011;8(4):e1000431. doi:10.1371/journal.pmed.1000431

36
Should Physicians or Health Organizations Be Environmentally Active?

Cheryl C. Macpherson and Leon Budrie

Key Points

- It is undeniable that the natural environment affects human health and well-being. In order for inroads to be made toward improving human health and flourishing, there needs to be a combined effort by healthcare organizations, individual physicians, medical schools, and professional associations to develop practices and policies that aim at reducing global emissions.
- Environmentalism and practicing environmental sustainability aligns with medical professionalism in multiple ways, notably in the forms of pro bono service and advocacy.
- Physicians and healthcare organizations have professional responsibilities to advance and implement environmentally sustainable policies and practices and should do so now. Given the urgency of meaningful actions, becoming environmentally sustainable should be a priority discussion in every clinical, academic, research, and policy workplace.

Healthcare Organizations and Climate Change

Countless news reports and sources document how the summer of 2022 devastated individuals, families, and populations with extreme heatwaves, droughts, and floods across North America, Europe, and elsewhere, straining their healthcare and housing. As global greenhouse gas emissions accumulate in the atmosphere, these events increase and intensify.[1] In addition to direct impacts on physical and mental health, emissions indirectly harm health by undermining agricultural productivity (and the ability to feed Earth's growing global population); damaging infrastructure for transportation and communication; causing displacement, migration, overcrowding, and infectious disease; and contributing to conflict and violence.

Climate change is a "threat multiplier" that precipitates extreme weather events and alters demand and supply of goods and services, including healthcare.[2] Altering resource distribution in locations that donate resources or provide care for those displaced by a climate-related event challenges healthcare organizations and contributes to burnout and moral distress among physicians and other health professionals. Becoming environmentally active is one way to alleviate such moral distress in healthcare.[3] Perhaps for this reason, increasing numbers of physicians are environmentally active.[4,5]

Around the world, public trust in medicine is upheld by physicians and healthcare organizations that help patients and communities recover from ill health or injury and promote the health of individuals and populations. This chapter explains why physicians and healthcare organizations have professional responsibilities to promote environmental sustainability within their workplaces. Talking about and incorporating environmentally sustainable practices within their workplaces is one means of meeting these responsibilities.

Being Environmentally Active Is a Professional Responsibility

That social and physical environments influence health and access to care is well known.[6] Many health impacts of climate change involve environmental disruptions. Direct health impacts of extreme events include heat stroke, injury, and the exacerbation of chronic conditions.[7,8] Indirect impacts precipitate or contribute to respiratory illness (wildfires); skin, gastrointestinal, and other infections (floods and contaminated water); and destroy crops that provide food and influence quality of life for humans, pets, and agricultural animals (drought, flood, or wildfire). Physicians and healthcare organizations routinely provide patient care and are often early responders to those impacted by such events. Providing patient care that is congruent with the goals of medicine helps fulfill these professional responsibilities, and these goals include promoting health and preventing disease and injury.[9] Given the causal relationship between human activities and environmental changes, including seasonal weather patterns and extreme weather events, one way to fulfill the goals of medicine (promoting health and preventing disease) is to advance environmental sustainability.

Physicians also have responsibilities to their communities and employers and in public health emergencies like extreme weather, pandemics, or war. These responsibilities vary with type and location of emergency and available resources and often justify providing a different approach to a standard of care than would be expected in other circumstances. The 2001 "Declaration of Professional Responsibility" calls on physicians to "combat natural and man-made assaults on the health and well-being of humankind." [10] While not directed at climate change, it commits physicians to responding to socioeconomic and physical environmental conditions. In 2022, the American Medical Association (AMA) called for reducing greenhouse gas emissions, aiming for carbon neutrality by 2050 and supporting incentivization of clean energy solutions.[11] This is consistent with the "Declaration of Professional Responsibility" and principles of medical ethics that highlight a physician's responsibility to actively contribute to improving community and public health.[12] Pediatricians accepted this responsibility when they worked to reduce exposure to lead paint; identified and tried to rectify water contamination in Flint, Michigan; and called attention to health impacts of climate change on children.[13,14] Arguably, other medical specialists and specialties have a responsibility to do similarly.

Some physicians hold that their professional duty is solely to deliver patient care, rejecting climate change as a legitimate concern in medicine or medical education.[15–17] This contradicts medical ethics and patient-centered care, which call on physicians to respond to the individuality of each patient and the circumstances and environments that shape their health needs. Consensus across medicine and medical ethics is that social and physical environments influence health and warrant physician engagement, and current standards of care make attending to patients' environments and circumstances a professional responsibility.[18–21] Failing to do so is hypocritical, as is *rejecting* scientific evidence about the health impacts of climate change while *accepting* scientific evidence that informs other types of diagnosis, management, and treatment decisions.

About 65% of global emissions result from industrial production and use of fossil fuels.[8,22] The healthcare industry is a heavy user of fossil fuels. While some hold that the need for high-quality healthcare justifies this heavy use, several healthcare organizations have attained or are working toward net zero emissions within their facilities and have done so without reducing quality or patient satisfaction and while attaining financial savings.[23] Examples described in this chapter were advanced by physicians and healthcare organizations.

The professional responsibilities of physicians and healthcare organizations include promoting health and preventing injury and illness, and as described in the paragraph below, they can make financial savings by becoming environmentally sustainable without compromising quality of care. Failing to embrace environmental sustainability worsens the health impacts of climate change and the existing injustices in access to healthcare and resources for health.[24–26] One way for physicians to fulfill their professional responsibilities is to advocate for and advance environmental sustainability within their workplaces and the wider healthcare industry. Physicians are positioned to influence health policy within their workplaces and might advocate within their organizations for establishing sustainability offices to audit their own emissions production; identify and negotiate for cost-effective changes in purchasing or transportation; and set internal targets for reductions. Examples from the US National Institutes of Health (NIH), British National Health Service (NHS), and two health systems in the United States are highlighted.

Successful Environmental Sustainability Initiatives in Healthcare

Rapid shifts to environmentally sustainable energy use, procurement, and waste management across the healthcare industry (and other industries) is critical to human health in the next decade. Whether and how rapidly and significantly these shifts are made will influence health and healthcare everywhere. As important recipients of public trust, medicine and healthcare should lead the way. Some healthcare organizations are doing so. For example, the NIH issued a notice of special interest (NOT-ES-22-006) calling for grant applications to investigate connections between health and climate change and made available a searchable portal for background literature (including some on bioethics).[27] Britain's NHS is the fifth largest global employer, has facilities across four countries, and accounts for 10% of British government spending; environmental sustainability measures within the NHS include policies and practices that eliminate single-use plastics where possible and leveraging purchasing power for negotiating environmentally sustainable products and services; consequently, the NHS is likely to attain 80% emissions reduction by 2028 and "net zero" by 2040.[28]

Kaiser Permanente serves 12 million members across California and other states, has been environmentally active since 1950, and in 2020 achieved carbon neutrality.[29] The Gundersen Health System in Wisconsin has been energy independent since 2014, produces more energy through renewables than it consumes, and innovates other ways to reduce its own emissions.[30] Gundersen has six affiliated hospitals that teach medical students and serve patients in Wisconsin and parts of Iowa and Minnesota; it was the first health system to replace its fossil fuel use with locally generated energy and remains repeatedly ranked among the top US hospitals for patient satisfaction.[31]

These significant accomplishments are not enough to stop the rise in global emissions that threatens health everywhere. Each physician and healthcare organization that advocates for or implements environmental sustainability is helping to protect health and life as we know it by bringing the healthcare industry closer to net zero and showing other industries that it can be done. The agricultural and food industries can make major contributions to health by becoming more environmentally sustainable and, as global suppliers to healthcare organizations and other consumers, might emulate or complement sustainability measures adopted by the healthcare industry and its organizations.[32] Financial and other benefits attained by the healthcare industry might encourage industries such as energy or transportation to do so, particularly as healthcare is a major consumer of their products and services.

Competing Responsibilities

Physicians have multiple professional responsibilities to patients and, depending on specialty and employment, to their employers, insurers, the medical profession, medical and other students, public health authorities, and human research participants and others in the research enterprise. Most physicians, regardless of specialty, are sometimes confronted by competing responsibilities. To what extent should they make time for meeting the responsibility to be environmentally active? There is no consensus answer, but, given globally rising emissions, it seems reasonable to propose that passively supporting environmental sustainability in their workplaces, or being environmentally active in their workplace or community, by, for example, joining one of the many physician or healthcare organizations addressing climate change, such as "Healthcare Without Harm," would fulfill this responsibility.[4]

Becoming environmentally active may begin with learning more about emissions produced by healthcare, the consequent health impacts, and how other health professionals are responding. Those reluctant to support environmental sustainability or unsure where to invest their time might reflect on criteria for determining their responsibility to act in response to climate change. These criteria are tabulated in Table 36.1 and, as more of these are met for a given physician or a given situation, the greater the responsibility to act becomes.[17]

Physicians and healthcare leaders and organizations can make significant improvements in global emissions and be role models for other professions and industries. Iterative clinical and scientific data documenting healthcare emissions and health impacts make it imperative for physicians and healthcare organizations to respond. Some are doing so with positive impacts.[33–37]

Table 36.1 Criteria for Health Professionals to Respond to Climate Change

Expertise	when having specific expertise makes it more likely that a physician's action will be beneficial, their responsibility to act increases
Proximity	when a physician is closer to an event or dilemma, their responsibility to act increases.
Effectiveness	when a physician's position gives them a greater likelihood of positive impact, their responsibility to act increases
Lower risk or cost	when a physician's safety or wellbeing is not harmed by acting, their responsibility to act increases
Unique	when there are few or no others available to act, physician's responsibility to act increases
Severity	when failing to act might cause a much worse outcome, physician's responsibility to act increases
Severity	when failing to act might cause a much worse outcome, physician's responsibility to act increases

Medical Schools and Associations

In medical education, determinants of health are generally defined and taught as being either social (economic status, level of education, and similar) or physical (built and natural environments that affect exposure to pollutants and toxins, and similar). In our experience, and others, social determinants receive the greatest emphasis in medical and healthcare teaching, research, practice, and policy.[38] The World Health Organization (WHO) recently described the built environment as a social determinant.[39] This shift may help others to recognize the overlapping and inseparable relationships between social and physical environments and is important because social environments exist within and are influenced dynamically by natural and physical ones and vice versa. The significance of these relationships for individual, community, and population health is reviewed elsewhere.[40] WHO's recent description of commercial determinants of health as "private sector activities impacting public health" opens new opportunities for interventions against a range of health challenges, including climate change and, arguably, commercial determinants also are social determinants.[41]

Environmental activity encompasses countless types of responses to environmental problems. Environmental activity to promote environmental sustainability tacitly acknowledges that medicine, health, and healthcare are dependent on resources extracted from natural environments, and that natural environments are diminishing globally as humans encroach on undeveloped land and "reclaim" land to develop roads or buildings. Unless governments and healthcare and other industries rapidly adopt environmentally sustainable policies and practices, the lifestyles enjoyed in North America today will undoubtedly be forced to change. Voluntary changes are already adopted by many, including reductions in meat consumption and conservation of water and energy. In June and July 2022 alone, thousands were displaced in the United States, United Kingdom, and around the world by unprecedented amounts of emissions in Earth's atmosphere, which steadily continue rising. Year round, leading news organizations document the increasingly frequent and severe consequences for populations in increasingly large geographic areas.

Like some physicians and healthcare organizations, medical educators are calling for integration of environmental sustainability into medical curricula. Some offer One Health (OH) as a vehicle for doing so.[42] OH aims to improve health through investigations of interactions between human and nonhuman species and their environments and to design interventions that prevent transmission or improve diagnosis and treatment. OH can help medical and veterinary students learn about environmental sustainability and its clinical value, provide opportunities to improve interprofessionalism, and strengthen professional competencies.[43,44] As OH encourages physicians and others to attend to reciprocal influences between environments, humans, and nonhuman species, it is a useful vehicle for teaching about environmental sustainability in medicine and healthcare and about medical professionalism and associated responsibilities.

Medical professionalism is integrated into medical curricula and evaluated for licensure and in practice. In North America, medical educators often draw from the late Ed Pellegrino and others describing attitudes, behaviors, and character as central to professionalism.[45] Professionalism makes possible strong and trusting doctor-patient relationships that facilitate patient-centered care, improves patient outcomes, and helps maintain public trust. In the United States, medical educators and licensing bodies require that students demonstrate "core Entrustable Professional Activities" (EPAs) focused on clinical competencies like history taking and physical exam and professional competencies like contributing to a culture of safety.[46] EPAs do not address health impacts of climate change, environmental activity, or environmental sustainability, but some medical curricula do address these topics.[17] Given the growing attention within medicine to health impacts of climate change, medical educators should perhaps consider adding related activities to EPAs.

As the websites of medical schools, licensing boards, and others often highlight their positions and policies, we explored the positions of influential medical schools and bodies on climate change and environmental sustainability by examining their websites. In the United States, student performance on the Medical Licensing Examination (USMLE) is an important criterion used by state medical boards to license physicians. Ten states credential approximately half of the total number of active physicians in the United States. None of those state websites or the USMLE website mentions climate change or environmental sustainability. In contrast, the website of the Medical Council of Canada (MCC), which licenses physicians in Canada, states that physicians should recognize causal relationships between the environment and a patient's clinical condition, communicate related risks to patients, partner with local and national agencies to address environmental risks, and respond to the disproportionate health impacts on some populations.[47,48] Canada's attention to climate change in physician licensure is likely facilitated by its having a single national healthcare system and regulatory environment and policy that treats healthcare delivery as a public service and good (rather than as a private or commercial service or good).

Some medical associations and societies in the United States address climate change with policies, statements on related responsibilities, or commitments to environmental activity. The American Academy of Family Physicians (AAFP) website commits to "providing strategies to help family physicians understand and recognize the impact of the environment on patient health" and developing resources with which physicians can better identify and address environmental influences on patients and patient care.[49] The AAFP Health Equity Curricular Toolkit addresses social and environmental determinants of health and includes a module on climate change.[50] The American Academy of

Pediatrics (AAP) "Policy Statement on Global Climate Change and Children's Health" emphasizes pediatricians responsibility to mitigate climate risks.[51] The American Psychiatric Association (APA), American College of Physicians (ACP), American Society of Anesthesiologists (ASA), and others in and beyond the United States also highlight professional responsibilities to respond to climate change.[52–54]

Medical societies articulate professional norms for their members and command an authoritative voice across medicine. Their acknowledgment of climate-related responsibilities suggests that medicine is increasingly attentive to environmental sustainability. Forty-one medical societies are members of the Medical Society Consortium on Climate Change and Health, which represents some 700,000 physicians in the United States and sixty-seven partner societies, like the American Lung Association, American Heart Association, and American Cancer Society; their environmental activities include educating the public and policymakers and advocating for environmentally sustainable policies.[55] The consortium's "United States Policy Action Agenda on Climate, Health, and Equity" is endorsed by over 200 professional societies and 500 hospitals calling for environmentally sustainable healthcare, including the AMA with its 250,000 members.[56,57]

The AMA acknowledged links between the environment, climate, and human health in its 1989 statement "Global Climate Change—The 'Greenhouse Effect'" endorsing research and congressional action and "Stewardship and the Environment" policy urging physician responsiveness.[58,59] Its 2008 statement "Global Climate Change and Human Health" called for educating the medical community on the health impacts and highlighted physicians' responsibilities to educate communities and policymakers.[60] The AMA 2019 policy "Climate Change Education Across the Medical Education Continuum" calls for integration of climate science, health impacts, and patient care into medical education and advocates for accreditation bodies to encourage associated curricular changes.[61] The AMA aims to improve understanding of and responses to health impacts of climate change, outlines reasons to adopt environmentally sustainable practices in medical facilities, and recommends immediate actions like resetting thermostats and reducing waste.[62–65]

Recent surveys by the US Liaison Committee on Medical Education (LCME) found that 125 of 140 medical schools offered required or elective courses on environmental health, and 60 of 155 did so on climate change.[66,67] These policy and curricular changes are examples of environmental activity. Interestingly, the websites of the AMA and LCME both omit information about environmental sustainability within their own facilities. The websites of many Ivy League and state universities and medical schools, however, document accomplishments of their environmental sustainability offices. The Sustainability Unit at Harvard Medical School (HMS), for example, reports a 40% reduction in waste, 12% reduction in water use, $20,000 of lab materials recycled, six LEED projects initiated, and other accomplishments since 2006.[68]

A Yale survey found that its community cares about improving sustainability and would be more environmentally active if its members could measure impacts of interventions and suggests ways to improve sustainability at Yale through materials management and energy and water use.[69] Medical schools at Penn State, Ohio State, University of Chicago, and others and universities in Alabama, Texas, Montana, and others provide information about their sustainability programs on their websites. In consultation with faculty and the local community, McGill University's Office of Sustainability recommends reducing air travel, decreasing printing and paper use, encouraging discussion of sustainability objectives with human resources and staff evaluation, and establishing related communication and partnerships.[70]

The National Medical Association (NMA) is the largest and oldest national organization representing African American physicians in the United States.[71] Its members have firsthand experience of the disproportionate impact of environmental disruptions on African Americans and other minority groups; its Environmental Health Task Force, established in 1999, was succeeded in 2014 by its Commission on Environmental Health.[72,73] A 2014 survey of NMA members documents their concern that climate change affects about 80% of their patients, and the NMA encourages members to adopt environmentally sustainable practices and lead by example.[74] Despite this, like the AMA, its website omits information about environmental sustainability within its own facilities.

The Planetary Health Report Card grades participating US medical schools on their inclusion of planetary health and environmental sustainability in their curricula, interdisciplinary research, community outreach and advocacy, support for student initiatives, and campus sustainability.[75] For 2021–2022 the overall grades for Emory University and University of California (UC) Berkeley's Joint Medical Program were respectively rated A and A minus, and the UC San Francisco and University of Arkansas Medical Sciences were respectively B plus and B minus.[75] HMS has a longitudinal series of required courses that address relationships between climate change, infectious disease, clinical practice, and health equity; Harvard's TH Chan School of Public Health offers the "Climate MD" program to better equip physicians to manage health impacts of climate change in patient care.[76,77] Numerous medical schools are expanding their curricula to address environmental sustainability.[78]

The American Association of Medical Colleges acknowledges that structural inequities exist in access to healthcare and advocates for physicians to reduce these inequities and thereby improve community health.[79] These inequities include disproportionate impacts of climate change and environmental disruption on communities comprising primarily people of color, low-income and low socioeconomic status, and the underserved.[80,81] Medicine and healthcare, and to a lesser degree bioethics, are increasingly attentive to climate change and the responsibilities of physicians and other health professionals and organizations to respond.[41,82,83]

Conclusion

Overwhelming clinical and scientific evidence affirms that environments significantly influence health. No single healthcare organization, physician, medical school, or association can independently reduce global emissions fast enough to stop or slow the extreme weather events confronting the world today. Combined, their efforts can make inroads, show that this can be done, and lead the way for others. If enough others follow rapidly enough, current standards of health and healthcare have a reasonable chance of surviving global climate change. Historically, physicians have honored their professional responsibility to provide pro bono service, often in the form of advocacy or activity for a disease or health issue of particular interest to them. Environmental sustainability in medicine and healthcare is of growing significance and warrants greater attention in medical education, research, policy, and practice. The more physicians are taught, learn about, and reflect on the necessity of advancing environmental sustainability in medicine, the more benefits will accrue to their patients, communities, and planetary health.

For this reason, medical schools and societies increasingly support environmental sustainability, and healthcare organizations are adopting associated policies and practices. These important steps in reducing global emissions model how other professions and industries can be environmentally active and environmentally sustainable. Physicians and healthcare organizations have professional responsibilities to advance and implement environmentally sustainable policies and practices and should do so now. Given the urgency of meaningful actions, becoming environmentally sustainable should be a priority discussion in every clinical, academic, research, and policy workplace.

References

1. The Royal Society. How does climate change affect the strength and frequency of floods, droughts, hurricanes, and tornadoes? Accessed November 04, 2022. https://royalsociety.org/topics-policy/projects/climate-change-evidence-causes/question-13/
2. Lubell J. How physicians can see health care through climate lens. American Medical Association. January 26, 2022. Accessed November 29, 2022. https://www.ama-assn.org/delivering-care/public-health/how-physicians-can-see-health-care-through-climate-lens
3. Jameton A. A reflection on moral distress in nursing together with a current application of the concept. *J Bioeth Inq*. 2013;10(3):297–308. doi:10.1007/s11673-013-9466-3
4. Healthcare Without Harm. Home page. Accessed June 18, 2022. https://noharm-uscanada.org/
5. Centre for Sustainable Healthcare. Home page. Accessed June 22, 2022. https://sustainablehealthcare.org.uk/
6. National Research Council (US); Institute of Medicine (US). Physical and social environmental factors. In: Woolf SH, Aron L, eds. *US Health in International Perspective: Shorter Lives, Poorer Health*. National Academies Press; 2013:7, Physical and Social Environmental Factors.
7. Health impacts of extreme weather—climate change and human health. National Institute of Environmental Health Sciences. Accessed November 29, 2022. https://www.niehs.nih.gov/research/programs/climatechange/health_impacts/weather_related_morbidity/
8. Romanello M, McGushin A, Di Napoli C, et al. The 2021 report of the Lancet Countdown on health and climate change: code red for a healthy future *Lancet*. 2021;398(10311):1619–1662. Published correction appears in *Lancet*. 2021;398(10317):2148. doi:10.1016/S0140-6736(21)01787-6
9. Anderson EE. What we talk about when we talk about goals. *Virtual Mentor*. 2007;9(6):407–409. doi:10.1001/virtualmentor.2007.9.6.fred1-0706
10. American Medical Association (AMA). AMA declaration of professional responsibility. December 4, 2001. Accessed: August 11, 2022. https://www.ama-assn.org/delivering-care/public-health/ama-declaration-professional-responsibility
11. American Medical Association (AMA). Press release. June 13, 2022. Accessed June 22, 2022. https://www.ama-assn.org/press-center/press-releases/ama-adopts-new-policy-declaring-climate-change-public-health-crisis

12. American Medical Association (AMA). Principles of medical ethics. Accessed June 22, 2022. https://www.ama-assn.org/about/publications-newsletters/ama-principles-medical-ethics

13. Ruckart PZ, Ettinger AS, Hanna-Attisha M, Jones N, Davis SI, Breysse PN. The Flint water crisis: a coordinated public health emergency response and recovery initiative. *J Public Health Manag Pract.* 2019;25(suppl 1, Lead Poisoning Prevention):S84–S90. doi:10.1097/PHH.0000000000000871

14. Council on Environmental Health. Global climate change and children's health. *Pediatrics.* 2015;136(5):992–997. doi:10.1542/peds.2015-3232

15. Parker CL. Slowing global warming: benefits for patients and the planet. *Am Fam Physician.* 2011;84(3):271–278.

16. Kotcher J, Maibach E, Miller J, et al. Views of health professionals on climate change and health: a multinational survey study. *Lancet Planet Health.* 2021;5(5):e316–e323. doi:10.1016/S2542-5196(21)00053-X

17. Macpherson CC, Wynia M. Should health professionals speak up to reduce the health risks of climate change? *AMA J Ethics.* 2017;19(12):1202–1210. doi:10.1001/journalofethics.2017.19.12.msoc1-1712

18. Thomasson C. Physicians' social responsibility. *AMA J Ethics.* 2014;16(9):753–757. doi:10.1001/virtualmentor.2014.16.9.oped1-1409

19. Lockwood AH. The physician's role in society: enhancing the health of individuals and the public. *AMA J Ethics.* 2004;6(4):189–190. doi:10.1001/virtualmentor.2004.6.4.msoc2-0404

20. Law A, Duff D, Saunders P, Middleton J, McCoy D. Medical organisations must divest from fossil fuels. *BMJ.* 2018;363:k5163. doi:10.1136/bmj.k5163

21. Thiel C, Richie C. Carbon emissions from overuse of US health care: medical and ethical problems. *Hastings Cent Rep.* 2022;52(4):10–16. doi:10.1002/hast.1404

22. UNEP. UN environment programme. Emissions gap report 2020. December 9, 2020. Accessed: June 16, 2022. https://www.unep.org/emissions-gap-report-2020

23. Healthcare. Net zero climate. Accessed November 9, 2022. https://netzeroclimate.org/sectors/healthcare/

24. Macpherson CC. Energy, emissions, and public health ethics. In: Mastroianni AC, Kahn JP, Kass NE, eds. *The Oxford Handbook of Public Health Ethics.* Online edition. Oxford Handbooks. Oxford Academic; 2January 8, 2019. Accessed November 29, 2022:739–753. https://doi.org/10.1093/oxfordhb/9780190245191.013.65

25. Resnik DB. Environmental justice and climate change policies. *Bioethics.* 2022;36(7):735741. https://doi.org/10.1111/bioe.13042

26. Dwyer J. Environmental migrants, structural injustice, and moral responsibility. *Bioethics.* 2020;34(6):562–569.

27. National Institutes of Health (NIH). Climate change and health initiative. Accessed June 16, 2022. https://www.nih.gov/climateandhealth

28. National Health Service (NHS). Delivering a "net zero" national health service. October 2020; one year on from the Net Zero Report. November 2021. Accessed June 7, 2022. https://www.england.nhs.uk/greenernhs/a-net-zero-nhs/

29. The road to carbon neutral. Kaiser Permanente. October 26, 2021. Accessed November 9, 2022. https://about.kaiserpermanente.org/community-health/improving-community-conditions/environmental-stewardship/the-road-to-carbon-neutral

30. Gundersen Envision. Gundersen Health System. Accessed November 9, 2022. https://www.gundersenenvision.org/

31. Gundersen Health System. Our system. Accessed November 9, 2022. https://www.gundersenhealth.org/our-system

32. Willett W, Rockström J, Loken B, et al. Food in the Anthropocene: the EAT-Lancet Commission on healthy diets from sustainable food systems [published correction appears in *Lancet.* 2019 Feb 9;393(10171):530] *Lancet.* 2019;393(10170):447–492. Published correction appears in *Lancet.* 2019;393(10191):2590. Published correction appears in *Lancet.* 2020;395(10221):338. Published correction appears in *Lancet.* 2020;396(10256):e56. doi:10.1016/S0140-6736(18)31788-4

33. Abbasi K, Godlee F. Investing in humanity: the *BMJ*'s divestment campaign. *BMJ.* 2020;368:m167. doi:10.1136/bmj.m167

34. Solomon CG, LaRocque RC. Climate change—a health emergency. *N Engl J Med.* 2019;380(3):209–211. doi:10.1056/NEJMp1817067

35. Cohen G. Is it possible to have healthy people on a sick planet?" Hastings Center Daniel Callahan Annual Lecture. April 19, 2022. https://www.thehastingscenter.org/callahan-lecture/

36. Mueller J, Lieber D. Decarbonizing the US health sector. *N Engl J Med.* 2022;386(10):1003–1004.

37. Law A, Duff D, Saunders P, Middleton J, McCoy D. Medical organisations must divest from fossil fuels. *BMJ.* 2018;363:k5163. doi:10.1136/bmj.k5163

38. Woolf SH, Braveman P. Where health disparities begin: the role of social and economic determinants—and why current policies may make matters worse. *Health Aff (Millwood).* 2011;30(10):1852–1859. doi:10.1377/hlthaff.2011.0685

39. Social determinants of health. World Health Organization. Accessed November 29, 2022. https://www.who.int/health-topics/social-determinants-of-health

40. Macpherson C. Can bioethics do for our planet what it's done for autonomy? *Perspect Biol Med.* 2022–2023;65(4):548–558.

41. Commercial determinants of global health. World Health Organization. Accessed November 29, 2022. https://www.who.int/health-topics/commercial-determinants-of-health

42. Allen-Scott LK, Buntain B, Hatfield JM, Meisser A, Thomas CJ. Academic institutions and one health: building capacity for transdisciplinary research approaches to address complex health issues at the animal–human–ecosystem interface. *Acad Med.* 2015;90(7):866.

43. Rabinowitz PM, Natterson-Horowitz BJ, Kahn LH, Kock R, Pappaioanou M. Incorporating one health into medical education. *BMC Med Educ.* 2017;17(1):1–7.

44. Walpole SC, Vyas A, Maxwell J, et al. Building an environmentally accountable medical curriculum through international collaboration. *Med Teach.* 2017;39(10):1040–1050.

45. Pellegrino ED. Professionalism, profession and the virtues of the good physician. *Mt Sinai J Med.* 2002;69(6):378–384.

46. American Association of Medical Colleges (AAMC). The core entrustable professional activities for entering residency. 2022. Accessed June 14, 2022. https://www.aamc.org/what-we-do/mission-areas/medical-education/cbme/core-epas

47. Environment 78-6. Medical Council of Canada. 2017. Accessed June 12, 2024. https://mcc.ca/wp-json/mcc/medical-expert-pdf/?id=9590

48. Health and the Climate Crisis 78-11. Medical Council of Canada. March 2022. Accessed June 12, 2024. https://mcc.ca/wp-json/mcc/medical-expert-pdf/?id=9608

49. Environmental health and climate change. American Academy of Family Practice (AAFP). February 20, 2020. Accessed May 18, 2022. https://www.aafp.org/family-physician/patient-care/prevention-wellness/social-determinants/environmental-health-and-climate-change.html.

50. American Academy of Family Practice (AAFP). AAFP Promotes health equity curricular toolkit. August 12, 2019. Accessed May 18, 2022. https://www.aafp.org/news/education-professional-development/20190812healtheqcurrictoolkit.html

51. Paulson JA, Ahdoot S, Baum CR, et al. Global climate change and children's health. Pediatrics. 2015;136(5):992–997. Accessed May 18, 2022. https://publications.aap.org/pediatrics/article/136/5/992/33836/Global-Climate-Change-and-Children-s-Health

52. Clayton S, Manning C, Krygsman K, Speiser M. *Mental Health and Our Changing Climate: Impacts, Implications and Guidance.* American Psychological Association and ecoAmerica; 2017.

53. Toolkit: Climate change and health. American College of Physicians. Accessed May 18, 2022. https://www.acponline.org/advocacy/advocacy-in-action/climate-change-toolkit.

54. Environmental sustainability. American Society of Anesthesiologists. October 2014. Accessed May 18, 2022. https://www.asahq.org/about-asa/governance-and-committees/asa-committees/environmental-sustainability.

55. Medical Society Consortium on Climate and Health. January, 2022. Accessed August 13, 2022. https://test.ms2ch.org/wp-content/uploads/2016/10/Consortium-Summary-2022-1.pdf.

56. US call to action on climate, health, and equity: a policy action agenda. Climate Health Action. 2019. Accessed May 18, 2022.https://climatehealthaction.org/cta/climate-health-equity-policy/

57. American Medical Association. AMA fact sheet on its decade of membership growth. June 2021. Accessed May 18, 2022. https://www.ama-assn.org/system/files/2021-06/ama-10-years-2021-fact-sheet.pdf

58. American Medical Association House of Delegates Proceedings, Annual Meeting v.1989 i.000. 1989. Accessed June 12, 2024. https://ama.nmtvault.com/jsp/PsImageViewer.jsp?doc_id=1ee24daa-2768-4bff-b792-e4859988fe94%2Fama_arch%2FHOD00001%2F00000128

59. American Medical Association House of Delegates Proceedings, Interim Meeting v.1989 i.000. 1989. Accessed June 12, 2024. https://ama.nmtvault.com/jsp/PsImageViewer.jsp?doc_id=1ee24daa-2768-4bff-b792-e4859988fe94%2Fama_arch%2FHOD00001%2F00000129

60. Global climate change and human health H-135.938. American Medical Association. 2019. Accessed May 18, 2022.https://policysearch.ama-assn.org/policyfinder/detail/climate%20change?uri=%2FAMADoc%2FHOD.xml-0-309.xml

61. Climate change education across the medical education continuum H-135.919. American Medical Association. 2019. Accessed May 18, 2022. https://policysearch.ama-assn.org/policyfinder/detail/climate%20change?uri=%2FAMADoc%2FHOD.xml-H-135.919.xml

62. American Medical Association House of Delegates Proceedings, Interim Meeting. November 16, 2019. Accessed June 12, 2024. https://www.ama-assn.org/house-delegates/interim-meeting/proceedings-2019-interim-meeting-house-delegates

63. Global climate change—the "greenhouse effect" H-135.977. American Medical Association. 2014. Accessed May 18, 2022. https://policysearch.ama-assn.org/policyfinder/detail/%22climate%20change%22?uri=%2FAMADoc%2FHOD.xml-0-348.xml

64. Stewardship of the environment H-135.973. American Medical Association. 2016. Accessed May 18, 2022. https://policysearch.ama-assn.org/policyfinder/detail/Environmental%20Health?uri=%2FAMADoc%2FHOD.xml-0-344.xml

65. Lower costs by going green. 2017. medsocietiesforclimatehealth.org. https://medsocietiesforclimatehealth.org/wp-content/uploads/2023/09/AMA-Office-Envir-Sustainability-Tool-Oct-2017.pdf

66. Association of American Medical Colleges. Number of medical schools including topic in required courses and elective courses: environmental health. Liaison Committee on Medical Education (LCME) Annual Questionnaire Part II, 2015–2019. Accessed May 18, 2022. https://www.aamc.org/data-reports/curriculum-reports/interactive-data/curriculum-topics-required-and-elective-courses-medical-school-programs

67. Association of American Medical Colleges. Number of medical schools including topic in required courses and elective courses: climate change. Liaison Committee on Medical Education (LCME) Annual Questionnaire Part II, 2015–2019. Accessed May 18, 2022. https://www.aamc.org/data-reports/curriculum-reports/interactive-data/curriculum-topics-required-and-elective-courses-medical-school-programs

68. HMS Green Initiative Highlights. 2022. Accessed August 14, 2022. https://green.harvard.edu/schools-units/medical-hms

69. Yale. Sustainability survey report. 2021. Accessed August 14, 2022. https://sustainability.yale.edu/

70. McGill. Climate and sustainability action plan. Accessed August 14, 2022. https://www.mcgill.ca/law/about/climate-and-sustainability-action-plan

71. National Medical Association (NMA). About Us. Accessed May 18, 2022. https://www.nmanet.org/page/About_Us

72. Resnik DB. Environmental justice and climate change policies. *Bioethics*. 2022;36(7):735–741. doi:10.1111/bioe.13042

73. EPA report shows disproportionate impacts of climate change on socially vulnerable populations in the United States. United States Environmental Protection Agency. September 2, 2021. Accessed June 20, 2022. https://www.epa.gov/newsreleases/epa-report-shows-disproportionate-impacts-climate-change-socially-vulnerable

74. Environmental Health. National Medical Association. Accessed May 19, 2022. https://www.nmanet.org/page/Environmental_Health

75. United States. Planetary Health Report Card. April 22, 2022. Accessed August 13, 2022. https://phreportcard.org/united-states/

76. Harvard Medical School. Planetary Health Report Card. Accessed May 18, 2022. https://phreportcard.org/wp-content/uploads/2022/04/Harvard-2021.pdfPublished 2022.

77. Climate MD. C-CHANGE. Harvard T.H. Chan School of Public Health. April 12, 2022. Accessed May 18, 2022. https://www.hsph.harvard.edu/c-change/issues/climate-md/

78. Abbott B. Medical schools are pushed to train doctors for climate change. *Wall Street J*. August 7, 2019. Accessed May 18, 2022. https://www.wsj.com/articles/medical-schools-are-pushed-to-train-doctors-for-climate-change-11565170205

79. American Association of Medical Colleges (AAMC). Advocacy and policy. 2022. Accessed June 14, 2022. https://www.aamc.org/advocacy-policy

80. Ray K. In the name of racial justice: why bioethics should care about environmental toxins. *Hastings Cent Rep.* 2021;51(3):23–26.

81. Galarneau C. Communities matter." *Hastings Cent Rep.* 2020;50(3):63–64.

82. Fins JJ. An evergreen metaphor: Strachan Donnelley, Dan Callahan, and environmental ethics. Hastings Center Bioethics Forum. 2021. Accessed June 22, 2022. https://www.the-hastingscenter.org/an-evergreen-metaphor-strachan-donnelley-dan-callahan-and-environmental-ethics/

83. Jameton A, Pierce J. Can clinical ethics survive climate change? *Perspect Biol Med.* 2021;64(4):511–540.

PART D: EPILOGUE

THIS IS NOT WHAT WE DO

Thomas S. Inui

I came into this world in the labor and delivery suite of Hopkins Hospital's Women's Clinic in July 1943. I have no conscious memories of that time, but I suspect that my subconscious harbors dark memories of the events surrounding my birth. My mother, a Hopkins-trained nurse, delivered me after a long labor complicated by a scopolamine delirium, forceps extraction, and a "generous" perineal incision ("Tommy, you gave me a rough time!"). She had come to Hopkins from a farming family in northwest Illinois, where she taught in the local one-room schoolhouse for several years in order to have enough money to support her BA from the University of Illinois, a prerequisite for admission to Hopkins School of Nursing in her day. The first child of her German and English immigrant family parents, her mother also contributed income from selling eggs and baked goods to finance the college education of all three of her daughters and one son.

My father, at the time of my birth the Halsted Fellow of Surgery and Surgical Pathology, had matriculated in, and graduated from, the Johns Hopkins University School of Medicine, after riding the train cross country from the University of California Los Angeles (UCLA). The son of Japanese immigrants from Fukushima, Japan, he had two older sisters who were born in Japan. His given name was Kazuo Inui until first grade in the hard-scrabble mining and railroad town of Helper, Utah, when the teacher decided that "Frank" would be easier to remember. The whole family worked in a laundry in Helper and then in a fruit stand in Los Angeles to support his education at University of California Berkeley and then UCLA. A perfect student, he applied to Hopkins, Harvard, and Columbia schools of medicine, was admitted to all three, but chose Hopkins. He continued to flourish in medical school, was admitted to the medical honor society Alpha Omega Alpha (AOA) and entered his surgery residency at Hopkins Hospital.

My parents met in the Hopkins Emergency Room (ER). The Halsted Fellow covered some weekend days in the ER. Mother was working in the ER, walked up to the Northeast Market to buy a chicken during her lunch break, but didn't have time to take it home. She slipped it into the ER refrigerator, just behind the tetanus vaccine vials, where she hoped it wouldn't be noticed until she finished her shift and took it home. An announcement over the ER intercom interrupted these plans: "Would whoever put a *chicken* in the ER refrigerator report to Dr. Inui now, please." "I'm sorry!" she said to the Japanese American resident, whom she did not know at all. "I just got it back here from the market with no time to go home and didn't want it to spoil." "What are you going to *do* with this *chicken*?" he asked, looking rather serious and not at all amused. "I'm cooking it for supper." Ah, said the resident, looking a little less severe. "I like chicken!"

And so they met. After inviting himself to supper that first evening, he kept visiting, not for the supper but for the friendship that grew with time. When they wrote to their families for permission to marry in 1942, an untimely Anglo/Japanese pairing during World War II, they got a supportive response from her farm family and an angry and disappointed response from his family, who by this time had been imprisoned behind barbed wire at the Heart Mountain relocation camp in the wilds of Wyoming.

In my own life, my parents made certain that I knew how much they loved their experiences at Hopkins. They were positively thrilled when I was admitted to medical school there and withdrew from other applications. My first real introduction to Hopkins Hospital was set up by my godmother, a member of the Hopkins School of Nursing faculty with lead responsibility for geriatrics. She arranged for me to meet with Lucky, an African American resident of East Baltimore and a linen restocking cart orderly. "He's worked here a long time and knows the place inside out!" Lucky met me at the feet of Jesus, an elegant large statue dominating the (then) main entrance to Hopkins Hospital. "Good to meet you, sir," I said not wanting to presume I could address him as "Lucky," as he stood before me, a short, thin, vigorous, smiling older Black man. He turned out to be a great teacher.

"Follow me, Mr. Inui" he said warming up his Socratic method: "But first, what do you notice about Jesus's feet?" pointing to the shiny area above the stigmata on the feet of the marble statue. "Patients come down here from the floors and want to pray. They touch Jesus where he was wounded." I knew the location. Godmother had told me that the nurses, including my mother, stood here for inspection of their long-sleeve uniform white cuffs by the chief of nursing before reporting for duty to their assigned floors. Then moving quickly, Lucky and I moved around Jesus into the low-ceiling entry hallway that merged into the main hospital corridor. 'What do you see here, Mr. Inui?" he asked. Looking around in some confusion, I said: "Well, two fountains on each side of the hallway and four doors, two on each side of the hall. One door says men's bathroom, one says women's bathroom and two doors with no signs." "Why do we need four fountains, Mr. Inui? Suppose I told you that behind those doors with no signs, there are full toilets. What do you suppose the doors used to say?" And on we sped, me having trouble keeping up with his fast pace. "Here's the surgery building. Your father used to work here. And through here the emergency room, where both your father and mother worked. Here's my favorite elevator operator—Eleanor, say hello to Mr. Inui. His parents used to work here." Down a level we entered different hallways—broad enough for carts, equipment storage (iron lungs!), kitchen food delivery. And here's the laundry room. "Say hi to Doris. You'll be bringing her your whites in another few years, but mainly they clean all the sheets, towels, and drapes. And here's the paging operators' room. And here's the medicine building, the ob/gyn building, and the morgue. Let's introduce you to Mr. Brown, who is the main diener. Mr. Brown, this is Mr. Inui, his father used to work here. Why don't you show him the morgue refrigerators, the two of them? Maybe you could explain to him why we need two cold rooms for the bodies. And Mr. Inui, these buckets you see are for the organs of patients who have had autopsies here. We've done thousands! Imagine that, and see if you can figure out why there are two different coloreds, did I say *colored*?—I meant color storage buckets." At this level, Mr. Brown, Eleanor, Doris, and most everyone else I saw was Black. Upstairs, downstairs. We seemed to be downstairs.

On a Saturday in December of 1945, Frank Inui was once again covering the ER as the resident in charge when he was called to the procedure room by a nurse who said they needed his help. In the room, a young doctor, probably an intern, was having trouble controlling an agitated Black kid with a bloody scalp laceration. The intern had wrestled the patient to the wall, pinning him into a hissing steam radiator, and was trying to wrap him into a sheet. Now the kid had rather significant burns on his back as well as the laceration. Dad intervened, and with the help of the nurse, got everyone calmed down. He dismissed the intern, telling him to go home, to think about what had just happened, and not to come back until Monday because: "This is not what we do."

On that next Monday, Frank Inui was called to Dr. Alfred Blalock's office. Dr. Blalock was a relatively new chairman of surgery, up from Vanderbilt. "Are you the resident who sent an intern home from the ER on Saturday?" asked Blalock. "You've made a mistake. That intern is my nephew, and I am dismissing you today from my surgery program. You are not my kind of man."

And so Frank Inui left Hopkins before he completed his residency. Joining a surgical pathology program in Salt Lake City, he became the chief resident in surgery when the incumbent chief resident there was drafted. He completed his residency and board of surgery requirements at Ohio State University Hospital and Mahoning County Tuberculosis Sanatorium in Youngstown, Ohio. During the Korean conflict, he was drafted and served as chief of surgery for the 46th Surgical Hospital, a "MASH" (Mobile Army Surgical Hospital) unit located four minutes behind the front lines in Korea. He was awarded a US Army Bronze Star for implementing a new repair procedure for major vessel repair in this MASH that reduced the rate of limbs lost to amputation from 62% to 7% (Inui FK, Shannon J, Howard JM. Arterial injuries in the Korean Conflict. Recent Adv Surg 17(5): 850-857; 1954). He practiced thoracic and general surgery in Youngstown, Ohio, where he served as chief of surgery for the city's two hospitals. His residency program in this system trained a generation of young surgeons from Thailand, including two individuals who became chiefs of surgery and directors for two national referral hospitals, one in Bangkok and another in Chiang Mai, Thailand. To finish his career, Frank Inui and his wife, Beulah, moved to Talihina, Oklahoma, where he worked as the surgeon in residence for the US Public Health Service Indian Health Service Hospital that served the Choctah Nation. His son, Thomas, received his MD from Johns Hopkins School of Medicine, his ScM from the Hopkins School of Public Health, completed an internal medicine residency and chief residency at Hopkins, and pursued a career in academic medicine. In some measure, he hopes his career is a fulfillment of his father's aspirations.

After reading this story, try using an exegesis method to explore its content.

1. Who in this story can I see as myself?
2. From the point of view of whomever you have chosen, what do you bring to the situation that makes these events possible?
3. Who else in this story (or its organizational or cultural context) influences this story?
4. Where/what in this story is "the good," the value, the virtue, the "North Star," or the principle we might seek to preserve?
5. What, then, ought I do?

37
Future Directions and Disruptive Innovations in Medical Professionalism[a]

Ariel Lefkowitz, Mantoa Mokhachane, Morag Paton, Pier Bryden, Cynthia R. Whitehead, Tasha R. Wyatt, Jerry M. Maniate, and Ayelet Kuper

Key Points

- Professionalism is defined in different ways by different people, and these definitions affect the loci of power in medicine, medical education, and the regulation of physicians.
- Professionalism can act as a force that not only protects patients and colleagues but also constrains what is or is not acceptable for a physician to say, do, or be.
- Grappling with the history of medicine is critical in allowing new ideas and new faces to thrive in Medicine.

Continuing Tensions in Medical Professionalism

A textbook on medical professionalism provides us a snapshot in time. If there is anything that the literature and history of medical professionalism tells us, it is that it is many things to many people,[1] that it evolves,[2] that it varies across cultures[3] and generations,[4] and thus it is difficult to define, demonstrate, or evaluate. Predictions regarding the future of medical professionalism therefore also represent a snapshot in time and are necessarily framed in current contextualized perspectives. We are a diverse group from countries with and without universal healthcare, from the Global North and the Global South, physicians and researchers, with a variety of personal and professional backgrounds. Our predictions and hopes for the future of medical professionalism reflect these backgrounds and are shaped by our social and political dispositions, by the concepts in the field that delight and dismay us, and, of course, by the times in which we write.

[a] **Disclaimer:** This work was prepared by a military or civilian employee of the US Government as part of the individual's official duties and therefore is in the public domain. The opinions and assertions expressed herein are those of the author(s) and do not necessarily reflect the official policy or position of the Uniformed Services University or the Department of Defense.

To highlight this point further, we look to the ways in which discussions around the important tensions in the medical professionalism literature have evolved even over the past two decades. In 2011, Hodges and colleagues described how professionalism grew into a major topic of concern, especially for medical educators, and, using discourse analysis, identified the tensions at the forefront of the professionalism literature.[1] At that time, these included whether professionalism is an individual characteristic, trait, behavior, or cognitive process; whether professionalism should be understood as belonging to an individual, to an interpersonal process, or as a societal or institutional phenomenon; and, to a lesser extent, whether professionalism is fixed and observable or whether it is evolving and culturally and historically informed. Eight years later, the author group reconvened to discuss the evolution of professionalism literature and found that there were significant shifts in the topics that sparked interest and inquiry among scholars. These included the interplay between professionalism and professional identity formation, ways in which professionalism can be used as a tool for social control, and a greater focus on differences in the conception of professionalism across cultures.[2] The current chapter is similarly informed by the trends in discourses around professionalism to this point, while also considering social, economic, political, and technological factors that are likely to influence the directions of professionalism in the coming years.

To this end, we have identified seven burgeoning tensions concerning medical professionalism that have been bubbling up in the literature and in the practice of medicine in evolving social and political landscapes. Some might call one or more of these tensions **future directions**, as they are likely to require addressing in the near future as they arise from topical challenges in modern medical practice. Others might see some of these tensions as **disruptive innovations**, those that we as a group recognize as essential to the profession becoming more inclusive, less restrictive, and, in doing so, providing better care to patients. In actuality, each of these tensions has features of these two categories, as each presents an ongoing and future challenge to the practice of medicine as we try to care for our patients and our populations in a world that is ever more complex. We discuss each of the seven tensions we identified in the literature in turn (for a complete list of the seven tensions, see Table 37.1).

Table 37.1 Seven Tensions

1. Professionalism as a universal truth vs. one that changes, evolves, and varies across cultures and contexts.
2. Professionalism as who we are vs. what we do at work.
3. Professionalism as promoting wellness vs. punishing un-wellness.
4. Professionalism as a force that is facilitated by technological innovation vs. one that is challenged by new technologies.
5. Professionalism as a force for protection of patients and colleagues vs. a tool for policing physicians.
6. Professionalism as promoting activism vs. forbidding engagement with controversial topics.
7. Professionalism as defining the "ideal doctor" vs. setting out guidelines that are inclusive of a diversity of ways of being.

Professionalism as a Universal Truth Versus One That Changes, Evolves, and Varies Across Cultures and Contexts

The tension between professionalism as a single concept that ignores culture and context and professionalism as a complex social construct that derives its various meanings from the understandings of those who use the word is ongoing. We saw how Hodges and colleagues' review of the literature in 2011 uncovered a multitude of differing opinions among scholars on the nature of professionalism: whether it is a trait or a pattern of behavior or whether it is a characteristic of individuals or of collectives.[1] This disagreement on *what professionalism is* extends to individuals within the profession, who also hold a multitude of understandings of professionalism so disparate that Burford and colleagues' wonder whether "It may be better to assume that 'professionalism' as a discrete construct does not exist per se, and to focus instead on specific skills. . . . If we are specifying the communication elements of professionalism, we should explicitly talk of those elements, if we mean adherence to standards, then we should say so."[5] Indeed, recently published evidence abounds documenting the ways in which professionalism differs across cultures.[3,6–9] In a globalized world, with a pluralistic outlook, the challenge posed to the possibility of a universally true conception of the nature of medical professionalism, by such context-specific descriptions of professionalism, grows increasingly persuasive.[10]

Thus, this tension remains unsettled. Professionalism is not simply an idea, but a tool, a way of differentiating between professional and unprofessional behavior, individuals, and perspectives. Therefore, this disagreement over the pluralistic social construct versus positivist binary nature of professionalism is not just abstract, but rather presents a practical quandary, given that the professionalism of medical trainees and physicians is assessed by medical schools, hospitals, regulatory colleges, and oversight boards. The challenge of assessing a construct that remains poorly defined continues to plague medical educators,[2] especially since most instruments used to measure professionalism are not methodologically sound.[11] If assessors, practitioners, trainees, and oversight bodies do not agree on how to define professionalism, then making judgments on the professionalism of trainees and physicians will continue to be an endeavor fraught with theoretical uncertainty and lack of construct specificity, no matter how confidently assessors carry out their work in practice.

One factor that further accentuates the tension of the evolving conceptions of professionalism is, simply, age. As with all generation gaps, older and younger physicians have different values, life experiences, goals, and challenges, and there are those in each group who may find the other at fault for unprofessionalism in medicine.[4] Some argue that these disparities in understandings of the world between generations may be widening further in recent years[12] (although others contend that every generation makes a variation on this claim[13]). With the changing cultural and political landscapes of our time, these disparities may make it still more difficult to agree on a meaningful conception of professionalism that allows satisfactory implementation. Future approaches to these challenges to medical professionalism will include the development of dialogue across generational gaps[14] and perhaps even education that directly addresses the different understandings of professionalism among different generations.

The disparity between evolving understandings of professionalism captures as a microcosm a greater philosophical tension between establishing a static standard of professionalism and accepting the fluid inchoateness of professionalism. This is highlighted most clearly in discourse that endeavors to establish professionalism as a competency that medical students and residents must demonstrate as part of their training,[15] one that comes on the heels of a surge in educators' zeal to establish competencies for every skill in medicine.[16] This school of thought, that professionalism is an observable behavior and therefore assessable as a competency, has consequences for how the behaviors of physicians are judged and disciplined since demonstrating a lack of "competence" in professionalism may result in the triggering of remediation and other consequences.[17] However, professionalism, like advocacy and collaboration, is not like some other skills in medicine that we call competencies. With anatomic knowledge, experience, and training, performing an appendectomy or a thoracentesis can become second nature for a skilled operator, rarely harder one day than the day before. In contrast, the challenges to maintaining professionalism as an individual, no matter how it is defined, involves the continuous navigation of myriad personal and institutional factors that can change in difficulty on a daily basis. In short, professionalism, even once "acquired" as a "competency," can be a daily struggle, shaped by interpersonal, institutional, and structural factors, no matter how experienced the clinician is. Addressing the philosophical tension of professionalism as competency versus daily struggle is one that will continue to beset leaders and educators in medicine hoping to assess and judge professionalism.

Professionalism as Who We Are Versus What We Do at Work

The increasing dominance of social media and the ability to record every moment on our phones with pictures, audio, and videos have introduced new challenges to the professionalism of physicians. Instead of one's professional behavior only being assessed while at the hospital or clinic, physicians' professionalism may be scrutinized wherever and whenever the internet can find them. Moreover, the standards of what is or is not professional are, as we have seen, not universal but rather specific to the observers' perspective. The #Medbikini scandal is an illustrative example, in which the *Journal of Vascular Surgery* published (and later retracted following an uproar of protest) a study called: "Prevalence of Unprofessional Social Media Content Among Young Vascular Surgeons."[18] In the study, three male investigators perused social media accounts and looked for what they felt was unprofessional behavior, which included "inappropriate attire [such as] pictures in underwear, provocative Halloween costumes, and provocative posing in bikinis/swimwear."[19] Beyond this sexism and puritanical voyeurism lies a belief that professionalism enacts a requirement to embody a set of institutionally defined values even while individuals are not doing anything remotely related to their care of patients.

Examples of "professionalism creep" like #Medbikini have led to calls to teach medical students how to carefully construct and cultivate digital professional identities that will not lead to professionalism calamities.[20] However, the overarching message to trainees and staff is clear—adhering to professionalism is more than just being professional at work; it includes adhering to a set of guidelines outside of work as well. One notable example that does not involve social media occurred when a surgeon driving in his car was cut off by another vehicle.[21] The two cars proceeded to a parking lot, and as the surgeon approached the other car to talk to the driver, the driver punched at the surgeon from the driver's seat.[22] The surgeon then punched the driver several times in the face and body.[21] The surgeon pled guilty to a charge of assault in criminal court and was disciplined by the College of Physicians and Surgeons of Ontario (CPSO) after he was found to have engaged in professional misconduct and "conduct unbecoming a physician."[22] This ruling demonstrates an extension of the jurisdiction of oversight bodies well beyond the walls of the hospital and clinic.

The members of this authorial team are fortunate that, in the countries in which we work, holding a particular religious or sexual orientation or gender identity is not currently seen as conduct unbecoming of a physician. However, the willingness of professional oversight bodies to extend their reach beyond the hospital and clinic is a clear example of the consequences that come from a lack of consensus around what constitutes unprofessional behavior. This hints at a future likely to challenge our notion of what is or is not acceptable for a physician to say, do, or be. Do promiscuity, nonmonogamy, or other expressions of sexuality constitute conduct unbecoming of a physician? Are activism or political engagement evidence of unprofessionalism? Is the provision of certain healthcare procedures in places that have legislated against them, such as abortion, evidence of unprofessionalism, or is it just providing healthcare? Are there still unspoken prohibitions on the level of self-expression that is acceptable as a physician, especially when one's background (ethnic, linguistic, religious, etc.) is not the same as the dominant culture? Are we allowed to express resistance and dissent within the system that supports and defines us as a community? We engage with these tough questions in relation to other tensions in the discussion that follows.

Professionalism as Promoting Wellness Versus Punishing Unwellness

There is an increasing focus on the wellness of physicians and physicians in training, driven by greater societal recognition of mental illness, by increased stresses on physicians from rising workloads and pandemics, and by proliferating evidence on the effect of burnout on patient care.[23,24] As a result, strong links have been drawn between wellness and professionalism. Since poor wellness is associated with a higher rate of self-reported medical errors,[25] it follows that a professional physician does everything they can to promote personal wellness, and it is incumbent on medical schools and institutions to promote wellness in their physicians and trainees.[26]

However, the flip side of this mandate is that, rather than fostering the normalization of mental illness among physicians, the drive to promote professionalism and weed out unprofessionalism may lead to the disparagement and disqualification of those with mental illness. A survey of state licensing body executive directors indicated that a significant number of them felt that a diagnosis of mental illness was sufficient grounds to sanction a physician.[27] The consequences of this policing of mental health results, ironically, in worse mental health care: In a study of over 5,000 physicians, almost 40% of physicians reported reluctance to seek medical treatment of a mental health condition for fear of losing their license to practice.[28] Even without a loss of licensure, fitness for duty evaluations investigating physicians with mental illness can cause harm through stigmatization and bias, through situating physicians with mental illness as unable to manage or monitor their own illness, and even placing stipulations on the type of therapy physicians must undergo to be allowed to return to work.[29] As we gain a greater understanding of the scope of the problem of mental illness and suicide among physicians,[30] we will have to grapple with the paradox of using professionalism to try to promote wellness and, in doing so, inadvertently worsening access to mental health resources and driving unwell physicians into hiding. Decoupling mental illness and unprofessional conduct will go a long way toward promoting disclosure of mental illness among physicians and allowing those in need to seek the care they require.

Professionalism as a Force That Is Facilitated by Technological Innovation Versus One That Is Challenged by New Technologies

New technologies are rapidly changing the approaches to how medicine is practiced, across all specialties and in a multitude of ways, including wearable technologies that send readings directly to physicians, artificial intelligence (AI) decision aids that help make diagnoses and advise on treatments, robotic surgical aids, and technologies that can monitor hand hygiene, hospital-acquired infections, and even the mental health of those using voice-activated software. Technological advances will continue to contribute to and complicate the provision of healthcare.[31] However, many have identified that while AI can extend our ability to provide care, it can also exacerbate and magnify existing inequities in healthcare. AI systems can contribute to inequity when they are constructed from data sets that do not accurately represent marginalized minority communities, when they are constructed to reflect the needs of those in power at the expense of marginalized communities, and when they are used to augment care for those who can afford technologies while leaving those who have barriers to participating in new technologies with inferior care.[32,33] Technologies are not neutral forces of progress, but rather are social artifacts that have the potential to amplify inequity. New technologies are not new toys to be blithely integrated into clinical practice, but rather challenge us as individuals and institutions to grapple with ethical and professional quandaries whose choices for paths forward will have ramifications for our patients and communities.

As technologies change the practice of medicine, the focus of professionalism in medicine must shift as well (as we saw in tension 1). For instance, some authors argue that with the potential benefits and inequities that new technologies bring, it is incumbent on physicians to increase their focus on compassionate care to ensure that new technologies are designed and distributed equitably and do not lead to depersonalization and distance in the way care is delivered.[34] One example of the risk of new technologies to eclipse person-centered care is in the increasing exaltation of point-of-care ultrasound (POCUS) and consequent de-emphasis of other sources of data, like clinical history taking or physical examination. Some argue that the perceived power of the ultrasound as a tool of obtaining "objective truth" from the physical body of the patient minimizes the importance of the subjective perspective of the patient, as competency in ultrasound use becomes incorporated into the identity of new physicians.[35] The use of POCUS does not in itself cause the devaluation of patients' perspectives, but Feilchenfeld and colleagues highlight how an overvaluation of its importance necessarily carries a risk of its "objective data" eclipsing the observations of the patient,[35] thus challenging the integrity of physicians' professional duty to center the patient's experience in clinical decision-making. Fenwick similarly argues that in the face of increasing technological innovation in medicine, the so-called core skills of "the professional" are those "that cannot be routinized including wise judgment, ethical decisions, action in unpredictable or ambiguous situations, creativity, and empathy."[36] It remains to be seen whether scholars, educators, and licensing bodies will codify these supratechnological traits as those that typify the professional in the age of technological medicine; failing to do so critically may result in the same old well-intentioned neglect of patients repackaged in shiny new trappings.[37]

Professionalism as a Force for Protection of Patients and Colleagues Versus a Tool for Policing Physicians

Professionalism is often framed as a force whose guidelines grant protection for others by making it unacceptable for physicians to engage in harassment and discrimination of patients and colleagues. However, those same professionalism guidelines, set by the institutions and organizations that hold the power, often limit professional speech to that which is "respectful," "civil," and respectful of "academic freedom." This can suppress the reporting of precisely the instances of harassment and discrimination that the tenets of professionalism purport to protect.[38] Sukhera and colleagues describe this in detail in their article, "Freedom From Discrimination or Freedom to Discriminate?" By framing professional discourse as "civil" and "respectful," those in power can arbitrate which discourse constitutes merely exercising one's academic freedom and which infringes on academic freedom and on the bounds of professionalism through its accusatory and uncivil nature. This is referred to as the "weaponization of professionalism," used to stifle dissent, as in the example of a medical student who was deemed unprofessional and ejected from the clinic when he suggested adding options for gender beyond male and female on the clinic's intake form.[39] While it is supposed to be unprofessional to engage in discrimination, in reality it can be deemed unprofessional to identify discrimination in practice, silencing advocacy.

Instances like this one, in which professionalism seems to reinforce inequity rather than foster positive change, are not anomalous but rather typify the power of "professionalism." In the early twentieth century, the American Medical Association (AMA) and other loci of medical power consolidated their control of the practice of medicine by defining what was and was not professional. Their consolidation of power in the hands of the dominant white male physicians was successful, as they wrested control of obstetric practice from midwives (resulting in worsening birth outcomes in that early period[40]) and forced most medical schools that admitted women and people of color to close.[41] This tradition has continued in how professionalism is defined and used to determine who is and is not adherent to the guidelines of professionalism since "white norms have become the standard of reference for what is considered professional."[42,43] The white, male, Christian, Western/Global North standard of professionalism not only operates in the Western World, but also in nations in the Global South, such as Ethiopia, where Indigenous traditions of medical professionalism continue to struggle against the "modern" Eurocentric and individualistic professionalism model.[44]

Professionalism constrains not only what physicians say but also what they can do and who they can be, and these restrictions again find their sources in white supremacy, heteronormativity, and the dominance of the Global North. Medical students undergo a socialization in medical school that pressures them to appear "neutral": "Student-physicians are encouraged to believe that the social class, 'race,' ethnicity, gender, sexual orientation of a physician is not—and should not be—relevant during physician-patient interactions."[45] The neutral to which medical students must default their behavior and identity is the one historically dominant in medical cultures, that of the Western, straight, white male. The construct of professionalism also allows physicians and physicians in training to be "more easily governable through a variety of self-disciplining mechanisms,"[46] thus policing their own behavior and identity expression. The indoctrination of doctors into this self-recriminating professionalism ensures that those who are not white, straight, male, or from the global North are made to feel that they intrinsically might be unprofessional and thus do not challenge the existing power structure. It is no wonder that those who do not look or act like "normal, neutral" doctors, such as those with tattoos,[47] black skin,[48] natural Black hair,[49] or a nonnormative sexuality[50] still do not feel welcome in medicine.

The future of professionalism will have to grapple with this abhorrent history and troubling present. Can professionalism be divested from its hegemonic history?[51] Can what it means to be professional be decoupled from an embodiment of professionalism that has resided only with the powerful? Can professionalism change from a tool of suppression of dissent to one that promotes progress and greater equity? Or does its history anchor it to the white man in the white coat? Is it unprofessional to even ask? These questions require answers or the entire enterprise of professionalism may need to be demolished and rebuilt on new foundations. The first steps may be in critically analyzing how the status quo in professionalism is maintained,[52] and in working to incorporate a greater focus in medical education on studying the white supremacist history of medicine that leads to the need for these questions to be asked.

Professionalism as Promoting Activism Versus Forbidding Engagement With Controversial Topics

Health advocacy is considered a core duty in many contemporary medical competency frameworks.[53,54] It mandates physicians to act and speak to promote health for their patients and their communities. Based on this core physician duty, it would be easy to conclude that physicians can and indeed should engage in political activism aiming to promote the health of patients and communities. However, there are those who argue that public activism is unprofessional because publicly taking up "controversial" positions that conflict with fundamental beliefs of certain groups of patients may make those patients feel unwelcome.[55] Others argue that advocacy may be a civic norm but is not a professional imperative.[56] Thus, major unanswered questions, especially in our increasingly politically polarized societies, are: is it a professional duty to engage in political activism that promotes the health of patients? Or, instead, is political activism inherently unprofessional?

These questions have come to the forefront in recent years after the National Rifle Association tweeted in response to gun control advocacy on the part of physicians: "Someone should tell self-important anti-gun doctors to stay in their lane."[57] While physicians have faced accusations of unprofessionalism over advocacy before,[58] and some have been silenced by authorities for speaking up against power structures,[59] #StayInYourLane galvanized a vociferous chorus of physician-activists with a volume that had not been heard before. Some based their professional responsibility to engage in social advocacy not only on their responsibility to treat the patient in front of them but also their responsibility to "public health" and to expose a "malignant normality"[60] in which harms to individuals have become so commonplace as to be unremarkable (e.g., frequent instances of gun violence).[61] This view has attracted both criticism and support; criticism for focusing on "social justice rather than treating illness"[62] and support for those who advocate for the promotion of health to do so from multiple angles, as long as it does not infringe on the rights of their patients.[63] The inclusion of advocacy in professional practice does have valid challenges, including whether patients who disagree with a physician's public positions will feel safe in their care; the effect of physician advocacy on public opinion of the profession; and whether the act of public advocacy could have adverse effects on patient care.

These concerns are highlighted by the arguments about whether it is unprofessional for physicians and physicians in training to strike. The South African #FeesMustFall movement, which aimed to decrease tuition costs to make education more affordable to disadvantaged students, in particular poor Black students,[64] was criticized because of the implications of a strike on patient care for its perceived impact on public opinion of the profession and for prioritizing physicians' finances over patient care.[65] However, a deeper understanding of this disagreement may be gained by learning that the students who did not initially participate in the protests were more likely to be white and financially well off: "The privileged students did not see the need to protest."[66] Many students who initially opposed the action later supported it "when they learnt about the looming financial exclusions of some of their classmates."[66] This highlights the crux of the danger of omitting public political advocacy from the sphere of professionalism—being "neutral" on issues of public importance is not harmless, but rather promotes the acceptability, through inaction, of the ongoing disadvantage and harm that befalls the underprivileged in society. "As such, physicians must be supported in breaking free from narrow notions of professional behaviour to engage with the work of racial justice. We cannot be neutral when the stakes are as high as the health and well-being of our patients."[67]

While this position seems straightforward in opposing racism, it is more fraught when physician advocacy is for causes that may not promote equity in the way it is usually understood. For example, in response to the perception of "bullying" of physicians who oppose abortions and gender reassignment surgeries, the US Department of Health and Human Services under the Trump administration tried to expand the "conscience rule" protecting doctors who refuse to treat certain patients based on self-affirmed religious beliefs.[68] This differs from the examples of advocacy above since discriminating against specific patients by excluding them from care is an abdication of the physician's duty to care. Physicians are allowed to engage in conscientious objection to performing procedures they find morally objectionable, such as medical assistance in dying and abortion, but the medical regulatory bodies of jurisdictions like Canada in which these procedures are legal may mandate that physicians who oppose providing this care refer patients to physicians who will.[69,70] Even scholars supporting the right of conscientious objection to performing abortions concede that these objections should not interfere with the provision of clinically indicated medical care to all patients.[71] Those grappling with politically charged issues of advocacy will have to decide how to ensure physician advocacy does not interfere with the day-to-day provision of patient care. With the polarization of opinions prevalent in contemporary society, taking a stand for something carries a risk of being construed as taking a stand against certain patients.

Professionalism as Defining the "Ideal Doctor" Versus Setting Out Guidelines That Are Inclusive of Diverse Ways of Being

The professionalism that emerged in the medical literature in the late twentieth century is thought to represent the views of the historic "ruling class of medicine," presenting a "nostalgic" view of what is and is not professional.[72] This nostalgic view dovetails with the scientific tradition of the neutral observer, the impartial physician whose adherence to the scientific method allows for objective data collection and objective conclusions.[73] However, as we saw in tension 6 on activism, neutrality has its pitfalls, with the potential to lionize the status quo and the current power structure. Therefore, the nostalgic view gives rise to a legacy of professionalism where a Christian, "[w]hite, cisgender, apolitical, heteronormative man not living with a disability has long been upheld as the model 'professional.'"[67] We also saw in tension 5 how understanding professionalism as neutrality has excluded and marginalized women, people of color, nonheterosexual individuals, and other disadvantaged groups. Professionalism's constraint on what physicians can do, say, and be extends even beyond marginalizing already minoritized groups. The hidden curriculum, unwritten lessons instilled in medical trainees by peers and teachers through words and role modeling about how to be a doctor,[74] teaches physicians and physicians in training what is and is not professional, often not through guidelines that can be referred to, but through subtle communication about what is and is not conduct becoming of a physician. This hidden curriculum gives rise to an understanding of medical professionalism that may never appear in written guidelines or textbooks yet informs our perceptions of what constitutes professional behavior.

One of us (AL) is an internal medicine physician with a background in theater and improvisational comedy, conferring on him skills that inform his educational style and practice of medicine. However, during his training, he received subtle and direct messaging that his natural style of communication, with an affinity for humor and emotional openness, was "too much," that while his conduct was socially appreciated and not inappropriate per se, it was not becoming for a physician. In his first year of residency, despite receiving a five out of five on his overall evaluation, his supervisor wrote in the comments section; "He has an admirable and strong clinical foundation which sometimes is left hidden behind his charming and effervescent personality." Years later, after AL completed his training, a first-year medical student sent him an email asking if they could shadow his practice, in which they wrote (emphasis theirs): "I'm particularly interested in learning from *you* because I'm eager to understand how physicians like yourself are able to toe the line between affability and professionalism in medicine." This example demonstrates that the restrictions on how a professional physician should behave may extend into a policing of personality and self-expression, even among those who may approve of deviations from the "norm."

Must professionalism delineate a specific archetype of the "ideal doctor"? If professionalism is to continue being a useful tool to guide physicians to engage in good practice, it must do more than act as a "bed of Procrustes" of Greek mythology, stretching those who are too short to fit its ideal or chopping the limbs off those who are too tall.[75] If professionalism can adapt to become a set of guidelines that are relevant to the community in which it acts, that is inclusive enough to welcome a variety of types of humans into the profession, that can allow many types of self-expression and ways of being, then it is worthy of ongoing consideration as a useful concept. Indeed, this question encompasses all the tensions that we have considered in this chapter. The medical professionalism of the future must evolve with a changing social landscape; must navigate new complicating factors (e.g., new technologies, social media, and political upheaval); must be a flexible force of good, protecting the disadvantaged and fostering speech and activism (the aim of which is to protect the vulnerable as well); and, perhaps at the same time, acknowledge its own troublesome past and its identity as a profession in a constant state of rediscovery. There are many challenges in our future, both inside and outside the practice of medicine. Shining a focused spotlight on medical professionalism and urging tough reflection on its legitimacy and the necessity for it to change will go a long way toward ensuring our profession serves its patients, its members, and its communities.

References

1. Hodges BD, Ginsburg S, Cruess R, et al. Assessment of professionalism: recommendations from the Ottawa 2010 Conference. *Med Teach.* 2011;33(5):354–363. doi:10.3109/0142159X.2011.577300
2. Hodges B, Paul R, Ginsburg S, The Ottawa Consensus Group M. Assessment of professionalism: from where have we come—to where are we going? An update from the Ottawa Consensus Group on the assessment of professionalism. *Med Teach.* 2019;41(3):249–255. doi:10.1080/0142159X.2018.1543862
3. Ho MJ, Lin CW, Chiu YT, Lingard L, Ginsburg S. A cross-cultural study of students' approaches to professional dilemmas: sticks or ripples. *Med Educ.* 2012;46(3):245–256. doi:10.1111/j.1365-2923.2011.04149.x
4. Smith LG. Medical professionalism and the generation gap. *Am J Med.* 2005;118(4):439–442. doi:10.1016/j.amjmed.2005.01.021
5. Burford B, Morrow G, Rothwell C, Carter M, Illing J. Professionalism education should reflect reality: findings from Three Health Professions. *Med Educ.* 2014;48(4):361–374.
6. Pan H, Norris JL, Liang YS, Li JN, Ho MJ. Building a professionalism framework for healthcare providers in China: a nominal group technique study. *Med Teach.* 2013;35(10):e1531–e1536. doi:10.3109/0142159X.2013.802299
7. Tsai SL, Ho MJ, Hirsh D, Kern DE. Defiance, compliance, or alliance? How we developed a medical professionalism curriculum that deliberately connects to cultural context. *Med Teach.* 2012;34(8):614–617. doi:10.3109/0142159X.2012.684913
8. Al-Rumayyan A, Van Mook W, Magzoub ME, et al. Medical professionalism frameworks across non-Western cultures: a narrative overview. *Med Teach.* 2017;39(suppl 1):S8–S14. doi:10.1080/0142159X.2016.1254740
9. Yasin L, Stapleton G, Sandlow L. Medical professionalism across cultures: a literature review. *MedEdPublish.* 2019;8(3). doi:10.15694/mep.2019.000191.1
10. Helmich E, Yeh HM, Kalet A, Al-Eraky M. Becoming a doctor in different cultures: toward a cross-cultural approach to supporting professional identity formation in medicine. *Acad Med.* 2017;92(1):58–62. doi:10.1097/ACM.0000000000001432
11. Li H, Ding N, Zhang Y, Liu Y, Wen D. Assessing medical professionalism: a systematic review of instruments and their measurement properties. *PLoS One.* 2017;12(5):e0177321. doi:10.1371/journal.pone.0177321

12. Frey WH. Old versus young: The cultural generation gap. Pew. January 25, 2018. Accessed May 31, 2022, https://www.pewtrusts.org/trend/archive/winter-2018/old-versus-young-the-cultural-generation-gap
13. Ruggeri A. People have always whinged about young adults. Here's proof. *BBC*. October 2, 2017. Accessed August 4, 2022. https://www.bbc.com/worklife/article/20171003-proof-that-people-have-always-complained-about-young-adults
14. Johnston SLLM, Peacock MA. Developing professionalism across the generations In: Creuss RL, Creuss SR, Steinert Y, eds. *Teaching Medical Professionalism*. Cambridge University Press; 2009:150–164.
15. Binder R, Friedli A, Fuentes-Afflick E. Preventing and managing unprofessionalism in medical school faculties. *Acad Med*. 2015;90(4):442–446. doi:10.1097/ACM.0000000000000592
16. Loftus S. Competencies in medical education: a trap for the unwary. *Med Sci Educ*. 2016;26:499–502.
17. Barnhoorn PC, Houtlosser M, Ottenhoff-de Jonge MW, Essers G, Numans ME, Kramer AWM. A practical framework for remediating unprofessional behavior and for developing professionalism competencies and a professional identity. *Med Teach*. 2019;41(3):303–308. doi:10.1080/0142159X.2018.1464133
18. Hardouin S, Cheng TW, Raulli S, et al. Prevalence of unprofessional social media content among young vascular surgeons. *J Vasc Surg*. 2019;69(3):e31.
19. Sosa JA. Editorial: doubling down on diversity in the wake of the #MedBikini controversy. *World J Surg*. 2020;44(11):3587–3588. doi:10.1007/s00268-020-05751-4
20. Jawed S, Mahboob U, Yasmeen R. Digital professional identity: dear internet! Who am I? *Educ Health (Abingdon)*. 2019;32(1):33–35. doi:10.4103/efh.EfH_232_17
21. Greenberg L. Ottawa surgeon convicted in road rage to face disciplinary hearing. *Ottawa Citizen*. January 30, 2008.
22. College of Physicians and Surgeons of Ontario (CPSO). *Between the College of Physicians and Surgeons of Ontario and Dr. Joel Bernard Freeman*. College of Physicians and Surgeons of Ontario; 2008.
23. Lemaire JB, Ewashina D, Polachek AJ, Dixit J, Yiu V. Understanding how patients perceive physician wellness and its links to patient care: a qualitative study. *PLoS One*. 2018;13(5):e0196888. doi:10.1371/journal.pone.0196888
24. Patel RS, Bachu R, Adikey A, Malik M, Shah M. Factors related to physician burnout and its consequences: a review. *Behav Sci (Basel)*. 2018;8(11):98–104. doi:10.3390/bs8110098
25. Hewitt DB, Ellis RJ, Chung JW, et al. Association of surgical resident wellness with medical errors and patient outcomes. *Ann Surg*. 2021;274(2):396–402. doi:10.1097/SLA.0000000000003909
26. West CP, Shanafelt TD. The influence of personal and environmental factors on professionalism in medical education. *BMC Med Educ*. 2007;7:29. doi:10.1186/1472-6920-7-29
27. Hendin H, Reynolds C, Fox D, et al. Licensing and physician mental health: problems and possibilities. *J Med Licens Discipline*. 2007;93(2):6–11.
28. Dyrbye LN, West CP, Sinsky CA, Goeders LE, Satele DV, Shanafelt TD. Medical licensure questions and physician reluctance to seek care for mental health conditions. *Mayo Clin Proc*. 2017;92(10):1486–1493. doi:10.1016/j.mayocp.2017.06.020
29. Bullock JL, Kimberg LS, Meeks LM. Trauma-informed transformation of evaluation and licensure for physicians with mental illness. *J Hosp Med*. 2021;16(7):434–437. doi:10.12788/jhm.3648

30. Harvey SB, Epstein RM, Glozier N, et al. Mental illness and suicide among physicians. *Lancet.* 2021;398(10303):920–930.

31. Amisha MP, Pathania M, Rathaur VK. Overview of artificial intelligence in medicine. *J Family Med Prim Care.* 2019;8(7):2328–2331. doi:10.4103/jfmpc.jfmpc_440_19

32. Leslie D, Mazumder A, Peppin A, Wolters MK, Hagerty A. Does "AI" stand for augmenting inequality in the era of COVID-19 healthcare? *BMJ.* 2021;372:n304. doi:10.1136/bmj.n304

33. Straw I. The automation of bias in medical artificial intelligence (AI): decoding the past to create a better future. *Artif Intell Med.* 2020;110:101965. doi:10.1016/j.artmed.2020.101965

34. Paton M, Naidu T, Richardson L, Kumagai A, Kuper A. Care in the real world: partial perspectives on compassion, technology, and equity. In: Hodges BD, Paech G, Bennett J, eds. *Without Compassion, There Is No Healthcare: Leading With Care in a Technological Age.* McGill-Queen's University Press; 2020:79–101.

35. Feilchenfeld Z, Kuper A, Whitehead C. Stethoscope of the 21st century: dominant discourses of ultrasound in medical education. *Med Educ.* 2018;52(12):1271–1287. doi:10.1111/medu.13714

36. Fenwick T. Pondering purposes, propelling forwards. *Stud Contin Educ.* 2018;40(3):367–380.

37. Benjamin R. *Race After Technology: Abolitionist Tools for the New Jim Code.* Polity; 2019.

38. Sukhera J, Goez H, Brown A, Haddara W, Razack S. Freedom from discrimination or freedom to discriminate? Discursive tensions within discrimination policies in medical education. *Adv Health Sci Educ Theory Pract.* 2022;27(2):387–403. doi:10.1007/s10459-022-10090-1

39. Lee JH. The weaponization of medical professionalism. *Acad Med.* 2017;92(5):579–580. doi:10.1097/ACM.0000000000001647

40. Wertz RW, Wertz DC. *Lying-in: A History of Childbirth in America.* Studies in the Life of Women. Schocken Books; 1979:xii.

41. Light DW. Ironies of success: a new history of the American health care "system." *J Health Soc Behav.* 2004;45(suppl):1–24.

42. Frye V, Camacho-Rivera M, Salas-Ramirez K, et al. Professionalism: the wrong tool to solve the right problem? *Acad Med.* 2020;95(6):860–863. doi:10.1097/ACM.0000000000003266

43. Goddard VCT, Brockbank S. Re-opening Pandora's box: who owns professionalism and is it time for a 21st century definition? *Med Educ.* 2022;57(1):66–75. doi:10.1111/medu.14862

44. Woldegiorgis ET. Decolonising a higher education system which has never been colonised. *Educ Philos Theory.* 2020;53(9):1–13.

45. Beagan BL. Neutralizing differences: producing neutral doctors for (almost) neutral patients. *Soc Sci Med.* 2000;51(8):1253–1265. doi:10.1016/s0277-9536(00)00043-5

46. Martimianakis MA, Maniate JM, Hodges BD. Sociological interpretations of professionalism. *Med Educ.* 2009;43(9):829–837. doi:10.1111/j.1365-2923.2009.03408.x

47. Janvier A. Tattoos, beer, and bow ties: the limits of professionalism in medicine. *JAMA Pediatr.* 2016;170(8):731–732. doi:10.1001/jamapediatrics.2016.0539

48. Wyatt TR, Rockich-Winston N, Taylor TR, White D. What does context have to do with anything? A study of professional identity formation in physician-trainees considered underrepresented in medicine. *Acad Med.* 2020;95(10):1587–1593. doi:10.1097/ACM.0000000000003192

49. Bizimungu S. Is this hair professional enough? *Can Med Assoc J.* 2021;193(7):E254–E255.

50. Frost HD, Regehr G. "I am a doctor": negotiating the discourses of standardization and diversity in professional identity construction. *Acad Med.* 2013;88(10):1570–1577. doi:10.1097/ACM.0b013e3182a34b05

51. Zaidi Z, Partman IM, Whitehead CR, Kuper A, Wyatt TR. Contending with our racial past in medical education: a foucauldian perspective. *Teach Learn Med.* 2021;33(4):453–462.

52. Wyatt T. "The sins of our forefathers": reimagining research in health professions education. *Adv Health Sci Educ.* 2022;27(4):1195–1206. doi:10.1007/s10459-022-10111-z

53. CanMEDS. Framework. Accessed November 23, 2019. http://canmeds.royalcollege.ca/en/framework

54. Dutch Framework medical leadership competences. DIRMInstitute. Accessed Jun 8, 2022. http://dirmi.eu/wp-content/uploads/2018/02/2016-DUTCH_Medical-Leadership-Framework.pdf

55. Vogel L. Should doctors talk politics with patients? *CMAJ.* 2018;190(16):E520–E521. doi:10.1503/cmaj.109-5589

56. Huddle T. Perspective: medical professionalism and medical education should not involve commitments to political advocacy. *Acad Med.* 2011;86(3):378–383.

57. Haag M. Doctors revolt after N.R.A. tells them to 'stay in their lane' on gun policy. *New York Times.* November 13, 2018. https://www.nytimes.com/2018/11/13/us/nra-stay-in-your-lane-doctors.html

58. Anderson CTM. Taking back our voices–#HumanityIsOurLane. *N Engl J Med.* 2020;383(17):1609–1611. doi:10.1056/NEJMp2021291

59. Patel NA, Rao A. Doctors have been whistleblowers throughout history. They've also been silenced. *Guardian.* April 8, 2020. https://www.theguardian.com/education/2020/apr/08/coronavirus-doctors-whistleblowers-history-silenced#maincontent

60. Lifton RJ. *The Nazi Doctors: Medical Killing and the Psychology of Genocide.* 4th ed., paperback ed. Basic Books; 2017:xvii.

61. Kopacz D. Medical activism: a foundation of professionalism. Closler. December 28, 2020. Accessed June 6, 2022. https://closler.org/passion-in-the-medical-profession/medical-activism-a-foundation-of-professionalism

62. Goldfarb S. Take two aspirin and call me by my pronouns. *Wall Street Journal.* Sep 12, 2019. Accessed 6/10/2024. https://www.wsj.com/articles/take-two-aspirin-and-call-me-by-my-pronouns-11568325291?mod=searchresults&page=1&pos=2

63. Jones N, Nguyen J, Strand NK, Reeves K. What should be the scope of physicians' roles in responding to gun violence? *AMA J Ethics.* 2018;20(1):84–90. doi:10.1001/journalofethics.2018.20.1.pfor2-1801.

64. Habib A. *Rebels and Rage: Reflecting on #FeesMustFall.* Jonathan Ball Publishers; 2019.

65. Stuart K. Of professionalism and health care strikes. *S Afr J Bioeth Law.* 2010;3(1):4–8.

66. Mokhachane M, George A, Wyatt T, Kuper A, Green-Thompson L. Rethinking professional identity formation amidst protests and social upheaval: a journey in Africa. *Adv Health Sci Educ Theory Pract.* 2022;28(2):427–452. doi:10.1007/s10459-022-10164-0

67. Sharda S, Dhara A, Alam F. Not neutral: reimagining antiracism as a professional competence. *CMAJ.* 2021;193(3):E101–E102.

68. Hull SC. Not so conscientious objection: when can doctors refuse to treat? *STAT*. November 8, 2019. https://www.statnews.com/2019/11/08/conscientious-objection-doctors-refuse-treatment/

69. College of Physicians and Surgeons of Ontario (CPSO). Advice to the profession: professional obligations and human rights. College of Physicians and Surgeons of Ontario. Accessed August 8, 2022. https://www.cpso.on.ca/Physicians/Policies-Guidance/Policies/Professional-Obligations-and-Human-Rights/Advice-to-the-Profession-Professional-Obligations

70. American College of Obstetricians and Gynecologists (ACOG). *The Limits of Conscientious Refusal in Reproductive Medicine*; 2007:1203–1208. ACOG Committee opinion no. 385.

71. Blackshaw BP, Rodger D. Questionable benefits and unavoidable personal beliefs: defending conscientious objection for abortion. *J Med Ethics*. 2020;46(3):178–182. doi:10.1136/medethics-2019-105566

72. Castellani B, Hafferty FW. The complexities of medical professionalism: a preliminary investigation. In: Aultman JM, Wear D, eds. *Professionalism in Medicine: Critical Perspectives* Springer Science & Business Media; 2006:3–23.

73. Hanan A. A view from somewhere: explaining the paradigms of educational research. *J Philos Educ*. 2006;40(2):205–221.

74. Hafferty FW, Castellani B. The hidden curriculum: a theory of medical education. In: Brosnan C, Turner B, eds. *Handbook of the Sociology of Medical Education*. Routledge; 2009:15–35.

75. Taleb NN. *The Bed of Procrustes: Philosophical and Practical Aphorisms*. Trade paperback ed. Random House; 2016:xiii.

Index

For the benefit of digital users, indexed terms that span two pages (e.g., 52–53) may, on occasion, appear on only one of those pages.

Page references followed by *b*, *f*, and *t* denote boxes, figures, and tables, respectively. References followed by n indicate notes.